Gastrointestinal Tract Cancer

SLOAN-KETTERING INSTITUTE CANCER SERIES

Series Editors:

ROBERT A. GOOD, Ph.D., M.D., and STACEY B. DAY, M.D., Ph.D., D.Sc.
Sloan-Kettering Institute for Cancer Research
New York, New York

GASTROINTESTINAL TRACT CANCER
Edited by Martin Lipkin, M.D., and Robert A. Good, Ph.D., M.D.

Gastrointestinal Tract Cancer

Edited by

Martin Lipkin, M.D., *and*
Robert A. Good, Ph.D., M.D.

Sloan-Kettering Institute for Cancer Research
New York, New York

Plenum Medical Book Company · New York and London

Library of Congress Cataloging in Publication Data

Main entry under title:

Gastrointestinal tract cancer.

(Sloan-Kettering Institute cancer series)
Includes bibliographies and index.
1. Alimentary canal – Cancer. 2. Oncology, Experimental. 3. Gastroenterology. I. Lipkin, Martin. II. Good, Robert A., 1922- III. Series: Sloan-Kettering Institute for Cancer Research, New York. Sloan-Kettering Institute cancer series. [DNLM: 1. Gastrointestinal neoplasms. WI149 G259]
RC280.A4G37 616.9'94'3 78-1964
ISBN 0-306-31098-8

227 West 17th Street, New York, N. Y. 10011

Plenum Medical Book Company is an imprint of Plenum Publishing Corporation

Printed in the United States of America

Contributors

M. Earl Balis	Memorial Sloan-Kettering Cancer Center, New York
Norman T. Berlinger	Memorial Sloan-Kettering Cancer Center, New York, New York
H. J. R. Bussey	St. Mark's Hospital, London, England
Edward H. Cooper	School of Medicine, The University of Leeds, Leeds, England
Thomas H. Corbett	Southern Research Institute, Birmingham, Alabama
Eleanor E. Deschner	Memorial Sloan-Kettering Cancer Center, New York, New York
Maria de Sousa	Memorial Sloan-Kettering Cancer Center, New York, New York
John A. Double	School of Medicine, The University of Leeds, Leeds, England
Cecilia M. Fenoglio	College of Physicians and Surgeons, Columbia University, New York, New York
Robert A. Good	Memorial Sloan-Kettering Cancer Center, New York, New York
Daniel P. Griswold, Jr.	Southern Research Institute, Birmingham, Alabama
J. U. Gutterman	M. D. Anderson Hospital and Tumor Institute, Houston, Texas
Joanna F. Haas	Cornell University Medical College, New York, New York
Steven I. Hajdu	Memorial Sloan-Kettering Cancer Center, New York, New York, and Cornell University Medical College, New York, New York
E. M. Hersh	M. D. Anderson Hospital and Tumor Institute, Houston, Texas
Takashi Kawachi	National Cancer Research Institute, Tokyo, Japan
Gordon I. Kaye	Albany Medical College, Albany, New York
Nancy Kemeny	Memorial Sloan-Kettering Cancer Center, New York, New York
John H. Kersey	University of Minnesota, Minneapolis, Minnesota
Nathan Lane	College of Physicians and Surgeons, Columbia University, New York, New York

Martin Lipkin	Memorial Sloan-Kettering Cancer Center, New York, New York
Henry T. Lynch	Creighton University School of Medicine, Omaha, Nebraska
Patrick M. Lynch	Creighton University School of Medicine, Omaha, Nebraska
Janet Marks	Royal Victoria Infirmary, Newcastle upon Tyne, England
Alain P. Maskens	Clinique Saint-Michel, Brussels, Belgium
G. M. Mavligit	M. D. Anderson Hospital and Tumor Institute, Houston, Texas
Basil C. Morson	St. Mark's Hospital, London, England
A. Munro Neville	School of Medicine, The University of Leeds, Leeds, England
Robert R. Pascal	Veterans Administration Hospital, Tampa, Florida
Jean-Claude Rambaud	Hôpital Saint-Lazare, Paris, France
David Schottenfeld	Memorial Sloan-Kettering Cancer Center, New York, New York, and Cornell University Medical College, New York, New York
Maxime Seligmann	Research Institute on Blood Diseases, Hôpital Saint Louis, Paris, France
Paul Sherlock	Memorial Sloan-Kettering Cancer Center, New York, New York, and Cornell University Medical College, New York, New York
Sam Shuster	Royal Victoria Infirmary, Newcastle upon Tyne, England
Beatrice D. Spector	University of Minnesota, Minneapolis, Minnesota
Maus W. Stearns, Jr.	Memorial Sloan-Kettering Cancer Center, New York, New York
Takashi Sugimura	National Cancer Research Institute, Tokyo, Japan
Jeremiah J. Twomey	Baylor College of Medicine, and Veterans Administration Hospital, Houston, Texas
Sidney J. Winawer	Memorial Sloan-Kettering Cancer Center, New York, New York, and Cornell University Medical College, New York, New York
Alan Yagoda	Memorial Sloan-Kettering Cancer Center, New York, New York
Morris S. Zedeck	Memorial Sloan-Kettering Cancer Center, New York, New York

Preface

In observing the development of modern scientific knowledge, many individuals have expressed concern over the rapid growth of information in various specialized disciplines. Over 100 years ago the first Secretary of the Smithsonian Institution, and more recently Dr. Vannevar Bush while proposing the modern expansion of the National Institutes of Health, both noted problems that prevented the proper utilization of information by individuals in medical and related scientific fields. These observations, together with concomitant implications of future difficulty, are particularly pertinent to the field of oncology. The rapid evolution of the latter discipline has largely been aided by the incorporation of concepts and methods developed over a long period of time, and drawn from a wide variety of other scientific fields.

The large body of discoveries that have contributed to our current understanding of neoplasia, however, cannot be viewed as being made up of equal parts. They bring to mind Claude Bernard's view "des déterminismes simples et complexes" in the physiological and biochemical regulation of bodily functions. He was able to observe that the most important and basic of physiologic processes were destined to be fewer in number than those of less fundamental and more highly specialized purpose. He understood that in the future development of medical science, studies of the latter would occupy much of the time and attention of investigators, and were likely to contribute much to scientific literature.

The emergence of oncology as a scientific discipline of major importance, and indeed those areas related to gastrointestinal cancer, have been accompanied by proliferations of literature having similar characteristics. Although science may be "built up with facts as a house is with stones,"* at this time new publications in the field should aid in the development of a milieu leading to new and incisive reasoning. Simultaneously, they should strengthen lines of communication that will improve our understanding both of basic mechanisms and the speedy and efficient application of new discoveries. "There are science and the applications of science, bound together."† These

*Henri Poincaré, 1908.
†Louis Pasteur, 1871.

points were major considerations in planning this volume, and in the creation of this series of books on neoplasia.

Recent advances in our understanding of gastrointestinal tract cancer have led to a fuller awareness of factors contributing to its pathogenesis, and have given new insights into methods of detection and treatment. When new findings from experimental disciplines as diverse as genetics, immunology, biochemistry, carcinogenesis, epidemiology, and pathology are brought together, an interesting view begins to emerge on the evolution of the disease, and on new approaches to its detection, prevention, and treatment. Increased susceptibility of specific population groups to disease and pathogenic elements including those of environmental origin can be viewed more clearly; an outline of programs that might well reduce the incidence of disease and its mortality begins to be seen.

In this volume, fundamental aspects of the biological organization of gastrointestinal mucosa are reviewed, and a number of areas are suggested for further development and integration among the specialized disciplines involved. The topic of individual and familial susceptibility to gastrointestinal malignancy is stressed, together with newer discoveries relating to environmental, genetic, and immunologic factors, highlighting their possible interactions. Experimental models and their contribution to our understanding of both gastric and colonic neoplasia and their treatment are reviewed. The concluding sections of the volume focus on future directions in the early diagnosis and detection of gastrointestinal cancer, and on its therapy; an attempt is made to present a critical appraisal of newer advances including those related to treatment.

Throughout the development of the book, emphasis has been placed on recent findings having the best potential for improving our understanding of fundamental processes in gastrointestinal neoplasia, and of equal importance for application to clinical oncology. The task at hand would have been easier had a single concept in neoplasia been sufficiently advanced to satisfy requirements proposed by Einstein: "A theory is the more impressive the greater the simplicity of its premises is, the more difficult kinds of things it relates, and the more extended is its area of applicability." At the present time, the accomplishments in biological research discussed in this volume are moving toward an objective of that type. The task underway however is still complex, the most important problems remain largely unsolved, and they have to be approached with even greater vigor in the future. In doing so, and in attempting to fulfill the goals referred to above, we are obliged to keep in mind the complexities of the biological sciences involved, and the slow but steady progress that has characterized the evolution of major advances in this area of human endeavor.

M. Lipkin
R. A. Good

Contents

Section I
Biological Organization of Gastrointestinal Mucosa

Section IIA
Individual and Familial Susceptibility to Gastrointestinal Malignancy: Immune Mechanisms

Chapter 3
Immunodeficiency Diseases and Malignancy
Beatrice D. Spector, Robert A. Good, and John H. Kersey

Chapter 4
Recognitive Immunity in Colon Cancer
Norman T. Berlinger

Chapter 5
Immunological Dysfunction with Atrophic Gastritis and Gastric Malignancy
Jeremiah J. Twomey

Chapter 17
Use of Experimental Models in the Study of Approaches to Treatment of Colorectal Cancer
Daniel P. Griswold, Jr., and Thomas H. Corbett

Section IV
Future Directions in Early Detection and Diagnosis

Chapter 18
Early Diagnosis and Detection of Colorectal Cancer in High-Risk Population Groups
Martin Lipkin, Paul Sherlock, and Sidney J. Winawer

Chapter 19
Logic and Logistics of Monitoring Large Bowel Cancer
Edward H. Cooper and A. Munro Neville

Chapter 20
Enzymes of Normal and Malignant Intestine

M. Earl Balis

Chapter 21
Cancer in Inflammatory Bowel Disease: Risk Factors and Prospects for Early Detection

Paul Sherlock and Sidney J. Winawer

Chapter 22
Cytopathology of Human Gastrointestinal Cancers

Steven I. Hajdu

Chapter 23
The Skin and Gastrointestinal Malignancy

Janet Marks and Sam Shuster

Section V
Future Directions in Therapy

Chapter 24
Early and Definitive Surgical Therapy for Colonic and Rectal Cancer
Maus W. Stearns, Jr.

Chapter 25
Chemotherapy of Colorectal Cancer: A Critical Analysis of Response Criteria and Therapeutic Efficacy
Alan Yagoda and Nancy Kemeny

Chapter 26
Adjuvant Chemotherapy and Immunotherapy in Colorectal Cancer
G. M. Mavligit, J. U. Gutterman, and E. M. Hersh

I

Biological Organization of Gastrointestinal Mucosa

1

Proliferation and Differentiation of Gastrointestinal Cells in Health and Disease

Eleanor E. Deschner and Martin Lipkin

1. Introduction

A comprehensive analysis of the structure and function of the gastrointestinal mucosa, bringing together various disciplines that include histology, cytochemistry, electron microscopy, and cell kinetics, has aided our present understanding of this tissue in normal and disease states. Related studies in other disciplines have broadened the scope of research currently under way.

Initially one may cite some of the newer developments that increase our understanding of the alimentary tract and its endocrine function. Findings in recent years have demonstrated the digestive tract to be the locale for the production or secretion of several hormones, thus expanding its role as an endocrine organ. Previously described epithelial cells with basal granules have since been defined as a network of endocrine cells whose product secretions are presumed to exist in a state of balance (Solcia and Sampietro, 1965). When in a state of imbalance, they may be responsible for diseases as widely divergent as migraine headaches and Zollinger-Ellison syndrome.

As a separate contribution, one may credit the cytological assessment of gastric and colonic biopsy and lavage specimens identifying the presence of neoplastic cells as leading to the development of simple diagnostic procedures for early cancer detection. These techniques (Raskin and Pleticka, 1971; Katz *et al.*, 1972) are expected to continue to increase significantly the cure rates for these cancers of high frequency both in the United States and in other countries.

Eleanor E. Deschner and Martin Lipkin • Memorial Sloan-Kettering Cancer Center, New York, New York 10021.

Another illustration of significant findings related to gastrointestinal cancer is the recognition of early biochemical abnormalities in normal-appearing gastric and colonic cells prior to the formation of polyps and cancer (Maskens and Deschner, 1977). Discoveries of this nature have been made possible by the development of microautoradiographic and chemical techniques which detect the presence of radioactive precursors incorporated into human or animal tissue (Deschner and Lipkin, 1975).

Lastly, critical analyses of adenomatous and hyperplastic polyps using histology, electron microscopy, and cell kinetics have shown some excrescences to have different modes of cell renewal and growth which can be related to their significance in future cancer development. Thus selective removal of adenomas rather than hyperplastic polyps has been regarded as having an important role in reducing the frequency of colon cancer (Gilbertsen, 1974; Lane *et al.,* 1971; Morson, 1974).

The details of these and other studies on the structure, function, and renewal of normal and diseased epithelial mucosa in various areas of the gastrointestinal tract will form the backbone of this chapter. Observations on preneoplastic and neoplastic cells will be compared with findings in normal mucosa in order to provide the most complete information on gastrointestinal epithelium in health and disease.

2. Stomach

2.1. Histology

The stomach is a tubular organ composed of three distinct histologically different regions: cardia, fundus, and pylorus. The esophagus with its stratified squamous cell epithelium leads directly into the cardia or esophageal-cardiac junction composed of simple columnar mucous epithelial cells thrown into pits or glands. This cell type also is indigenous to the other two regions of the stomach (Table 1).

The body or the fundus is more complex in structure and composes the largest portion of the stomach. Here the gastric pits are lined with cuboidal or low columnar mucous cells at the isthmus or neck of the gland, the region in which mitotic figures are seen. These cells have the primary purpose of renewing themselves. Such undifferentiated cells give rise to daughter cells which migrate to the surface or lumen, where they mature into tall columnar epithelial cells with the capability of secreting mucus.

Below the isthmus are the fundic glands, which are lined with chief or zymogen cells and parietal or acid-secreting cells (Table 1). Mucous neck cells are believed to act as stem cells for both of these specialized cell types as well as for the population of endocrine polypeptide cells located in this organ (Cheng and Leblond, 1974; Matsuyama and Suzuki, 1970).

These cells are interspersed among the mucous cells but occur primarily in the midzone of the gastric glands; they synthesize, store, and secrete hor-

Table 1. Gastric Epithelial Cell Types and Their Functions

Area of stomach	Epithelial cell type	Function or secretory product
Cardia	Surface mucous	Mucus
	Undifferentiated mucous	Cell renewal
Fundus	Surface mucous	Mucus
	Mucous neck	Cell renewal
	Parietal	HCl, intrinsic factor
	Zymogen or chief	Pepsinogen
	A cell	Enteroglucagon
	G cell	Gastrin
	Argentaffin	Serotonin, histamine, motilin (?)
	Argyrophil	Secretin (?)
Pylorus	Surface mucous	Mucus
	Parietal	HCl
	G cell	Gastrin

mones such as gastrin and enteroglucagon (Table 1). These endocrine cells are thought to have a neural crest origin (Pearse, 1973) and to respond to autonomic, mechanical, and intraluminal stimuli by discharging their specific granule content directly into the circulation. Such endocrine cells have been seen to extend their apical processes to reach a gland lumen, where they terminate in microvilli (Kobayashi *et al.,* 1970).

While electron microscopists agree that there are at least 11 different types of endocrine cells present in the gastrointestinal mucosa, the primary ones in the fundus are the A cell or enteroglucagon-secreting cell, the G cell or gastrin cell, and the argentaffin cell, which secretes serotonin and histamine.

The mucosa of the pyloric antrum has gastric pits which are deeper than in the fundic region, and is lined primarily with a cell type that appears similar to the mucous neck cell. Recent studies have demonstrated the presence of two other cell types in the region; they are the parietal cell (Tominaga, 1975) or acid-secreting cell and the G cell or endocrine cell secreting gastrin. The most concentrated gastrin activity has been found to be localized in the middle third of this antral mucosa (Tominaga, 1975).

2.2. *Proliferation Kinetics of Normal Stomach*

Gastric cell turnover in man has been studied using several different approaches. Most studies have employed the techniques of isotopic labeling and autoradiography which photographically detects biochemical events involving the radioactive precursor. The isotope frequently in use is [^{3}H]thymidine (TdR^{3}H), which becomes incorporated into newly synthesized DNA. The radionuclide may be injected into patients with limited life expectancy—the *in vivo* approach—or biopsies may be obtained and incubation of the specimens with TdR^{3}H in nutrient media may allow for incorporation of the label—the *in vitro* approach. After suitable exposure, the slides may be read to learn the number and location of the labeled cells.

If the frequency of labeled mitoses is followed over an extended period such as 48–72 hr, and repeated biopsies have been taken, then the total cell cycle may be estimated directly. A pulse injection of TdR^3H will label a cohort of cells, which at that precise time are in the S or DNA synthesis phase of the cell cycle. Immediately following the injection, there is a period at which labeled mitoses slowly increase in frequency, then approach a maximum value, and then decline in number. A smaller second wave very often follows. The midpoint of the ascending limb to the midpoint of the descending limb of the first wave is a measure of the duration of S or DNA synthesis phase for this cohort of cells. The duration of G_1 is obtained from the time of the midpoint of the descending limb to the midpoint of the ascending limb of the second wave. Obviously the total cell cycle time can be obtained from the midpoint of the first ascending limb to the midpoint of the second ascending limb, or the midpoint of the first maximum to the midpoint of the second peak of labeled mitoses.

In vitro studies with biopsy specimens and a double-label procedure employing [^{3}H]thymidine and [^{14}C]thymidine or a low (*l*) and a high (*h*) dose of TdR^3H may also provide one with a value for S phase (T_S) : $N_h/N_l = S/t$. The total cell cycle time is derived when one provides the labeling index and S phase duration: $T_c = (T_s/\text{LI}) \times 100$ (Bleiberg *et al.*, 1971; Galand *et al.*, 1968).

Undifferentiated cells in the isthmus area incorporate TdR^3H and therefore are the progenitor cells for the replacement of epithelial cells lost at the surface (Bell *et al.*, 1967). The turnover time for epithelial cells of the gastric mucosa has been reported to range from 2 days (Bleiberg *et al.*, 1971; Lipkin *et al.*, 1963*b*) to 4–6 days (MacDonald *et al.*, 1964). The undifferentiated cells are also believed to be the stem cells for the parietal, chief, and endocrine cells, which differ only in that these newly formed cells migrate in a downward direction (Willems and Lehy, 1975).

The durations of some of the phases of the gastric epithelial cell cycle are known (Table 2); the T_{G_1} phase is obviously the longest and most variable in duration and may account for differences in the value of T_c and turnover

Table 2. Kinetic Parameters in Normal Human Gastric Mucosa

	LI (%)	MI (%)	T_{G_2} (hr)	T_S (hr)	T_{G_1} (hr)	T_c or turnover time (hr)	References
Cardia	13.1	1.3	—	—	—	—	Tanaka (1968)
Fundus	—	—	2–4	10	—	48	Lipkin *et al.* (1963*b*)
	9.3	1.0	—	—	—	—	Tanaka (1968)
	14	—	—	9	—	48	Bleiberg *et al.* (1971)
	11.7	—	—	—	—	—	Lipkin *et al.* (1963*b*)
	7.7	—	—	—	—	—	
	4.2	—	—	—	—	—	Bell *et al.* (1967)
	10.0	0.8	1	7.1	62	72	Castrup *et al.* (1975)
Antrum	12.8	—	—	—	—	—	Hansen *et al.* (1975)
	15.2	1.4	—	—	—	—	Tanaka (1968)

time. The labeling index is a measure of the proliferative activity of the epithelial cells of the stomach, and is seen to vary between 4.2% and 11.7%, a range obtained by the *in vivo* technique. *In vitro* studies have shown reasonably good agreement, with a range of 9.3–11.0% (Table 2). The mucosa of the antrum and cardia appeared to have slightly higher labeling and mitotic indices. Unfortunately, not many kinetic studies have involved these specific areas of the stomach, although the antrum is a frequent site of cancer and information concerning it would be of value.

2.3. *Proliferation Kinetics of Gastric Mucosa in Disease*

Benign and malignant diseases of the stomach are accompanied by definite alterations in the size and chromosome content of epithelial cell nuclei. Ninety percent of cells in normal mucosa have a diploid ($2n$) nucleus containing 46 chromosomes. Preneoplastic diseases such as ulcers, polyps, atrophic gastritis, and pernicious anemia (PA) show an increase in nuclear ploidy, with approximately 25–50% of cells between the triploid and tetraploid chromosome number ($3n$–$4n$). Gastric carcinomas also show this shift in ploidy number; however, no correlation has been found between the degree of increase in chromosome number and the type or extent of disease (Wiendl *et al.*, 1974).

This increase in chromosome content is, however, related to an increase in the size of nuclei. Normal $2n$ epithelial cell nuclei have a range of size or diameter from approximately 5.8 to 7.9 μm, while the nuclei in PA mucosa range from 7.9 to 10.5 μm and in gastric cancer from 8.00 to 10.54 μm. These observations confirm the larger size of epithelial cell nuclei in premalignant and malignant diseases of the gastric mucosa.

Labeling indices in the various disease states of the stomach demonstrate marked elevations over normal ranges (Table 3). The contribution that intestinal metaplasia makes to these higher values (12.9–23.0) cannot be assessed completely, but it definitely has some impact on the labeling and mitotic indices since it very often is present in these gastric diseases.

Cell cycle times (T_c) have been found to be approximately 2 days in epithelial cells of gastric mucosa of patients with atrophic gastritis and Zollinger-Ellison (Z-E) syndrome, the latter a disease in which there is hyperplasia of the parietal and peptic cell populations. Although differences in the values for the duration of S phase were found, the percentage of cells involved in epithelial cell renewal (LI) did not appear to differ markedly. The atrophic gastritis data were obtained from an *in vivo* study of one patient, while the Z-E data are a composite of *in vitro* double label study of three patients (Castrup *et al.*, 1975). A decided reduction in the duration of G_1 appears to be most responsible for a short T_c when observed.

Clearly the proliferative activity of cells in these tissues not only is increased but also has a more diverse pattern than that found in the normal stomach mucosa. While the cells from which parietal and chief cells originate have not been firmly established, it is quite possible that in Z-E both cell types may reproduce their own cell type rather than be derived from mucous neck

Table 3. Kinetic Parameters in Diseased Human Gastric Mucosa

	LI (%)	MI (%)	T_{G_2} (hr)	T_S (hr)	T_{G_1} (hr)	T_c or turnover time (hr)	References
Atrophic gastritis							
Fundus	14.0		1–6	16		>30	Winawer and Lipkin (1969)
	19						Hansen *et al.* (1975)
Antrum	12.9						Hansen *et al.* (1975)
		12.9					Liavag (1968)
Gastric cancer							
Fundus	19.3						Hansen *et al.* (1975)
	16.4	1.2					Tanaka (1968)
	9.9	2.3					Hoffman and Post (1967)
Antrum	15.8						Hansen *et al.* (1975)
	23.0	1.8					Tanaka (1968)
Gastric ulcer							
Cardia	20.1	2.1					Tanaka (1968)
Fundus	13.4						Hansen *et al.* (1975)
Antrum	16.2						Hansen *et al.* (1975)
Zollinger-Ellison syndrome	15.7	0.8	1	6.7	36	45 ± 4.0	Castrup *et al.* (1975)

cells as is believed to be the case under normal conditions (Willems and Lehy, 1975). Similarly, in severe atrophic gastritis this pluripotent quality or diversity of cell production is maximally demonstrated by the formation of intestinal cell types including goblet, columnar epithelial, and Paneth cells.

In addition to faster cell proliferation with the production of a remarkably wide spectrum of cell types, rapid migration of epithelial cells to the gastric surface (Bell *et al.*, 1975; Winawer and Lipkin, 1969) was shown in atrophic gastritic mucosa. But perhaps the most unusual observation in this tissue has been the recognition of DNA-synthesizing mature gastric and intestinal epithelial cells at or near the luminal surface of the mucosa (Winawer and Lipkin, 1969 Deschner *et al.*, 1972). This is believed to indicate an early event in a sequence leading to the formation of neoplastic excrescences. When it is seen in well-differentiated intestinal-type epithelial cells within the stomach, it is doubtless related to the developing metaplasia and/or the possible lesion which may form concurrently or following this event (Deschner *et al.*, 1972).

A progressive sequence of morphological and biochemical changes has been reported in *in vitro* labeled precursor studies which correlate with the pathological staging of atrophic gastritis. The earliest event is the appearance of TdR^{3}H-labeled cells at the surface and upper one-third of normal-appearing gastric pits, a time when minimal superficial gastritis is seen. DNA synthetic activity continues in this area within cuboidal-appearing gastric cells when the mucosa has mild to moderate atrophic gastritis. A third proliferative pattern appears when well-differentiated intestinal cells incorporate TdR^{3}H in the upper one-third of intestinalized pits and the mucosa is moderately atrophic. When severe gastritis is present, a fourth proliferative pattern occurs and may be seen concurrently with that previously mentioned. The incorporation of TdR^{3}H takes place only in the lower two-thirds of the intestinalized pits, and not at the surface, a pattern which is normal for intestinal mucosa.

The gastric cells have now undergone complete transformation to small intestine, morphologically, biochemically, and enzymatically. They are, for all intents and purposes, small bowel mucosa. The consequences of this transformation may be thought of in terms of the effect of the presence of acidic mucin, rather than neutral mucin, on the mucous barrier which acts to protect the mucosa from autodigestion. So too the altered character of this abnormal mucosa within the stomach may allow absorbed dietary carcinogens to gain access to and function within this tissue.

3. Small Intestine

3.1. Histology

The tubelike digestive tract continues after the stomach with the small intestine, which is subdivided into three portions: duodenum, jejunum, and ileum. The basic substructure is the same throughout the small intestine. The mucous membrane is thrown up into crypts and villi which act to increase the surface area for absorption of nutrients into the lymphatics and blood vessels. The number of cells which compose the crypts of Lieberkühn in all three portions of the small bowel does not differ, nor does age affect this factor (Fry *et al.*, 1963). Only the length and shape of the villi change in the three portions of the small intestine; they are longest and broadest in the duodenum and shortest and most fingerlike in the ileum. In the mouse, a further difference reported was the number of crypts surrounding a villus, which was greater in the duodenum than the number surrounding a jejunal villus (Fry *et al.*, 1963). A decreasing cephalocaudal ratio of the number of crypts per villus was confirmed by Clarke (1970).

Four main differentiated cell types are present in the small bowel mucosa; these include columnar epithelial cells, goblet cells, enteroendocrine cells, and Paneth cells. It is believed that they all originate from the same precursor or stem cell (Cheng and Leblond, 1974), called a crypt base columnar cell. Daughter cells of this stem cell often acquire characteristics which make it possible to forecast the particular cell type being formed. For example, intermediate cells, called oligomucous cells, upon division are presumed to give rise to mature goblet cells, while crypt base columnar cells with a granule may form mature Paneth or endocrine cells (Cheng and Leblond, 1974). The endocrine cells of the small intestine are scattered diffusely in the mucosa, where they synthesize, store, and secrete various hormones. Cells producing secretin are most numerous in the duodenum and only occasionally occur in the jejunum. This distribution is reasonable since the function of secretin is to decrease the acidity of the duodenum and neutralize its contents (Polak *et al.*, 1971*a*). Epithelial cells immunohistochemically identified as storing cholecystokinin have a distribution in the small bowel similar to that of secretin-storing cells (Buffa *et al.*, 1976).

Epithelial cells secreting enteroglucagon are most often found in the mid to terminal jejunum as well as fundic mucosa (Polak *et al.*, 1971*b*). These enteroglucagon-producing cells usually lie along the basement membrane, and evidence that they reach the lumen of the gland has not been reported.

Motilin-producing cells are most numerous in the duodenum and upper jejunum, where they are primarily situated in the lower portion of the crypts. More than 85% of motilin cells proved via immunocytochemistry to be argentaffin cells (Pearse *et al.*, 1974). The localization of this hormone in the enterochromaffin cells of the small intestine has since been confirmed (Polak *et al.*, 1975) by immune electron cytochemistry, which identifies the endocrine cells at the ultrastructural level, as well as by staining and immune response. A fourth hormone, gastric inhibitory polypeptide, has been found to be present in cells situated predominantly in the midzone of glands in the duodenum and less frequently in the jejunum (Polak *et al.*, 1973). The function of this hormone, which is to inhibit gastric acid production and stimulate insulin release, correlates well with the distribution of this cell type and overlaps in function with previously mentioned gut hormones.

3.2. Proliferation Kinetics of Normal Small Intestine

Microscopic examination of the small bowel reveals the zone from which cells are renewed. Mitotic figures move out toward the lumen and are seen with ease in the lower two-thirds of crypts. The frequency of the appearance of mitoses in the duodenum was used as the basis for estimating the renewal time for epithelial cells and found to be approximately 2 days (Bertalanffy and Nagy, 1961). A similar duration was obtained by Wright *et al.* (1973*a,b*) using a metaphase accumulation technique involving vincristine. Isotopic labeling studies have given a range of values for the replacement time of from 48 to 144 hr (Lipkin *et al.*, 1963*b*; MacDonald *et al.*, 1964).

Cell cycle parameters for epithelial cells of the small bowel are presented in Table 4. A large fraction of cells are observed to be involved in proliferation as evidenced by the high labeling and mitotic index, as well as the large growth fraction (GF). A labeled mitotic wave of ileal mucosa used as a urinary conduit provided a total cell cycle time or generation time of 36 hr (Deschner *et al.*, 1976), with values for several phases of the cell cycle (Table 4) similar to durations previously reported (Lipkin *et al.*, 1963*b*).

Indeed, this portion of the gastrointestinal tract has a somewhat faster rate of renewal than the stomach or large bowel. It is probably a reduced duration of G_1 rather than a shorter G_2 or S which contributes most to this faster generation time demonstrated by small bowel mucosa.

3.3. Diseases of Small Intestine

When the small intestine becomes diseased, it is easily recognizable by a decline in the height or even complete loss of villi. Marked alterations in the proliferative characteristics of the mucosa also accompany this change in architecture. A decreased epithelial cell population and a shortening of villi with a concomitant reduction in absorptive surface occur in patients with severe pernicious anemia. In addition, there is a decline in the number of mitoses as well as an increase in nuclear size that accompanies this vitamin B_{12} deficiency (Foroozan and Trier, 1967). The mechanism whereby this deficiency interfers with proliferation to produce a reduced size of the villi and a decreased mitotic frequency is not well understood. However, if DNA synthesis were selectively impaired or inhibited by a lack of vital nutrients and the duration of mitosis were unaltered, then a reduction of dividing cells would occur in crypts. This hypothesis can be tested easily in an *in vitro* system utilizing radioactive isotopes and autoradiography.

3.3.1. Sprue

Gluten enteropathy or celiac sprue is a condition marked in its most severe state by a loss of villi and a hypertrophy of the crypts. Excessive cell loss has been measured in untreated patients (Croft *et al.*, 1968), and increased numbers of mitoses have been observed in intestinal crypts (Padykula *et al.*, 1961).

Table 4. *Kinetic Parameters in Normal and Diseased Human Small Intestine*

	T_{G_2} (hr)	T_M (hr)	T_S (hr)	T_c (hr)	T_{G_1}	LI	MI (%)	Growth fractions	References
Normal									
Duodenum		1.09		54			2.36	0.83	Wright *et al.* (1973*a*)
Jejunum		1.10		42					Wright *et al.* (1973*a*)
							3.05	0.72	Wright *et al.* (1973*b*)
Duodenum				48					Bertalanffy and Nagy (1961)
Jejunum	1.5			48					Shorter *et al.* (1966)
						27.4	2.1		Bell *et al.* (1967)
Ileum conduit	2	1	11	>24					Lipkin *et al.* (1963*b*)
	1–2	1	11	36	22				Deschner *et al.* (1976)
Diseased									
Duodenum-jejunum		1.31		22			5.09	0.61	Wright *et al.* (1973*a*)
		1.55		21					Wright *et al.* (1973*a*)
Sprue							5.22	0.55	Wright *et al.* (1973*b*)

Isotopic labeling studies have revealed that approximately a three-fold increase over normal values for labeled cells occurred in untreated patients with sprue. The withdrawal of gluten from the diet for 6–12 weeks nevertheless left a twofold elevation over normal values. Migration of the leading edge of labeled cells was 3 times faster in sprue patients than in control biopsies, and migration in treated patients was intermediate between that seen in the untreated and that in normals (Trier and Browning, 1970).

In addition to the above evidence for accelerated proliferation, migration, and cell loss in sprue, further studies have quantitated the depth and width of crypts and shown that there is a four fold increase in the total number of cells composing the gland of a patient with celiac sprue. This is made possible by an increase not only in the length but also in the width of crypts. The mitotic index is nearly double the control value in the sprue patient (Table 4), while the number of proliferating cells is increased threefold (Wright *et al.*, 1973*b*) from a mean of 780 to 3050 in the sprue patient. Cells in the maturational compartment, directly above the proliferative compartment, were increased 6 times the number normally found in the control crypt.

It can be seen in Table 4 that the growth fraction, that is, the number of cells participating in cell proliferation, is lower in sprue patients than in control patients. Keeping in mind the increased number of proliferating cells in these patients, this percentage, while lower, nevertheless involves a greater number of epithelial cells in the entire crypt.

The total cell cycle time of the epithelial cells in the untreated sprue patient was also found to be markedly shorter than that in the unaffected patient. On this basis alone, a doubling of the cell production rate would occur (Wright *et al.*, 1973*a*).

The mucosa of the sprue patient, in summary, shows an increased rate of cell production, which balances its high rate of cell loss. To accommodate the large number of proliferating cells recognized by the high mitotic index, there is a compensatory increase in the depth and width of these crypts, a finding that agrees with the deep and convoluted glands often seen in sprue mucosa.

3.3.2. *Gastric Heterotopia in Small Bowel Mucosa*

Patients with longstanding regional enteritis or Crohn's disease commonly have pyloric gland metaplasia present in the small bowel mucosa. However, only occasionally do patients with regional enteritis also have metaplastic glands with parietal and chief cells (Lechago *et al.*, 1976). No endocrine cells were observed in the latest report on gastric heterotopia in the small intestine.

Trier *et al.* (1973) did observe several types of endocrine cells by electron microscopy as well as the presence of parietal and zymogen cells in small bowel tissue from a patient with celiac sprue. The origin of this heterotopic gastric mucosa is of great interest and can be speculated about in several ways. If, as stated by several investigators, a stem cell gives rise to all cell types (Cheng and Leblond, 1974; Matsuyama and Suzuki, 1970), then the simplest explanation has been provided. Alternatively, if endocrine cells of the gut originate from the neural crest and migrate to the primitive gut during embryogenesis, then they should be present as a congenital condition. The lack of endocrine cells in the case reported by Lechago *et al.* (1976) would suggest the acquisition of a heterotopic mucosa.

4. Large Intestine

4.1. Histology

The tubelike alimentary tract becomes the large bowel immediately following the appendix and caecum and is composed of several portions: ascending or left colon, transverse colon, descending or right colon, sigmoid colon, and rectum. The basic architecture of the large intestine is the same throughout, with the mucosa structured into glands called crypts of Lieberkühn. These are lined with epithelial cells of four types: columnar, mucous, enteroendocrine, and Paneth cell, the last two occurring in relatively small numbers. For example, human rectal mucosa contains approximately two argentaffin cells per crypt (Deschner, 1965) and Paneth cells are only rarely found in the ascending colon. Verity *et al.* (1962) reported the number to be four Paneth cells per 100 crypts in normal human ascending colon, whereas a 200-fold increase occurred in mucosa of ulcerative colitis.

Because of the wide dispersion of enteroendocrine cells, their specific type and function have not been easily worked out. However, cells showing glucagon immunoreactivity have been found in the middle and deeper parts of the crypt with a mean frequency of 3.3 cells per crypt (Knudsen *et al.*, 1975). The stem cells for these four cell types of the colonic mucosa are the vacuolated crypt-base columnar cells. After one mitosis and the formation of some intermediate cell types, endocrine and mucous cells have a limited capacity to undergo mitosis and form their own cell type (Chang and Nadler, 1975; Nabeyama, 1975).

4.2. Proliferation Kinetics of Normal Large Bowel Mucosa

The colon and rectum of man were among the earliest regions of the human gastrointestinal tract to be examined with detailed kinetic measurements of cell renewal. Repeated biopsies were obtained from patients who were intravenously injected with tritiated thymidine. Samples of the same area were taken at intervals which made it feasible to learn the zone of DNA synthesis, the duration of S phase, the speed of migration of labeled cells, and the turnover rate of the tissue (Cole and McKalen, 1961; Lipkin *et al.*, 1963*a;* MacDonald *et al.*, 1964). These studies showed the replacement time for these tissues to range from 3–4 days (Lipkin *et al.*, 1963*a*) to 6–8 days (Cole and McKalen, 1961) (Table 5). Cell proliferation occupied about 65% of the lower crypt column, and about 15–25% of the crypt cells were in the S phase which

Table 5. Kinetic Parameters of Normal Large Bowel

	T_{G_2} (hr)	T_S (hr)	T_M (hr)	T_{G_1} (hr)	T_c	Turnover time (hr)	LI (%)	References
Colon,								
in vivo	1, 2	14, 14				72–96	17, 18	Lipkin *et al.* (1963*a*)
	<6	20	1	14	40			Lipkin *et al.* (1963*a*)
	2	11				72–96	12	Lipkin *et al.* (1963*b*)
Rectum								
In vivo	2	9–10			24–48	144	25	Lipkin *et al.* (1963*b*)
		14					18.8	Shorter *et al.* (1966)
						144–192		Cole and McKalen (1961)
						96–132		MacDonald *et al.* (1964)
In vitro					82 ± 14			Camplejohn *et al.* (1973)
		7.2–8.9			77.2–129.9		5.9–9.4	Galand *et al.* (1968)
		8, 8.6				74, 86	10, 10.8	Bleiberg *et al.* (1972)
						58.56 ± 6.48 (S.E.)		Spencer *et al.* (1969)
						87.84 ± 10.08	1.53 ± 0.12	Shorter *et al.* (1966)
		7.9			90		9.5	Bleiberg *et al.* (1970)
		11.2				73	17.0	Bleiberg and Galand (1976)

lasted 10–15 hr (Lipkin *et al.*, 1963*a,b*). Additional studies of the duration of S in the various areas of the large bowel have not shown them to have more than a twofold variability (i.e., 9–20 hr), although some *in vitro* studies of normal rectum have reported S phase to be as short as 7.2 hr (Galand *et al.*, 1968). In addition to shorter duration of S phase, these *in vitro* experiments reported a significantly lower percentage of labeled cells after short exposure of the tissue to the radioactive precursor. In this instance, incorporation of the isotope throughout the specimen may have been prevented since adequate penetration is oxygen dependent and a point of anoxia is rapidly reached within specimens larger than about 170 μm (Thomlinson and Gray, 1955).

Studies on the descending colon of mice have shown diurnal variation to be present and to influence proliferative activity (Chang and Nadler, 1975). Almost a twofold range of values for labeling indices was demonstrated within a 24-hr period. The lowest values for the appearance of labeled cells occurred at 1600 hr, i.e., late afternoon. Obviously, should diurnal variation characterize colonic epithelial cells in man, then greater care will be required in experiments and their interpretation.

The existence of diurnal variability can possibly explain data recently obtained from a patient with multiple polyposis who was studied with both *in vitro* and *in vivo* techniques. A labeling index of 19.4% was obtained when fragments of a biopsy of normal-appearing mucosa were incubated at 11:30 A.M. in nutrient media with tritiated thymidine added (Deschner, unpublished observations). Diffusion of the isotope under these *in vitro* conditions was maximal, with similar grain densities evident throughout each fragment. In contrast, a labeling index of 2.9% occurred when the radionuclide was injected at 9 P.M. (Lipkin *et al.*, unpublished observations).

In addition to replication of the epithelial cells which line the crypts, fibroblasts which provide the collagenous sheath that surrounds each crypt also have been shown to undergo DNA synthesis and mitosis (Kaye *et al.*, 1968). These cells have been demonstrated to migrate in an upward direction and differentiate close to the surface. Possibly the intimate contact which exists between epithelial and mesenchymal cell components enables them not only to be associated but also to interact in a close relationship.

4.3. Diseases of Large Intestine

4.3.1. Ulcerative Colitis

Inflammatory bowel disease has been analyzed for chromosomal abnormalities and found to show a modal chromosome number in the diploid range but with cells in the hypotetraploid range also present (Xavier *et al.*, 1973). In addition, chromatid breaks were demonstrated in over 10% of the metaphase plates analyzed.

This disease state marked by continued ulceration and regeneration of the mucosa is seen to have its earliest changes at the surface beneath the columnar epithelial layer when foci of degeneration of the reticular, fibrillar, or collagen membrane occur (Donnellan, 1966). This degeneration spreads laterally and later extends into the lamina propria, where the collagen fibers become altered and plasma cells and lymphocytes are increased in number. Adenomatous polyps have been reported in 3% and inflammatory polyposis in 17% of cases assessed by colonoscopy (Teague and Read, 1975).

The morphology of the surface epithelium also becomes changed in time, with characteristic shrinkage of the cells, increase in intercellular spaces, and stunting or decrease in the microvilli taking place. Occlusion of blood vessels occurs and eventually causes necrosis of the epithelium followed by the formation of abscesses and ulceration of the mucosa, and various stages of regeneration.

This continued process of damage and repair, the causation of which is unknown, has serious consequences which include a higher risk for colon cancer. The transformation of this injured mucosa to adenomatous epithelium is thought to be an early stage in its progression to cancer (Fenoglio and Pascal, 1973). Nineteen percent of biopsy and colectomy specimens from patients with ulcerative colitis have been found to contain foci of adenomatous epithelium. It is believed that cancer evolves by the further action of unknown promoting agents on this noninvasive neoplastic mucosa (Fenoglio and Pascal, 1973). Lane and his associates (1971) as well as Morson (1974) have suggested that any carcinoma of the large bowel arises from adenomatous epithelium, and its existence in ulcerative colitis specimens would provide support for this mode of pathogenesis.

4.3.2. *Kinetic Measurements*

Estimates of the renewal time of epithelial cells in specimens of rectal mucosa from patients with ulcerative colitis have been carried out using different parameters; those employing mitotic indices have shown decreased cell proliferation in rectal mucosa (Shorter *et al.*, 1966; Spencer *et al.*, 1969) in this tissue. Completely divergent results have been obtained using isotopic labeling techniques with this same tissue. Cultured rectal biopsies from patients with ulcerative colitis showed faster migration of labeled epithelial cells to the luminal surface as well as a twofold increase in the number of cells involved in DNA synthesis (Eastwood and Trier, 1973).

These findings correlate with those of Bleiberg *et al.* (1970), who used a double-labeling technique that enabled them to obtain a value for S phase, which may be altered in this disease state. Two different dilutions of $TdRH^3$, one heavy and one weak, were used to selectively label cells with a brief interval between. The ratio $N_h/N_w = S/t$ provides a value for T_S. With a known S phase and labeling index, one may substitute numerical values in the following formula to derive the turnover time: $T = (T_S/\mathrm{LI}) \times 100$.

The duration of T_S was not altered (normal 7.9 hr, ulcerative colitis 9.2 hr), but the labeling index was found to be 2½ times that of the normal rectal mucosa. The turnover time in normal rectal mucosa using this technique was

90 hr while in mucosa from ulcerative colitis it was 40% of that, indicating an extremely fast proliferation rate (Bleibert *et al.*, 1970).

An additional abnormality reported by investigators (Bleiberg *et al.*, 1970; Eastwood and Trier, 1973) was the presence of a zone of DNA synthesis extended toward the surface, a phenomenon often seen in mucosa adjacent to polyps (Deschner *et al.*, 1966). The degree of severity of the cell loss at the surface undoubtedly acts by a feedback mechanism to govern the extent of the crypt needed to produce new epithelial cells so that the more severely affected and friable the mucosa, the more extensive the zone of DNA synthesis. Simultaneously a defect in the regulation of DNA synthesis in this tissue associated with the transformation of cells to adenomatous neoplasia may also lead to this abnormal zone of DNA synthesis. Fenoglio and Pascal (1973) have indicated the not too frequent appearance of foci of adenomatous epithelium, which may correlate with these areas' displaying an extended zone of proliferation.

4.3.3. *Polyps*

Adenomatous or tubular polyps as well as villous adenomas occur in the asymptomatic population over 40 years of age with an incidence that has been found to vary from 0.5% to 7.9% (Corman *et al.*, 1974). Patients with a colorectal polyp also demonstrate a high frequency of metachronous polyps and future carcinomas in this portion of the alimentary canal (Prager *et al.*, 1974). Although there is an increased susceptibility to polyp formation in this population, the factors which act to initiate and accelerate the polyp-to-cancer sequence are not well understood, and are now being investigated in several ways, including kinetic analysis.

Cell renewal within these polyps has been shown to occur along the luminal surface as well as along the length of the crypt columns (Kaye *et al.*, 1971; Deschner *et al.*, 1966). This can be quantitated and expressed graphically (Fig. 1) to show that in the adenoma over 60% of the cells undergoing DNA synthesis are located in the upper one-third of the neoplastic glands. Villous adenomas show a similar proliferative pattern (Deschner *et al.*, 1966).

This is in contrast to the hyperplastic polyp, which has epithelial cells primarily in the lower two-thirds of the crypts incorporating TdR^3H and undergoing cell proliferation (Kaye *et al.*, 1971). Both the epithelial cells and the fibroblastic sheath at the surface are well differentiated in the case of the hyperplastic polyp, whereas an immature sheath underlies the luminal cells of the adenoma. No differences have been found to characterize the single isolated adenoma from the adenomas found in patients with multiple or familial polyposis. Neither the microscopic or submicroscopic appearance nor the kinetic behavior of the cells in these neoplasms can discriminate the disease in which they arise; only the criteria of their frequency separate the two conditions.

Bleiberg *et al.* (1972) have obtained values for some kinetic parameters in the polyp and flat mucosa of patients with familial polyposis using the double-

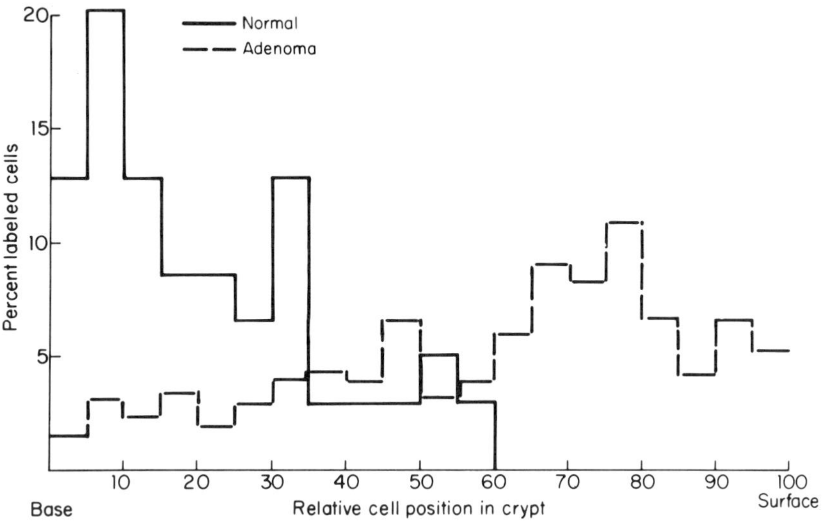

Fig. 1. Percent of labeled cells in five cell positions, in normal colonic mucosa and adenomas of an individual with inherited adenomatosis of colon and rectum, after intravenous pulse injection of tritiated thymidine. In normal mucosa, thymidine is incorporated into proliferating cells located in the lower two-thirds of the colonic crypts. In adenomas, epithelial cells incorporating thymidine into DNA are mainly located near the surfaces of the crypts.

label technique. No difference in the durations of S phase of 7–8 hr was found, but labeling indices in polyp specimens were twice those in the normal-appearing mucosa. A lower value for the estimate of the polyp turnover time was obviously reflected (Table 6). While cell production proceeds rapidly in this tissue, cell loss may also be high, so that the net retention of cells may be small and the size of the lesion only relatively slowly increases.

4.3.4. Flat Mucosa of Patients with Polyps

Histologically normal-appearing mucosa of patients with a single isolated polyp and mucosa between polyps in patients with multiple or familial polyposis often have epithelial cell proliferation beyond the lower two-thirds of crypts (Deschner *et al.,* 1963, 1966; Deschner and Lipkin, 1975; Cole and McKalen, 1963; Bleiberg *et al.,* 1972). Well-differentiated cells that incorporate TdR in the upper third and along the surface can be found. This finding appears to indicate a loss of the regulatory control that terminates DNA synthesis as matured cells reach this region of the gland. In addition to patients with one or more polyps, symptom-free members of polyposis families and even symptom-free patients in the general population have been shown to have this abnormal zone of DNA synthesis in some crypts of their rectal mucosa (Deschner and Lipkin, 1975). This abnormality is believed to be an early event in the formation of neoplasms since it has been seen with greatest frequency in patients with familial polyposis and patients with a previous history of polyps.

Table 6. Kinetic Parameters of Preneoplastic and Neoplastic Conditions of the Large Bowel

	L.I. (%)	M.I. (%)	S (hr)	Turnover time (hr)	References
Rectum, *in vitro*					
Ulcerative colitis in remission	7.0 ± 2.6				Deschner *et al.* (1966)
Active ulcerative colitis	25.9		9.2	34.2	Bleiberg *et al.* (1970)
Polyp, villous adenoma			12	>24	Lipkin *et al.* (1970)
Polyp, adenoma of familial polyposis	22.9		7.4	32.6	Bleiberg *et al.* (1972)
In vivo polyps, adenoma of familial polyposis	2.0		15	>40	Lipkin *et al.* (unpublished observations)
Carcinoma					
In vivo	21.7	2.9			Hoffman and Post (1967)
In vitro	15.4	0.3		51.9	Lieb and Lisco (1966)
	32.5		19.4	61.9	Bleiberg and Galand (1976)
In vivo		1.17		159–244	Camplejohn *et al.* (1973)
In vivo	23.1	2.2	14	26	Terz *et al.* (1971)
Carcinoma					
Rectosigmoid *in vitro*	4.5	1.2		177.7	Lieb and Lisco (1966)
Sigmoid *in vitro*	10.9, 26.5	2.8, 1.4		30.2–73.4	Lieb and Lisco (1966)
Colon					
In vivo	13, 14.5	2.1, 2.9			Hoffman and Post (1967)
In vivo				75	Baserga *et al.* (1962)
Caecum, *in vitro*	20.2	0.7		39.6	Lieb and Lisco (1966)

4.3.5. Colonic Carcinoma

Relatively few studies have successfully been carried out on the growth characteristics of colonic carcinomas, undoubtedly because of the difficulty and inconvenience in obtaining repeated specimens, as well as the reluctance of investigators to use the nuclear-incorporated isotopic precursor TdR^3H. As might be expected, labeling indices of tissues that were tagged *in vitro* provide the lowest values for the percent of cells in DNA synthesis phase (4.5% and 10.9%) as well as the lowest mitotic indices (0.3% and 0.7%). Several observations emerge from the data presented in Table 6. Wide differences in labeling and mitotic indices were reported among the tumors studied even when handled by the same investigators. Replicates from a different area of the tumor also showed marked variability, with some having a threefold difference in the percent of labeled cells in the center (11.9%) vs. the periphery (38%) of the lesion (Lieb and Lisco, 1966). This difficulty in characterizing kinetic parameters of tumors was also experienced by Camplejohn *et al.* (1973), who attempted to correlate mitotic indices with the Duke stage of each cancer. No correlation between the degree of differentiation and spread could be found with the rate of mitotic activity. These authors believe the variability within an individual tumor to be of the same order as the variability between tumors.

A productive study of a colonic carcinoma was carried out by Terz *et al.* (1971) over a 6-day span. The cell cycle parameters were obtained with several methods, including the percent labeled mitoses curve and grain count halving technique. The total cell cycle time was found to be approximately 26 hr, with an S phase of 14 hr and G_1 of 5 hr. It is the latter phase which had proved most difficult to obtain in previous studies since secondary waves are so depressed as to make the midpoint of the ascending limb unreadable (Lipkin *et al.*, 1970). The lack of a clear secondary wave stems from the loss of synchrony of the labeled population of cells.

Values for the duration of G_2 in adenocarcinomas range from 4 hr (Lipkin *et al.*, 1970) to 5.7 hr (Terz *et al.*, 1971). However, it was extended to a 15-hr duration in a villous papilloma reported by Lipkin *et al.* (1970). Likewise, a long duration of mitosis was calculated by Camplejohn *et al.* (1973) using an *in vivo* technique in which the interphase blocking agent vincristine sulfate was intravenously injected. Epithelial cells of the 19 carcinomas studied had a mean mitotic duration of 2.3 hr compared with a value of 1.2 hr for cells in the normal rectal tissue. The importance of this finding lies in relationship to the observation made by investigators that tumors proliferate rapidly by virtue of the frequent occurrence of mitoses in that tissue. Obviously, instead of an increased number of dividing cells, there appears to be a prolongation of that stage of the cell cycle.

Epithelial cells of carcinomas of the large bowel have cell cycle times which are reported to vary from 26 to 244 hr (Table 6). The percentage of cells engaged in proliferative activity, known as the growth fraction, can be estimated, and only 13–25% was derived for the renewal of the 19 carcinomas studied by Camplejohn *et al.* (1973). This is a smaller fraction than that reported by Terz, which, depending on the formula he followed, was 42–49% of the cells. Frindel *et al.* (1968) showed a similar twofold variability in growth fractions among five cases of different solid tumors. However, differences may exist within a tumor since poorly oxygenated tumor areas have lower growth fractions than do well-oxygenated ones (Tannock and Steel, 1970).

Doubling times of colon cancers using radiological techniques have been reported to range from 111 to 3430 days (Welin *et al.*, 1963). Cell kinetic studies have usually estimated this factor; for example, Terz *et al.* (1971) calculated 45 days for this parameter. Other values have been in the range of 3 days (Lieb and Lisco, 1966; Hoffman and Post, 1967; Baserga *et al.*, 1962) to ten days (Camplejohn *et al.*, 1973). Steel (1967) calculated the potential doubling time of 31 colon tumors to be 13.5 days, a value which again differed drastically with measurements of the actual volume doubling times. Thus it is valuable to combine cell kinetic studies and radiological measurements on the same tumors, to assess doubling time in relation to other kinetic parameters.

There is a need to reconcile the durations of the cell cycle time, which are relatively short, and the values for the growth fraction with the slow growth of these tumors. One factor which may contribute to this difference is the high rate of cell loss which affects the tumor population. Estimates of this value range from the extremely high rate of over 90% (Camplejohn *et al.*, 1973) to between 36% and 49% (Terz *et al.*, 1971). Undoubtedly wide variability exists based on such considerations as the size of the tumor, the blood supply, and the degree of abnormality expressed within the genetic material and proliferative characteristics of the neoplastic cells.

Rather than cell loss, one may consider the reverse situation, that is, estimate the fraction of proliferating epithelial cells retained in the tumor. This can be calculated from the kinetic parameter or growth coefficient (k_g/k_b) when values are estimated in cells per hour per cell for the birth rate of cells (k_b) and growth rate of adenomatous lesions (k_g). In a patient with familial polyposis the value for this parameter indicated that 25% of cells were retained in the expanding colonic polyps while 75% of the newly formed cells died or were extruded from the tumor mass (Lipkin *et al.*, unpublished observations).

The important kinetic concept within tumors of a nonproliferating pool of cells also is important. This has been borne out by continuous infusion of tritiated thymidine into patients with leukemia (Clarkson *et al.*, 1970). Seven to twelve percent of leukemic cells were unlabeled after 8–10 days of constant infusion, indicating either the presence of cells with cell cycle times longer than this or the presence of cells which were no longer capable of proliferation. Quastler (1963) proposed that cells in G_1 which did not reenter S phase, but instead had an extended interval in this G_1 phase, were in a reserve state he termed G_0. The size of this nonproliferating pool is essentially unknown in solid tumors, yet it is undoubtedly one of the most important parameters to investigate since it is of therapeutic concern. Such cells as are outside the proliferating pool are presumed to be resistant to both radiation and chemotherapy and may be the nucleus of cells from which tumors regrow after such treatments. Procedures which recall these nonproliferating cells back into the proliferating pool are a necessary adjunct to therapy if a cure rather than a relapse is to be expected.

5. Conclusion

In conclusion, it is evident that a reasonably large body of information has been developed about proliferation and differentiation of normal and abnormal cells of the gastrointestinal tract. These studies have begun to offer a rational description of cell growth in disease states and of the areas in cell cycle analysis where metabolic abnormalities should be studied to further elucidate biochemical changes in the affected cells. Information of this type also should contribute to new approaches to the therapy of disease.

In continuance of the various approaches to the topics mentioned above, two general types of investigation are under way. One involves attempts to elucidate intracellular factors that function during various stages of proliferation and differentiation, and includes analysis of events that are involved in DNA metabolism, transcription, and translation during cell maturation. Another involves analyses of extracellular elements that may contribute to cell proliferation and differentiation, including hormonal, neural, and nutritional factors, together with interactions that may initially involve the cell membranes. Stimulatory and inhibitory properties contained in the extracellular environment have been shown to influence cell proliferation and differentiation.

With studies in these areas under way, attempts are being made to elucidate mechanisms contributing to gastrointestinal disease. For example, studies of the evolution of neoplastic transformation of gastrointestinal cells and of the mechanisms involved in gastrointestinal carcinogenesis are dependent on accurate measurements of proliferation and differentiation-specific events occurring in the cells. It has been found that the proliferative changes involved in the progression of neoplastic transformation of gastrointestinal cells in man are similar to those in rodent after the administration of chemical carcinogens. These studies have led to the development of programs to identify humans that have cytological and related biochemical abnormalities denoting aberrant proliferative activity and cell transformation. Current and future considerations of factors that contribute to the cause and to the prevention of gastrointestinal neoplasia must focus on identification of human population groups having early proliferative abnormalities in their cells. Relationships between inherited and environmental elements, and means to modify the evolution of proliferative errors during neoplasia, will be addressed. Classification of individuals on the basis of aberrant cell proliferation, measurement of the progression of cell transformation within them, and determination of the susceptibility of their cells to tumorigenesis are some of the topics that will occupy the attention of investigators.

ACKNOWLEDGMENTS

The authors' original work reported in this chapter was carried out in the Laboratory of Gastrointestinal Research of the Sloan-Kettering Institute, and the Cornell University Medical College, and was aided by NCI Contract 1-CP-43366 and Grants CA 14991 and 08748 from the National Cancer Institute, Department of Health, Education and Welfare.

6. *References*

Baserga, R., Henegar, G. C., Kisieleski, W. E., and Lisco, H., 1962, Uptake of tritiated thymidine by human tumors in vivo, *Lab. Invest.* **11**:360–364.

Bell, B., Almy, T. P., and Lipkin, M., 1967, Cell proliferation kinetics in the gastrointestinal tract of man. III. Cell renewal in esophagus, stomach, and jejunum of a patient with treated pernicious anemia. *J. Natl. Cancer Inst.* **38**:615–628.

Bertalanffy, F. D., and Nagy, K. P., 1961, Mitotic activity and renewal of the epithelial cells of human duodenum, *Acta. Anat.* **45**:362–370.

Bleiberg, H., and Galand, P., 1876, *In vitro* autoradiographic determination of cell kinetic parameters in adenocarcinomas and adjacent healthy mucosa of the human colon and rectum, *Cancer Res.* **36**:325–328.

Bleiberg, H., Mainguet, P., Galand, P., Chreteen, J., and Dupont-Mairesse, N., 1970. Cell renewal in the human rectum: *In vitro* autoradiographic study on active ulcerative colitis, *Gastroenterology* **58**:851–855.

Bleiberg, H., Mainguet, P., and Vandenhende, J., 1971, Mesure autoradiographicque de la prolifération cellulaire á différente niveaux du tractus digestif normal et pathologique: Utilisation de biopsies incubées *in vitro, Rev. Eur. Etud. Clin. Biol.* **16**:233–239.

Bleiberg, H., Mainguet, P., and Galand, P., 1972, Cell renewal in familial polyposis: Comparison between polyps and adjacent healthy mucosa, *Gastroenterology* **63**:240–245.

Buffa, R., Solcia, E,, and Go, V. L. M., 1976, Immunohistochemical identification of the cholecystokinin cell in the intestinal mucosa, *Gastroenterology* **70**:528–532.

Camplejohn, R. S., Bone, G., and Aherne, W., 1973, Cell proliferation in rectal carcinoma and rectal mucosa: A stathmokinetic study, *Eur. J. Cancer* **9**:577–581.

Castrup, H. J., Fuchs, K., and Peiper, H. J., 1975, Cell renewal of gastric mucosa in Zollinger-Ellison syndrome, *Acta Hepato-Gastroenterol.* **22**:40–43.

Chang, W. W. L., and Nadler, N. J., 1975, Renewal of the epithelium in the descending colon of the mouse. IV. Cell population kinetics of vacuolated-columnar and mucous cells, *Am. J. Anat.* **144**:39–56.

Cheng, H., and Leblond, C. P., 1974, Origin, differentiation, and renewal of the four main epithelial cell types in the mouse small intestine. V. Unitarian theory of the origin of the four epithelial cell types, *Am. J. Anat.* **141**:537–548.

Clarke, R. M., 1970. A new method of measuring the rate of shedding of epithelial cells from the intestinal villus of the rat, *Gut* **11**:1015–1019.

Clarkson, B. S., Strife, A., Fried, J., Sakai, Y., Ota, K., Ohkita, T., and Masuda, R., 1970, Studies of cellular proliferation in human leukemia. IV. Behavior of normal hematopoietic cells in 3 adults with acute leukemia given continuous infusions of ^{3}H-thymidine for 8 or 10 days, *Cancer* **26**:1–19.

Cole, J. W., and McKalen, A., 1961, Observations of cell renewal in human rectal mucosa *in vivo* with thymidine-H^{3}, *Gastroenterology* **41**:122–125.

Cole, J. W., and McKalen, A., 1963, Studies on the morphogenesis of adenomatous polyps in the human colon, *Cancer* **16**:998–1002.

Corman, M. L., Veidenheimer, M. C., and Coller, J. A., 1974, Barium-enema findings in asymptomatic patients with rectal polyps, *Dis. Col. Rect.* **17**:325–330.

Croft, D. W., Loehry, C. A., and Creamer, B., 1968, Small bowel cell-loss and weight-loss in the celiac syndrome, *Lancet* **2**:68–70.

Deschner, E. E., 1965, Argentaffin cell incidence in the rectal mucosa of man, mouse and hamster, *Nature (London)* **207**:873–874.

Deschner, E. E., and Lipkin, M., 1975, Proliferative patterns in colonic mucosa in familial polyposis, *Cancer* **35**:413–418.

Deschner, E. E., Lewis, C. M., and Lipkin, M., 1963, *In vitro* study of human epithelial cells. I. Atypical zone of H^3-thymidine incorporation in mucosa of multiple polyposis, *J. Clin. Invest.* **42**:1922–1928.

Deschner, E. E., Lipkin, M., and Solomon, C., 1966, *In vitro* study of human epithelial cells. II H^3-Thymidine incorporation into polyps and adjacent mucosa, *J. Natl. Cancer Inst.* **36**:849–857.

Deschner, E. E., Winawer, S., and Lipkin, M., 1972, Patterns of nucleic acid and protein synthesis in normal human gastric mucosa and atrophic gastritis, *J. Nat. Cancer Inst.* **48**:1568–1574.

Deschner, E. E., Goldstein, M. J., Melamed, M. R., and Sherlock, P., 1976, Autoradiographic observations of a nineteen month old ileal conduit, *Gastroenterology* **71**:832–834.

Donnellan, W. L., 1966, Early histological changes in ulcerative colitis, *Gastroenterology* **50**:519–540.

Eastwood, G. L., and Trier, J. S., 1973, Epithelial cell renewal in cultured rectal biopsies, *Gastroenterology* **64**:383–390.

Fenoglio, C. M., and Pascal, R. R., 1973, Adenomatous epithelium, intraepithelial anaplasia, and invasive carcinoma in ulcerative colitis, *Digest. Dis.* **18**:556–562.

Foroozan, P., and Trier, J. S., 1967, Mucosa of the small intestine in pernicious anemia, *N. Eng. J. Med.* **277**:553–559.

Frindel, E., Malaise, E. P., Alpen, E., and Tubiana, M., 1968, Kinetics of cell proliferation of an experimental tumor, *Cancer Res.* **27**:1122–1130.

Fry, R. J. M., Lesher, S., Kisieleski, W. E., and Sacher, G., 1963, Cell proliferation in the small intestine, in: *Cell Proliferation* (L. F. Lamerton and R. J. M. Fry, eds.), pp. 213–233, F. A. Davis, Philadelphia.

Galand, P., Mainguet, P., Arguello, M., Chretien, J., and Douxfils, N., 1968, *In vitro* autoradiographic studies of cell proliferation in the gastrointestinal tract of man, *J. Nucl. Med.* **9**:37–39.

Gilbertsen, V. A., 1974, Proctosigmoidoscopy and polypectomy in reducing the incidence of rectal cancer, *Cancer* **34**:936–939.

Grable, E., Zamcheck, N., Jankelson, O., and Shipp, F., 1957, Nuclear size of cells in normal stomachs, in gastric atrophy, and in gastric cancer, *Gastroenterology* **32**:1104–1112.

Hansen, O. H., Pedersen, T., and Larsen, J. K., 1975, A method to study cell proliferation kinetics in human gastric mucosa, *Gut* **16**:23–27.

Hoffman, J., and Post, J., 1967, *In vivo* studies of DNA synthesis in human normal and tumor cells, *Cancer Res.* **27**:898–902.

Katz, S., Sherlock, P., and Winawer, S. J., 1972, Rectocolonic exfoliative cytology: A new approach. *Am. J. Digest. Dis.* **12**:1109–1116.

Kaye, G. I., Lane, N., and Pascal, R. R., 1968, Colonic pericryptal fibreoblast sheath: Replication, migration, and cytodifferentiation of a mesenchymal cell system in adult tissue. II. Fine structural aspects of normal rabbit and human colon, *Gastroenterology* **54**:852–865.

Kaye, G. I., Pascal, R. R., and Lane, N., 1971, The colonic pericryptal fibroblast sheath: Replication, migration, and cytodifferentiation of a mesenchymal cell system in adult tissue. III. Replication and differentiation in human hyperplasia and adenomatous polyps, *Gastroenterology* **60**:515–536.

Knudsen, J. B., Holst, J. I., Asmoes, S., and Johansen, A., 1975, Identification of cells with pancreatic-type and gut-type glucagon immunoreactivity in the human colon, *Acta Pathol. Microbiol. Scand. Sec. A* **83**:741–743.

Kobayashi, S., Fujita, T., and Sasagawa, T., 1970, The endocrine cells of human duodenal mucosa: An electron microscope study, *Arch. Histol. Jpn.* **31**:477–494.

Lane, N., Kaplan, H., and Pascal, R. R., 1971, Minute adenomatous and hyperplastic polyps of the colon: Divergent patterns of epithelial growth with specific associated mesenchymal changes, *Gastroenterology* **60**:537–551.

Lechago, J., Black, C., and Samloff, I. M., 1976, Immunofluorescence studies of gastric heterotopia of the small intestine in Crohn's disease, *Gastroenterology* **70**:429–432.

Liavag, I., 1968, Mitotic activity of gastric mucosa, *Acta Pathol. Microbiol. Scand.* **72**:43–63.

Lieb, L. M., and Lisco, H., 1966, *In vitro* uptake of tritiated thymidine by carcinoma of the human colon, *Cancer Res.* **36**:733–740.

Lipkin, M., and Bell, B., 1967, Cell proliferation, in: *Handbook of Physiology,* Vol. 5, Sect. 6: *Alimentary Canal* (C. F. Code, ed.), pp. 2861–2879, American Physiological Society, Washington, D.C.

Lipkin, M., Bell, B., and Sherlock, P., 1963*a,* Cell proliferation kinetics in the gastrointestinal tract of man. I. Cell renewal in colon and rectum, *J. Clin. Invest.* **42**:767–776.

Lipkin, M., Sherlock, P., and Bell, B., 1963*b,* Cell proliferation kinetics in the gastrointestinal tract of man. II. Renewal in stomach, ileum, colon, and rectum, *Gastroenterology* **45**:721–729.

Lipkin, M., Bell, B., Stadler, G., and Troncale, F., 1970, The development of abnormalities of growth in colonic epithelial cells of man, in: *Carcinoma of the Colon and Antecedent Epithelium* (H. Burdette, ed.), pp. 213–221, Thomas, Springfield, Ill.

MacDonald, W. C., Trier, J. S., and Everrett, N. B., 1964, Cell proliferation and migration in the stomach, duodenum, and rectum of man: Radioautographic studies, *Gastroenterology* **46**:405–417.

Maskens, A. P., and Deschner, E. E., 1977, Tritiated thymidine incorporation into epithelial cells of normal-appearing colorectal mucosa of cancer patients, *J. Natl. Cancer Inst.* **58**:1221–1224.

Matsuyama, M., and Suzuki, H., 1970, Differentiation of immature mucous cells into parietal, argyrophil and chief cells in stomach grafts, *Science* **169**:385–387.

Morson, B. C., 1974, The polyp–cancer sequences with the large bowel, *Proc. R. Soc. Med.* **67**:451–457.

Nabeyama, A., 1975, Presence of cells combining features of two different cell types in the colonic crypts and pyloric glands of the mouse, *Am. J. Anat.* **142**:471–484.

Padykula, H. A., Strauss, E. W., Ladman, A. J., and Gardner, E. H., 1961, A morphologic and histochemical analysis of the human jejunal epithelium in nontropical sprue, *Gastroenterology* **40**:736–765.

Pearse, A. G. E., 1973, Cell migration and the alimentary system: Endocrine contributions of the neural crest to the gut and its derivatives, *Digestion* **8**:372–385.

Pearse, A. G. E., Polak, J. M., Bloom, S. R., Adams, C., Dryburgh, J. R., and Brown, J. C., 1974, Enterochromaffin cells of the mammalian small intestine as a source of motilin, *Virchows Arch. B. Cell Pathol.* **16**:111–120.

Polak, J. M., Bloom, S., Coulling, I., and Pearse, A. G. E., 1971*a,* Immunofluorescent localization of secretin in the canine duodenum, *Gut* **12**:605–610.

Polak, J. M., Bloom, S., Coulling, I., and Pearse, A. G. E., 1971*b,* Immunofluorescent localization of enteroglucagon cells in the gastrointestinal tract of dog, *Gut* **12**:311–318.

Polak, J. M., Bloom, S. R., Kuzio, M., Brown, J. C., and Pearse, A. G. E., 1973, Cellular localization of gastric inhibitory polypeptide in the duodenum and jejunum, *Gut* **14**:284–288.

Polak, J. M., Pearse, A. G. E., and Heath, C. M., 1975, Complete identification of endocrine cells in the gastrointestinal tract using semithin-thin sections to identify motilin cells in human and animal intestine, *Gut* **16**:225–229.

Prager, E. D., Siventon, N. W., Young, J. L., Veidenheimer, M. C., and Corman, M. L., 1974, Follow-up study of patients with benign mucosal polyps discovered by proctosigmoidoscopy, *Dis. Col. Rectum* **17**:322–324.

Quastler, H., 1963, The analysis of cell population kinetics, in: *Cell Proliferation* (L. F. Lamerton and R. J. M. Fry, eds.), pp. 18–34, F. A. Davis, Philadelphia.

Raskin, H. F., and Pleticka, S., 1971, Exfoliative cytology of the colon, *Cancer* **28**:127–130.

Shorter, R. G., Spencer, R. J., and Hallenbeck, G. A., 1966, Kinetic studies of the epithelial cells of the rectal mucosa in normal subjects and patients with ulcerative colitis, *Gut* **7**:593–596.

Solcia, E., and Sampietro, R., 1965, Cytologic observation on the pancreatic islets with reference to some endocrine-like cells of the gastrointestinal mucosa, *Z. Zellforsch. Mikrosk. Anat.* **68**:689–698.

Spencer, R. J., Huizenga, K. A., Hammer, C. S., and Shorter, R. G., 1969, Further studies of the kinetics of rectal epithelium in normal subjects and patients with ulcerative or granulomatous colitis, *Dis. Colon Rectum* **12**:406–408.

Steel, G. G., 1967, Cell loss as a factor in the growth rate of human tumors, *Eur. J. Cancer* **3**:381–387.

Tanaka, J., 1968, Autoradiographic studies on the cell proliferation of the human gastric mucosa in supravital condition, *Acta. Pathol. Jpn.* **18**:307–318.

Tannock, I. F., and Steel, G. G., 1970, Tumor growth and cell kinetics in chronically hypoxic animals, *J. Natl. Cancer Inst.* **45**:123.

Teague, R. H., and Read, A. E., 1975, Polyposis in ulcerative colitis, *Gut* **16**:792–795.

Terz, J. J., Curatchet, H. P., and Lawrence, W., 1971, Analysis of the cell kinetics of human solid tumors, *Cancer* **28**:1100–1110.

Thomlinson, R. H., and Gray, L. H., 1955, The histological structure of some human lung cancers and the possible implications for radiotherapy, *Br. J. Cancer* **9**:539–549.

Tominaga, K., 1975, Distribution of parietal cells in the antral mucosa of human stomachs, *Gastroenterology* **69**:1201–1207.

Trier, J. S., and Browning, T. H., 1970, Epithelial-cell renewal in cultured duodenal biopsies in celiac sprue, *N. Eng. J. Med.* **283**:1245–1250.

Trier, J. S., Moxley, P. C., and Fordtran, J. S., 1973, Ectopic gastric mucosa in celiac sprue, *Gastroenterology* **65**:712–727.

Verity, M. A., Mellinkoff, S. M., Frankland, A. B., and Greipel, M., 1962, Serotonin content and argentaffin and Paneth cell changes in ulcerative colitis, *Gastroenterology* **43**:24–31.

Welin, S., Youker, J., and Spratt, J. S., 1963, The rates and patterns of growth of 375 tumors of the large intestine and rectum observed serially by double contrast enema study (Malmo technique), *Am. J. Roetgenol.* **90**:673–687.

Wiendl, H. J., Schwabe, M., Becker, G., and Kowatsch, J., 1974, Feulgencrytophotometric studies of gastric mucosal smears in malignant and benign diseases of the stomach, *Acta Cytol.* **18**:222–230.

Willems, G., and Lehy, T., 1975, Radiographic and quantitative studies on parietal and peptic cell kinetics in the mouse: A selective effect of gastrin on parietal cell proliferation, *Gastroenterology* **69**:418–427.

Winawer, S. J., and Lipkin, M., 1969, Cell proliferation kinetics in the gastrointestinal tract of man. IV. Cell renewal in the intestinalized gastric mucosa, *J. Natl. Cancer Inst.* **42**:9–17.

Wright, N., Watson, A., Morley, A., Appleton, D., Marks, J., and Douglas, A., 1973*a*, The cell cycle time in the flat (avillous) mucosa of the human small intestine, *Gut* **14**:603–606.

Wright, N., Watson, A., Morley, A., Appleton, D., and Marks, J., 1973*b*, Cell kinetics in flat (avillous) mucosa of the human small intestine, *Gut* **14**:701–710.

Xavier, R. G., Prolla, J. C., Bemvenuti, G. A., and Kirsner, J. B., 1973, Further tissue cytogenetic studies in inflammatory bowel disease, *Gastroenterology* **62**:189–875.

2

T- and B-Cell Populations in Gut and Gut-Associated Lymphoid Organs: Arrangement, Migration, and Function

Maria de Sousa and Robert A. Good

1. Introduction

The need to clarify the interface between gastrointestinal malignancy and the arrangement of lymphoid cell populations in the gut is well illustrated by the frequent finding of GI tumors in immunodeficient patients (reviewed in Chapter 3). Ironically, however, most of the experimental studies on the definition of the lymphatic system in the gut have focused on small intestine, Peyer's patches, and appendix (Parrott, 1976), whereas most of the tumours associated with immunodeficiency are located in the stomach (Chapter 3).

This is a further illustration of how the historical development of a subject influences the experiments one elects to do (de Sousa, 1976). First interest in the gut-associated lymphoid tissue (GALT), in modern immunological terms, was prompted by the search for a bursa-equivalent system in the mammal (Cooper *et al.,* 1966); the separate interest in IgA synthesis prompted the search for the tissue distribution of IgA-producing plasma cells (Tomasi *et al.,* 1965, Crandall *et al.,* 1967). Both motivating historical forces led to numerous studies of the intestinal lamina propria, the Peyer's patches, the appendix, and the mesenteric lymph node (reviewed by Parrott, 1976).

In the present chapter we summarize the conclusions of those studies, in the hope that the present climate of interest in cancer (Goodfield, 1975, 1977;

Maria de Sousa and Robert A. Good • Memorial Sloan-Kettering Cancer Center, New York, New York 10021.

Table 1. Chronology of Definition of Gut-Associated Lymphoid Populations

Year	Author(s)	Tissue	Procedure	Observation
1964	Gowans and Knight	Rat small intestine	Autoradiography	Large lymphocytes from the thoracic duct migrate to intestinal mucosa
1965	Tomasi *et al.*	Human parotid tissue	Immunofluorescence	Cells containing anti-11 S γA found in interstitial tissue
	Crabbe *et al.*	Human duodenal and jejunal mucosa	Immunofluorescence	Mean population density of γA-type cells: 181,000/mm^3 of interstitial tissue, against 18,000 for γG and 30,000 for γM cells
1967	Crandall *et al.*	Duodenum and ileum from *Trichinella spiralis*-infected rabbits	Immunofluorescence	Uniformly high proportion of IgA-containing cells found throughout infection
1968	Mandel and Asofsky	Mouse ileum, jejunum, and thoracic duct lymphocytes	Immunoglobulin synthesis *in vitro*	IgA synthesis by ileum, jejunum, and thoracic duct lymphocytes
1969	Crabbe *et al.*	Germ-free mouse duodenum, ileum, and colon	Detection of Ab-producing cells after subcutaneous, intraperitoneal, or enteric immunization with ferritin	Highest concentration of IgA-producing cells in lamina propria of small and large intestine
	de Sousa *et al.*	Nude mouse Peyer's patches	Light microscopy of histological sections	Selective lymphocyte (T) depletion of interfollicular areas
	Griscelli *et al.*	Rat Peyer's patches and small intestine mucosa	Autoradiography after transfer of [^{3}H]thymidine-labeled mesenteric or peripheral lymph node dividing cells	Preferential migration of the mesenteric and thoracic duct lymphoblasts to gut and gut-associated lymphoid tissue

1971	Craig and Cebra	Rabbit ileum	Cell transfer into animals of different allotype	Peyer's patches cells have the potential to proliferate and differentiate into IgA-producing cells; confirmation of Griscelli *et al.*'s discovery of preferential migration of "central lymph" lymphoid cells to gut
	Raff *et al.*	Mouse Peyer's patch	Immunofluorescence	
1972	Ferguson and Parrott	Mouse small intestine	Counts of intraepithelial lymphocytes in normal-sited and fetal small intestine grafted under the kidney capsule	Appearance of thymus-dependent and thymus-independent lymphocytes in epithelium is independent of antigen stimulation, but higher numbers are found after antigen stimulation
1973	Chanana *et al.*	Peyer's patches of newborn mice	Indirect immunofluorescence	Increase of Thy 1^+ cells from 60% in 1-day-old mice to 90% in 4-day-old mice
	Waksman	Calf and mouse Peyer's patches	Autoradiography following intrathymic labeling with $[^3H]$thymidine	Calf: heavily labeled cells found exclusively in TDA (thymus-dependent areas); newborn mouse: preponderance of labeled cells in TDA but also in adjacent dome epithelium
1974	Guy Grand *et al.*	Mouse small bowel, caecum, large bowel	Tracing the fate of ^{51}Cr-labeled or $[^3H]$thymidine-labeled peripheral and gut-associated lymphoid cells quantitatively and qualitatively by use of specific antisera	Highest amount of recovered radioactivity following injection of ^{51}Cr-labeled gut-associated cells in small bowel (4.9–6%); smaller amounts in caecum (1–3.2%) and large bowel (0.9–2.9%); all of intraepithelial lymphocytes appear to be T lymphocytes
	Rudzik and Bienenstock	Rabbit ileum	Passage of intestinal cell suspensions through glass bead column and BSA gradient for separation of lymphocytes	1% of lymphoid cells in epithelium contain intracytoplasmic IgA; 25% contain metachromatic granules that stain at low pH with Alcian blue, functional nature unknown
	Parrott and de Sousa	Nude mouse Peyer's patches	Autoradiography and light microscopy	No germinal centers in the absence of T cells; recovery after thymus grafting

Glasser, 1976) will prompt further studies to clarify the exact significance of the lymphoid structure and arrangement of lymphoid populations in the gut to the development, initial location, and spread of GI tumors.

2. *Experimental Animals and Procedures*

A list of the experimental animals and procedures whose use led to the present views on the distribution of T- and B-lymphocyte populations in the gut, Peyer's patches, and appendix is given in Table 1. The original immunofluorescent studies of Tomasi's and Hermann's groups established that the majority of plasma cells found associated with the acini of the salivary glands (Tomasi *et al.,* 1965) and in the intestinal lamina propria (Crabbe *et al.,* 1965) in man were synthesizing IgA.

Specific antiallotype antisera and immunofluorescence were used by Craig and Cebra (1971) to define for the rabbit the distribution of allotype-marked clones of IgA-producing cells transferred into allogeneic recipients of a different allotype. Specific anti-T- and anti-B-cell antisera have been used by Guy Grand *et al.* (1974*a*) to determine the exact positioning of transferred radioisotopically labeled T or B blasts in syngeneic recipient mice. Morphological studies of the structure of Peyer's patches in congenitally athymic nude mice led also to definition of T and B areas in Peyer's patches (de Sousa *et al.,* 1969), and quantitative morphological analysis of the numbers of lymphocytes associated with epithelial cells was done in the gut of nude mice raised in germ-free (Ferguson and Parrott, 1972) or conventional (Parrott and de Sousa, 1974) conditions.

In recent years, a considerable number of studies centered around the question of migration patterns of small and large lymphocyte populations to the gut. Most of these experiments have been done in rats, mice, and rabbits using autoradiography as the detection method for transferred radioisotopically labeled cells. $UdR^{125}I$ became the radioisotope of choice in experiments tracing the fate of blast cells, for it enables the simultaneous quantitative analysis of distribution of radioactivity in the recipient and autoradiographic analysis of the precise location of the labelled cells in tissues.

Regrettably, experimental studies of traffic of lymphoid cell populations to the stomach and the colon are lacking (Table 1).

3. *Morphological Aspects*

The evidence in favor of considering the mammalian gut-associated lymphoid system a peripheral lymphoid organ has been reviewed by Parrott (1976). Briefly, the work of Owen *et al.* (1974) on the differentiation of B cells in mouse fetal tissues demonstrated that B lymphocytes develop in the yolk sac, liver, spleen, and bone marrow before they can be detected in the gut. Moreover, following antigen stimulation morphological and cell traffic changes occur in the Ag-draining regions of the gut which are essentially similar to those occurring in other peripheral lymphoid organs, i.e., the lymph nodes. It must be said, however, that the close interactions of lymphocytes, epithelium, and antigens, which result from the basic anatomical arrangement of the gut, make this vast peripheral lymphoid organ intriguingly unique and complex. Only for the purpose of clarity shall we describe the distribution of the two main lymphocyte populations in the gut as if it were a simpler organ.

3.1. Positioning of T Cells

Knowledge of the positioning of T cells in the intestinal epithelium, the lamina propria, and the organized gut-associated lymphoid organs, i.e., Peyer's patches and appendix, has been derived from morphological studies of tissues of animals selectively depleted of T cells (Veldman, 1970; Nieuwenhuis, 1971; de Sousa *et al.*, 1969; Ferguson and Parrott, 1972; Parrott and de Sousa, 1974), from autoradiographic analysis of the distribution of radioisotopically labeled T cells derived from a [^{3}H]thymidine-infused thymus or following intravenous injection of T cells in syngeneic recipients

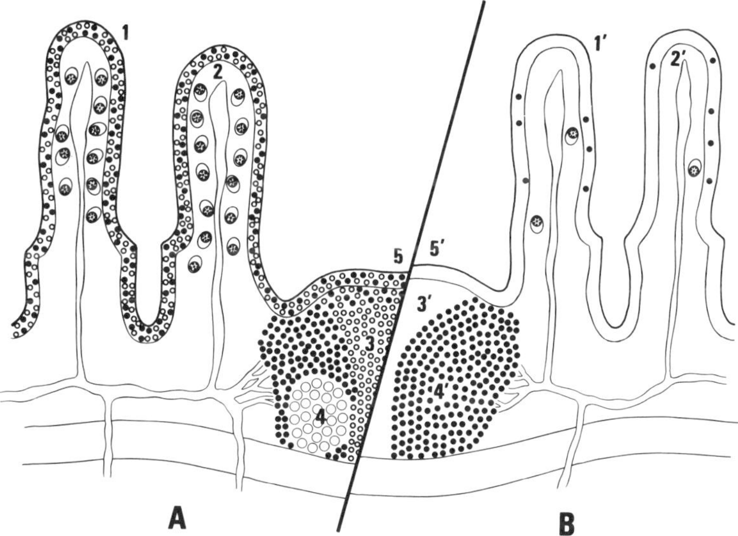

Fig. 1. Schematic representation of the distribution of T (○, 3) and B (•, 4′) lymphocytes, plasma cells (⊛), and germinal centers (◯,4) in the gut. Numerous T lymphocytes and variable numbers of B lymphocytes have been observed in the gut epithelium (1). The numbers of intraepithelial lymphocytes are markedly reduced in thymus-deprived animals (1′). Numerous IgA-containing plasma cells are normally present in the lamina propria (2). In the absence of T cells, the numbers of IgA-containing cells are reduced (2′). Thymus-dependent (3,3′) and thymus-independent (4,4′) areas have been delineated in the Peyer's patches. In thymus-deprived animals, germinal center development is impaired. Interaction between antigen and immunologically competent cells occurs most extensively in the dome areas (5,5′) of the Peyer's patches.

Table 2. Reported Percentages of T and B Lymphocytes in Gut Mucosa and Peyer's Patches

Section	Species	Marker	T	B	Null	Author(s)
Peyer's patch	Mouse (newborn)	T: anti-Thy 1 antiserum	60 (1 day) 90 (4 days)	ND ND	ND ND	Chanana *et al.* (1973)
	Mouse (adult)	T: anti-Thy 1 antiserum B: antiimmunoglobulin	20–40	67–68	—	Raff *et al.* (1971)
	Guinea pig (adult)	T: rosette formation with rabbit erythrocytes	33	68	—	Müller-Schoop and Good (1975)
	Mouse (adult)	T: heterologous rabbit antithymus antiserum B: anti-Peyer's patch cells	21	61	13	Veldkamp *et al.* (1974)
Epithelium	Mouse	T: rabbit anti-mouse specific antiserum (anti-MSLA) Immunofluorescence	100	0	0	Guy Grand *et al.* (1974*a,b*)
Gut mucosa	Rabbit	T: goat anti-rabbit thymus lymphocyte (cytotoxic test) B: anti-IgM, anti-IgG, anti-IgA antisera Immunofluorescence	11	16	70	Rudzik *et al.* (1975)

(Waksman, 1973; Parrott, 1976), from immunofluorescence analysis of tissue sections stained with specific anti-T antisera (Guy Grand *et al.*, 1974*a*), and from ultrastructural studies of intraepithelial lymphoblasts (Marsh, 1975*a*).

In the Peyer's patches, T cells are found in the interfollicular and dome areas and in the zone close to the external muscle layer (Fig. 1). Frequently in B mice which have been thymectomized, irradiated, and reconstituted with bone marrow cells, plasma cells are found in the T-cell-depleted areas, particularly in the outer and interfollicular zones.

In the rabbit appendix, T cells are distributed in the diamond-shaped areas between the upper ends of adjacent lymphoid nodules (Parrott, 1976).

T cells in the gut are not confined to organized lymphoid organs; their presence in the lamina propria and among villi epithelial cells has been detected with great precision in sections of mouse small intestine stained with specific rhodamine-labeled anti-T antiserum (Guy Grand *et al.*, 1974*a*). Furthermore, lymphoblasts with a large nucleus, a prominent nucleolus, and a cytoplasm packed with polyribosomes but no rough endoplasmic reticulum have been described by Marsh (1975*a*) in mouse epithelium. These are the characteristic features of T lymphoblasts in the mouse (Janossy *et al.*, 1973). In Marsh's study the lymphoblasts (both T and B) constituted approximately 5% of the total population of lymphocytes found associated with the epithelial cells. In an ultrastructural study without the simultaneous use of some surface marker, it is not possible to discern the origin of other-size lymphocytes (90% medium, 5% small), hence the significance of Guy Grand's first immunofluorescence studies in the mouse. From these studies it seems that the majority of epithelial lymphocytes are thymus derived, although some B lymphocytes are also present in this region (Table 2).

3.2. Positioning of B Cells

The positioning of B cells in the intestinal epithelium, lamina propria, and organized gut-associated lymphoid organs has been defined in part in the same work that led to the definition of T-cell distribution. In addition, interest in IgA synthesis (Mestecky and Lawton, 1974) was paralleled by an early interest in B cells in the gut and gut-associated lymphoid tissues, reflected in the studies published between 1965 and 1971 (Tomasi *et al.*, 1965; Crabbe *et al.*, 1965, 1969; Crandall *et al.*, 1967; Craig and Cebra, 1971). More recent work on traffic of B lymphocytes in the rabbit (Durkin *et al.*, 1975) and of thoracic duct lymphocytes with surface IgA in the rat (Williams and Gowans, 1975) has enlarged our understanding of the migration patterns of the gut-associated lymphoid populations involved in immune responses and immunoglobulin production.

In the Peyer's patches, B lymphocytes constitute the large nodular areas within which germinal centers develop in normal experimental animals raised in conventional conditions (Fig. 1). In axenic mice germinal centers do not develop in Peyer's patches but can be induced when bacteria are added to the germ-free diet (Pollard and Sharon, 1970). Germinal center development in

Peyer's patches does not seem to be related exclusively to antigen stimulation. Morphological studies of the peripheral lymphoid organs of congenitally athymic nude mice (Mitchell *et al.*, 1973; de Sousa and Pritchard, 1974) have revealed a failure to form germinal centers in the absence of T lymphocytes, even following stimulation with thymus-independent antigens (de Sousa and Pritchard, 1974; Parrott and de Sousa, 1974). Peyer's patch development has been observed in fetal grafts of small intestine implanted under the kidney capsule of mice kept in conventional conditions, in which the graft lumen remains antigen free; Peyer's patches under these conditions were about 1/10 or 1/20 the size of the Peyer's patches in the recipient's intestine and did not develop germinal centers even after 15 weeks *in situ* (Ferguson and Parrott, 1972). Similar examples of the influence of antigen "access" on the development of gut-associated lymphoid organs have been observed in studies of the rabbit appendix (Perey and Good, 1968; Stramignoni *et al.*, 1969; Blythman and Waksman, 1973) in which continuity of the appendix with the gut lumen was interrupted.

Under these conditions the size of the appendix is reduced considerably. The major morphological change consists in the loss of the sizable germinal centers usually found in this organ. Germinal centers reappear once continuity with the gut lumen is reestablished.

Each segment of the appendix contains a large germinal center surrounded by small B lymphocytes. B lymphocytes, however, are not confined to organized gut-associated lymphoid organs. Immunoblasts with ultrastructural features of B immunoblasts, i.e., densely staining cytoplasm containing abundant ribosomes and prominent collections of rough endoplasmic reticulum, have been observed among epithelial cells in the mouse jejunum (Marsh, 1975*a*). The majority of B cells in the intestine are IgA-containing cells in the lamina propria. Heremans and co-workers estimated a figure of 181,000 IgA-containing cells/mm^3 of lamina propria in a study of human intestine (Table 1). In the rabbit and mouse intestinal mucosa, the IgA-containing cells constitute 80–90% of the total population of plasma cells.

4. Quantitative Data on the Distribution of T and B Lymphocytes in Peyer's Patches and Intestinal Mucosa

Examination of tissue sections under the light, the fluorescence, or the electron microscope is a way of mapping the distribution of cells, but it does not give an exact measure of the proportions of cells present in the tissues. This can be achieved only by the analysis of cell suspensions for specific markers. The markers most frequently utilized to characterize the two major lymphocyte populations are surface immunoglobulin for the B cells, Thy 1 antigen on the surface of mouse T cells, and the presence of other T-cell antigens detected by specific anti-T antisera in other species. In the guinea pig, T cells have also been characterized by their ability to form rosettes with rabbit erythrocytes (Stadecker *et al.*, 1973; Müller-Schoop and Good, 1975).

The results of different groups studying the proportions of T and B cells in Peyer's patches of different experimental animals are remarkably close (Table 2). With the exception of the newborn mouse, in which there is a singularly high percentage (85–90%) of T cells (Chanana *et al.*, 1973), in the adult animals studied, namely the mouse (T: 20–40%, B: 67–69%, Raff *et al.*, 1971), the guinea pig (T: 33%, B: 68%, Müller-Schoop and Good, 1975), and the rabbit (T: 21%, B: 61%, Veldkamp *et al.*, 1974), the percentage of T cells in the Peyer's patches ranged from 20% to 40% and the percentage of B cells from 61% to 69%.

Studies attempting to mark the lymphoid cells found in the intestinal mucosa are more variable. Guy Grand *et al.* (1974*b*) found in mouse tissue sections stained with a specific anti-T antiserum that *all* intraepithelial lymphocytes were of thymus origin.

Rudzik *et al.* (1975), in a study of suspensions of rabbit intraepithelial lymphocytes isolated from the gut mucosa by the method of Rudzik and Bienenstock (1974), found a much lower proportion of T cells (11%), 17% B lymphocytes, and a very high proportion of "null" cells (65–70%), i.e., lymphoid cells with no detectable T or B marker on the surface. Mowatt (1975, quoted in Parrott, 1976), using the same technique for separation of intraepithelial lymphocytes in the mouse, detected a higher percentage of T cells (33%), no B cells, and a similar high proportion of "null" cells (Table 2).

5. Migration Patterns

Unlike the heart, the liver, or the kidney, the peripheral lymphoid organs consist basically of "nomad" populations. By preparing a cell suspension or looking at a still tissue section, one is running the risk of thinking that the populations of small lymphocytes in the Peyer's patches on the appendix are "sedentary." Like small lymphocytes in the spleen and lymph nodes, however, the small lymphocytes in the gut-associated lymphoid organs are in transit as part of their continuous process of circulation between blood and lymph (Gowans and Knight, 1964; Ford, 1975; de Sousa, 1976). In addition, from the morphological studies referred to above, we learned that numerous T lymphoblasts are present in the intestine epithelium, and numerous T and B lymphoblasts are found in the lamina propria. What is the molecular basis of their "attraction" to these sites? What are the functional consequences, if any, of their positioning? What influence does the presence of a "nomad" lymphoid population have on the transit of the intestine's own "nomad" epithelial cell population (Chapter 1)?

In the present section we shall review work on the patterns of migration of small and large lymphocytes in the intestine, and relate it to the development of local immune responses and production of IgA.

5.1. Small T and B Lymphocytes

Experiments delineating the traffic of small T and B lymphocytes through the Peyer's patches and appendix have been done mostly in rodents.

The general design of most experiments is similar to the one adopted originally by Gowans and Knight (1964) to trace the fate of rat thoracic duct lymphocytes. Cells labeled *in vitro* with a tritiated RNA (uridine) or DNA and RNA precursors (adenosine) are transferred into syngeneic recipients and their fate in the recipient's lymphoid organs is traced by means of autoradiography. With the use of pure suspensions of thymus cells, T cells, or peripheral B lymphocytes in mice and rats (Parrott and de Sousa, 1969; Howard *et al.*, 1972; Parrott and Ferguson, 1974) it has been shown that both T and B cells enter the Peyer's patches through postcapillary venules in the main interfollicular thymus-dependent area (Fig. 1) and ultimately ecotax to distinct T or B sites. B lymphocytes are found in the large nodular areas, whereas T cells are present in the interfollicular zones. Both small T and B lymphocytes are found in the dome area (Parrott, 1976). Definition of the sites of traffic of thymus-derived lymphocytes has also been attained from the study of the fate of labeled cells leaving the thymus after intrathymic infusion of [^{3}H]thymidine in the calf (Waksman, 1973). A similar distribution of the labeled thymus-derived cells in the interfollicular thymus-dependent areas and in the subepithelial dome area was found.

T- and B-lymphocyte traffic areas have also been defined in the rabbit appendix. Tritiated adenosine-labeled thymocytes migrate to the diamond-shaped intranodular zones, found depleted of T lymphocytes after thymectomy, irradiation, and reconstitution with bone marrow cells (Parrott, 1976). Tritiated adenosine-labeled bone marrow cells, on the other hand, migrate preferentially to the nodular appendix areas (Durkin *et al.*, 1975); moreover, Durkin *et al.* (1975) showed that pretreatment of labeled B cells *in vitro* with antiimmunoglobulin prevented the cells from reaching their normal territory in the appendix.

Traffic experiments with labeled appendix lymphoid cell populations have demonstrated that the appendix, like the spleen and the lymph nodes, contains a mixed T- and B-lymphocyte population which after transfer is found distributed over T and B areas of the spleen and lymph nodes (Durkin *et al.*, 1975). These experiments provide further support for the notion that the appendix is a peripheral lymphoid organ.

5.2. *T and B Lymphoblasts: Maturation of IgA-Producing Cells*

Large lymphoblasts migrate in large numbers to the small intestine mucosa. However, the first observations of this fact were made at a time (Gowans and Knight, 1964; Hall *et al.*, 1972; Halstead and Hall, 1972) when the significance of the distinction between T- and B-cell traffic was not widely acknowledged (Parrott *et al.*, 1966; Parrott and de Sousa, 1969, 1971), and the discovery of Griscelli *et al.* (1969) that mesenteric and peripheral lymph node blasts differ in their ultimate destinations stood unnoticed in its singular and crucial conclusion.

The assumptions then were that *all* lymphoblasts migrate to the intestinal mucosa, and that *all* lymphoblasts in the intestine are plasma cell precursors. Neither proved to be entirely correct.

The assumption that all lymphoblasts migrate to the intestine is incorrect, for the numbers of labeled lymphoblasts from peripheral lymph and peripheral lymph nodes found in the gut are negligible (Griscelli *et al.*, 1969; Guy Grand *et al.*, 1974*b*; Parrott and Ferguson, 1974; Parrot *et al.*, 1975; Rose *et al.*, 1976; McWilliams *et al.*, 1975; Hopkins and Hall, 1976). The assumption that lymphoblasts in the intestinal mucosa are plasma cell precursors has been challenged by morphological analysis of the intestine of congenitally athymic nude mice (Ferguson and Parrott, 1972; Parrott and de Sousa, 1974) and by the elegant work of Guy Grand, Griscelli, and Vassalli using combined autoradiography and immunofluorescence to demonstrate that both T and B lymphoblasts migrate to the lamina propria and that large numbers of T blasts are present among the intestinal epithelial cells. This has been confirmed directly by the more recent work or Rose in Parrott's laboratory on migration of $UdR^{125}I$-labeled T lymphoblasts from the mesenteric lymph node draining the site of *T. spiralis* injection in the mouse (Parrott *et al.*, 1975; Rose *et al.*, 1976*a,b*). The earlier work of Ferguson in the same laboratory (Ferguson and Parrott, 1973) on the histopathology of small intestine allograft rejection in the mouse, however, already indicated that large numbers of T cells penetrate the small intestine mucosa.

What factor or factors influence the destination of blast cells?

Mesenteric, Peyer's patch, and thoracic duct lymph blasts show a preferential migration to the intestine lamina propria and epithelium, in striking contrast to blasts obtained from peripheral lymph nodes, which do not (Griscelli *et al.*, 1969).

In a comparative study of the fate of $UdR^{125}I$-labeled mesenteric and auricular lymph node blast cells in *Trichinella spiralis*-infected or skin-sensitized mice, it was confirmed that mesenteric blasts preferentially migrate to the gut (Rose *et al.*, 1976*b*). A significant increase in the amount of radioactivity recovered in the gut of the infected mice was observed at 4 days of infection, which could be attributed to the T blast component of the inoculum, for when a population of B blast cells was injected no significant differences were observed between recovery in infected and noninfected mice. Moreover, when T blast cells from the mesenteric lymph node were traced in mice that had been previously sensitized with oxazolone, a powerful contact-sensitizing agent in mice (de Sousa and Parrott, 1969), the recovery of blast cells in the skin was negligible (0.7–0.6% of injected dose) compared to the amount recovered from the small intestine (12–13%). The reverse situation is not so clear-cut; peripheral lymph node T blast cells can be found in significantly higher numbers in the gut of *T. spiralis*-infected mice, although the numbers are always much smaller than those of mesenteric node T blast cells.

Thus the existence of a dichotomy of circulation of peripheral and central lymph lymphoblasts, originally discovered by Griscelli *et al.* (1969), has been confirmed (Guy Grand *et al.*, 1974*a;* Parrott *et al.*, 1975; Rose *et al.* 1976*a,b;* McWilliams *et al.*, 1975). Intestinal inflammation, however, seems to create local conditions which enhance extravasation of at least peripheral T blast cells (Rose *et al.*, 1976*b*).

The existence of a more fundamental dichotomy of circulation of peripheral and central T lymphoblasts has been proposed on the basis of similar findings with ^{51}Cr-labeled lymphocytes obtained from the drainage of peripheral or central lymph in the sheep (Cahill *et al.*, 1977). This observation awaits confirmation in other species.

One of the important features of the preferential migration of mesenteric lymph node blast cells to the intestine is that it is not antigen dependent. A similar pattern of migration has been observed to "antigen-free" fetal gut grafts implanted under the skin (Moore and Hall, 1972) or the kidney capsule (Parrott and Ferguson, 1974; Guy Grand *et al.*, 1974*b*). Thus some other more subtle "territorial recognition" process must be in operation, possibly related to the close interaction of the large lymphoblast, the intestinal epithelial cell, and the basement membrane (Marsh, 1975*b*). Do the blast cells found in the epithelium stay there indefinitely? Do they die? Or do they reenter the circulation?

Partial answers to these questions can be found in a sequential quantitative autoradiographic study of intraepithelial and intralymphatic labeled lymphocytes in mouse jejunum following a 6-hr dose of 150 μCi TdR^{3}H (Marsh, 1975*b*). Two peaks of labeled epithelial lymphocytes were seen between 6 and 60 hr and 72 and 168 hr. Between 60 and 96 hr after TdR^{3}H administration the total population of labeled and unlabeled lymphocytes fell at an estimated rate of three epithelial lymphocytes/1000 epithelial cell nuclei/hour. The symmetrical distribution of the labeled epithelial lymphocytes in the three main villous segments, proximal, middle, and distal, indicates that lymphocytes are not migrating along the villi, in contrast to the migration of the epithelial cells themselves (Fig. 2).

Moreover, the finding of a similar fall in labeled lymphocytes between 48 and 80 hr after TdR^{3}H paralleled closely the biphasic pattern of epithelial lymphocyte labeling. This impressive high-resolution autoradiography study in which over 10^4 epithelial lymphocytes were counted and none was seen extending through the tight junctions of adjacent columnar epithelial cells suggests that intraepithelial lymphocytes are more likely to enter the villous lymphatics than to be shed in the intestinal lumen. Once in the villous lymphatics they will join the pool of circulating cells that seem to travel through the Peyer's patches into the mesenteric lymph node and the thoracic duct lymph in a journey whose first steps were defined by the work of Craig and Cebra (1971) in the rabbit.

In the search for the lymphoid sources of IgA plasma cells and of the cells capable of populating the lamina propria, Craig and Cebra transferred allogeneic peripheral blood, popliteal node, and Peyer's patch lymphocytes from rabbits of one Ig allotype (*b5*, κ chain) into lethally irradiated recipients of *b4* allotype, and found that only Peyer's patch cells generated plasma cells in the lamina propria (Craig and Cebra, 1971). Peyer's patch cells also generate large numbers of IgA-producing cells in the spleen, following allogeneic transfer.

The sequential maturation steps of IgA-producing cells are presently

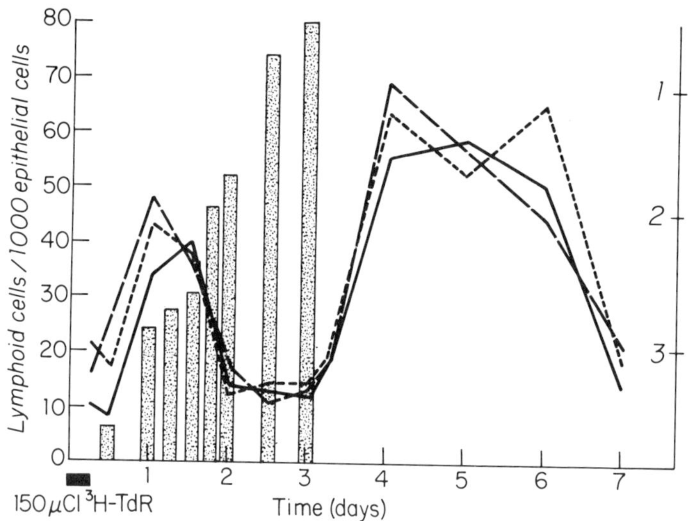

Fig. 2. Number of labeled epithelial lymphocytes in proximal (——), middle (- -), and one-third (— —) sections of villi found at various intervals after an initial 6-hr dose of 150 μCi TdR^{3}H. The shaded bars represent progressive migration of labeled epithelial cells with time along proximal (3), middle (2), and distal (1) segements of villi. At each time point, the proportion of labeled lymphocytes is identical in each villi segment; this finding indicates that intraepithelial lymphocytes, unlike epithelial cells, do not migrate along the villi. Modified from Marsh (1975*b*).

thought to involve (1) a Peyer's patch stage, in which a negligible percentage of blast cells (2%) have surface and intracellular IgA, (2) a mesenteric lymph node stage, where a much higher percentage (50%) of the blast cells have both surface and intracytoplasmic IgA, and (3) the thoracic duct lymph stage, where 75% of the blasts have both surface and intracytoplasmic IgA. From the thoracic duct, IgA blasts find their way into the lamina propria where they differentiate into IgA-secreting plasma cells.

The process of differentiation of IgA-producing cells is not a straightforward sequence of B-cell migration and lodging, as it appeared to be at first.

The nomad repopulation of the lamina propria with IgA-producing plasma cells is dependent on presence of normal numbers of T lymphocytes.

In nude mice (Guy Grand *et al.*, 1974*a*) surface IgA-bearing lymphocytes are present in the Peyer's patches; without T cells, however, they fail to migrate, lodge, and mature into lamina propria plasma cells. The number of IgA plasma cells in the lamina propria of the athymic mice is 10–15 times below normal; this is reflected in the failure to detect IgA in the serum (Pritchard *et al.*, 1973). The thymus dependency of IgA synthesis has also been demonstrated in rats, rabbits and chickens (reviewed by Cooper *et al.*, 1974).

Correction of the IgA deficiency in the nude mice is achieved with thymus grafts (Pritchard *et al.*, 1973).

6. Conclusion: Significance to Disease in Man

What does this all mean beyond the obvious satisfaction of understanding?

If it means that at the end of reading the other sections immunologists go back to their little worlds to complete their elegant experiments and gastroenterologists go back to changing patients' diets and resecting patients' colons, then the writing of this chapter will have been pointless.

In conclusion, we shall raise two questions that are of relevance to both groups of workers:

1. What is the significance to the clinician of the fact that there are two separate circuits of circulation of peripheral and central lymph blasts?

2. What is the significance to the GI oncologist of the basic anatomical fact that the most considerable amount of lymphoid tissue in the gut is associated with the small intestine and *not* the colon?

6.1. Clinical Significance of the Existence of Two Separate Circuits of Circulation of Blast Cells

Assuming that the migration to the gut of blast cells obtained from the thoracic duct lymph is the expression of the existence of some unidentified molecular component of the intestinal epithelium (presumably in the basement membrane) shared by other epithelia, the prediction is that all gut diseases characterized by heavy lymphocyte infiltration of the mucosa should have concomitant skin or bronchial lesions of the same type.

Conversely, patients with skin diseases characterized by heavy lymphocyte infiltrates, e.g., mycosis fungoides, would be expected to have severe intestinal lesions. This is not the case.

Concomitant skin and intestinal lesions occur in graft vs. host disease, where the allogeneic cells are responding to antigens common to all recipient tissues.

Concomitant skin and jejunal lesions occur also in dermatitis herpetiformis (DH). This suggests that in patients with DH skin and jejunum share antigenic components not present in normal people. Alternatively, in these patients T cells may have a failure of the normal "territorial sensory" ("ecotaxing") mechanism. Once T cells reach the intestinal mucosa in large numbers, their presence therein is reflected in considerable morphological changes of the villi and crypts.

It has been postulated by Ferguson (1974) that the villous atrophy observed in celiac disease is the consequence of the development of a local cell-mediated immunity reaction resulting from the presence of large numbers of T cells in the area. The numbers of intraepithelial and lamina propria lymphocytes, and of lamina propria plasma cells, appear to vary from study to study.

It has been argued that "alterations in plasma cell and lymphocyte numbers might implicate humoral or cell-mediated mechanisms respectively" (Lancaster-Smith *et al.*, 1975). However, as the studies of the intestinal mucosa of athymic nude mice show, and the finding of exceptionally high levels of serum IgA in some celiac disease patients suggests, the presence of plasma cells in the lamina propria is in fact a thymus-dependent event, and therefore it is meaning very much the same as the finding of intraepithelial lymphocytes. The variation in the numbers of lamina propria lymphocytes found at different times and with different doses of gluten challenges is also of interest in the light of the observations of Marsh (1975*b*) (Fig. 2). If lymphocytes circulate through the villous epithelium and the lamina propria in a cyclic fashion, a considerable variation in the numbers of lymphocytes found in jejunal biopsies with the time of the biopsy should be expected.

A more intriguing question is why the presence of large numbers of T cells should be associated with villous atrophy. It will be of interest to redefine the T-lymphocyte populations present in the epithelium and the lamina propria in the light of current immunological evidence of the existence of suppressor and helper T-cell subpopulations. It is appealing to think that the intraepithelial lymphocytes have a suppressor activity resulting in control of eptithelial cell division, whereas the lamina propria lymphocytes are mostly helper cells thus influencing the appearance of IgA-producing plasma cells in that area.

Kinetic studies of the kind described in Chapter 1 of the intestinal epithelium of nude mice will most certainly help to clarify the issue of the exact significance of the positioning of T lymphocytes within the epithelium.

6.2. *Significance of the Presence of Lymphoid Tissue in the Small Intestine*

As mentioned in the introduction to this chapter, it is somewhat ironic that initially all the studies of the gut have been confined to the small intestine when cancer in the GI tract is most frequently found in the stomach and the colon. The question of a possible relationship between the high concentration of lymphoid tissue in the small bowel and low frequency of adenocarcinoma in this region seems inescapable.

From experimental studies of lymphoid cell traffic in nematode infections it has been recently shown that T lymphoblasts are attracted to the actual intestine sites affected at the various stages of progression of the infection (Rose and Parrott, personal communication). For instance, with *Trichuris muris* infection in mice, T lymphoblasts have been found to migrate to the colon (Rose and Parrott, personal communication), indicating that under certain circumstances of intestinal infection increased numbers of lymphoid cells can be "persuaded" to migrate to sites otherwise poor in their lymphoid cell component.

These findings raise the possibility that variation in incidence of gut infection may be related to the known geographical variation in incidence of colon cancer (Wynder *et al.*, 1976). The high incidence of colon cancer in countries with the lowest incidence of gastrointestinal infection and its low frequency in South America, Africa, and Asia make one wonder how valuable a study of numbers of intraepithelial lymphocytes in age- and sex-matched groups from a high- and a low-incidence country could be.

It seems to us that any epidemiological approach to the question of cancer of the gastrointestinal tract that leaves out the geography of lymphocyte distribution within the intestine itself is likely to prove fundamentally incomplete.

ACKNOWLEDGMENTS

The original work by Dr. de Sousa and Dr. Good has been supported by Grants CA-08748 and CA-17404 from the National Cancer Institute, by the Special Projects Committee MSKCC, by the American Cancer Society, and by the Zelda R. Weintraub Cancer Fund

7. *References*

Blythman, H. E., and Waksman, B. H., 1973, Effect of irradiation and appendicostomy on appendix structure and responses of appendix cells to mitogens, *J. Immunol.* **111**:171.

Cahill, R. N. P., Poskitt, D. C., Frost, H., and Trnka, Z., 1977, Two distinct pools of recirculating T lymphocytes: Migratory characteristics of nodal and intestinal T lymphocytes, *J. Exp. Med.* **145**:420.

Cebra, J. J., Craig, S. W., and Jones, P. P., 1974, Cell types contributing to the biosynthesis of IgA, in: *The Immunoglobulin A System* (J. Mestecky and A. R. Lawton, eds.), p. 25, Plenum, New York.

Chanana, H. D., Schaedeli, J., Hess, M. W., and Cottier, H., 1973, Predominance of theta-positive lymphocytes in gut associated and peripheral lymphoid tissues of newborn mice, *J. Immunol.* **110**:283.

Cooper, M. D., Perey, D. Y., McKneally, M. F., Gabrielson, A. E., Sutherland, D. E. R., and Good, R. A., 1966, A mammalian equivalent of the avian bursa of Fabricius, *Lancet* **1**:1388.

Cooper, M. D., Kincade, P. W., Bockman, D. E., and Lawton, A. R., 1974, Origin, distribution and differentiation of IgA producing cells, in: *The Immunoglobulin A System* (J. Mestecky and A. R. Lawton, eds.), p. 13, Plenum, New York.

Crabbe, P. A., Carbonara, A. O., and Heremans, J. F., 1965, The normal human intestinal mucosa as a major source of plasma cells containing γA-immunoglobulin, *Lab. Invest.* **14**:235.

Crabbe, P. A., Nash, D. R., Bazin, H., Eyssen, H., Heremans, J. F., 1969, Antibody of the IgA type in intestinal plasma cells of germfree mice after oral or parenteral immunization with ferritin, *J. Exp. Med.* **130**:723.

Craig, S. W., and Cebra, J. J., 1971, Peyer's patches: An enriched source of precursors of IgA producing immunocytes in the rabbit, *J. Exp. Med.* **134**:188.

Craig, S. W., and Cebra, J. J., 1975, Rabbit Peyer's patches, appendix and popliteal lymph node B lymphocytes: A comparative analysis of their membrane immunoglobulin components and plasma cell precursor potential, *J. Immunol.* **114**:492.

Crandall, R. B., Cebra, J. J., and Crandall, C. A., 1967, The relative proportions of IgG, IgA and IgM-containing cells in rabbit tissues during experimental trichinosis, *Immunology* **12**:147.

de Sousa, M., 1973, The ecology of thymus-dependency, in: *Contemporary Topics in Immunobiology*, Vol. 2 (A. J. S. Davies and R. L. Carter, eds.), p. 119, Plenum, New York.

de Sousa, M., 1976, Cell traffic, *Receptors Recognition Ser. A* **2**:105.

de Sousa, M. A. B., and Parrott, D. M. V., 1969, Induction and recall in contact sensitivity, *J. Exp. Med.* **130**:671.

de Sousa, M. A. B., and Pritchard, H., 1974, The cellular basis of immunological recovery in nude mice after thymus grafting, *Immunology* **26:**769.

de Sousa, M. A. B., Parrott, D. M. V., and Pantelouris, E. M. 1969, The lymphoid tissues in mice with congenital aplasia of the thymus, *Clin. Exp. Immunol.* **9:**371.

Durkin, H. G., Caporale, L., and Thorbecke, G. J., 1975, Migratory patterns of B lymphocytes. I. Fate of cells from central and peripheral lymphoid organs in the rabbit and its selective alterations by anti-immunoglobulin. *Cell Immunol.* **16:**285.

Ferguson, A., 1974, Lymphocytes in coeliac disease, in: *Coeliac Disease: Proceedings of the Second International Coeliac Symposium* (W. T. J. H. Hekkens and A. S. Pena, eds.), p. 265, Stenfert Kroese, Linden.

Ferguson, A., and Parrott, D. M. V., 1972, The effects of antigen deprivation on thymus-dependent and thymus-independent lymphocytes in the small intestine of the mouse, *Clin. Exp. Immunol.* **12:**477.

Ferguson, A., and Parrott, D. M. V., 1973, Histopathology and time course of rejection of allografts of mouse small intestine, *Transplantation* **15:**546.

Ford, W. L., 1975, Lymphocyte migration and immune responses. *Progr. Allergy* **19:**1.

Glasser, R. J., 1976, *The Greatest Battle,* Random House, New York.

Goodfield, J. G., 1975, *The Siege of Cancer,* Random House, New York.

Goodfield, J. G., 1977, To each and everyone, his own pestulence, *Skeptic.*

Gowans, J. L., and Knight, E. T., 1964, The route of recirculation of lymphocytes in the rat, *Proc. R. Soc. (London) Ser. B* **159:**257.

Griscelli, C., Vassalli, P., and McCluskey, R. T., 1969, The distribution of large dividing lymph node cells in syngeneic recipient rats after intravenous injection, *J. Exp. Med.* **130:**1427.

Guy Grand, D., Griscelli, C., and Vassalli, P. 1974*a*, Gut associated lymphoblasts and intestinal IgA plasma cells, in: *The Immunoglobulin A System* (J. Mestecky and A. R. Lawton, eds.), p. 41, Plenum, New York.

Guy Grand, D., Griscelli, C., and Vassalli, P., 1974*b*, The gut associated lymphoid system: Nature and properties of the large dividing cell, *Eur. J. Immunol.* **4:**435.

Hall, J. G., Parry, D. M., and Smith, M. E., 1972, The distribution and differentiation of lymph borne immunoblasts after intravenous injection into syngeneic recipients, *Cell Tissue Kinet.* **5:**269.

Halstead, T. G., and Hall, J. G., 1972, The homing of lymph borne immunoblasts to the small gut of neonatal rats, *Transplantation* **14:**342.

Hopkins, J., and Hall, J. G., 1976, Selective entry of immunoblasts into gut from intestinal lymph, *Nature (London)* **259:**308.

Howard, J. C., Hunt, S. V., and Gowans, J. C., 1972, Identification of marrow derived and thymus-derived small lymphocytes in the lymphoid tissue and thoracid duct lymph of normal rats, *J. Exp. Med.* **135:**200.

Janossy, G., Shoat, M., Greaves, M. F., and Dourmarshkin, R., 1973, Lymphocyte activation. IV. The ultrastructural pattern of the response of mouse T and B cells to mitogenic stimulation *in vivo*, *Immunology* **24:**211.

Lancaster-Smith, M., Kumar, P. J., and Dawson, A. M., 1975, The cellular infiltrate of the jejunum in adult coeliac disease and dermatitis herpetiformis following the reintroduction of dietary gluten, *Gut* **16:**683.

Mandel, M. A., and Asofsky, R., 1968, Studies of thoracic duct lymphocytes in mice. I. Immunoglobulin synthesis *in vitro*, *J. Immunol.* **100:**363.

Marsh, M. N., 1975*a*, Studies of intestinal lymphoid tissue. I. Electron microscope evidence of "blast transformation" in epithelial lymphocytes of mouse small intestinal mucosa, *Gut* **16:**665.

Marsh, M. N., 1975*b*, Studies of intestinal lymphoid tissue. II. Aspects of proliferation and migration of epithelial lymphocytes in the small intestine of mice, *Gut* **16:**674.

McWilliams, M., Phillips-Quagliata, J. M., and Lamm, M. E., 1975, Characteristics of mesenteric lymph node cells homing to gut associated lymphoid tissue in syngeneic mice, *J. Immunol.* **115:**54.

Mestecky, J., and Lawton, A. R., 1974, *The Immunoglobulin A System,* Plenum, New York.

Mitchell, J., Pye, J., Holmes, M. C., and Nossal, G. J. V., 1973, Antigens in immunity: Antigen localisation in congenitally athymic nude mice, *Aust. J. Exp. Biol. Med. Sci.* **50:**637.

Moore, A. R., and Hall, J., 1972, Evidence for a primary association between immunoblasts and small gut, *Nature (London)* **239:**161.

Müller-Schoop, J. W., and Good, R. A., 1975, Functional studies of Peyer's patches: Evidence for their participation in intestinal immune responses, *J. Immunol.* **114:**1757.

Nieuwenhuis, P., 1971, On the origin and fate of immunologically competent cells, doctorate thesis, Groningen University, Groningen.

Owen, J. J. T., Cooper, M. D., and Raff, M. C., 1974, *In vitro* generation of B lymphocytes in mouse foetal liver, a mammalian "bursa equivalent," *Nature (London)* **249:**361.

Parrott, D. M. V., 1976, The gut as a lymphoid organ, *Clin. Gastroenterol.* **5:**211.

Parrott, D. M. V., and de Sousa, M. A. B., 1969, The source of cells within different areas of lymph nodes draining the site of primary stimulation with a contact sensitizing agent, in: *Lymphatic Tissue and Germinal Centres in Immune Responses* (L. Fiore Donati and M. G. Hanna, eds.), p. 293, Plenum, New York.

Parrott, D. M. V., and de Sousa, M. A. B., 1971, Thymus-dependent and thymus-independent populations: Origin, migratory patterns and lifespan, *Clin. Exp. Immunol.* **8:**663.

Parrott, D. M. V., and de Sousa, M. A. B., 1974, B cell stimulation in nude (*nu/nu*) mice, in: *First International Workshop in Nude Mice* (J. Rygaard and C. O. Polvsen, eds.), p. 61, Gustav Fisher, Stuttgart.

Parrott, D. M. V., and Ferguson, A., 1974, Selective migration of lymphocytes within the mouse small intestine, *Immunology* **26:**571.

Parrott, D. M. V., de Sousa, M. A. B., and East, J., 1966, Thymus-dependent areas in the lymphoid organs of neonatally thymectomized mice, *J. Exp. Med.* **123:**191.

Parrott, D. M. V., Rose, M. L., Sless, F., Freitas, A. A., and Bruce, R. G., 1975, Factors which determine the accumulation of immunoblasts in gut and skin, in: *Future Trends in Inflammation II,* Burkause, Basel.

Perey, D. Y. E., and Good, R. A., 1968, Experimental arrest and induction of lymphoid development in intestinal lympho-epithelial tissue of rabbits, *Lab. Invest.* **18:**15.

Pollard, M., and Sharon, N., 1970, Responses of Peyer's patches in germ-free mice to antigen stimulation, *Infect. Immun.* **2:**96.

Pritchard, H., Riddaway, J., and Micklem, H. S., 1973, Immune responses in congenitally thymus-less mice. II. Quantitative studies of serum immunoglobulins, the antibody response to sheep erythrocytes and the effect of thymus allografting, *Clin. Exp. Immunol.* **15:**125.

Raff, M. C., Nase, S., and Mitchison, N. A., 1971, Mouse-specific B lymphocyte antigen (MBLA) a marker for thymus-independent lymphocytes, *Nature (London)* **230:**50.

Rose, M. L., Parrott, D. M. V., and Bruce, R. G., 1976*a*, Migration of lymphoblasts to the small intestine. I. Effect of *Trichinella spiralis* infection on the migration of mesenteric lymphoblasts and mesenteric T lymphoblasts in syngeneic mice, *Immunology* **31:**723.

Rose, M. L., Parrott, D. M. V., and Bruce, R. G., 1976*b*, Migration of lymphoblasts to the small intestine. II. Divergent migration of mesenteric and peripheral immunoblasts to sites of inflammation in the mouse, *Cell. Immunol.* **27:**36.

Rudzik, O., and Bienenstock, J., 1974, Isolation and characteristics of gut mucosal lymphocytes, *Lab. Invest.* **30:**260.

Rudzik, O., Clancy, R. L., Perey, D. Y. E., Bienenstock, J., and Singal, D. P., 1975, The distribution of a rabbit thymic antigen and membrane immunoglobulins in lymphoid tissue, with special reference to mucosal lymphocytes, *J. Immunol.* **114:**1.

Stadecker, M. J., Bishop, G., and Wortis, H. H., 1973, Rosette formation by guinea pig thymocytes and thymus derived lymphocytes with rabbit red blood cells, *J. Immunol.* **111:**1834.

Stramignoni, H., Mollo, F., Riea, J., and Palestro, G., 1969, Development of the lymphoid tissue in the rabbit appendix isolated from the intestinal tract, *J. Pathol.* **99:**265.

Tomasi, T. B., Jr., Tan, E. M., Solomon, A., and Prendergast, R. A., 1965, Characteristics of an immune system common to certain external secretions, *J. Exp. Med.* **121:**101.

Veldkamp, J., de Renver, M. J., and Willers, J. M. N., 1974, Distribution of different cell types in the lymphoid organs of the mouse, as determined with sera against thymus and Peyer's patches, *Immunology* **25**:761.

Veldman, J. E. 1970, Histophysiology and electron microscopy of the immune response, doctorate thesis, Groningen University, Groningen.

Waksman, B. H., 1973, The homing pattern of thymus-derived lymphocytes in calf and neonatal mouse Peyer's patches, *J. Immunol.* **111**:878.

Williams, A. F., and Gowans, J. L. 1975, The presence of IgA on the surface of rat thoracic duct lymphocytes which contain internal IgA, *J. Exp. Med.* **141**:335.

Wynder, E. L., Reddy, B. S., McCoy, G. D., Weisburger, J. H., and Williams, G. M., 1976, Diet and gastrointestinal cancer, *Clin. Gastroenterol.* **5**:463.

IIA

Individual and Familial Susceptibility to Gastrointestinal Malignancy: Immune Mechanisms

3

Immunodeficiency Diseases and Malignancy

Beatrice D. Spector, Robert A. Good, and John H. Kersey

1. Introduction

This review of immunodeficiency diseases and malignancy is based primarily on evidence provided by over 200 cases of cancer occurring in patients with diagnosed primary immunodeficiency diseases. The cases were collected by the Immunodeficiency-Cancer Registry, a tumor registry established in 1971 under the aegis of the World Health Organization Committee on Primary Immunodeficiencies (Fudenberg *et al.,* 1971). Compilation of case reports provides evidence that immunodeficiency diseases predispose to malignancy, since mortality rates for cancer in immunodeficiency groups exceed by 100 times the expected rates for the general population (Kersey *et al.,* 1974). An intimate association between an abnormal immune system and subsequent development of malignancy also exists among renal transplant recipients on immunosuppressive regimens, who have developed lymphomas at significantly higher rates than expected for an age- and sex-matched population during a comparable period (Penn, 1975; Hoover and Fraumeni, 1973). Another condition, the actual presence of a malignancy, demonstrates the effect of cancer on the immune system in persons with Hodgkin's disease, chronic lymphatic leukemia, and multiple myeloma (Schier, 1954; Kelly *et al.,* 1958; Southam, 1961; Cone and Uhr, 1964; Dent *et al.,* 1968).

Evaluation of immunocompetence and its relationship to malignancy has been actively pursued in experimental animal models, and results from these studies have provided additional insights into the interrelationship between immunodeficiency and malignancy in human populations (Kersey *et al.,* 1973*a*). In addition, epidemiological studies may provide clues to the origins

Beatrice D. Spector and John H. Kersey • Department of Laboratory Medicine and Pathology, University of Minnesota, Minneapolis, Minnesota 55455. ***Robert A. Good*** • Memorial Sloan-Kettering Cancer Center, New York, New York 10021.

of malignancies by testing hypotheses developed through laboratory experimentation and by generating hypotheses through descriptive studies and identification of high-risk groups (Miller, R. W., 1967; Fraumeni *et al.,* 1971).

2. *Identification of Primary Immunodeficiencies Which Predispose to Malignancy*

Immunologists have identified a wide range of immunodeficiency disorders which have been classified according to several criteria: inheritance, association with certain well-defined clinical abnormalities, and estimation of circulating antibodies, immunoglobulins, B cells, and T cells (Cooper *et al.,* 1973). A list of primary immunodeficiency disorders associated with relatively well characterized features and classified according to the suggested nature of the cellular defect as ascertained by enumeration and function of T and B cells was published by Cooper *et al.* (1973). Criteria for this list provided the Immunodeficiency-Cancer Registry (ICR) with a means of classifying each case report into an appropriate primary immunodeficiency disease category. The 205 cases registered in the ICR at present fit into seven primary immunodeficiency categories: X-linked (Bruton's) agammaglobulinemia (12 cases), IgA deficiency (13 cases), IgM deficiency (7 cases), variable immunodeficiency (58 cases), severe combined immunodeficiency (11 cases), ataxia–telangiectasia (70 cases), and Wiskott–Aldrich syndrome (34 cases).

For a number of years, it appeared that each of these disorders was associated with an increased cancer risk, ranging from 2 to 10%, depending on the primary immunodeficiency disease (Table 1) (Gatti and Good, 1971; Good, 1972; Kersey *et al.,* 1973*b*). Newly obtained data from a nationwide survey of over 800 cases of various immunodeficiency diseases provide additional insight into this problem (Spector *et al.,* unpublished). The data suggest that X-linked (Bruton's) agammaglobulinemia and IgA deficiency may not be associated with an increased predisposition to develop cancer, and

Table 1. Estimated Incidence of Malignancy in Primary Immunodeficiency Syndromes[a]

Disease	Incidence	Estimated Risk (%)
X-linked (Bruton's) agammaglobulinemia	6/≈ 100	6
IgM deficiency	6/≈ 70	8
Variable immunodeficiency	41/≈ 500	8
Severe combined immunodeficiency	9/≈ 400	2
Ataxia–telangiectasia	52/≈ 500	10
Wiskott–Aldrich syndrome	24/≈ 300	8
TOTAL	138/≈1870	7

[a]From Kersey *et al.* (1973*b*).

that other immunodeficiency diseases such as ataxia-telangiectasia and Wiskott-Aldrich syndrome may have higher cancer risks than previously estimated. These preliminary conclusions are currently undergoing further evaluation and analysis.

A brief, general description of each of the seven immunodeficiency diseases follows. An excellent review is available for more comprehensive readings on each disorder (Bergsma, 1975).

X-linked (Bruton's) agammaglobulinemia, isolated IgA deficiency, and *isolated IgM deficiency* are examples of immunodeficiency diseases in which the primary defect lies in the humoral B-cell system.

Boys with X-linked agammaglobulinemia are compromised immunologically, since they generally have very few B lymphocytes and no Ig-secreting plasma cells (Kersey and Gajl-Peczalska, 1975). They have an inordinately high susceptibility to infections with encapsulated organisms, e.g., *Hemophilus influenzae, Pseudomonas aeruginosa,* and *Diplococcus pneumoniae.* These clinical problems have been aided somewhat by the use of γ-globulin or plasma therapy. A total of 12 cancer cases have been identified in this disorder.

Isolated IgA deficiency is a clinically heterogeneous disorder which may produce no symptoms in some persons, while in others, the effect may be sinopulmonary infections, autoimmune disease, or GI problems, such as sprue-linked disorders and GI cancer (Amman and Hong, 1971). The incidence of isolated IgA deficiency may be as high as 1 in 700 persons, which is considerably higher than the frequency of lethal, recessively inherited diseases such as X-linked agammaglobulinemia, Wiskott-Aldrich syndrome, and ataxia-telangiectasia (Amman and Hong, 1971). A total of 13 patients with IgA deficiency developed malignancies; 2 had at least one additional primary tumor (see Table 2).

Isolated IgM deficiency occurs in approximately 1 in 1000 persons tested (Hobbs, 1975). It produces a range of clinical severity similar to isolated IgA deficiency in that some persons remain free of any clinical evidence of disease, while others are highly susceptible to bacterial infections, particularly gram-negative organisms (Hobbs, 1975). To date, malignancies have been found in 7 persons with IgM deficiency.

Variable immunodeficiency, severe combined immunodeficiency, ataxia-telangiectasia, and *Wiskott-Aldrich syndrome* each involve defects of both B- and T-cell immune components. Patients with these disorders have increased susceptibility to infection of varying types, including bacterial, viral, fungal, and protozoal organisms (Kersey and Gajl-Peczalska, 1975).

Variable immunodeficiency probably encompases several syndromes which have not yet been clearly defined. Included are cases previously classified as "congenital" and non-X-linked (or sporadic) hypogammaglobulinemia, primary dysgammaglobulinemia of both childhood and adult life, and "acquired" primary hypogammaglobulinemia (Good, 1972). Enumeration of Ig-bearing lymphocytes in such patients has led to the delineation of at least two different patterns, which probably reflect different underlying mechanisms (Cooper *et al.,* 1973). In general, cell-mediated responses are usually intact until late in the course of the disease (Kersey and Gajl-Peczalska, 1975). Further delineation of these syndromes awaits further analysis of variables such as time of onset of condition, immunoglobulin patterns, family studies, and studies of associated disorders (Cooper *et al.,* 1973). Cancer diagnoses have been reported in 58 patients with this disease classification; 13 had developed their malignancy before the age of 20, 43 after 20 years, and 2 at an unknown age. One patient had multiple primaries.

Severe combined immunodeficiency consists of a heterogeneous group of disorders which begins in the newborn period or infancy. Some of these patients appear to have abnormal differentiation from stem cells to fully functional T and B cells (Kersey and Gajl-Peczalska, 1975). It is often considered that the different degrees of severity of severe combined immunodeficiency reflect abnormalities at different points in T- and B-cell differentiation. Affected children usually die within the first 2 years of life without immunological reconstitution through organ transplantation (e.g., bone marrow, fetal liver). Of children with this disorder, 11 have succumbed to malignancy.

Ataxia-telangiectasia is a multisystem disease which presents as cerebellar ataxia, ocular telangiectasia, and recurrent sinopulmonary infections (Sedgwick and Boder, 1972). The thymus of children affected with this disease is found to be small and hypoplastic at autopsy. Cell-mediated responses are abnormal during life. Concomitant hormonal abnormalities have been observed in many girls who reach puberty (Boder, 1975). IgA levels are frequently low or zero, as are IgE levels (Good, 1972). Ataxia-telangiectasia is transmitted in an autosomally recessive pattern, and the gene frequency for this disorder has been estimated to be as high as 1 in 100 (Swift *et al.,* 1976). Family studies of cancer history indicate higher than expected frequencies of cancer of several sites, including lymphomas, gallbladder and biliary carcinomas, and pancreatic carcinoma (Swift *et al.,* 1976). The largest number of cancers reported in any immunodeficiency is in ataxia-telangiectasia, in which 70 cases have been identified.

Wiskott-Aldrich syndrome is also a multisystem disorder, inherited in an X-linked pattern. It is characterized by eczema, low platelet counts, and increased susceptibility to infections. Patients with this disease have frequent and progressive deficit of cell-mediated immunity, deficiency in the concentration of circulating IgM, and frequently elevated concentrations of IgA and IgE. They fail to respond with antibody production or with development of cellular immunity to polysaccharide antigens—e.g., *Pneumococcus* polysaccharide, Vi antigen, and blood group antigens—but they make both IgM and IgG antibodies to protein antigens very well (Good, 1972). Immunoglobulin catabolism is enhanced in this disorder, and isohemagglutinin titers are almost always low or zero (Krivit and Good, 1959; Blaese *et al.,* 1975). Boys with Wiskott-Aldrich syndrome usually die of severe infections or cerebral hemorrhage by the second decade. There have been 34 cases of cancer reported to date.

3. Malignancy Patterns in the Primary Immunodeficiencies

3.1. Tumor Histology

Table 2 groups the 205 cases by immunodeficiency diagnosis and pathological diagnosis of the tumor. Each of the 4 cases with multiple primaries is grouped by the histology of the initially diagnosed cancer. The immunodeficiencies are listed in increasing order of the proportion of lymphoid tumors obtained for each disorder. The total number of cases, ranging from 7 in IgM deficiency to 70 in ataxia-telangiectasia, represents 26 years of experience, the year of cancer diagnosis being from 1949 to 1975.

Each primary immunodeficiency disease is associated with a significant number of lymphoreticular tumors. Not only does the total number of lymphoreticular tumors (117) dominate the overall proportions of cancer when they are analyzed by general histological type (57% of total cases), but also lymphoreticular tumors account for the majority of cell types in five of the seven primary immunodeficiencies; variable immunodeficiency (49%), severe combined immunodeficiency (55%), ataxia-telangiectasia (60%), IgM deficiency (71%), and Wiskott-Aldrich syndrome (82%) (Table 2). Furthermore, lymphoreticular tumors accounted for 4 of 13 and 4 of 12 cancers each for IgA deficiency and X-linked agammaglobulinemia (31 and 33.5% of the total, respectively).

Differences in malignancy patterns are found in the distribution of epithelial cancers (carcinomas) and leukemias (all types). Epithelial tumors or leukemias accounted for the majority of cancer in two diseases; 54% of all cancers in IgA deficiency were epithelial, and 58% of all reported cancers in X-linked agammaglobulinemia were leukemias (Table 2). Epithelial cancers occurred almost as frequently as lymphoreticular tumors in variable immunodeficiency (42 vs. 49%), and they occurred to a lesser extent in ataxia-telangiectasia (13%) and IgM deficiency (14.3%). Similarly, leukemias accounted for a large percentage of cancers in severe combined immunodeficiency (45%), less in ataxia-telangiectasia (23%), and considerably less for Wiskott-Aldrich syndrome (6%, 2 cases) and variable immunodeficiency (7%, 4 cases). Mesenchymal tumors (sarcomas, etc.) and nervous system tumors (neuroblastoma, primary tumors of the brain) were reported in very small numbers (i.e., 1-3 cases) for all primary immunodeficiency diseases; mesenchymal and nervous system tumors represented 2 and 4%, respectively, of all reported tumors in the registry file.

Recent epidemiological studies on childhood leukemias and lymphomas in the general population have related cell type to sibship aggregates and congenital defects (Fraumeni and Miller, 1967; Fraumeni *et al.*, 1971; Grundy *et al.*, 1973). These approaches provide direction for future studies of lymphoreticular tumors and other malignancies in primary immunodeficiencies, particularly since immunodeficiency diseases and cancer have been reported in at least 14 sibling groups (Kersey *et al.*, 1973*b*). In 12 of the 14 families,

Table 2. Immunodeficiency-Cancer Registry: Summary of Cases

Primary immunodeficiency disease	Histological type										Total cases
	Lymphoreticular		Leukemia		Epithelial		Mesenchymal		Nervous system		
	%	*N*	%	*N*	%	*N*	%	*N*	%	*N*	
IgA deficiency	31	4	—	—	54	7	7.5	1	7.5	1	13
X-linked (Bruton's) agammaglobulinemia	33.5	4	58	7	—	—	—	—	8.5	1	12
Variable immunodeficiency	49	28	7	4	42	24	1	1	1	1	58
Severe combined immunodeficiency	55	6	45	5	—	—	—	—	—	—	11
Ataxia–telangiectasia	60	42	23	16	13	9	1	1	3	2	70
IgM deficiency	71.4	5	—	—	14.3	1	—	—	14.3	1	7
Wiskott–Aldrich syndrome	82	28	6	2	—	—	3	1	9	3	34
Totals	57	117	17	34	20	41	2	4	4	9	205

Table 3. Lymphoreticular Malignancies by Cell Type Reported in 117 Patients with Seven Primary Immunodeficiency Diseases (Year of Cancer Diagnosis: 1949–1975)[a]

Tumor type reported[b]	Number of cases
Reticulum-cell sarcoma	22
Lymphosarcoma	21
Lymphoma, NOS	18
Hodgkin's disease	18
Malignant reticuloendotheliosis	8
Malignant lymphoma	7
Lymphoreticular, NOS	5
Undifferentiated lymphoma	2
Lymphoblastic lymphosarcoma	2
Other (1 case each)	14
Reticular lymphosarcoma	
Lymphoepithelial thymoma	
Malignant reticulosis	
Small-cell lymphosarcoma	
Generalized reticuloendotheliosis	
Reticulum-cell lymphoma	
Malignant lymphosarcoma	
Histiocytosarcoma	
Undifferentiated round-cell sarcoma	
Malignant lymphogranulomatosis	
Histocytosis reticulosis	
Thymoma with lymphocytic lymphoma	
Burkitt's lymphoma	
Histiocytic lymphoma	

[a]Collected by the ICR, 1972–1975.
[b](NOS) Not otherwise specified.

tumors were of the same histological type, and in all cases, the primary immunodeficiency diagnoses were identical.

The classification of all 117 lymphoreticular tumors by reported cell type appears in Table 3. The most frequently reported cell type was reticulum-cell sarcoma (22 cases), followed by lymphosarcoma (21 cases), lymphoma, NOS, and Hodgkin's disease (18 cases each), malignant reticuloendotheliosis (8 cases), malignant lymphoma (7 cases), lymphoreticular, NOS (5 cases), undifferentiated lymphoma and lymphoblastic lymphosarcoma (2 cases each), and a large group (14 cases) of cell types that appeared only once each. The observed spectrum of pathological diagnoses of lymphoreticular tumors in immunodeficient patients is of interest. This distribution is clearly different from that of lymphoreticular malignancy in patients without immunodeficiency (Williams *et al.*, 1972). The reasons for the difference are not clear, but probably relate to the pathogenetic mechanisms involved. There is evidence to suggest that lymphoreticular tumors which develop in immunodeficient patients behave differently from similar tumors in nonimmunodeficient persons; e.g., a significant number of lymphoreticular tumors have been found at autopsy despite the close medical surveillance of these individuals. The spectrum of cell-type diagnoses of lymphoreticular tumors in immunodeficient patients may also be a reflection of varied diagnostic criteria, where different morphological, functional, and cytological characteristics have been used (Lukes and Collins, 1974).

Functional problems, such as repeated assaults of the immune system due to recurrent infections and abnormal regulation of T and B cells due to inborn immunological defects, likely play a major role in determining the appearance of these malignancies. The morphological characteristics of lymphoreticular tumors in immunodeficiency diseases are similar to the lymphoid tumor characteristics in renal transplant recipients (Penn, 1975; Hoover and Fraumeni, 1973).

3.2. Sex and Age

Cancers in an immunodeficiency population, as in the general population, have unique sex- and age-specific characteristics which provide additional etiological clues to oncogenesis. Table 4 lists 171 cases by sex, age at cancer diagnosis, and primary site of the tumor, and 34 cases by sex or age or both unknown and primary site of the tumor. Grouped with lymphoreticular tumors are a few cases in which the lymphoma originated in nonlymphoid organs, e.g., skin, bladder, bone, small intestine, brain. The highest incidence of tumors for both sexes occurs in childhood and is comprised mainly of lymphoreticular malignancies and leukemias which developed in patients with immunodeficiencies that have early ages of onset—e.g., X-linked (Bruton's) agammaglobulinemia, severe combined immunodeficiency, Wiskott–Aldrich syndrome, and ataxia-telangiectasia (Kersey *et al.*, 1973*b*)—and which is reflected in Table 2 in the proportional rates for these sites with the four diseases. Similarly, the bulk of epithelial malignancies, e.g., stomach, other digestive organs, occurred later in life and correlate with the frequency of this histological type in IgA deficiency and variable immunodeficiency, which have a more varied age of onset (Table 2).

The high male–female ratio, 2 : 1, overall, can be attributed to the X-linked disorders of childhood. Sex becomes a less significant variable beyond childhood.

The distribution of cancers by age and primary site indirectly supports the conclusion that immunodeficient patients are at greatly increased risk for developing cancer. Despite a shortened life span (2–20 years), these patients frequently develop cancer. Two years ago, a survey of physicians was done to estimate the prevalence of childhood immunodeficiency diseases. The results showed that approximately 700 children, up to 15 years of age, had been diagnosed with various primary immunodeficiency diseases during a 12-year period, 1960–1972, when 69 immunodeficient children had died of cancer. It was estimated that the median life span was 10 years. These figures indicated that the cancer mortality rate for children with primary immunodeficiency diseases is about 0.8 per 100 per year (Kersey *et al.*, 1974). R. W. Miller (1969)

Table 4. Immunodeficiency-Cancer Registry: Distribution of Cancers by Sex and Age, 171 Cases, and by Sex or Age or Both Unknown, 34 Cases

Primary site	Age (yr):	Males										Females										Sex and/or age unk.
		0–9	10–14	15–19	20–29	30–39	40–49	50–59	60–74	Age unk.	Total	0–9	10–14	15–19	20–29	30–39	40–49	50–59	60–74	Age unk.	Total	
Lymphoreticular		34	14	6	5	3	—	3	1	11	77	13	6	2	—	1	6	1	3	1	33	7
Leukemias		12	5	—	1	—	—	2	—	5	25	5	1	—	—	—	—	—	1	—	7	2
Stomach		—	—	1	1	2	2	4	1	—	11	—	—	2	1	—	—	3	1	—	7	—
Other digestive organs		—	—	—	—	—	—	—	—	—	—	—	1	1	—	—	1	1	1	—	5	—
Lung		—	—	—	—	—	—	1	1	1	3	—	—	—	—	—	—	1	—	—	1	1
Breast		—	—	—	—	—	—	—	—	—	—	—	—	—	—	1	1	—	—	—	2	1
Genitourinary		—	—	—	—	—	—	—	—	—	—	—	—	2	—	—	1	—	—	—	3	—
Nervous system		2	1	—	—	—	—	—	—	3	6	1	2	—	—	—	—	—	—	—	3	—
Skin		—	—	—	1	1	1	—	1	—	4	—	—	1	—	—	—	—	—	—	1	—
Other sites		—	—	—	—	—	—	—	—	1	1	1	—	—	—	1	—	1	1	—	4	1[a]
TOTALS		48	20	7	8	6	3	10	4	21	127	20	10	8	1	3	9	7	7	1	66	12

[a]Liposarcoma.

Table 5. Mortality from Cancer of Various Types in Children Less Than 15 Years of Age[a]

Tumor type	Unselected children[b]	Primary immunodeficiency children[c]	
		All countries	U.S. only
Leukemias	48%	27% (16)	26% (10)
Central nervous system	16%	3% (2)	2.5% (1)
Lymphoreticular (e.g., reticulum cell sarcoma, lymphosarcoma, Hodgkin's disease)	8%	67% (40)	69% (27)
Bone	4%	1.5% (1)	0%
Other	24%	1.5% (1)	2.5% (1)
TOTALS:		60	39

[a]From Kersey *et al.* (1974).
[b]Death certificates of 29,457 children in the United States, 1960–1966 (Miller, R. W., 1969).
[c]ICR; number of cases in parentheses.

noted that the national childhood cancer mortality rate is 0.007 per 100 per year. The relative cancer mortality risk for immunodeficient children is, then, approximately 100 times that of the general childhood population. A comparison of malignancy patterns for immunodeficient children and "unselected" children in the general population who died of cancer appears in Table 5. The data show the significantly different patterns of tumors between the two groups. Most significantly, while only 8% of tumors were lymphoreticular in origin in unselected children, 67% were lymphoreticular in immunodeficient persons. While leukemias accounted for 48% of malignancies in unselected children, they accounted for 25% of cancer in our cases. Single cases of Wilms's tumor and neuroblastoma have been reported in association with IgA deficiency and IgM deficiency, respectively. These tumors occur quite frequently in the general childhood population (Young and Miller, 1975).

3.3. Gastrointestinal Tumors in Primary Immunodeficiencies

The data presented in Table 4 point out an additional fact in the complex association between immunodeficiency and cancer—the surprisingly large number of primary immunodeficiency patients who developed gastrointestinal malignancies, particularly stomach cancers. The series of GI tumors, comprised of literature reports and unpublished cases submitted to the ICR, is presented in Table 6. There are 18 stomach cancer cases (Case Nos. 1–18) and 5 cases of primary malignancies of other digestive organs, including 3 sigmoid colon tumors (Case Nos. 20, 22, 23) and 1 each of the parotid gland (Case No. 19) and the buccal cavity (Case No. 21). Stomach cancers occurred in 3 females with ataxia-telangiectasia (Case Nos. 1-3), ages 16, 21, and 19; in 4 females (Case Nos. 10, 12, 14 15) and 8 males (Case Nos. 4-9, 11, 13) with variable immunodeficiency, ages 15-67; and in 3 males with IgA deficiency (Case Nos. 16-18), ages 40, 53, and 72. Age-specific incidence rates obtained from published results of the Third National Cancer Survey for stomach cancer indicate that this tumor occurs more frequently later in life than has been observed in our registry group (Cutler and Young, 1975). Our series is too small to draw conclusions on this point, except to suggest that since immunodeficiency is generally associated with a shortened survival period, stomach cancers in immunodeficient patients likely require a shorter latency period than in nonimmunodeficient patients who develop this malignancy.

As indicated in Table 6, several clinical problems, besides immunodeficiency, preceded the development of stomach carcinomas, including nodular lymphoid hyperplasia, 4 cases (Nos. 6, 10, 12, 20); pernicious anemia, 4 cases (Nos. 8, 12, 16, 18); malabsorption or atrophic gastritis or both, 4 cases (Nos. 5, 12, 13, 17); and *Giardia lamblia* or *Trichomonas hominis* cysts, 5 cases (Nos. 4, 6, 11-13). Symptoms of several clinical problems were found in several cases (Nos. 6, 12, 13). Recent studies on autoimmune disorders in immunodeficiency diseases indicate that pernicious anemia occurs earlier than in persons without a history of immunological abnormalities (Twomey *et al.*, 1970). IgA levels were low or zero in several cases; these data may have etiological significance (Walker and Hong, 1973). Cancer was reported in families of 3 cases, including stomach cancer in the mother of Cases Nos. 2 and 3 and nonspecified tumors in the mother and 2 siblings in Case No. 15. An interesting association between immunodeficiency and cancer obtains for Case No. 22, in which the brother of this female, who had several primary tumors in addition to the adenocarcinoma of the large bowel, died of a recticulum-cell sarcoma. He was found to have no quantitative IgA in his serum (Hamoudi *et al.*, 1974). In summary, in an age-matched population, we would expect bowel cancers to occur more frequently than stomach tumors (Cutler and Young, 1975). The opposite situation obtains in our series. It is possible that subclinical immunological abnormalities play a role in the development of gastric carcinomas in both the immunodeficient and the general population. A recent study of surviving members of a large kindred in which 12 members in 4 generations had died of gastric cancer showed that in at least 5 relative members, immunological abnormalities were present (Creagan and Fraumeni, 1973). Although any cancer in an immunodeficient patient could be related in an intimate manner to the prior immunological abnormalities, it may be that breast and cervical cancers, lung tumors, and skin carcinomas, which have been reported to date in small numbers, were more influenced by other, nonimmunological factors. Accumulation of more cases of these and other common tumors of adulthood in immunodeficiency diseases will undoubtedly increase their interpretive significance. The occurrence of a series of GI tumors suggests, however, that an intimate association does exist between immunodeficiency and carcinomas of this site.

Table 6. Gastrointestinal Tumors in Immunodeficiency Diseases

		Immunodeficiency		Malignancy			
Case No.	Sex	Age of onset[a]	Dx[b]	Age at Dx	Cell type[c]/ primary site	Associated conditions/comments	Ref. No.[d]
1	F	NB	AT	16	Colloid cancer, pylorus	Absent serum IgA	1
2	F	2	AT	21	Mucin adenocarcinoma, stomach	Maternal history of adenocarcinoma of stomach; sister of Case 3	2
3	F	EC	AT	19	Adenocarcinoma, stomach	Sister of Case No. 2	2
4	M	8	V	15	Adenocarcinoma, stomach	*Giardia lamblia* cysts; serum IgA nil	3
5	M	12	V	27	Carcinoma, NOS, stomach	Nontropical sprue, age 12; poliomyelitis, age 22; furunculosis, atrophic gastritis, malabsorption	4
6	M	22	V	31	Scirrhous adenocarcinoma, stomach	Nodular lymphoid hyperplasia, small bowel; splenomegaly; *G. lamblia* in stools	5
7	M	Inf.	V	33	Carcinoma, NOS, stomach	Steatorrhea; brother has similar immunodeficiency	6
8	M	41	V	47	Carcinoma, NOS, stomach	Pernicious anemia, age 28	7, 8
9	M	Unk.	V	50	Carcinoma, NOS, stomach		9
10	F	39	V	54	Carcinoma, NOS, stomach	Diarrhea, steatorrhea, nodular lymphoid hyperplasia, small bowel	5
11	M	29	V	55	Adenocarcinoma, stomach	*Giardia lamblia*	10
12	F	31	V	56	Adenocarcinoma, stomach	Pernicious anemia; malabsorption, atrophic gastritis; nodular lymphoid hyperplasia; *G. lamblia;* splenomegaly	5

13	M	26	V	59	Scirrhous adenocarcinoma, stomach	Mild malabsorption; myexedema; *T. hominis* in stool; emphysema	5
14	F	24	V	53	Carcinoma, NOS, stomach	Persistent diarrhea from age 41; serum IgA nil	6
15	F	16	V	67	Carcinoma, NOS, stomach	Steatorrhea; serum IgA nil; mother, 2 siblings died of cancer, >60 years	6
16	M	Unk.	IgA	40	Carcinoma, NOS, stomach	Pernicious anemia, age 25; repeated infections 4 years before cancer; serum IgA nil	11
17	M	Unk.	IgA	53	Anaplastic cancer, stomach	Malabsorption, age 55; vitiligo, 57; IgA nil at autopsy	12
18	M	Unk.	IgA	72	Adenocarcinoma, stomach	Pernicious anemia, 64	13
19	F	Unk.	AT	17	Mucoepidermoid, parotid gland		14
20	F	27	V	47	Carcinoma, NOS, sigmoid colon	Diarrhea, nodular lymphoid hyperplasia, small bowel; toxic thyroid nodule	5
21	F	Unk.	V	59	Carcinoma, NOS, buccal cavity		15
22	F	3	IgA	12	Adenocarcinoma, sigmoid colon	Hereditary spherocytic anemia; recurrent polyps, age 10; benign cavernous hemangioma, 14; malignant thymoma, 15.5; epidermoid carcinoma, scalp, 17; primary malignant astrocytoma, 20; brother with IgA deficiency and histiocytic lymphoma	16
23	F	Unk.	IgA def.	46	Carcinoma, sigmoid colon	Serum IgA nil 14 years post cancer diagnosis	17

[a](NB) Newborn; (EC) early childhood; (Inf.) infancy; (Unk.) unknown.
[b](At) Ataxia-telangiectasia; (V) variable immunodeficiency; (IgA) IgA deficiency.
[c](NOS) Not otherwise specified.
[d]References: (1) Schuler *et al.* (1971); (2) Haerer *et al.* (1969); Jackson (1972); (3) Shackelford and McAlister (1975); (4) Forssman and Herner (1964); (5) Hermans *et al.* (1976); (6) Medical Research Council (1970); (7) Rolles (1973); (8) Rees-Jones (1976); (9) Morell (1973); (10) Chaplin (1975); (11) Leikola *et al.* (1973); (12) Fraser and Rankin (1970); (13) Hanson (1975); (14) Ochs (1973); (15) Kirkpatrick (1976); (16) Hamoudi *et al.* (1974); (17) W. V. Miller *et al.* (1970).

4. *Possible Mechanisms Linking Human Immunodeficiency and Malignancy: Hypotheses*

Primary immunodeficiency diseases likely provide one of the more dramatic examples of the influence of genetic factors on malignancy, since the lymphoid apparatus in individuals with these diseases is both the site of genetic aberration and the principal site of cancer development (Kersey and Spector, 1975). Epidemiological data collected on this series, such as the association among primary disease, age, and tumor histology, strongly implicate abnormalities of the immune system as a major factor in oncogenesis. Hypotheses of the mechanisms of oncogenesis of the lymphoid system fall into at least two general categories: (1) the immune system in primary immunodeficiencies is subject to the formation of too many malignant cells; and (2) the immune system in these diseases has a decreased ability to get rid of malignant cells when they do develop (Kersey and Spector, 1975).

Several pathogenic mechanisms may be responsible for the increased malignant transformation of lymphoid cells, including (1) intrinsic defects in lymphoid cells and (2) chronic antigenic stimulation (including graft-host diseases), resulting in enhanced lymphoid proliferation with increased opportunity for development of malignant cells; (3) the activation of endogenous viruses or infection with exogenous oncogenic viruses; and (4) the lack of regulatory feedback mechanisms resulting in enhanced lymphoid proliferation. Evidence of an etiological role in oncogenesis of intrinsic defects in lymphoid cells is available on at least one primary immunodeficiency disease, ataxia-telangiectasis, in which chromosomal instability of lymphoid populations has been observed in several patients (Hecht *et al.*, 1973; Bochkov *et al.*, 1974; McCaw *et al.*, 1975). In both fibroblasts and lymphocytes from these patients, chromosome 14 was most often the site of aberration, particularly translocation of the long-arm portion with most often the 14 homologue or chromosome 6, 7, or X. Other chromosomal abnormalities have been observed in ataxia-telangiectasia, including increased breakage, as well as gain or loss of chromatid material. In one case report, a 19-year-old male with ataxia-telangiectasia, who had 2 siblings who died of ataxia-telangiectasia and acute lymphocytic leukemia, was found to have 1% of lymphoid cells with a translocation at chromosome 14. Over the next 4 years, the number of cells with this karyotypic abnormality increased to 80% at time of death at 23 years. No malignancy was observed prior to or at autopsy (Hecht *et al.*, 1973). Another case, a woman in her 20's with the same disease, was found to have lymphocyte clones with a balanced translocation of chromosome 14. She developed chronic lymphatic leukemia a few years later. When the leukemia was diagnosed, the leukemic lymphocytes had the same karyotypic abnormalities. Eventually, 100% of her lymphocytes examined had the 14:14 translocation (McCaw *et al.*, 1975). In other studies, chromosome banding has revealed an extra band on chromosome 14 in several patients with a variety of lymphoproliferative malignancies, including Burkitt's lymphoma, multiple myeloma, plasma-cell leukemia, Hodgkin's disease, and lymphocytic lymphoma (Manolova and Manolova, 1972; Petit *et al.*, 1972; Wurster-Hill *et al.*, 1973; Reeves, 1973). It is of interest that many of these lymphoproliferative malignancies have frequently been observed in patients with ataxia–telangiectasia and other primary immunodeficiencies (see Table 2).

Other evidence for the role of intrinsic defects of lymphoid cells in the pathogenesis of malignancy is from a recent study that shows that DNA-repair mechanisms in ataxia–telangiectasia (AT) are likely impaired (Paterson *et al.*, 1976). In this study, fibroblasts from 3 AT donors and 2 normal controls were used to measure DNA-repair properties after exposure to γ radiation. The results showed that the level of DNA repair attained in the AT fibroblast strains was about half that found in the normal strains. These data may provide an explanation for the enhanced radiosensitivity of AT patients with tumors. For example, 3 AT patients had developed unusually severe complications, e.g., radiation dermatitis, following conventional radiotherapy for lymphoreticular malignancies (Morgan *et al.*, 1968; Gotoff *et al.*, 1967; Cunliffe *et al.*, 1975). Another AT patient developed basal-cell carcinoma of the scalp following radiation treatment to the area for a *Tinea* infection (Levin and Perlov, 1971). Impaired DNA-repair mechanisms have been found for a genetic disorder which predisposes to skin tumors, xeroderma pigmentosum (XP). Like AT, this disorder, is inherited as an autosomal recessive trait; persons with XP have high skin sensitivity to ultraviolet (UV) light, and fibroblasts from these persons are defective in UV-stimulated DNA repair (Cleaver, 1968). It is possible that defective DNA repair due to either UV or γ radiation has an etiological role in some forms of neoplastic transformation in patients with these genetic disorders.

Some evidence exists for the role of exogenous or endogenous viruses as a pathogenic mechanism of malignancies in primary immunodeficiencies. In a recent study, virological and cell analysis was performed on tissue from a reticulum-cell sarcoma of the brain in a boy with Wiskott–Aldrich syndrome; a virus was isolated that resembled the papovavirus BKV previously found by others (Takemoto *et al.*, 1974). BKV has also been isolated from the urine of several renal-transplant recipients on immunosuppressive therapy and from the brains of 2 patients with progressive multifocal leukoencephalopathy, a demyelinating disorder with concomitant immunlogical abnormalities (Gardner *et al.*, 1971; Padgett *et al.*, 1971; Weiner *et al.*, 1972). The relationship between the new virus (called MMV by the authors) and BKV was established morphologically and immunologically; MMV produced hemagglutin when tumor cells were cultivated with human fetal brain tissue and a continuous line from African green monkey kidney (VERO), and the hemagglutin could be inhibited by the addition of anti-BKV rabbit serum to the brain isolate culture. MMV was also isolated from urine pellets, and papovavirus particles from brain and urine were observed by electron microscopy. Serum from the patient had high antiviral antibody at least 1 year before the tumor was detected. In this Wiskott–Aldrich syndrome case, it is possible that the MMV was a passenger virus having no causative role in tumor production. However, viruses which were serologically identical to BKV were isolated from 2 additional patients with Wiskott–Aldrich syndrome, although neither of these 2 boys had a malignancy at the time the virus studies were performed (Takemoto *et al.*, 1974). The various papovavirus studies suggest that papovaviruses may be common in renal-transplant recipients and in patients with immunodeficiency diseases. The role of viruses in the increased incidence of malignancies in these disorders needs further investigation.

Data supporting the role of impaired regulatory feedback mechanisms in oncogenesis are available from studies on experimental animals. Suppressor T lymphocytes have been shown to act as regulators of proliferative responses to several antigens in the mouse. The New Zealand mouse, an inbred strain which spontaneously develops autoimmune disease, i.e., Coombs-positive hemolytic anemia and immune complex glomerulonephritis as well as lymphoreticular malignancies (Gershwin and Steinberg, 1973), appears to be defective in generation of suppressor cells. By analogy, in humans with abnormal immune systems, a lack of suppressor function could allow an increased lymphoproliferative response due to any one of a variety of mechanisms. This in turn could result in increased risk of mutation and abnormal lymphoid clones that would lead to a malignant cell population.

The second category of hypotheses—i.e., that suggesting decreased ability of the lymphoid system to recognize and destroy malignant lymphoid cells—includes several possibilities, including the possibility of defective recognition or defective response following recognition. Defective recognition of malignant cells may be due to deficient receptors for tumor cells. Defective response could be a result of inability to generate effector mechanisms which normally destroy malignant lymphoid cells.

These various hypotheses of the pathogenic mechanisms involved in oncogenesis in human immunodeficiencies refine and complement the immunological surveillance theory, which predicts that a major role of the immune system (especially the cell-mediated system) is host defense against malignant cells. A premise of the theory is that malignant cells develop frequently, and that under normal conditions, cells are destroyed by immunological mechanisms. Therefore, immunodeficiency, which is due to abnormal immune function, should be associated with earlier and more frequent cancers of all types (Kersey *et al.*, 1973*a*). However, most epithelial tumors common to the general adult population, i.e., breast, lung, colon, have not occurred in excess numbers in comparable age-matched immunodeficient patients. Soft-tissue sarcomas common to the general childhood population—e.g., Wilms's tumor, retinoblastoma, Ewing's sarcoma, and nervous system tumors—have rarely been reported in immunodeficient children. The proportion of tumors which arise in the lymphoid system (lymphoreticular tumors and leukemias, 74% of total tumors) is simply too large and, in comparison with the general population, significantly greater than expected. If the immune surveillance theory explains the increased malignancy rate in primary immunodeficiencies (Melief and Schwartz, 1975), multiple primaries would be a frequent event. In the registry series, only 4 patients have developed multiple primaries, and 2 of them had lymphoreticular tumors as one of their tumors. These 4 included Case No. 22 in Table 6; a patient with IgA deficiency who developed squamous-cell carcinoma of the lung and esophogeal cancer; a 72-year-old male with variable immunodeficiency with multiple skin cancers who developed a fibrosarcoma and a reticulum-cell sarcoma; and a 31-year-old woman with ataxia–telangiectasia who developed multiple leiomyosarcomas of the uterus, malignant lymphoma, and acute lymphatic leukemia.

Finally, it seems that much work remains to define the nature of the association between immunodeficiency and cancer. Patients with primary immunodeficiency who develop cancer, while useful in the development of models for the role of the immune system in cancer control, are of such complexity as to defy precise analysis. Future studies will undoubtedly be directed at more subtle forms of immune deficiency which are more commonly found in the general population and which could account for a large number of malignancies, especially those of the lymphoreticular system.

ACKNOWLEDGMENTS

The original research discussed in this chapter was aided by Grant CA-17404 from the National Cancer Institute, from the American Cancer Society, and from the National Foundation–March of Dimes.

5. References

Amman, A. J., and Hong, R., 1971, Selective IgA deficiency: Presentation of 30 cases and a review of the literature, *Medicine (Baltimore)* **50:**223–236.

Bergsma, D. (ed.), 1975, *Immunodeficiency in Man and Animals, Birth Defects: Orig. Artic. Ser.* **11,** Sinauer Associates, Sunderland, Massachusetts.

Blaese, R. M., Strober, W., and Waldmann, T. A., 1975, Immunodeficiency in the Wiskott–Aldrich syndrome, in: *Immunodeficiency in Man and Animals* (D. Bergsma, ed.), *Birth Defects: Orig. Artic. Ser.* **11:**250–254, Sinauer Associates, Sunderland, Massachusetts.

Bochkov, N. P., Lopukhin, Y. M., Kuleshov, N. P., and Kovalchuk, L. V., 1974, Cytogenetic study of patients with ataxia–telangiectasia, *Humangenetik* **24:**225–238.

Boder, E., 1975, Ataxia–telangiectasia: Some historic, clinical, and pathologic observations, in: *Immunodeficiency in Man and Animals* (D. Bergsma, ed.), *Birth Defects: Orig. Artic. Ser.* **11:**255–270, Sinauer Associates, Sunderland, Massachusetts.

Chaplin, H., 1975, personal communication to the Immunodeficiency-Cancer Registry.

Cleaver, J. E., 1968, Defective repair replication of DNA in xeroderma pigmentosum, *Nature (London)* **218:**652–656.

Cone, L., and Uhr, J. W., 1964, Immunological deficiency diseases associated with chronic lymphatic leukemia and multiple myeloma, *J. Clin. Invest.* **43:**2241–2248.

Cooper, M. D., Faulk, W. P., Fudenberg, H. H., Good, R. A., Hitzig, W., Kunkel, H., Rosen, F., Seligmann, M., Soothill, J., and Wedgwood, R. J., 1973, Classification of primary immunodeficiencies, *N. Engl. J. Med.* **288:**966–967.

Creagan, E. T., and Fraumeni, J. R., Jr., 1973, Familial gastric cancer and immunologic abnormalities, *Cancer* **32:**1325–1331.

Cunliffe, P. N., Mann, J. R., Cameron, A. H., and Roberts, K. D., 1975, Radiosensitivity in ataxia–telangiectasia, *Br. J. Radiol.* **48:**374–376.

Cutler, S. J., and Young, J. L., Jr., 1975, *Third National Cancer Survey: Incidence Data,* National

Cancer Institute Monograph 41, U.S. Department of Health, Education, and Welfare, Washington, D.C.

Dent, P. B., Peterson, R. D. A., and Good, R. A., 1968, The relationship between immunologic function and oncogenesis, in: *Immunologic Deficiency Diseases in Man* (R. A. Good and D. Bergsma, eds.), Vol. 4, pp. 443–453, National Foundation Press, New York.

Forssman, O., and Herner, B., 1964, Acquired agammaglobuilinemia and malabsorption, *Acta Med. Scand.* **176**:779–786.

Fraser, K. J., and Rankin, J. G., 1970, Selective deficiency of IgA immunoglobulins associated with carcinoma of the stomach, *Aust. Ann. Med.* **19**:165–167.

Fraumeni, J. F., Jr., and Miller, R. W., 1967, Epidemiology of human leukemia: Recent observations, *J. Natl. Cancer Inst.* **38**:593–605.

Fraumeni, J. F., Jr., Manning, M. D., and Mitus, W. J. 1971, Acute childhood leukemia: Epidemiologic study by cell type of 1,263 cases at the Children's Cancer Research Foundation in Boston, 1947–65, *J. Natl. Cancer Inst.* **46**:461–470.

Fudenberg, H. H., Good, R. A., Goodman, H. C., Hitzig, W., Hunkel, H., Roitt, I., Rosen, F., Rowe, D., Seligmann, M., and Soothill, J., 1971, Primary immunodeficiencies: Report of a World Health Organization Committee (Special article), *Pediatrics* **47**:927–946.

Gardner, S. D., Field, S. M., Coleman, D., and Hulme, B., 1971, New human papovavirus (B.K.) isolated from urine after renal transplantation, *Lancet* **1**:1253–1257.

Gatti, R. A., and Good, R. A., 1971, Occurrence of malignancy in immunedeficiency diseases, *Cancer* **28**:89–98.

Gershwin, M. E., and Steinberg, A. D., 1973, Loss of suppressor function as a cause of lymphoid malignancy, *Lancet* **2**:1174–1176.

Good, R. A., 1972, Relations between immunity and malignancy, *Proc. Natl. Acad. Sci. U.S.A.* **69**:1026–1032.

Gotoff, S. O., Amirmokri, E., and Liebner, E. J., 1967, Ataxia-telangiectasia: Neoplasia, untoward response to X-irradiation and tuberous sclerosis, *Am. J. Dis. Child.* **114**:617–625.

Grundy, G. W., Creagan, E. T., and Fraumeni, J. F., Jr., 1973, Non-Hodgkin's lymphoma in childhood: Epidemiologic features, *J. Natl. Cancer Inst.* **51**:767–776.

Haerer, A. F., Jackson, J. F., and Evers, C. G., 1969, Ataxia-telangiectasia with gastric carcinoma, *J. Am. Med. Assoc.* **210**:1884–1887.

Hamoudi, A. B., Ertel, I., Newton, W. A., Jr., Reiner, C. B., and Clatworthy, H. W., 1974, Multiple neoplasms in an adolescent child associated with IgA deficiency, *Cancer* **33**:1134–1144.

Hanson, L. A., 1975, personal communication to the Immunodeficiency-Cancer Registry.

Hecht, F., McCaw, B., and Koler, R. D., 1973, Ataxia-telangiectasia: Clonal growth of translocation lymphocytes, *N. Engl. J. Med.* **289**:286–291.

Hermans, P. E., Diaz-Buxo, J. A., and Stobo, J. D., 1976, Idiopathic late-onset immunoglobulin deficiency: Clinical observations in 50 patients, *Am. J. Med.* **61**:221–237.

Hobbs, J., 1975, IgM deficiency, in: *Immunodeficiency in Man and animals* (D. Bergsma, ed.), *Birth Defects: Orig. Artic. Ser.* **11**:112–116, Sinaur Associates, Sunderland, Massachusetts.

Hoover, R., and Fraumeni, J. F., Jr., 1973, Risk of cancer in renal-transplant recipients, *Lancet* **2**:55–57.

Jackson, J. F., 1972, Ataxia-telangiectasia, in: *Skin, Heredity, and Malignant Neoplasma* (H. T. Lynch, ed.), pp. 94–103, Medical Examination Publishing Co., Flushing, New York.

Kelly, W. D., Good, R. A., and Varco, R. L., 1958, Anergy and skin homograft survival in Hodgkin's disease, *Surg. Gynecol. Obstet.* **107**:565–570.

Kersey, J. H., and Gajl-Peczalska, K. J., 1975, T and B lymphocytes in humans: A review, *Am. J. Pathol.* **81**:446–458.

Kersey, J. H., and Spector, B. D., 1975, Immune deficiency diseases, in: *Persons at High Risk of Cancer: An Approach to Cancer Etiology and Control* (J. F. Fraumeni, Jr., ed.), pp. 55–67, Academic Press, New York.

Kersey, J., Spector, B. D., and Good, R. A., 1973*a*, Immunodeficiency and cancer, in: *Advances in Cancer Research* (S. Weinhouse and G. Klein, eds.), Vol. 18, pp. 211–230, Academic Press, New York.

Kersey, J. H., Spector, B. D., and Good, R. A., 1973*b*, Primary immunodeficiency diseases and cancer: The Immunodeficiency-Cancer Registry, *Int. J. Cancer* **12**:333–347.
Kersey, J. H., Spector, B. D., and Good, R. A., 1974, Cancer in children with primary immunodeficiency diseases, *J. Pediatr* **84**:263–264.
Kirkpatrick, C., 1976, personal communication to the Immunodeficiency-Cancer Registry.
Krivit, W., and Good, R. A., 1959, Aldrich's syndrome (thrombocytopenia, eczema, and infection in infants), *AMA J. Dis. Child.* **97**:137–153.
Leikola, J., Koistinen, J., Lehtinen, J., and Virolainen, M., 1973, IgA-induced anaphylactic transfusion reactions: A report of 4 cases, *Blood* **42**:111–119.
Levin, S., and Perlov, S., 1971, Ataxia-telangiectasia in Isreal with observations on its relationship to malignant disease, *Isr. J. Med. Sci.* **7**:1535–1541.
Lukes, R. J., and Collins, R. D., 1974, Immunologic characteristics of malignant lymphomas, *Cancer* **34** (Suppl. 4):1488–1503.
Manolova, G., and Manolova, Y., 1972, Marker band in one chromosome 14 from Burkitt's lymphomas, *Nature (London)* **237**:33–34.
McCaw, B. K., Hecht, F., Harnden, D. G., and Teplitz, R., 1975, Somatic rearrangement of chromosome 14 in human lymphocytes, *Proc. Natl. Acad. Sci. U.S.A.* **72**:2071–2075.
Medical Research Council, 1970, *Hypogammaglobulinemia in the United Kingdom,* Her Majesty's Stationery Office, London.
Melief, C. J. M., and Schwartz, R. S., 1975, Immunocompetence and malignancy, in: *Cancer: A Comprehensive Treatise* (F. F. Becher, ed.), Vol. 1, pp. 121–160, Plenum Press, New York.
Miller, R. W., 1967, Persons at exceptionally high risk of leukemia, *Cancer Res.* **27**:2420–2423.
Miller, R. W., 1969, Fifty two forms of childhood cancer: United States mortality experience, 1960–1966, *J. Pediatr.* **75**:685–689.
Miller, W. V., Holland, P. V., Sugarbaker, E., Strober, W., and Waldmann, T. A., 1970, Anaphylactic reactions to IgA: A difficult transfusion problem, *Am. J. Clin. Pathol.* **54**:618–621.
Morell, A., 1973, personal communication to the Immunodeficiency-Cancer Registry.
Morgan, J. L., Holcomb, T. M., and Morrissey, R. W., 1968, Radiation reaction in ataxia-telangiectasia, *Am. J. Dis. Child.* **116**:537–538.
Ochs, H., 1973, personal communication to the Immunodeficiency-Cancer Registry.
Padgett, B. L., Walker, D. L., Zurhein, G. M., and Eckroade, R. J., 1971, Cultivation of papova-like virus from human brain with progressive multifocal leucoencephalopathy, *Lancet* **1**:1257–1260.
Paterson, M. C., Smith, B. P., Lohman, P. H. M., Anderson, A. K., and Fishman, L., 1976, Defective excision repair of gamma ray-damaged DNA in human (ataxia-telangiectasia) fibroblasts, *Nature (London)* **260**:444–446.
Penn, I., 1975, The incidence of malignancies in transplant recipients, *Transplant. Proc.* **7**:323.
Petit, P., Verhest, A., Lecluse van der Bilt, F., and Jengsma, A., 1972, The chromosomes of the EB virus-positive Burkitt cell line PsJ.HRJK studied by the fluorescent staining technique, *Pathol. Eur.* **7**:17–21.
Rees-Jones, A., 1976, personal communication to the Immunodeficiency-Cancer Registry.
Reeves, B. R., 1973, Cytogenetics of malignant lymphomas: Studies using a Giemsa-banding technique, *Humangenetik* **20**:231–250.
Rolles, T. E., 1973, personal communication to the Immunodeficiency-Cancer Registry.
Schier, W. W., 1954, Cutaneous anergy and Hodgkin's disease, *N. Engl. J. Med.* **250**:353–361.
Schuler, D., Schöngut, L., Cserhati, E., Siegler, J., and Gacs, G., 1971, Lymphoblastic transformation, chromosome pattern and delayed-type skin reaction in ataxia-telangiectasia, *Acta Paediatr. Scand.* **60**:66–72.
Sedgwick, R. P., and Boder, E., 1972, Ataxia-telangiectasia, in: *Handbook of Clinical Neurology* (P. J. Vinken and G. W. Bruyen, eds.), pp. 267–339, North-Holland, Amsterdam.
Shackelford, G. D., and McAlister, W. H., 1975, Primary immunodeficiency disease and malignancy, *Am. J. Roentgenol. Radium Ther. Nucl. Med.* **123**:144–153.
Southam, C. J., 1961, Application of immunology to clinical cancer: Past attempts and future possibilities, *Cancer Res.* **21**:1302–1361.

Spector, B. D., Kersey, J. H., and Perry, G. S., III, 1978, Immunodeficiency cancer registry (in preparation).

Swift, M., Sholman, L., Perry, M., and Chase, C., 1976, Malignant neoplasma in the families of patients with ataxia-telangiectasia, *Cancer Res.* **36**:209–215.

Takemoto, K. K., Rabson, A. S., Mullarkey, M. F., Blaese, R. M., Garon, C. F., and Nelson, D., 1974, Isolation of papovavirus from brain tumor and urine of a patient with Wiskott-Aldrich syndrome, *J. Natl. Cancer Inst.* **53**:1205–1207.

Twomey, J. J., Jordan, P. H., Laughter, A. H., Meuwissen, H. J., and Good, R. A., 1970, The gastric disorder in immunoglobulin patients, *Ann. Intern. Med.* **72**:499–504.

Walker, W. A., and Hong, R., 1973, Immunology of the gastrointestinal tract, Part I, *J. Pediatr.* **83**:517–530.

Weiner, L. P., Herndon, R. M., Narayan, O., Johnson, R. T., Shar, K., Rubinstein, L. J., Preziosk, T. J., and Conley, F. K., 1972, Isolation of virus related to SV40 from patients with progressive multifocal leukoencephalopathy, *N. Engl. J. Med.* **286**:385–390.

Williams, W. J., Beutler, E., Erslev, A., and Rundles, R. W. (eds.), 1972, *Hematology*, McGraw-Hill, New York.

Wurster-Hill, D. H., McIntyre, O. R., Cornell, G. G., and Maurer, L. H., 1973, Marker-chromosome 14 in multiple myeloma and plasma-cell leukaemia, *Lancet* **2**:1031.

Young, J. L., and Miller, R. W., 1975, Incidence of malignant tumors in U.S. children, *J. Pediatr.* **86**:254–258.

4

Recognitive Immunity in Colon Cancer

Norman T. Berlinger

1. Possible Antigenicity of Colon Carcinomas

1.1. Serological Evidence

The possibility of controlling cancer by immunological means continues to provoke the interest and excitement of many workers. Such a possibility, however, is entirely dependent on the fact that tumors express antigens which are associated with those tumors. Efforts have been made to demonstrate tumor antigenicity by serological methods. As early as 1930, Witebsky produced in guinea pigs a putative antiserum to a human stomach cancer. After adsorption of this antiserum with extracts of normal human stomach, he found that it was still capable of producing a precipitation reaction with the cancer extract. This work suggested that an antigen was present in a cancerous stomach which was not present in a normal stomach. Other serological evidence followed. Graham and Graham (1955) claimed the ability to demonstrate positive complement fixation reactions for some patients using extracts of autologous tumors. Other claims were made (Finney *et al.*, 1960) for the demonstration of precipitating antibody in the sera of cancer patients against extracts of their own tumors.

1.2. Evidence from Delayed Hypersensitivity Skin Testing

Workers then explored the possibility of whether a malignant tumor exhibited sufficient antigenic differences from its host to be considered as a

Norman T. Berlinger • Research Associate, Memorial Sloan-Kettering Cancer Center, New York, New York 10021, and Fellow, Clinical Immunology Service, Memorial Hospital for Cancer and Allied Diseases, New York, New York 10021.

malignant homograft. This approach found basis in the early observation (Brent *et al.,* 1958) that a skin homograft reaction in outbred guinea pigs manifested itself as a delayed hypersensitivity reaction of the tuberculin type, transferable by activated lymphoid cells but not by serum. This tuberculinlike reaction correlated well with the presence of a satisfactory graft rejection immune mechanism. Hughes and Lytton (1964) injected 50 patients having carcinomas of the lung, breast, stomach, or colon with cell-free extracts of their own tumors and demonstrated delayed cutaneous hypersensitivity reactions, with normal tissue extracts as controls, in 27% of these patients. Herberman and Oren (1969) demonstrated delayed cutaneous hypersensitivity reactions to membrane extracts of autochthonous tumor cells in 38 of 53 patients with lymphoid or solid tumors. Histological examination of biopsies from the skin test sites showed perivascular infiltration of mononuclear cells, a picture consistent with an antigen-directed delayed hypersensitivity reaction. Stewart (1969) demonstrated delayed hypersensitivity reactions in 26% of 142 patients to extracts of their tumors. He further investigated the possibility that these positive reactions were directed against components of contaminating bacteria in the extracts. In patients with carcinoma of the breast, bacterial antigen could be relatively well excluded as the cause of this phemonenon, and the same conclusion seemed to hold for patients with carcinoma of the gastrointestinal tract, although the possibility that bacterial products contributed to some of the reactions could not be firmly excluded. In addition, the majority of the patients showed the strongest reaction to the skin test material present in the supernatant of extracts centrifuged at 14,000*g*, the fraction which probably contained external cellular membranes.

It was appreciated, however, that such skin testing procedures may not in fact reveal the patient's true immune status to his tumor. Fass *et al.* (1970) tested eight patients for delayed hypersensitivity reactions to antigens on autologous tumor cells. The three patients with localized tumors demonstrated positive reactions, whereas the five patients with metastatic disease did not. These latter negative reactions could not be explained by a general state of anergy existing in these patients, for each demonstrated at least one positive delayed hypersensitivity reaction to tuberculin, mumps antigen, *Candida albicans* extract, *Tricophyton* extract, or *Brucella* antigen. This apparent relationship of skin reactivity to clinical status could be due to antigenic differences on metastatic tumors. Also, however, it is known that an excess of tumor antigen in patients with widespread disease could attenuate the specific host immune response to the tumor. Wang (1968) observed that all rats with benzpyrene-induced tumors produced delayed hypersensitivity reactions to their own ultrasonically prepared tumor extracts only after complete removal of the tumor. If the tumors were only partially removed, delayed hypersensitivity reactions were uniformly negative.

It was earlier suggested (Mikulska *et al.,* 1966) that such a phenomenon was due to the exhaustion of the supply of lymphocytes specifically reactive against the tumor. Such a formulation was not so tenable after the report of

Hoy and Nelson (1969) which showed that mice bearing methylcholanthrene-induced tumors which showed no delayed hypersensitivity reactions to the tumor cells also showed depressed delayed immune reactions to sheep erythrocytes. Among others, Eilber and Morton (1970) showed that patients bearing solid tumors could display depressed delayed cutaneous reactivity to an immunogen unrelated to tumor antigens, namely dinitrochlorobenzene (DNCB). After surgical removal of the tumor, many patients recovered their ability to respond do this chemical antigen. Berlinger *et al.* (1976*a*) showed that patients bearing tumors displayed significantly impaired capacities to respond to allogeneic lymphocytes in the mixed leukocyte culture reaction (MLC), an *in vitro* analogue of a delayed hypersensitivity reaction. Interestingly, if an adherent population of these patients' cells was removed from the reaction, the lymphocytes could demonstrate normal proliferative capacities. These and other findings strongly suggest that the tumor-bearing patient may not have exhausted certain populations of immunocompetent cells, but rather may have paradoxically suppressed immune capacity as a natural concomitant of the malignant situation. Therefore, the demonstration of the antigenicity of colon carcinomas by such skin testing procedures may not be incisive, for the patient with a tumor may possess a general immune hyporesponsiveness to many types of antigens.

1.3. In Vitro Evidence

In vitro methods have also been employed to attempt the demonstration of the antigenicity of human colon carcinoma. In particular, many of these methods have attempted the demonstration of delayed, or cellular, hypersensitivity to tumors, since the cellular immune system appears to be the major immunological component addressing malignancy. A significant disadvantage of intracutaneous testing is that the influence of circulating antibodies against the tumor cannot be excluded, and certain cutaneous reactions manifested may not be truly of the delayed type. For instance, Buchanan *et al.* (1958) showed in patients with Hashimoto's thyroiditis, a disease of autoimmune etiology, that skin reactions against an extract of thyroid tissue could be induced. The nature of these reactions, considered together with the fact that the patients who demonstrated positive reactions also showed circulating precipitating antibody to a saline extract of thyroid tissue, strongly suggested that they were not of the cellular, delayed type but rather antibody-dependent Arthus reactions.

The inhibition of migration of sensitized immunocompetent cells in response to the sensitizing antigen has been developed as a specific *in vitro* test of cellular immunity. Søborg (1967) was one of the first to employ this test in the study of human immunity, showing that the migration of immunocompetent cells from *Brucella*-positive persons was significantly inhibited in the presence of *Brucella* antigens, whereas this was not the case for *Brucella*-negative persons. Evidence was subsequently presented that this macrophage migration inhibition technique was a suitable *in vitro* assay to demonstrate cellular immunity to tumor antigens. Bloom *et al.* (1969) showed the inhibition of migration of peritoneal exudate cells or lymph node cells in response to the soluble antigens of chemically induced sarcomas in guinea pigs which had been immunized with this same extract. This assay for the determination of cellular hypersensitivity to tumor components was then applied in humans. Andersen *et al.* (1969) showed that in patients with carcinoma of the breast an extract of the autologous tumor induced inhibition of *in vitro* leukocyte migration. Extracts of the patient's normal mammary tissue yielded no inhibition, and no inhibition of normal leukocyte migration could be detected in response to malignant or normal breast tissue. Other reports followed (Wolberg and Goelzer, 1971; Segall *et al.,* 1972) indicating that immunocompetent cells sensitized to tumor-associated antigens could be detected in many patients with solid tumors. Guillou and Giles (1973), using the leukocyte migration inhibition test, demonstrated that 15 of 22 patients with adenocarcinoma of the colon or rectum possessed circulating leukocytes sensitized to autologous tumor extracts. These results were confirmed and amplified by Bull *et al.* (1973), Elias and Elias (1975), and House *et al.* (1975). The significance of leukocyte migration inhibition lay in the fact that this phenomenon is dependent on the release of a soluble lymphocyte mediator, or lymphokine, called migration inhibitory factor (MIF), from sensitized lymphocytes upon specific exposure to the sensitizing antigen (Pick and Turk, 1972). In addition to revealing a state of cellular immunity to carcinoma in affected patients, such positive tests strongly indicate that the tumors are indeed antigenic.

1.4. Specificity of Colon Carcinoma Antigens

The evidence from *in vivo* and *in vitro* analyses strongly suggests that human colon carcinomas are antigenic in their hosts. The question remains as to how specific this antigen is for colon carcinoma. The Hellströms' colony inhibition technique has been used extensively for the detection of immunity against tumor antigens. This test is predicated on the killing or growth inhibition of tumor cells by specifically immune lymphocytes. By comparison of the number of colonies of tumor cells formed in a tissue culture vessel when immune lymphocytes are admixed, the percentage of tumor cells killed or inhibited by the immune lymphocytes can be determined and the demonstration of tumor antigenicity can be appreciated. Hellström *et al.* (1968) studied eight patients with adenocarcinoma of the colon. Autochthonous lymphocytes from each of these patients inhibited colony formation of his own explanted tumor cells, whereas this effect was not found with lymphocytes from normal individuals or from individuals with nonneoplastic diseases. Normal fibroblasts from the patient were not inhibited by his lymphocytes, indicating that the antigen being recognized was probably expressed preferentially on the malignant tissue. More significantly, lymphocytes from patients with adenocarcinoma of the colon inhibited explanted colon carcinoma cells from other patients as well but did not inhibit other histological types of tumor cells, suggesting that colon neoplasms may have common tumor antigens which are not found in other types of neoplasms. Nairn *et al.* (1971) likewise found evidence of some tumor specificity. Using lymphocytotoxicity and complement-dependent cytotoxicity assays, they determined that patients with carcinoma of the colon could express antitumor immunoreactivity against their own cultured tumor cells and not against target cells derived from malignant melanomas or cutaneous squamous cell carcinomas. When an individual was tested for immunoreactivity against cultured colonic tumor cells from another patient, some degree of reactivity was often seen, but it was sometimes weaker than the autologous response, perhaps suggesting a degree of specificity in individual colon tumors. Notably, this has not been the experience of other investigators.

Hellström *et al.* (1971*a,b*) later extended their observations with a large number of solid tumor patients. Employing both colony inhibition and cytotoxicity tests of cell-mediated immunity, they showed that patients with colonic carcinoma were reactive against their autochthonous tumor cells and also against allogeneic colon tumor cells, indicating that colon carcinomas possessed identical or cross-reacting antigens against which the patient's lymphocytes were immune. Lymphocytes from patients with breast or lung carcinomas, malignant melanomas, or sarcomas were not reactive against colon carcinoma cells, and lymphocytes from patients with colon carcinomas were not inhibitory to a variety of other neoplasms. These and other findings imply that several groups of tumors exist within which immunological cross-reactions occur. These include not only colon carcinoma but also Burkitt's lymphoma, neuroblastoma, bladder carcinoma, malignant melanoma, breast carcinoma, ovarian and testicular tumors, and sarcomas.

There are a number of reasonable hypotheses to entertain to explain why tumors of the same histological type seem to possess cross-reacting antigens. One could speculate that tumors of different histological types are induced by different viruses which specify in the malignantly transformed tissue antigens which are unique to that virus. There are currently no data to confirm or deny this hypothesis. It is also possible that cross-reactions among colon carcinomas are due to normal colon-specific antigens against which a patient with colonic carcinoma could have developed immunity. This possibility seems to have been conclusively ruled out by the demonstration that blood lymphocytes from patients with adenocarcinomas of the colon can inhibit colony formation of plated malignant colon cells but not cells from normal adult colon mucosa (Hellström *et al.*, 1970). A third possibility is that the tumor-associated antigen which is recognized as foreign and results in such cross-reactivity among colon carcinomas is an organ- or tissue-specific antigen not present on normal adult colon cells but expressed on embryonic colon cells. Evidence for this last possibility comes from the finding that lymphocytes from patients with colon carcinoma which inhibit colony formation of plated colon carcinoma cells also inhibit fetal gut epithelial cells but not normal adult colon epithelial cells or fetal kidney cells. These data suggest that the antigen(s) associated with colon carcinoma which are recognized as foreign and evoke an immune response could be of embryonal origin.

1.5. Nature of Colon Carcinoma Antigens

The natural question to consider at this point is what is the nature of the colon carcinoma-associated antigen(s). This antigen behaves like a true immunogenic substance. The above-cited evidence speaks to the fact that cell-mediated immune reactions against this antigen can be readily observed *in vitro*. Lymphocytes from patients who have had their tumors surgically extirpated are just as effective in the colony inhibition assay as are lymphocytes of patients with tumors. In fact, such immunoreactive lymphocytes have been detected in an individual 29 years after tumor removal (Hellström *et al.*, 1971*a*), suggesting a phenomenon similar to vaccination. The humoral immune system likewise seems to be activated, for complement-dependent cytotoxic antibodies to colon carcinoma cells can be detected in the tumor-bearing host, and these toxic sera can be rendered neutral by adsorption with autologous or homologous colonic tumor cells (Nairn *et al.*, 1971). In addition, patients with colorectal carcinoma can demonstrate complement-dependent cytotoxic antibodies to established cell lines from colonic tumors (Schultz *et al.*, 1975). This type of analysis has been quite revealing, for cell lines could be identified against which there was or was not immunoreactivity. Interestingly, cell lines against which serum cytotoxicity could not be demonstrated produced carcinoembryonic antigen (CEA) in amounts comparable to those of cell lines for which cytotoxicity could be shown. Thus it could be concluded that the cytotoxic response was not necessarily directed against CEA.

1.5.1. Skin Testing

Studies of cellular immunity have also failed to disclose any convincing evidence that CEA is the primary antigen against which the immune attack is generated. Hollinshead *et al.* (1970) prepared soluble fractions of tumors of colorectal carcinoma patients for use in autologous delayed hypersensitivity skin testing. They found that 17 of 19 patients so tested developed characteristic cutaneous reactions with one of the soluble fractions (III), but only four gave equivocally positive reactions to a lower molecular weight fraction (II). Interestingly, CEA was detected by radioimmunoassay in both fractions, thus questioning whether the delayed hypersensitivity responses were indeed directed against a tumor-associated antigen distinct from CEA. A number of these patients were tested with material from gut tissues of first- and second-trimester fetuses, and positive reactions were elicited. CEA was present in detectable quantities only in the first-trimester preparations, again underscoring the possibility that the immune reactions were not necessarily directed against CEA but possibly against an embryonal antigen different from CEA.

Hollinshead *et al.* (1972) subsequently ascertained the relation of the above-described skin-reactive antigen to CEA. Using fractionation by polyacrylamide gel electrophoresis, it was apparent that the skin-reactive antigen extractable from colorectal carcinomas was found in a region of the gels different from that of the antigen which produced cutaneous delayed hypersensitivity reactions.

1.5.2. *In Vitro Immunological Studies*

Employing *in vitro* lymphocyte transformation as an index of cell-mediated immunity, Lejtenyi *et al.* (1971) obtained no evidence for this type of immune reactivity against CEA either in patients with digestive system cancer or in pregnant women. Straus *et al.* (1975) used *in vitro* inhibition of leukocyte migration to study cell-mediated immune responses to purified CEA in patients with Crohn's disease, active ulcerative colitis, and colonic or pancreatic carcinoma. No significant leukocyte migration inhibition was detected in response to CEA, with the exception of one patient with carcinoma of the pancreas.

1.5.3. *Nephrotic Syndrome*

An interesting line of inquiry has also questioned whether an antigen distinct from CEA provokes the immune response. Although the association of the nephrotic syndrome with cancer is uncommon, in some of the cases which have been studied the renal pathology could not be attributed to renal amyloidosis or renal vein thrombosis. Cantrell (1969) reported the development of the nephrotic syndrome in a patient with an unsuspected adenocarcinoma of the stomach, and, once the cancer was discovered and surgically removed, the nephrotic syndrome spontaneously remitted. Such cases, along with the observations that cancer seemed to occur 10 times more frequently in patients with the nephrotic syndrome than in an age-matched population (Lee *et al.*, 1966) and that the nephrotic syndrome may actually be a prodrome to lymphoma (Ghosh and Muehrcke, 1970), supported the notion of more than just a chance association of these two conditions. Such a suspicion was further supported by the peculiarities of nephritis in NZB mice that is coincident with the development of lymphomas of putative viral etiology. Not only can viral antigens be found in extracts of both the lymphoma tissue and the kidney, but also they can be identified in the glomerular lesions immunofluorescently (Mellors *et al.*, 1968). Intriguingly, the development of the membranous glomerulonephritis in these mice correlates temporally well with the appearance of specific antibody to at least one of these virus-associated antigens.

Although the nephrotic syndrome concomitant with malignancy is not always of immunopathological origin, as is the case with lipoid nephrosis in Hodgkin's disease (Sherman *et al.*, 1972), deposits of IgG can be found in the kidneys of patients with both the nephrotic syndrome and concurrent malignancy (Loughridge and Lewis, 1971; Froom *et al.*, 1972). Such findings suggest that glomerulonephritis can result from the deposition within the glomeruli of immune complexes (antigen–antibody complexes) formed in the circulation. Such is the case with lupus nephritis, a glomerular disease in which complexes of native DNA and antibody of corresponding specificity are of major importance (Koffler *et al.,* 1971). Thus the presence of immune complexes in the glomeruli of a patient with a neoplasm may give a clue as to the nature of the antigen which could be recognized and be provoking the immune response. Lewis *et al.* (1971) described a patient with a bronchial squamous cell carcinoma and the nephrotic syndrome. Immunoglobulins eluted from the glomeruli reacted specifically with the cell surfaces of the bronchial tumor cells. Adsorption of this eluate with tumor cells removed this reactivity. In immunodiffusion, the patient's serum and kidney eluate showed a line of identity with a crude extract of the tumor. These studies suggested that the patient's serum contained an antibody capable of reacting with an antigen associated with the bronchial carcinoma and that immune complexes of this nature were deposited in the kidneys. No investigations into the nature of the tumor-associated antigen in the kidneys were made.

Costanza *et al.* (1973) studied a patient with carcinoma of the colon and the nephrotic syndrome. Sections of a kidney biopsy revealed granular deposits of immunoglobulins and complement components along the glomerular basement membranes. Using a comparable immunofluorescent technique, deposits of CEA were likewise detected in a similar pattern, suggesting that the renal pathology was generated by immune complexes of CEA and antibody directed against CEA. Although this study indicated that the nephrosis in this patient could certainly have been a complication of the immune response to the tumor, it still could not be construed as having defined the colon tumor antigen which is the major object of the immune response. Couser *et al.* (1974) similarly studied a patient with the nephrotic syndrome, colon carcinoma, and elevated serum levels of CEA. They could not demonstrate CEA in the glomerular immune deposits. However, the patient's serum contained an antibody which reacted with an antigen in the immune deposits. That this antigen was associated with the colon tumor was demonstrated by the removal of the antibody activity with homogenates of the patient's colon tumor but not with normal colon. These studies unfortunately have yielded no substantial information as to the nature of the tumor-associated antigen which provokes an immune response in patients with colon carcinoma. Whether the antigen is CEA is at present unknown. However, the accumulation of such immune complexes in the kidney provides a unique source for the further study of the nature of human colon carcinoma antigens.

2. *Tests of Recognitive Immunity in the Colon Carcinoma Patient*

Since immune recognition (afferent events) must of necessity proceed before an immune attack (efferent events) can be mounted, the determination of a cancer patient's ability to recognize a foreign antigen is crucial for the assessment of the patient's immunocompetence. However, the tumor antigen(s) associated with colon carcinoma has yet to be rigorously defined, and so it becomes impossible precisely to test whether a patient with colon cancer is immunologically recognizing his tumor. As a consequence, diverse tests of recognitive immune function to various stimuli have been developed. If the patient is hyporesponsive in this regard, it may be logical to consider his tumor defense mechanisms (recognitive, effector, or both) to be deficient.

2.1. *Morphological Tests*

2.1.1. *Lymphocytic Infiltration of Tumors*

Infiltration by immunocompetent cells is a frequent histological feature of many human neoplasms, particularly testicular seminomas, medullary carcinoma of the breast, and malignant melanoma. Although in the nineteenth century this was considered to reflect the origin of cancer at sites of previous chronic inflammation, the widely held modern opinion is that infiltration of tumors represents a defensive immunological response to tumor antigens. More than 30 reports in this century have documented a positive correlation between survival and lymphoreticular infiltration of many types of nonlymphoid tumors. Most of these reports have been collated by Underwood (1974).

a. Infiltration of Gastrointestinal Tumors. Takahashi (1961) studied 128 cases of squamous cell carcinoma of the esophagus. Although in his series no complete correlations were found between length of survival and stage or grade of the tumors, the degree of inflammatory cell infiltration at the periphery of the tumor exhibited good correlation with longevity after surgery. The infiltrating cells were composed of lymphocytes, mononuclear phagocytes, plasma cells, and sometimes eosinophils. An interesting finding was that the tumor cells at the site of the inflammatory infiltration demonstrated some degree of retrogressive change such as distortion with cytoplasmic vacuolization, fragmentation, or karyorrhexis.

Originally, Steiner *et al.* (1948) and Black *et al.* (1954) reported that a lymphoid reaction at the periphery of gastric cancers was associated with a prolonged survival. This was also the experience of Monafo *et al.* (1962) in studying 222 patients with gastric carcinoma. This type of positive correlation was amplified by Inokuchi *et al.*, (1967), who showed that for cases of metastatic gastric cancer the presence of an inflammatory infiltrate at the metastases was also important for prognosis. Hawley *et al.* (1970) showed that a marked infiltrate of lymphocytes and plasma cells at the margins of gastric cancers was not a very frequent finding (19 of 120 patients), but the 5-year survival for these 19 patients was 40% as compared to 18% for the remaining patients with scanty or no evidence of such an infiltrate.

Concerning colorectal carcinoma, as early as 1922 McCarty forwarded the proposition that lymphocytic infiltration of the tumor was associated with increased survival. He gleaned this impression from 102 cases of carcinoma of the rectum, all of which eventuated in death due to recurrence or metastasis.

Increased survival was associated with better differentiation of the tumor cells or with lymphocytes in intimate contact with tumor cells. The longest survival time was seen with both factors. Yoon (1959) studied 108 cases of carcinoma of the colon or rectum and discerned a trend toward better prognosis with lymphoreticular infiltration of the tumor.

b. Significance of Lymphoreticular Infiltration. Despite these numerous positive correlations, many investigators considered such an infiltration to have more trivial explanations such as a response to necrosis or to infection. These explanations are not to be wholly discounted, for necrosis and infection are powerful stimuli for the infiltration of polymorphonuclear leukocytes. Nevertheless, a substantial proportion of neoplasms elicit a lymphoid infiltrate independently of these factors. There is also little agreement concerning which lymphoreticular cell type is of importance. Cells to which defensive abilities have been attributed on histological bases include lymphocytes (Hawley *et al.,* 1970), mononuclear phagocytes (Evans, 1972), plasma cells (Berg, 1959), mast cells (Graham and Graham, 1966), and eosinophils (Yoon, 1959).

Survival rates for patients with carcinoma of the breast have been reported to be higher in Japan than in the United States (Morrison *et al.,* 1972). Interestingly, one study (Morrison *et al.,* 1973) showed that breast tumors with marked degrees of lymphoid infiltration were more common in Japan than in the United States. However, critical review of the data from this multicenter study could not relate the increased survival of Japanese women to this characteristic.

c. Experimental and Ultrastructural Aspects of Lymphoid Infiltration. Probably the best situation in which to evaluate the significance of tumor infiltration by lymphoid cells would be to examine a spontaneously regressing neoplasm. Since this is quite a rare event, some investigators have focused attention on the halo nevus, a spontaneously regressing mole which develops an enlarging halo of depigmentation. As the regression and depigmentation proceed, an inflammatory infiltrate can be detected, causing some investigators to believe that this is morphological evidence for an immunological attack on the nevus cells (Lerner, 1971), especially since circulating antibodies to malignant melanoma cells have been demonstrated in patients with regressing halo nevi (Lewis and Copeman, 1972) and since *in vitro* cellular immunity to melanoma antigens in melanoma patients with regressing halo nevi has been observed (Epstein *et al.,* 1973). Jacobs *et al.* (1975) have studied the ultrastructure of the interaction of inflammatory cells with halo nevi in various stages of regression. They described the infiltration of lymphocytes, plasma cells, and monocytes into and around nevus cell nests in early stages of regression, and nevus cell degeneration and phagocytosis by macrophages in late stages of regression. They defined a scheme of events to suggest that the nevus regression was immunologically mediated and that the lymphoid infiltration was significant in this regard.

The animal studies of Carr *et al.* (1974) are relevant to the investigations with halo nevi. These workers studied the ultrastructure of immunocompetent cells in a nonlymphoid experimental rodent tumor at the time of likely rejection. Lymphocytes were usually closely related to the tumor cells and sometimes protruded fine processes into them. Macrophage processes were closely applied to tumor cells and sometimes completely surrounded them. Interestingly, dead tumor cells were not seen in large numbers outside macrophages, suggesting that the macrophages were specifically engulfing live tumor cells rather than merely scavenging necrotic material. This work implies that the infiltration of immunocompetent cells is a specific defensive response to a tumor.

2.1.2. *Lymph Node Histology*

a. Sinus Histiocytosis. The varied clinical behavior of human tumors of the same histological type cannot be wholly accounted for by the grade or the stage of the tumor. This has prompted many investigators to consider that factors other than those intrinsic to the tumor are operative for the eventual outcome of an individual patient. In other words, the biological behavior of a tumor can well be considered the net result of the aggressive properties of the tumor and the defensive capacities of the patient.

Black and his co-workers have specifically investigated the relationship between the survival of cancer patients and various structural features of the lymph nodes regional to the tumor. They found that breast cancer patients (Black *et al.* 1953) and gastric cancer patients (Black *et al.*, 1954) who demonstrated a marked reaction of sinus histiocytosis in the lymph nodes regional to the tumor enjoyed prolonged survivals. This correlation appeared independent of the microscopic structure of the tumor or the presence of lymph node metastases. Wartman (1959) reported that sinus histiocytosis present in the lymph nodes regional to colon carcinomas was not related to necrosis in the primary tumor. In addition, it was determined that sinus histiocytosis was only rarely encountered in the lymph nodes of noncancer patients (Black and Speer, 1958). The interpretation of these various data was that sinus histiocytosis could be interpreted as an immune defensive reaction in response to tumor antigen(s). The validity of this type of morphological analysis of immune response was questioned by Berg (1956) and by DiRe and Lane (1963).

b. Lymph Node Morphology in Relation to Immunological Function. It is well established that the morphological appearance of a stimulated lymph node represents an immunological response to the presence of foreign antigen in the area of tissue being drained. The first cytological reaction in draining lymph nodes of normal intact animals to skin grafts (Scothorne and McGregor, 1955) and in contact hypersensitivity (Oort and Turk, 1965) is the appearance of lymphoblasts in the deep cortex of the node. In studying the lymph node manifestations of cellular immunity, Parrott (1967) showed that this type of reactive lymphocyte proliferation was absent in the regional lymph nodes of neonatally thymectomized C3H mice which had received allogeneic skin grafts and which could not therefore reject them. In other words with a deficient cellular immune system, such histological evidence of antigenic stimulation was not apparent in the draining lymph nodes. Concerning the humoral component of the immune system, patients with infantile X-linked agammaglobulinemia fail to form germinal centers in the draining lymph nodes after antigenic stimulation, unlike individuals with intact humoral immunity. Thus, by extrapolation, these defined histological patterns of lymph node stimulation have a special relevance for malignancy since the capacity of a patient's lymph node lymphocytes to show morphological responses to inciting tumor antigens may be evaluated. Those who do not show such evidence may be considered as not having mounted an optimal immune response to the tumor, whereas those who do may be considered to have initiated immune events.

There is sound functional evidence for such a formulation. Mice inoculated with isogeneic or allogeneic sarcoma cells demonstrate immunocompetent cells in the regional lymph nodes which are sensitized to the sarcoma cells as demonstrated in colony inhibition assays (Barna and Deodhar, 1975). Lymph nodes other than regional nodes show no colony inhibition activity. Ambus *et al.* (1974) showed that patients with gastrointestinal neoplasms or with other cancers have a population of lymph node cells capable of *in vitro* blastogenic responses to autochthonous tumor cells, indicating that recognitive immune events to tumor antigens have occurred in these regional nodes. In addition, employing a leukocyte migration inhibition assay, Guillou *et al.* (1975) have demonstrated the sensitization of regional lymph node lymphocytes to colorectal tumor extracts.

c. Lymph Node Morphology and Colon Cancer. Tsakraklides and coworkers have formulated a morphological analysis of the immunological activity of lymph nodes regional to cancer of the cervix (1973) or breast (1974). This analysis stresses not the presence of sinus histiocytosis but rather the presence of reactive proliferation of lymphocytes either as an expanded deep cortex with numerous lymphoblasts or as an active outer cortex with the presence of active germinal centers. In these retrospective studies, there was a strong positive correlation between survival and evidence of immunological stimulation in the regional nodes. Berlinger *et al.* (1976*b*) confirmed this association in patients with squamous cell carcinomas of the upper aerodigestive tract. This particular type of analysis could not, however, be fully extended to patients with colon or rectal cancer (Tsakraklides *et al.*, 1975). Although there was a higher survival rate in patients whose mesenteric nodes showed active germinal centers, the results were not statistically significant. Interestingly, Patt *et al.* (1975) obtained different results. They studied a group of patients with carcinoma specifically of the sigmoid colon, since the resected mesocolic lymph nodes drain only the colon and not more distal pelvic organs. They showed that patients whose lymph nodes demonstrated an active and expanded deep cortex or sinus histiocytosis survived significantly longer than those patients whose nodes did not. Patients whose nodes showed both phenomena had the best survival of all. These relationships appeared independent of the Dukes's classification.

Thus the sum total of the evidence seems to indicate that morphological patterns suggestive of an immune response can portend a more favorable outcome for a given patient. Although this evidence can lead to the conclusion that recognitive immune events have transpired, the morphological assessment of immune vigor is but a crude measure, and functional analyses of recognitive immunity are more incisive.

2.2. *Functional Tests in Vivo*

To test cellular immune function, the ability to mount a cutaneous delayed hypersensitivity reaction to intradermally injected, commonly encountered antigens has been employed. Of course, the assumption here is that the patient has had sufficient prior exposure to one of these antigens. As a consequence, a battery of common microbial antigens is used, or tuberculin testing can be used in areas where BCG vaccination is common. This mode of testing is more a test of immunological memory and the integrity of the effector arm of the immune system than only a test of recognitive immunity. Nevertheless, impaired reactivity to common recall antigens does indicate a perturbation somewhere in the immune arc and does provide information as to how a patient may interact immunologically with a foreign antigenic challenge in the form of a tumor. The sum of the findings in patients with colon cancer is that they often show defective cellular immunity to common recall antigens, and the degree of depression is more severe with more widespread disease (Hughes and Mackay, 1965; Kronman *et al.*, 1972). The most logical conclusion to draw from this type of data is that immunodepression may be secondary to malignancy since immunodepression worsens as the tumor progresses. Therefore, any prognostic significance attached to such findings may merely be an indirect reflection of the stage of disease. This in no way negates the fact that immune mechanisms restrict neoplastic proliferation, for, on the other hand, one may postulate that certain neoplasms may owe their aggressiveness to their ability to perturb protective immunological functions.

Bolton *et al.* (1975) compared Mantoux reactions among patients with carcinoma of the breast, stomach, or colon and found that impaired immune reactivity appeared earliest in patients with carcinoma of the colon and that normal reactivity tended to be retained until a late stage in breast cancer. Since, from a broad outlook, prognoses tend to be similar for breast cancer and colon cancer, they felt that these findings underscore the notion that immunocompetence is not the sole or major parameter for prognosis. The binary perspective for cancer must be emphasized: the host to a tumor does indeed possess defense mechanisms, but the tumor also has peculiar aggressive characteristics. The outcome for a given patient is not determined by either one or the other of these factors but rather by the net influence of the two.

Skin testing with DNCB is a better alternative to testing with common antigens which relies on adequate prior exposure because DNCB testing measures the ability to recognize a new antigen and to become sensitized to it. Nearly all normal individuals can be sensitized to this chemical (Eilber and Morton, 1970). Histologically, the cellular response to DNCB is a characteristic delayed response of lymphocytes and monocytes just as is the response to common antigens which evoke a delayed hypersensitivity response.

DNCB testing has likewise shown that patients with colorectal cancers have impaired cell-mediated immunity and the degree of impairment is greater with more advanced tumors (Chakravorty *et al.*, 1973; Bone and Lauder, 1974). It has also been shown that there is no correlation between the rate of proliferation of rectal carcinoma cells and the cellular immunocompetence of the patient as measured by DNCB reactivity (Bone and Camplejohn, 1973). Although cellular immune mechanisms adversely affect neoplastic growth, this finding suggests that this effect is not mediated by a restriction of the proliferation rate of the tumor cells.

2.3. Functional Tests in Vitro

On a theoretical basis, a mixed leukocyte culture (MLC) assay of cellular immunity appears to be a test which is particularly relevant for the tumor patient. Lymphocyte reactivity in MLC represents the response to foreign histocompatibility antigens, which, like tumor antigens, are only subtly different from those of the patient. As such, the lymphocyte response in MLC represents the recognition phase of the *in vivo* allograft response (Bach, 1974). The MLC possesses the characteristics of a true cell-mediated immune reaction in that lymphocytes, macrophages, and soluble factors all must participate (Twomey *et al.*, 1970; Rode and Gordon, 1974; Miller and Mishell, 1975). The magnitude of the MLC is related to the survival of allografts between the leukocyte donor pairs (Oppenheim *et al.*, 1965). T lymphocytes which have undergone blastogenesis in MLC are specifically cytotoxic for lymphocytes from the donor who provided the culture with the stimulating cells (Wagner, 1972). These qualities suggest that the MLC is particularly suited to the study of the integrity of the recognition phase of cellular immunity in patients who bear tumors.

When deficiencies of cell-mediated immunity are detected in MLC, the MLC can be adapted to become a test of either lymphocyte or macrophage function, thus having the desirable result of providing some understanding of the nature of the immunopathology. By appropriately adapted MLC testing, it has been shown that patients with herpes zoster infections have an apparent functional macrophage deficit rendering these macrophages unable to mediate the MLC reaction. In certain cases of lymphosarcoma the patient's purified lymphocytes do not respond normally in MLC to an allogeneic stimulus despite the presence of normal allogeneic macrophages, implying a functional lymphocyte abnormality (Twomey and Sharkey, 1972). Similarly, lymphocytes obtained from patients during the lymphoproliferative phase of infectious mononucleosis are hyporesponsive in MLC (Twomey, 1974).

Clinically, the MLC as a measure of the integrity of cell-mediated immunity in patients with solid tumors is just beginning to be used. Depressed MLC responses have been observed in patients with bronchogenic carcinoma (Han and Takita, 1972) and in patients with squamous cell carcinoma of the upper aerodigestive tract (Berlinger and Good, 1976). In most cases, the degree of depression correlates well with the clinical stage of the tumor. The *in vitro* measurement of cellular immunity by MLC testing is quite appropriate, for Golub *et al.* (1974) have shown for carcinoma patients that MLC reactivity is an *in vitro* measurement which correlates especially well with *in vivo* measurements such as skin testing with common antigens or with DNCB.

As mentioned above, the MLC can be adapted to test differentially the integrity of lymphocyte or macrophage in cell-mediated immune responses. In a series of patients with carcinoma of the breast, colon, ovary, or head and neck areas, it has been demonstrated that those who showed significantly depressed MLC responses could usually show normal responses if their macrophages were removed from the cultures (Berlinger *et al.,* 1976*a*). These data strongly suggest that carcinoma patients experience a perturbation of macrophage function whereby there occurs a paradoxical suppressive influence *in vitro* during the response to foreign histocompatibility antigens, and this functional perturbation can mask apparently normal lymphocyte blastogenic abilities. These data find foundation in the work of Kirchner *et al.* (1974) and Pope *et al.* (1976), who demonstrated an adherent population of spleen cells from tumor-bearing mice which suppressed mitogenic responses of lymphocytes and the replication of lymphoma cells. Furthermore, these studies indicated that the adherent cells demonstrated macrophage characteristics.

To confirm that such findings indicative of defective recognitive immunity were not artifactual, Lopez and Berlinger (submitted) have developed an animal model in which the same type of immunopathology could be induced with the inoculation of syngeneic tumor cells. The tumor cells used in this mouse model were BALB/c fibroblasts which had been transformed with the Kirsten sarcoma virus (Todaro and Aaronson, 1969). A clone of transformed cells which were not producing virus was used in order to obviate any possible immunosuppressive effects of viremia and to establish a model which most closely parallels the human situation. In these studies it was found that 13 days after subcutaneous inoculation with tumor cells (tumors were palpable at this time), and at all times thereafter, splenic cells from these tumor bearing BALB/c mice exhibited significantly depressed MLC responses to allogeneic cells (C57BL/6). If the macrophages of these mice were removed from the cultures, the splenic lymphocytes demonstrated normal proliferative capacities in MLC. In addition, after the tumors were surgically extirpated, the mice showed recovery of normal MLC responses. These findings confirm the earlier observations that macrophages were involved in the suppression of normal lymphocyte capacities in an *in vitro* test of cellular immunity. There also obtains the suggestion that diminished cellular immunocompetence can develop secondary to the presence of a growing tumor. This adverse effect could be due to inhibitory substances liberated by the tumor cells. It is also possible that the putatively normal immune system of the BALB/c mouse will experience a pathological perturbation of immunological homeostasis when confronted with an antigen (tumor cell) which possesses both self and non-self characteristics. In other words, the BALB/c mouse may not be truly normal in the immunological sense, but may possess an easily perturbable immune system such as could be the case with the human cancer patient. Studies with other strains of allegedly immunologically normal mice will confirm or deny this hypothesis.

Some light may have been shed on these speculations by a study of members of family aggregates of colon carcinoma (Berlinger *et al.*, 1976*c*). None of these families demonstrated any of the findings characteristic of polyposis coli, Gardner's syndrome, or Turcot's syndrome. Rather, they fulfilled the stringent criteria set forth by Lynch (1974) describing authenticated hereditary colon carcinoma without any detectable precancerous condition. Each of these five families met at least two of these criteria: (1) adenocarcinoma of the colon appearing in three successive generations; (2) adenocarcinoma of the colon appearing with a higher than expected frequency in the family or in an individual sibship; (3) the occurrence of multiple primary adenocarcinomas of the colon; (4) the occurrence of multiple primary cancers of diverse histological type; (5) the appearance of adenocarcinoma of the colon in the third or fourth decade of life. The question was asked whether any carcinoma-free offspring of a parent with colon carcinoma might show a deficit of cell-mediated immunity to explain possibly this underlying diathesis to colon carcinoma.

Seven of 16 (44%) unaffected blood relatives of the affected family members showed significantly decreased cell-mediated immune capacities as measured by MLC responsiveness. Provocatively, six of these seven individuals could exhibit normal MLC responses when their macrophages were removed from the cultures. These findings indicate that deficits of recognitive immunity appear to aggregate in families in which colon carcinoma aggregates. Furthermore, this deficit appeared to be a perturbation of macrophage function similar to that demonstrated in patients with established cancer and in mice bearing tumors. These findings are reminiscent of the work of Creagan and Fraumeni (1973) which disclosed a high frequency of immune deficits in cancer-free members within a family aggregate of gastric cancer. It is appropriate to speculate that the immunopathology detected in these cancer-free individuals takes the form of an easily perturbable recognitive mechanism in that confrontation with an allogeneic stimulus results in inappropriate suppression of the immune response.

3. Escape Mechanisms

Although the subject of escape from immune attack is too lengthy to treat here, some comment seems appropriate concerning how tumors continue to grow in patients who have demonstrated immune reactivity to tumor cells *in vitro*.

One postulate is that cells of certain tumors may be only weakly antigenic and may not provide a strong enough stimulus to provoke optimal recognitive and effector responses. Pihl *et al.* (1975) have found in 132 cases of colonic carcinoma that *in vitro* antitumor immunoreactivity was inversely correlated with the histological degree of differentiation of the tumor, thus suggesting that poorly differentiated tumors may provoke less frequent and less intense immune responses and therefore can become more widely spread due to this poor degree of immunological restriction.

Alternatively, it is possible that the infrequent antitumor immunoreactivity observed in cases of poorly differentiated tumors may be due to the fact that these tumors are more widely spread and are, by some unknown mechanism, leading to immunological paralysis. Support for this formulation derives from the work of Baldwin *et al.* (1973*a*), who showed that papain-solubilized tumor membrane extracts of pooled colon carcinomas inhibited the cytotoxic effect of sensitized lymphocytes from patients with colon carcinoma. This inhibitory effect was not observed with similar extracts of normal colon or melanoma cells, suggesting that an antigen associated with colon carcinoma was involved. All the colon carcinoma extracts employed in this study contained CEA, but it was not established whether CEA *per se* was responsible for the inhibitory activity, although the colon carcinoma extract which was the least inhibitory contained escessively high levels of CEA. In an animal model involving chemically induced hepatomas or sarcomas, Zöller *et al.* (1976) similarly showed that tumor cell extracts likewise inhibited lymphocyte cytotoxicity for cultured tumor cells. Interestingly, in this study, soluble extracts of tumors containing embryonic antigens or soluble extracts of embryos themselves inhibited lymphocyte cytotoxicity, indicating that one of the targets for the sensitized cells was an embryonic antigen.

Such inhibitory reactions no doubt represent a complex array of events and do not at this time easily lend themselves to clear explanations. It is possible that the expression of embryonic antigens on tumor cells may actually evoke a population of suppressor cells which coincidentally then restrict the immune attack on tumor cells that bear these antigens. It is also possible that circulating tumor antigens, be they embryonic or otherwise, may block lymphocyte activity by binding to the receptor sites on the effector lymphocytes.

A role for antibody has also been postulated in the mechanism by which tumors escape immune attack. Numerous studies originally proposed the phenomenon of the blocking antibody since sera of tumor-bearing hosts could inhibit the cytotoxicity *in vitro* of sensitized lymphocytes for cultured tumor cells (Hellström *et al.*, 1971*b*; Sjögren *et al.*, 1972). It was postulated that this antitumor antibody was bound to the antigenic site(s) of the tumor cell and thus these sites were masked for recognition by effector lymphocytes. However, Baldwin *et al.* (1973*b*) showed with a rat hepatoma model that sera taken from the animals after excision of the tumor still contained complement-dependent cytotoxic antibody, but the antibody alone showed no ability to block the attack of sensitized lymphocytes. When, however, soluble tumor-specific antigen was added to these seara, blocking activity was exhibited, suggesting that the blocking phenomenon was due to immune complexes of tumor antigen and antitumor antibody (Baldwin *et al.*, 1972). The tumor specificity of this blocking phenomenon was confirmed since hepatoma extracts blocked only the lymphocyte immunoreactivity to homologous tumors and since the isolated tumor antigens could adsorb tumor-specific antibody. If immune complexes block antitumor immunity, they may do so by masking of the target cell antigen(s) by the antibody portion or by ineffectual combination with the antigen portion to the receptor on the effector lymphocyte. Not to be discounted is a more positive type of response which may be the seemingly paradoxical elicitation of a population of suppressor cells. In this regard, abnormally high levels of α-fetoprotein (AFP) have been reported in gastric carcinoma (Mehlman *et al.,* 1971) and in other tumors. Murgita and Tomasi (1975) have reported that AFP has the capacity to suppress the responses of T lymphocytes to mitogens and to allogeneic cells in the MLC. They have made the intriguing speculation that the immunosuppressive phenomena seen in malignant diseases may be due to elevated levels of AFP either circulating in the serum or produced locally in the microenvironment around tumor cells.

Since AFP is synthesized during embryonic life and appears to serve an immunoregulatory function, this thesis proposes that AFP has a natural role in protecting an allograft in the form of a fetus from possible harmful effects of the maternal immune mechanism and a perverted role in protecting a malignant allograft from the effector events of antitumor immunity.

4. References

Ambus, U., Mavligit, G. M., Gutterman, J. U., McBride, C. M., and Hersh, E. M., 1974, Specific and non-specific immunologic reactivity of regional lymph node lymphocytes in human malignancy, *Int. J. Cancer* **14:**291–300.

Andersen, V., Bendixen, G., and Schiødt, T., 1969, An *in vitro* demonstration of cellular immunity against autologous mammary carcinoma in man, *Acta Med. Scand.* **186:**101–103.

Bach, F. H., 1974, Normal histocompatibility antigens as a model for tumors, *Am. J. Clin. Pathol.* **62:**173–183.

Baldwin, R. W., Price, M. R., and Robins, R. A., 1972, Blocking of lymphocyte-mediated cytotoxicity for rat hepatoma cells by tumour-specific antigen–antibody complexes, *Nature (London) New Biol.* **238:**185–187.

Baldwin, R. W., Embleton, M. J., and Price, M. R., 1973*a,* Inhibition of lymphocyte cytotoxicity for human colon carcinoma by treatment with solubilized tumor membrane fractions, *Int. J. Cancer* **12:**84–92.

Baldwin, R. W., Embleton, M. J., and Robins, R. A., 1973*b,* Cellular and humoral immunity to rat hepatoma-specific antigens correlated with tumour status, *Int. J. Cancer* **11:**1–10.

Barna, B., and Deodhar, S. D., 1975, The activity of regional nodes in the evolution of immune responses to allogeneic and isogeneic tumors, *Cancer Res.* **35:**920–926.

Berg, J. W., 1956, Sinus histiocytosis: A fallacious measure of host resistance to cancer, *Cancer* **9:**935–939.

Berg, J. W., 1959, Inflammation and prognosis in breast cancer, *Cancer* **12:**714–720.

Berlinger, N. T., and Good, R. A., 1976, Concomitant immunopathology with squamous cell carcinomas of the head and neck regions, *Trans. Am. Acad. Ophthalmol. Otolaryngol.* **82:**ORL 588–594.

Berlinger, N. T., Lopez, C., and Good, R. A., 1976*a*, Facilitation or attenuation of mixed leukocyte culture responsiveness by adherent cells, *Nature (London)* **260:**145–146.

Berlinger, N. T., Tsakraklides, V., Pollak, K., Adams, G. L., Yang, M., and Good, R. A., 1976*b,* Immunologic assessment of regional lymph node histology in relation to survival in head and neck carcinoma, *Cancer* **37:**697–705.

Berlinger, N. T., Lopez, C., Vogel, J. E., Lipkin, M., and Good, R. A., 1977. Defective recognitive immunity in family aggregates of colon carcinoma, *J. Clin. Invest.* **59:**761–769.

Black, M. M., and Speer, F. D., 1958, Sinus histiocytosis of lymph nodes in cancer, *Surg. Gynecol. Obstet.* **106:**163–175.

Black, M. M., Kerpe, S., and Speer, F. D., 1953, Lymph node structure in patients with cancer of the breast, *Am. J. Pathol.* **29:**505–521.

Black, M. M., Opler, S. R., and Speer, F. D., 1954, Microscopic structure of gastric carcinomas and their regional lymph nodes in relation to survival, *Surg. Gynecol. Obstet.* **98:**725–734.

Bloom, B. R., Bennett, B., Oettgen, H. F., McLean, E. P., and Old, L. J., 1969, Demonstration of delayed hypersensitivity to soluble antigens of chemically induced tumors by inhibition of macrophage migration, *Proc. Natl. Acad. Sci. USA* **64:**1176–1180.

Bolton, P. M., Mander, A. M., Davidson, J. M., James, S. L., Newcombe, R. G., and Hughes, L. E., 1975, Cellular immunity in cancer: Comparison of delayed hypersensitivity skin tests in three common cancers, *Br. Med. J.* **3:**18–20.

Bone, G., and Camplejohn, R., 1973, The role of cellular immunity in control of neoplasia, *Br. J. Surg.* **60:**824–827.

Bone, G., and Lauder, I., 1974, Cellular immunity, peripheral blood lymphocyte count, and pathological staging of tumors in the gastrointestinal tract, *Br. J. Cancer* **30:**215–221.

Brent, L., Brown, J., and Medawar, P. B., 1958, Skin transplantation immunity in relation to hypersensitivity, *Lancet* **2:**561–564.

Buchanan, W. W., Anderson, J. R., Goudie, R. B., and Gray, K. G., 1958, A skin test in thyroid disease, *Lancet* **2:**928–931.

Bull, D. M., Leibach, J. R., Williams, M. A., and Helms, R. A., 1973, Immunity to colon cancer assessed by antigen-induced inhibition of mixed mononuclear cell migration, *Science* **181:**957–959.

Cantrell, E. G., 1969, Nephrotic syndrome cured by removal of gastric carcinoma, *Br. Med. J.* **2:**739–740.

Carr, I., Underwood, J. C. E., McGinty, F., and Wood, P., 1974, The ultrastructure of the local lymphoreticular response to an experimental neoplasm, *J. Pathol.* **113:**175–182.

Chakravorty, R. C., Curutchet, H. P., Coppolla, F. S., Park, C. M., Blaylock, W. K., and Lawrence, Jr., W., 1973, The delayed hypersensitivity reaction in the cancer patient: Observations on sensitization by DNCB, *Surgery* **73:**730–735.

Costanza, M. E., Pinn, V. P., Schwartz, R. S., and Nathanson, L., 1973, Carcinoembryonic antigen-antibody complexes in a patient with colonic carcinoma and nephrotic syndrome, *N. Eng. J. Med.* **289:**520–522.

Couser, W. G., Wagonfeld, J. B., Spargo, B. H., and Lewis, E. J., 1974, Glomerular deposition of tumor antigen in membranous nephropathy associated with colonic carcinoma, *Am. J. Med.* **57:**962–970.

Creagan, E. T., and Fraumeni, J. F., Jr., 1973, Familial gastric cancer and immunologic abnormalities, *Cancer* **32:**1325–1331.

DiRe, J. J., and Lane, N., 1963, The relation of sinus histiocytosis in axillary lymph nodes to the surgical curability of carcinoma of the breast, *Am. J. Clin. Pathol.* **40:**508–515.

Eilber, F. R., and Morton, D. L., 1970, Impaired immunologic reactivity and recurrence following cancer surgery, *Cancer* **25:**362–367.

Elias, E. G., and Elias, L. L., 1975, Some immunologic characteristics of carcinoma of the colon and rectum, *Surg. Gynecol. Obstet.* **141:**715–718.

Epstein, W. L., Sagabeil, R., Spitler, L., Wybran, J., Reed, W. B., and Blois, M. S., 1973, Halo nevi and melanoma, *J. Am. Med. Assoc.* **225:**373–377.

Evans, R., 1972, Macrophages in syngeneic animal tumors, *Transplantation* **14:**468–473.

Fass, L., Ziegler, J. L., Herberman, R. B., and Kiryabwire, J. W. M., 1970, Cutaneous hypersensitivity reactions to autologous extracts of malignant melanoma cells, *Lancet* **1:**116–118.

Finney, J. W., Byers, E. H., and Wilson, R. H., 1960, Studies in tumor auto-immunity, *Cancer Res* **20:**351–356.

Froom, D. W., Franklin, W. A., Hano, J. E., and Potter, E. V., 1972, Immune deposits in Hodgkin's disease with nephrotic syndrome, *Arch. Pathol.* **94:**547–553.

Ghosh, L., and Muehrcke, R. C., 1970. The nephrotic syndrome: A prodrome to lymphoma, *Ann. Intern. Med.* **72:**379–382.

Golub, S. H., O'Connell, T. X., and Morton, D. L., 1974, Correlation of *in vitro* and *in vivo* assays of immunocompetence in cancer patients, *Cancer Res.* **34:**1833–1837.

Graham J. B., and Graham, R. M., 1955, Antibodies elicited by cancer in patients, *Cancer* **8:**409–416.

Graham, R. M., and Graham, J. B., 1966, Mast cells and cancer of the cervix, *Surg. Gynecol. Obstet.* **123:**3–9.

Guillou, P. J., and Giles, G. R., 1973, Inhibition of leukocyte migration by tumor-associated antigens of the colon and rectum, *Gut* **14:**733–738.

Guillou, P. J., Brennan, T. G., and Giles, G. R., 1975, A study of lymph nodes draining colorectal cancer using a two-stage inhibition of leukocyte migration technique, *Gut* **16:**290–297.

Han, T., and Takita, H., 1972, Impaired lymphocyte responses to allogeneic cultured lymphoid cells in patients with lung cancer, *N. Eng. J. Med.* **286:**605–606.

Hawley, P. R., Westerholm, P., and Morson, B. C., 1970, Pathology and prognosis of carcinoma of the stomach, *Br. J. Surg.* **57:**877–883.

Hellström, I., Hellström, K. E., Pierce, G. E., and Yang, J. P. S., 1968, Cellular and humoral immunity to different types of human neoplasms, *Nature (London)* **220:**1352–1354.

Hellström, I., Hellström, K. E., and Shepard, T. H., 1970, Cell-mediated immunity against antigens common to human colonic carcinomas and fetal gut epithelium, *Int. J. Cancer* **6:**346–351.

Hellström, I., Hellström, K. E., Sjögren, H. O., and Warner, G. A., 1971*a,* Demonstration of cell-mediated immunity to human neoplasms of various histological types, *Int. J. Cancer* **7:**1–16.

Hellström, I., Sjögren, H. O., Warner, G., and Hellström, K. E., 1971*b,* Blocking of cell-mediated tumor immunity by sera from patients with growing neoplasms, *Int. J. Cancer* **7:**226–237.

Herberman, R. B., and Oren, M. E., 1969, Delayed cutaneous hypersensitivity reactions to membrane extracts of human tumor cells, *Clin. Res.* **17:**403.

Hollinshead, A., Glew, D., Bunnag, B., Gold, P., and Herberman, R., 1970, Skin-reactive soluble antigen from intestinal cancer cell membranes and relationship to carcinoembryonic antigens, *Lancet* **1:**1191–1195.

Hollinshead, A., McWright, C. G., Alford, T. C., and Glew, D. H., 1972, Separation of skin reactive intestinal cancer antigen from the carcinoembryonic antigen of Gold, *Science* **177:**887–889.

House, A. K., Wisniewski, S., and Woodings, T. L., 1975, Immunity in colonic tumor patients after operation: Determination of leukocyte migration inhibition, *Dis. Col. Rect.* **18:**100–106.

Hoy, W. E., and Nelson, D. S., 1969, Delayed-type hypersensitivity in mice after skin and tumour allografts and tumour isografts, *Nature (London)* **222:**1001–1003.

Hughes, L. E., and Lytton, B., 1964, Antigenic properties of human tumors: Delayed cutaneous hypersensitivity reactions, *Br. Med. J.* **1:**209–212.

Hughes, L. E., and Mackay, W. D., 1965, Suppression of the tuberculin response in malignant disease, *Br. Med. J.* **2:**1346–1348.

Inokuchi, K., Inutsuka, S. Furusawa, M., Soejima, K., and Ikeda, T., 1967, Stromal reaction around tumor and metastasis and prognosis after curative gastrectomy for carcinoma of the stomach, *Cancer* **20:**1924–1929.

Jacobs, J. B., Edelstein, L. M., Snyder, L. M., and Fortier, N., 1975, Ultrastructural evidence for destruction in the halo nevus, *Cancer Res.* **35:**352–357.

Kirchner, H. T. M., Chused, T. M., Herberman, R. B., Holden, H. T., and Laurin, D. H., 1974, Evidence of suppressor cell activity in spleens of mice bearing primary tumors induced by Moloney sarcoma virus, *J. Exp. Med.* **139:**1473–1484.

Koffler, D., Agnello, V., Thoburn, R., and Kunkel, H. G., 1971, Systemic lupus erythematosus: Prototype of immune complex nephritis in man, *J. Exp. Med.* **134:**169s–179s.

Kronman, B. S., Shapiro, H. M., and Localio, S. A., 1972, Newer concepts of cancer of the colon and rectum: Delayed hypersensitivity responses of patients with carcinoma of the colon and other solid tumors, *Dis. Col. Rect.* **15:**106–110.

Lee, J. C., Yamauchi, H., and Hopper, J., 1966, The association of cancer and the nephrotic syndrome, *Ann. Intern. Med.* **64**:41–51.

Lejtenyi, M. C., Freedman, S. O., and Gold, P., 1971, Response of lymphocytes from patients with gastrointestinal cancer to the carcinoembryonic antigen of the human digestive system, *Cancer* **28**:115–120.

Lerner, A. B., 1971, On the etiology of vitiligo and gray hair, *Am. J. Med.* **51**:141–147.

Lewis, M. G., and Copeman, P. W. M., 1972, Halo naevus: A frustrated malignant melanoma, *Br. Med. J.* **2**:47–48.

Lewis, M. G., Loughridge, L. W., and Phillips, T. M., 1971, Immunological studies in nephrotic syndrome associated with extrarenal malignant disease, *Lancet* **2**:134–135.

Loughridge, L. W., and Lewis, M. G., 1971, Nephrotic syndrome in malignant diseases of non-renal origin, *Lancet* **1**:256–258.

Lynch, H. T., 1974, Familial cancer prevalence spanning eight years, *Arch. Intern. Med.* **134**:931–938.

MacCarty, W. C., 1922, Factors which influence longevity in carcinoma, *Ann. Surg.* **76**:9–12.

Mehlman, D. J., Bulkley, B. H., and Wiermk, P. H., 1971, Serum alpha-fetoglobulin with gastric and prostatic carcinomas, *N. Eng. J. Med.* **285**:1060–1061.

Mellors, R. C., Aoki, T., and Huebner, R., 1968, Further implication of murine leukemia-like virus in the disorders of NZB mice, *J. Exp. Med.* **129**:1045–1061.

Mikulska, Z. B., Smith, S., and Alexander, P., 1966, Evidence for an immunological reaction of the host directed against its own actively growing primary tumor, *J. Natl. Cancer Inst.* **36**:29–35.

Miller, C. L., and Mishell, R. F., 1975, Differential regulatory effects of accessory cells in the generation of cell-mediated immune reactions, *J. Immunol.* **114**:692–695.

Monafo, W. W., Jr., Krause, G. L., Jr., and Medina, J. G., 1962, Carcinoma of the stomach: Morphological characteristics affecting survival, *Arch. Surg.* **85**:754–763.

Morrison, A. S., Lowe, C. R., MacMahon, B., Yuasa, S., and Warram, J. H., 1972, Survival of breast cancer patients related to incidence risk factors, *Int. J. Cancer* **9**:470–476.

Morrison, A. S., Black, M. M., Lowe, C. R., MacMahon, B., and Yuasa, S., 1973, Some international differences in histology and survival in breast cancer, *Int. J. Cancer* **11**:261–267.

Murgita, R. A., and Tomasi, Jr., T. B., 1975, Suppression of the immune response by alpha-fetoprotein. II. The effect of mouse alpha-fetoprotein on mixed lymphocyte reactivity and mitogen induced lymphocyte transformation, *J. Exp. Med.* **141**:440–452.

Nairn, R. C., Nind, A. P. P., Guli, E. P. G., Davies, D. H., Rolland, J. M., McGiven, A. R., and Hughes, E. S. R., 1971, Immunological reactivity in patients with carcinoma of the colon, *Br. Med. J.* **4**:706–709.

Oort, J., and Turk, J. L., 1965, A histological and autoradiographic study of lymph nodes during the development of contact sensitivity in the guinea pig, *Br. J. Exp. Pathol.* **46**:147–154.

Oppenheim, J. J., Wang, T., and Frei, E., 1965, The effect of skin homograft rejection on recipient and donor mixed leukocyte cultures, *J. Exp. Med.* **122**:651–654.

Parrott, D. M. V., 1967, The response of draining lymph nodes to immunological stimulation in intact and thymectomized animals, *Symp. Tissue Org. Transpl. Suppl. J. Clin. Pathol.* **20**:456–465.

Patt, D. J., Brynes, R. K., Vardiman, J. W., and Coppelson, L. W., 1975, Mesocolic lymph node histology is an important prognostic indicator for patients with carcinoma of the sigmoid colon: An immunomorphologic study, *Cancer* **35**:1388–1397.

Pick, E., and Turk, J. L., 1972, The biological activities of soluble lymphocyte products, *Clin. Exp. Immunol.* **10**:1–23.

Pihl, E., Hughes, E. S. R., Nind, A. P. P., and Nairn, R. C., 1975, Colonic carinoma: Clinocopathological correlation with immunoreactivity, *Br. Med. J.* **3**:742–743.

Pope, B. L., Whitney, R. B., Levy, J. G., and Kilburn, D. G., 1976, Suppressor cells in the spleens of tumor-bearing mice: Enrichment by centrifugation on hypaque-ficoll and characterization of the suppressor population, *J. Immunol.* **116**:1342–1346.

Rode, H. N., and Gordon, J., 1974, Macrophages in the mixed leukocyte culture reaction (MLC), *Cell. Immunol.* **13**:87–94.

Schultz, R. M., Woods, W. A., and Chirigos, M. A., 1975, Detection in colorectal carcinoma patients of antibody cytotoxic to established cell strains derived from carcinoma of the human colon and rectum, *Int. J. Cancer* **16:**16–23.

Scothorne, R. J., and McGregor, I. A., 1955, Cellular changes in lymph nodes and spleen following skin homografting in the rabbit, *J. Anat.* **89:**283–292.

Segall, A., Weiler, O., Genin, J., Lacour, J., and Lacour, F., 1972, *In vitro* study of cellular immunity against autochthonous human cancer, *Int. J. Cancer* **9:**417–425.

Sherman, R. L., Susin, M., Weksler, M. E., and Becker, E. L., 1972, Lipoid nephrosis in Hodgkin's disease, *Am. J. Med.* **52:**699–706.

Sjögren, H. O., Hellström, I., Bansal, S. C., Warner, G. A., and Hellström, K. E., 1972, Elution of "blocking factors" from human tumors capable of abrogating tumor cell destruction by specifically immune lymphocytes, *Int. J. Cancer* **9:**274–283.

Søborg, M., 1967, *In vitro* detection of cellular hypersensitivity in man: Specific migration inhibition of white blood cells from brucella-positive persons, *Acta Med. Scand.* **182:**167–174.

Straus, E., Vernace, S., Janowitz, H., and Paronetto, F., 1975, Migration of peripheral leukocytes in the presence of carcinoembryonic antigen: Studies in patients with chronic inflammatory diseases of the intestine and carcinoma of the colon and pancreas, *Proc. Soc. Exp. Biol. Med.* **148:**494–497.

Steiner, P. E., Maimon, S. N., Palmer, W. L., and Kirsner, J. B., 1948, Gastric cancer: Morphologic factors in 5-year survival after gastrectomy, *Am. J. Pathol.* **24:**947–969.

Stewart, T. H. M., 1969, The presence of delayed hypersensitivity reactions in patients toward cellular extracts of their malignant tumors, *Cancer* **23:**1368–1379.

Takahashi, K., 1961, Squamous cell carcinoma of the esophagus: Stromal inflammatory cell infiltration as a prognostic factor, *Cancer* **14:**921–933.

Todaro, G. J., and Aaronson, S. A., 1969, Properties of clonal lines of murine sarcoma virus transformed Balb/3T3 cells, *Virology* **38:**174–179.

Tsakraklides, V., Anastassiades, O. T., and Kersey, J. H., 1973, Prognostic significance of regional lymph node histology in uterine cervical cancer, *Cancer* **31:**860–868.

Tsakraklides, V., Olson, P., Kersey, J. H., and Good, R. A., 1974, Prognostic significance of regional lymph node histology in cancer of the breast, *Cancer* **34:** 1259–1267.

Tsakraklides, V., Wanebo, H. J., Sternberg, S. S., Stearns, M., and Good, R. A., 1975, Prognostic evaluation of regional lymph node morphology in colorectal cancer, *Am. J. Surg.* **129:**174–180.

Twomey, J. J., 1974, Abnormalities in the mixed leukocyte reaction during infectious mononucleosis, *J. Immunol.* **112:**2278–2281.

Twomey, J. J., and Sharkey, O., 1972, An adaptation of the mixed leukocyte culture test for use in evaluating lymphocyte and macrophage function, *J. Immunol.* **108:**984–990.

Twomey, J. J., Sharkey, O., Jr., Brown, J. A., Laughter, A. H., and Jordan, P. H., Jr., 1970, Cellular requirements for the mitotic response in allogeneic mixed leukocyte cultures, *J. Immunol.* **104:**845–853.

Underwood, J. C. E., 1974, Lymphoreticular infiltration in human tumours: Prognostic and biological implications: A review, *Br. J. Cancer* **30:**538–548.

Wagner, H., 1972, The correlation between the proliferation and cytotoxic responses of mouse lymphocytes to allogeneic cells *in vitro*, *J. Immunol.* **109:**630–637.

Wang, M., 1968, Delayed hypersensitivity to extracts from primary sarcomata in the autochthonous host, *Int. J. Cancer* **3:**483–490.

Wartman, W. B., 1959, Sinus cell hyperplasia of lymph nodes regional to adenocarcinoma of the breast and colon, *Br. J. Cancer* **13:**389–397.

Wolberg, W. H., and Goelzer, M. L., 1971, *In vitro* assay of cell mediated immunity in human cancer: Definition of leukocyte migration inhibitory factor, *Nature (London)* **229:**632–633.

Yoon, I. L., 1959, The eosinophil and gastrointestinal carcinoma, *Am. J. Surg.* **97:**195–200.

Zöller, M., Price, M. R., and Baldwin, R. W., 1976, Inhibition of cell-mediated cytotoxicity to chemically induced rat tumours by soluble tumour and embryo cell extracts, *Int. J. Cancer* **17:**129–137.

5

Immunological Dysfunction with Atrophic Gastritis and Gastric Malignancy

Jeremiah J. Twomey

1. Introduction

Atrophic gastritis is an indolent disease of the stomach of unknown etiology. Histologically normal glandular gastric mucosa is replaced by flat colonic-type endothelium and the submucosa is heavily infiltrated with immune reactive cells (Fenwick, 1870; Coghill, 1960; Wood *et al.,* 1964). The stomach loses its ability to secrete hydrochloric acid, pepsin, and intrinsic factor (Levine and Ladd, 1921; Castle, 1929) and serum gastrin levels are elevated when antral mucosa is preserved (McGuigan and Trudeau, 1970; Strickland and Mackay, 1973; Hughes *et al.,* 1972). The lack of intrinsic factor secretion due to atrophic gastritis causing vitamin B_{12} malabsorption is the basic lesion of pernicious anemia (Castle, 1929). Patients with pernicious anemia require lifelong parenteral vitamin B_{12} replacement. Much still remains to be learned about the etiology and pathophysiology of atrophic gastritis. It is not known whether atrophic gastritis results from one or more pathogenetic mechanisms. It is not understood why (1) various autoimmune phenomena, (2) other immunological disorders, and (3) outwardly unrelated diseases involving other organs frequently coexist with atrophic gastritis. Patients with atrophic gastritis have an increased risk of developing cancer of the stomach. It is not known whether this association is an unexplained coincidence or whether atrophic gastritis is a precancerous condition. The primary objectives of this chapter

Jeremiah J. Twomey • Baylor College of Medicine, and Veterans Administration Hospital, Houston, Texas 77031.

are to review current information about immunological perturbations with atrophic gastritis and gastric carcinoma and to discuss the potential significance of these perturbations.

2. *Epidemiology*

The epidemiology of atrophic gastritis is a difficult subject. It is difficult to obtain the cooperation needed for direct gastroscopic surveys of biopsy material because of discomfort to the subject during the procedure. Autolysis of gastric mucosa renders autopsy material unsuitable for histological examination. Thus estimates on the incidence of atrophic gastritis are usually acquired indirectly from data on pernicious anemia and gastric carcinoma. Patients with pernicious anemia or cancer of the stomach are usually hospitalized on at least one occasion. Therefore, the incidence of either disease in the general population is likely to be overestimated from reviews of hospital records. Conversely, population surveys that include all age groups distort the public health significance of atrophic gastritis and related disorders because these conditions usually develop after the fourth age decade. Since atrophic gastritis is rarely recognized before systemic reserves of vitamin B_{12} are depleted, surveys pertaining to pernicious anemia underestimate the actual incidence of atrophic gastritis. Elderly individuals who develop atrophic gastritis may die from unrelated causes before the gastric lesion is identified. Epidemiological surveys from different locations should be analyzed individually because the incidence of pernicious anemia and gastric carcinoma is influenced by geographical location, race, and socioeconomic conditions (McConnell, 1966).

These observations are supported by published experience. Siurala *et al.* (1968), in Finland, performed gastric biopsies on 50 unselected volunteers over the age of 50 years; 4% had severe atrophic gastritis. The hospital records of 23,231 U.S. patients who died after the age of 45 years contained clinical evidence that 0.5% had pernicious anemia and autopsy material indicated that 4.1% had cancer of the stomach (Kaplan and Regler, 1945). It has been estimated that <0.2% of the overall population of Britain (Scott, 1960) and Denmark (Bisgaard Pedersen and Mosbech, 1968) has pernicious anemia. About 10 per 100,000 Americans develop carcinoma of the stomach annually at the present time (Krain, 1973).

Autopsy material collected prior to 1955 indicated that the risk of developing carcinoma of the stomach is increased about threefold in patients with pernicious anemia (Kaplan and Regler, 1945; Zamcheck *et al.,* 1955). This risk may be greatest in patients with pernicious anemia who are less than 65 years of age (Zamcheck *et al.,* 1955) and in patients with antral gastritis (Strickland and Mackay, 1973). In recent years, there has been a remarkable decline in new cases of stomach cancer (Krain, 1973). It is not known whether atrophic gastritis is also occurring less frequently in recent years.

3. Genetics

There is convincing evidence that pernicious anemia and cancer of the stomach occur more often among relatives of patients with these diseases than in the population at large. A history of a blood relative having pernicious anemia was elicited from 19% of 1600 patients with that disease (Zamcheck *et al.*, 1955). In other surveys, 20% of 106 relatives of patients with pernicious anemia had impaired vitamin B_{12} absorption (McIntyre *et al.*, 1959) and 19% of 220 other relatives had parietal cell autoantibody detected in their serum (TeVelde *et al.*, 1964). Parietal cell autoantibody is about 3 times more prevalent among relatives of patients with pernicious anemia than in an age-matched, control population (Doniach and Roitt, 1964). First-degree relatives of patients with gastric carcinoma also have a threefold higher risk of developing the same neoplasm than the general population (McConnell, 1966).

These surveys indicate that there is a familial incidence with a minority of cases of pernicious anemia or gastric carcinoma. Usually, only a few members of these families are affected and a pattern of genetic transmission has not emerged. However, occasional families have been reported in which atrophic gastritis (Ardeman *et al.*, 1966) or carcinoma of the stomach (Cruze *et al.*, 1961) has been identified with remarkable frequency. Clearly, these diseases of adult onset are not classical inborn pathophysiological disorders. Perhaps some individuals are genetically predisposed to these gastric lesions and develop them after exposure to other etiological factors, the identity of which is not known. Genetic factors may include other disorders that have been coincidentally related to atrophic gastritis and do not primarily involve the stomach. It has, for example, been reported that thyroid disorders, diabetes mellitus, and vitiligo are particularly prevalent in families with more than one member known to have pernicious anemia (Hippe and Jensen, 1969). In contrast to kindred members genetically unrelated cohabitants of patients with cancer of the stomach do not have an increased incidence of gastric carcinoma (McConnell, 1966).

The frequency of blood type A in series of patients with pernicious anemia or carcinoma of the stomach is about 20% higher than in the general population (McConnell, 1966). Blood group substances are antigenic glycoproteins (Morgan, 1970) that are also present in many normal tissues including gastric mucosa (Glynn *et al.*, 1957; Szulman, 1960). These substances are secreted into the lumen of the gastrointestinal tract by some genetically determined individuals (Kabat *et al.*, 1947; Schiff and Saskai, 1932). There is no evidence that the local presence of group A substance predisposes to atrophic gastritis or neoplastic change. Perhaps a group A locus is linked to another genetic locus that predisposes to these gastric disorders. A genetic locus relevant to pernicious anemia may also be linked to a locus that determines HLA-B7 specificity (Zittoun *et al.*, 1975).

The relationship between tissue blood group substances and atrophic gastritis is complex. Blood group antigens are often not demonstrable in gastric mucosa involved with atrophic gastritis (Sheahan *et al.*, 1971) or in tumor tissue from patients with carcinoma of the stomach (Sheahan *et al.*, 1971; Davidsohn *et al.*, 1966; Hakkinen, 1974; Denk *et al.*, 1974). When blood group antigen is identified in tumor tissue, it may differ in antigenic specificity from that of blood from the same patient (Denk *et al.*, 1974). Carcinoembryonic antigens are molecularly similar to blood group substances (Simons, 1971) and may be the result of defective assembly of blood group molecules. Carcinoembryonic antigens are found in serum (Gefro *et al.*, 1971) and tumor tissue (Denk *et al.*, 1974) from patients with various neoplasms, including carcinoma of the stomach. Likewise, changes in phenotype of blood group antigens in tumor tissue (Denk *et al.*, 1974) may result from altered glycoprotein synthesis by diseased mucosal cells. Such biochemical changes are also present in cells from atrophic gastric mucosa (Sheahan *et al.*, 1971).

Carcinoembryonic antigens are normally produced only during early embryonic life (Gold and Freedman, 1965). α-Fetoprotein is another molecule whose normal production is limited to early fetal life; this globulin is also produced by neoplastic tissues, including carcinoma of the stomach (Montplaisir *et al.*, 1973; Bierfeld *et al.*, 1973). Carcinoembryonic antigens and α-fetoprotein have been identified in cells from the same tumor (Bierfeld *et al.*, 1973). The synthesis of these primitive substances probably reflects alteration of the genetic code within cells where they are produced (Luderitz *et al.*, 1966; Simons and Perlmann, 1973). Replacement of normal gastric mucosa with atrophic gastritis and some gastric neoplasms by colonic-type, mucus-secreting cells is also compatible with cellular dedifferentiation at the mucosal level (Lipkin, 1973).

The significance of these observations to the pathophysiology of gastric disease is not known. These phenomena may be consequences of cancerous or precancerous changes within affected cells. However, they do present evidence that the synthesis of antigenic matter is altered within these cells. Altered antigenicity of substances produced by gastric mucosal cells may be pertinent to the various autoimmune phenomena that usually accompany atrophic gastritis.

4. Gastric Antigens

This discussion will be limited to gastric antigens with a degree of organ specificity. The study of gastric antigens was introduced through efforts to induce atrophic gastritis in experimental animals by immunization with gastric mucosa or gastric juice. Additional information was derived from autoimmune responses recognized in patients with pernicious anemia. In general, gastric antigens that may be relevant to atrophic gastritis have been identified through antibody rather than cell-mediated immune responses. This does not imply that gastric antigens, identified in this fashion, have pathophysiological importance, or imply greater importance to humoral or cell-mediated autoimmune phenomena that occur with pernicious anemia.

An antibody response to the microsomal fraction of canine parietal cells occurs following immunization with an extract from gastric mucosa (Walder, 1968) or gastric juice (Krolin and Finlayson, 1973). The antigenicity of gastric juice seems to be independent of intrinsic factor (Krolin and Finlayson, 1973) and may be derived from mucosal cells or cell products released into the stomach. Antiserum to canine parietal cell antigens cross-reacts with parietal cell antigens from other species, including man, and is, after appropriate adsorption, relatively target organ specific (Walder, 1968). Serum antibody from patients with pernicious anemia also reacts with parietal cell microsomal antigens from normal subjects (Baur *et al.*, 1965) and from other species (Fisher *et al.*, 1965). These clinical and experimental studies indicate that the cytoplasmic contents of gastric parietal cells of man and other species share antigenic determinants that are not demonstrable in many other tissues.

Intrinsic factor is a glycoprotein secreted by normal gastric mucosa and is essential for adequate adsorption of dietary vitamin B_{12} (Castle, 1929; Glass, 1963). Autoantibodies against intrinsic factor have been identified in serum (Schwartz, 1958; Taylor, 1959) and gastric juice (Goldberg and Bluestone, 1970; Rose and Chanarin, 1969) from patients with pernicious anemia. Intrinsic factor has at least two antigenic determinants, one that blocks the binding of vitamin B_{12} to intrinsic factor and a second that does not block this reaction and is identified by radioimmunoprecipitation techniques (Irvine, 1965). These intrinsic factor antigens are distinct from other antigens that are identified with the microsomal fraction of parietal cells.

The relevance of parietal cell and intrinsic factor antigens to the pathogenesis of atrophic gastritis remains to be determined. There is no reason to believe that antigens from gastric mucosa or secretions are more accessible to the immune system in patients who develop atrophic gastritis than in individuals who do not. Antigenic determinants of parietal cells or intrinsic factor are not appreciably altered with pernicious anemia. However, the antigenicity of gastric mucosal cells is otherwise altered (e.g., in blood group substances and the reappearance of carcinoembryonic antigen) in patients with atrophic gastritis (Sheahan *et al.*, 1971; Simons, 1971). Perhaps normal parietal cell and intrinsic factor antigens are unappreciably altered with these gastric disorders, thereby inducing autoimmune responses that crossreact with normal antigenic counterparts.

5. *Humoral Autoimmunity*

Autoantibody responses in patients with pernicious anemia and related diseases have been the subject of extensive investigation. Techniques used to detect and quantitate these unusual antibody responses have been discussed elsewhere (Doniach and Roitt, 1964). The findings from representative surveys on the frequency of parietal cell, intrinsic factor, and thyroid autoantibodies in serum from patients with pernicious anemia, thyroid disorders, and gastric carcinoma are compared in Table 1 with their frequency in appar-

Table 1. Incidence of Gastric and Thyroid Autoantibodies in Serum

References	Subjects tested	Parietal cell antibody (% of subjects seropositive)	Intrinsic factor antibody (% of subjects seropositive)	Thyroid-hemagglutinating antibody (% of subjects seropositive)
1. Pernicious anemia:				
Doniach and Roitt (1964)	189	89	60	55
Irvine (1965)	130	73	55	41
Fisher and Taylor (1965)	86	85	56	44
2. Thyroiditis:				
Doniach and Roitt (1964)[a]	394	32	—	87
Irvine (1965)	258	30	3	78
3. Gastric carcinoma:				
Ungar *et al.* (1971)	60	22	<1	—
4. Normal blood donors:				
Irvine (1965), 15–60[b]	629	5	<1	13
Ungar *et al.* (1971), <60[b]	≥400	7	<1	—
>60[b]	≥200	20	<1	—

[a]Series includes patients with thyroiditis and hypothyroidism.
[b]Age range in years.

ently healthy blood donors (Doniach and Roitt, 1964; Irvine, 1965; Fisher and Taylor, 1965; Ungar *et al.*, 1971). These autoantibodies are uncommon in the general population through the sixth age decade, after which these and other autoimmune phenomena are more prevalent (Hooper *et al.*, 1972). Parietal cell antibody is present in serum from most patients with pernicious anemia; intrinsic-factor-blocking antibody and thyroid-hemagglutinating antibody are detected somewhat less often. The incidence of nonblocking antibodies to intrinsic factor is somewhat lower (Goldberg and Bluestone, 1970; Herbert, 1967; Odgers and Wangel, 1968). Intrinsic-factor-blocking antibody is also present in gastric juice from about 50% of patients with pernicious anemia (Goldberg and Bluestone, 1970; Rose and Chanarin, 1969; Odgers and Wangel, 1968), where it complexes with intrinsic factor and compromises intrinsic-factor-mediated vitamin B_{12} absorption (Schade *et al.*, 1966; Rose and Chanarin, 1971). Although these studies do not refer to the age of the patient populations or to their overall immunological competence, it is apparent that the incidence of all three classes of autoantibodies is greatly increased with pernicious anemia.

The frequency of thyroid-hemagglutinating antibody with thyroiditis or hypothyroidism is about comparable to the high frequency of parietal cell antibody with pernicious anemia (Doniach and Roitt, 1964; Irvine, 1965; Fisher and Taylor, 1965). About one-third of patients with thyroiditis, hypothyroidism, or hyperthyroidism are seropositive for parietal cell antibody (Doniach and Roitt, 1964; Irvine, 1965). Although microsomal antigens of parietal cells and thyroid glandular cells are quite similar (Roitt *et al.*, 1964), serum autoantibodies to these antigens are target organ specific (Irvine *et al.*, 1962; Taylor *et al.*, 1962).

The slightly increased or normal incidence of gastric and thyroid autoantibodies with cancer of the stomach (Ungar *et al.*, 1971) is in striking contrast to experience with pernicious anemia. This observation supports other evidence that, while overlap occurs, the gastric mucosa of many patients with cancer of the stomach and that of patients with pernicious anemia may be intrinsically different (Strickland and Mackay, 1973). The rate of cell proliferation and extrusion into the lumen may also be greater from atrophic than from neoplastic gastric mucosa (Winawer and Lipkin, 1969; Cooper and Lipkin, 1973). Alternatively, the relatively low incidence of gastric autoantibodies with cancer of the stomach may reflect reduced immunological responsiveness. It remains to be determined whether the likelihood of developing gastric carcinoma with pernicious anemia is highest in patients without autoantibody responses to gastric antigens.

Circulating gastric autoantibody usually has IgG specificity, while autoantibody in gastric juice is likelier to have IgA specificity and may be attached to secretory piece (Goldberg *et al.*, 1968; Strickland *et al.*, 1971). A dissociation has been observed in the occurrence and also in Ig specificity of autoantibodies in serum and gastric juice from individual patients with pernicious anemia (Goldberg and Bluestone, 1970; Strickland *et al.*, 1971). The majority of antibody-producing cells in normal gastric mucosa contain IgA while there is a predominance of IgG-containing cells in the inflammatory infiltrates of atrophic gastritis (Odgers and Wangel, 1968). Antibody activity has been demonstrated in the cytoplasm of these immune reactive cells against intrinsic factor–vitamin B_{12} complexes (Baur *et al.*, 1968). It is not known whether change in Ig specificity of antibody-producing cells in the wall of the stomach is pertinent to the pathogenesis of atrophic gastritis or whether gastric autoantibody is also produced by patients with pernicious anemia in lymphoid tissues remote from the stomach.

6. *Cell-Mediated Autoimmunity*

Cell-mediated autoimmunity has been studied less extensively than have humoral manifestations of gastric autoimmunity. Most reports concern lymphocyte proliferation and lymphokine production by leukocytes in response to stimulation *in vitro* with gastric antigens. These *in vitro* responses normally correlate with the presence or absence of delayed hypersensitivity *in vivo* to soluble microbial antigens (Kerby, 1968; David, 1966). Apart from the minority of patients with coexistent immune deficiency disorders and a report of low [^{3}H]thymidine incorporation by cultured leukocytes when stimulated with phytohemagglutinin (MacCuish *et al.*, 1974), there is little evidence that leukocytes from patients with pernicious anemia are hyporesponsive to antigenic challenge (Tai and McGuigan, 1969; Salupere *et al.*, 1972; Twomey and Laughter, unpublished data).

There are some technical difficulties with methods used to study cell-mediated gastric autoimmunity. The antigenic specificity of heterologous mucosal extracts remains open to some question (Ramsey and Herbert, 1965; Goldberg *et al.,* 1969; Twomey *et al.,* 1972). Human gastric juice is usually concentrated and otherwise manipulated before it is used as antigen (Tai and McGuigan, 1969; Chanarin and James, 1974); these gastric juice preparations exceed physiological requirements (Twomey *et al.,* 1972) and secretory capacity (Twomey *et al.,* 1971*b*) in their intrinsic factor content and may not be representative of antigenic circumstances on the systemic side of the luminal surface of the stomach. In lymphoproliferative studies, the duration of the culture period has varied considerably (Tai and McGuigan, 1969; Chanarin and James, 1974; Fixa and Thiele, 1969); in some instances, incubation may have been too brief for the development of optimal responses to antigenic stimulation. Nevertheless, there is substantial evidence to indicate that cell-mediated autoimmunity to gastric antigens is present in many patients with pernicious anemia. Similar tests, performed on healthy young individuals, are rarely positive (Chanarin and James, 1974; Finlayson *et al.,* 1972; Goldstone *et al.,* 1973; Zittoun *et al.,* 1975).

Some (Tai and McGuigan, 1969; Chanarin and James, 1974), but not all (Strickland and Mackay, 1973), studies have demonstrated lymphoproliferative responses to gastric antigens by cultured leukocytes from a minority of patients with pernicious anemia (Table 2). Responses of this type were recorded most often when cultures were incubated through 7 days (Tai and McGuigan, 1969). Leukocytes from more than 50% of patients with pernicious anemia have been shown, with conventional laboratory techniques, to produce macrophage migration inhibitory factor when incubated with gastric antigens (Chanarin and James, 1974; Fixa and Thiele, 1969; Finlayson *et al.,* 1972; Goldstone *et al.,* 1973). It has been suggested (Weisbart *et al.,* 1975) that, with more sensitive tests for detecting lymphokines (Weisbart *et al.,* 1973), cell-mediated autoimmunity to gastric antigens may occur at least as often as humoral autoimmunity with pernicious anemia. There is no apparent coincidental relationship between the different expressions of antibody and cell-mediated gastric autoimmunity in individual patients with pernicious anemia.

Similar lymphokine responses are observed with leukocytes from only 20% of patients with atrophic gastritis whose ability to absorb vitamin B_{12} is not impaired (Goldstone *et al.,* 1973; James *et al.,* 1974). This lower incidence than with classical pernicious anemia could reflect less aggressive gastric immunopathology. It could also reflect a relatively early phase of the disease (Fenwick, 1870; Siurala *et al.,* 1966). However, such a sequence would imply that cell-mediated autoimmunity to gastric antigens has a consequential rather than an etiological relationship to atrophic gastritis. In many instances histologically established atrophic gastritis does not progress to a stage where vitamin B_{12} absorption is impaired (Siurala *et al.,* 1966). Perhaps patients with autoimmunity to gastric antigens are those who are likeliest to develop vitamin B_{12} malabsorption while those who do not manifest these immunological perturbations are at greatest risk of developing cancer of the stomach (Strickland and Mackay, 1973). While the incidence of gastric autoantibodies is considerably lower with cancer of the stomach than with pernicious anemia (Table 1),

Table 2. Cell-Mediated Immune Responses to Gastric Antigens with Pernicious Anemia

Lymphoproliferative responses					MIF[a] production			
References	Days in culture	Antigen[a]	Patients tested	Percent positive	References	Antigen[a]	Patients tested	Percent positive
Fixa and Thiele (1969)	4	Hog	15	0	Same	Hog	15	80
Chanarin and James (1974)	3	HGJ	51	20	Same	HGJ	39	44
						Hog	39	56
Tai and McGuigan (1969)	7	HGJ	16	38	Finlayson *et al.* (1972)	HGJ	9	67
					Goldstone *et al.* (1973)	HME	18	50
					Weisbart *et al.* (1975)	Hog[b]	17	65

[a]MIF, macrophage migration inhibitory factor; Hog, hog mucosal extract; HGJ, concentrated human gastric juice; HME, human mucosal extract.
[b]At 50 μg/ml; with 25 μg/ml and recording of enhanced as well as inhibited macrophage migration, 17/18 patients' leukocytes gave positive results.

the incidence of cell-mediated autoimmunity to gastric antigens among patients with carcinoma of the stomach remains to be determined.

7. Can Immune Reactivity Cause Atrophic Gastritis?

There is considerable experimental evidence that immunization with gastric antigens can induce atrophic changes in the mucosa of the stomach. Animals immunized with gastric juice or mucosal extract develop atrophy and secretory failure of their gastric mucosa (Walder, 1968; Krolin and Finlayson, 1973; Brunschwig *et al.*, 1939; Hennes *et al.*, 1962). These changes are induced with autologous as well as with homologous or heterologous antigens (Krolin and Finlayson, 1973; Hennes *et al.*, 1962) and the effects appear to be target organ specific (Walder, 1968). In addition to structural and secretory changes in gastric mucosa, sensitized animals develop delayed hypersensitivity and autoantibodies to gastric antigens (Walder, 1968; Krolin and Finlayson, 1973; Hennes *et al.*, 1962). The onset of atrophic changes in gastric mucosa is temporarily related to the development of delayed hypersensitivity to gastric antigens; autoantibody appears a few weeks later (Krolin and Finlayson, 1973). Furthermore, transfer of thoracic duct lymphocytes from sensitized to nonsensitized animals induces atrophy of gastric mucosa in the recipients (Fixa *et al.*, 1970); heterologous serum antibody to gastric antigens has also been shown to cause acute inflammation in gastric mucosa of recipient experimental animals (Hauseman *et al.*, 1969). Thus experimentally induced immune responses to gastric antigens are causally related to gastric atrophy.

Experimental gastric atrophy differs histologically in one respect from atrophic gastritis in man. The heavy infiltration of the stomach wall with immune reactive cells, which is a characteristic of human atrophic gastritis (Wood *et al.*, 1964), does not occur in the experimental model. Perhaps this difference reflects the systemic route of sensitization used to achieve experimental gastric atrophy. Since (presumably normal) autologous gastric antigens can cause experimental gastric atrophy (Krolin and Finlayson, 1973; Hennes *et al.*, 1962), the location and dose of immunogen may be more relevant to gastric autoimmunity than alteration of antigenic specificity. Altered specificity of gastric antigens has, likewise, not been identified with atrophic gastritis in man.

Immunological reactivity is greatly increased in the stomach wall with human atrophic gastritis. This increased reactivity is manifested by deposition of immunoglobulins (Jeffries and Sleisenger, 1965) and accumulation of immune reactive cells (Wood *et al.*, 1964), particularly in the submucosa. This local immune response must be considered abnormal because of its intensity and the switch from a predominance of IgA- to IgG-containing cells (Odgers and Wangel, 1968). The intracellular immunoglobulin acquires antibody activity against intrinsic factor–vitamin B_{12} complexes (Baur *et al.*, 1968). Both humoral and cell-mediated autoimmunity to gastric antigens (Tables 1 and 2) are present within the circulation of patients with pernicious anemia. Therefore, gastric autoimmunity in these patients must be considered to be a systemic as well as a local phenomenon.

Clinical observations suggest that autoimmune responses that accompany pernicious anemia contribute to the pathogenesis of atrophic gastritis. Gastric autoantibodies have been detected for a brief period in serum from infants born of mothers with pernicious anemia (Bar-Shany and Herbert, 1967; Goldberg *et al.,* 1967; Charache *et al.,* 1968). This transient seropositivity, which probably reflects transplacental transfer of antibody from the mother's circulation, may be accompanied by transient impairment of gastric secretion (Bar-Shany and Herbert, 1967; Goldberg *et al.,* 1967). Conversely, it has been reported that immunosuppression of patients with pernicious anemia using adrenocorticosteroids is accompanied by improvement in secretory capabilities (Ardeman and Chanarin, 1965) and in the histology (Jeffries, 1965) of gastric mucosa and a lowering of circulating levels of intrinsic-factor-blocking antibody (Charache *et al.,* 1968). Circulating IgG from seropositive patients with pernicious anemia has also been reported to lower gastric secretion and reduce parietal cell mass when infused into rats (Tanaka and Jerzy Glass, 1970). It therefore seems that autoimmune responses can cause, and may perpetuate, atrophic gastritis.

Autoimmune phenomena that occur with pernicious anemia are themselves unusual and may reflect an intrinsic functional derangement of the immune system. The autoimmune responses that occur with pernicious anemia are not limited in specificity to gastric antigens. These patients also have an increased incidence of autoantibody responses to other tissue antigens that include the thyroid (Doniach and Roitt, 1964) and adrenal (Irvine *et al.,* 1967) glands and red cell (Pirofsky and Vaughn, 1968) and lymphocyte membranes (Goldberg *et al.,* 1972).

A coincidental relationship has been established between pernicious anemia and other diseases that do not seem to involve the stomach but may include an immunological component of their own (Table 3). These diseases include various thyroid disorders (Doniach and Roitt, 1964; Chanarin, 1972), hypoparathyroidism (Blizzard *et al.,* 1966), adrenocortical insufficiency (Blizzard *et al.,* 1967), probably diabetes mellitus (Ungar *et al.,* 1968; Munichoodappa and Kozak, 1970; Irvine *et al.,* 1970), and vitiligo (Bor *et al.,* 1969; Howitz and Schwartz, 1971). It is not clear why endocrine disorders, including the polyendocrine syndrome (Morse *et al.,* 1961), figure so prominently in this relationship. Immunological abnormalities have been implicated in the pathogenesis of these other diseases. The evidence that incriminates the immune system in the pathogenesis of these other disorders includes the high rate of autoimmunity identified against antigenic determinents of target tissues and the ability to induce similar lesions in experimental animals by immunization with appropriate antigens. Patients with these disorders that have been coincidentally related to pernicious anemia are often seropositive for gastric autoantibodies, thereby extending the relationship from the clinical to the immunopathological level.

Both pernicious anemia and endocrinopathies have been associated more

Table 3. Pernicious Anemia with Other Diseases Believed to Have an Autoimmune Component

Disease	Percent of patients with pernicious anemia	Autoimmune phenomena related to primary disease[a]
1. Thyroiditis	12–20 (Doniach and Roitt, 1964; Chanarin, 1972)	Autoantibody (Chanarin, 1972); MIF (Calder *et al.*, 1972); Imm. (Witebsky and Rose, 1956); humoral (Penhale *et al.*, 1975) and cell-mediated (Wick *et al.*, 1970); passive transfer (Wall *et al.*, 1973; McMaster and Lerner, 1967)
Hypothyroidism	10–12	
Hyperthyroidism	1–3	
2. Hypoparathyroidism	9 (Blizzard *et al.*, 1966)	Autoantibody (Blizzard *et al.*, 1966); Imm. (Lupulescu *et al.*, 1965)
3. Adrenocortical insufficiency	6 (Blizzard *et al.*, 1967)	Autoantibody (Blizzard *et al.*, 1967); MIF (Nerup *et al.*, 1969); Imm. (Witebsky and Milgrom, 1962; Shulman *et al.*, 1965)
4. Diabetes mellitus	≤4 (Ungar *et al.*, 1968; Munichoodappa and Kozak, 1970; Irvine *et al.*, 1970)	Autoantibody (Mancini *et al.*, 1964); MIF (Richens *et al.*, 1974; Nerup *et al.*, 1971); Imm. (LeCompte *et al.*, 1966)
5. Vitiligo	3–8 (Bor *et al.*, 1969; Howitz and Schwartz, 1971)	Indirect; clinical associations
6. General population	<0.2 (Scott, 1960; Bisgaard Pedersen and Mosbech, 1968)	

[a]Autoantibody, target organ-specific autoantibody; MIF, lymphokine response (diabetes mellitus: liver mitochondrial antigens, Richens *et al.*, 1974); Imm., target organ lesion in experimental animals after specific immunization.

directly with dysfunction of the immune system. These disorders have been coincidentally associated with chronic mucocutaneous candidiasis (Quie and Chilgren, 1971; Kirkpatrick *et al.*, 1971; Higgs and Wells, 1972; Wuepper and Fudenberg, 1967; Twomey *et al.*, 1975; Olin and Poindexter, 1972) as well as with each other. A variety of immunodeficiencies, primarily involving cell-mediated immunity, have been identified with chronic mucocutaneous candidiasis (Quie and Chilgren, 1971; Kirkpatrick *et al.*, 1971; Higgs and Wells, 1972; Lehner *et al.*, 1972; Twomey *et al.*, 1975). The occurrence of various autoantibody responses has also been identified with this indolent syndrome (Wuepper and Fudenberg, 1967).

8. Pernicious Anemia and Antibody Deficiency Syndromes

A coincidental relationship has been clearly established between atrophic gastritis and immunoglobulin deficiency. At least 35 cases of pernicious anemia plus immunoglobulin deficiency have been reported (James *et al.*, 1974; Hermans and Huizenga, 1972; Cowling *et al.*, 1974; Douglas *et al.*, 1970; Manigand *et al.*, 1974; Hughes *et al.*, 1972; Twomey *et al.*, 1969, 1970; Gelfand *et al.*, 1972; Clinicopathological Conference, 1965; Larsson *et al.*, 1961; Lee *et al.*, 1964; Hoskins *et al.*, 1967). These reports present a relatively uniform syndrome that has the following characteristics:

1. Fewer than 1% of patients with pernicious anemia but without apparent immunodeficiency (henceforth referred to as classical pernicious anemia) are diagnosed before the age of 30 years (Twomey *et al.*, 1969; Wintrobe, 1961). In contrast, the median age at diagnosis of atrophic gastritis in 23 patients with the pernicious anemia–immunoglobulin deficiency (PA-IgDef) syndrome was 25 years; 65% of these patients were less than 30 years of age when the gastric lesion was identified (Twomey, 1975; Cowling *et al.*, 1974; Douglas *et al.*, 1970; Manigand *et al.*, 1974; Gelfand *et al.*, 1972; Clinicopathological Conference, 1965; Larsson *et al.*, 1961). Pernicious anemia was recognized in both of a pair of monozygotic twins at the age of 14 years (Gelfand *et al.*, 1972). Pernicious anemia has also been reported in relatives of patients with PA-IgDef who were not themselves believed to be immunodeficient (Gelfand *et al.*, 1972; Larsson *et al.*, 1961; Lee *et al.*, 1964).

2. Serum gastrin levels are usually elevated with classical pernicious anemia (McGuigan and Trudeau, 1970; Hughes *et al.*, 1972). This finding has been related to preservation of normal antral mucosa (Strickland and Mackay, 1973). When atrophic gastritis involves antral mucosa, serum gastrin levels are not elevated, vitamin B_{12} malabsorption is less frequent, and the risk of developing cancer of the stomach may be particularly high (Strickland and Mackay, 1973). Serum gastrin levels are in the low normal range with PA-IgDef (Hughes *et al.*, 1972). This suggests that these patients have antral gastritis. Antral gastritis was established histologically in one of our patients and in another patient reported by Cowling *et al.* (1974). Two of our patients with histological evidence of advanced atrophic gastritis had normal vitamin B_{12}

absorption by Schilling test. At least five cases of immunoglobulin deficiency with coexistent cancer of the stomach have been reported (Hermans and Huizenga, 1972; Twomey *et al.,* 1969; Forssman and Homer, 1964). These observations support the possibility that atrophic gastritis with PA-IgDef may be of the variety that frequently involves antral mucosa. Stimulated gastric secretion aspirated from patients with immunoglobulin deficiency (even from patients without histological evidence of atrophic gastritis) is unusually viscous (Twomey *et al.,* 1970). Perhaps these patients have an intrinsic disorder of gastric mucosa that predisposes them to develop atrophic gastritis with extensive mucosal involvement. Such a predisposition may explain the unusually early age at which atrophic gastritis is recognized in immunoglobulin-deficient patients.

3. Intestinal absorption is usually normal with treated pernicious anemia, although malabsorption has been reported in untreated patients with megaloblastic hematopoiesis (Brody *et al.,* 1966). This absorptive defect may be related to "megaloblastoid" changes in rapidly proliferating cells of intestinal mucosa (Foroozan and Trier, 1967). Intestinal dysfunction occurs in over 50% of patients with common variable immunoglobulin deficiency (Hughes *et al.,* 1971; Twomey, 1975). Bowel dysfunction is equally prevalent, regardless of the presence or absence of atrophic gastritis. The severity of the intestinal disorder varies from mild or episodic diarrhea to a florid malabsorption syndrome (Twomey *et al.,* 1969; Huizenga *et al.,* 1961). Intestinal dysfunction in immunoglobulin-deficient patients has been associated with nodular dysplasia of intestinal lymphoid tissue (Hughes *et al.,* 1971; Hermans *et al.,* 1966) and giardiasis (Ochs *et al.,* 1975). Intestinal dysfunction complicates the evaluation of vitamin B_{12} absorption with immunoglobulin deficiency as exemplified by the fact that urinary excretion of labeled vitamin B_{12} ingested with exogenous intrinsic factor was abnormally low in tests on 16 of 23 patients with PA-IgDef (Hughes *et al.,* 1972; Twomey *et al.,* 1969, 1970; James *et al.,* 1974). Pancreatic insufficiency has been demonstrated in two of six patients with common variable immunoglobulin deficiency (Hughes *et al.,* 1971), and coexistent PA-IgDef plus ulcerative colitis has been reported (Twomey *et al.,* 1969). It seems, therefore, that atrophic gastritis is but one of a number of gastrointestinal disorders that occur unusually often in immunoglobulin-deficient patients.

4. Increased susceptibility to bacterial infections became apparent in all of 23 PA-IgDef patients after an interval of at least 2 years of life with apparent good health (Cowling *et al.,* 1974; Douglas *et al.,* 1970; Manigand *et al.,* 1974; Gelfand *et al.,* 1972; Clinicopathological Conference, 1965; Larsson *et al.,* 1961; Twomey, 1975). The male–female sex ratio of 26 patients with PA-IgDef was 1.36:1. The pair of identical twins (Gelfand *et al.,* 1972) was the only instance in which more than one member of individual kindreds had the complete syndrome. Serum IgG, IgA, and IgM levels were usually severely depressed (Douglas *et al.,* 1970; Manigand *et al.,* 1974; Gelfand *et al.,* 1972; Twomey, 1975; Hughes *et al.,* 1972); one patient had a serum IgG level of 932 mg % (Cowling *et al.,* 1974), another had a modest pan-Ig deficiency (Gelfand *et al.,* 1972), and a third had 99 mg % of serum IgM (Twomey, 1975). It

seems, therefore, that the immunoglobulin deficiency usually associated with atrophic gastritis is of the common variable type. This type of immunoglobulin deficiency is pathophysiologically heterogeneous (Waldmann *et al.*, 1974; Geha *et al.*, 1974) and may include some derangement of cell-mediated immunity (Kopp *et al.*, 1968; Tormey *et al.*, 1967). None of the 35 cases of PA-IgDef had clinical evidence that would suggest impaired cell-mediated immunity. However, one patient was anergic to nine microbial antigens and could not be sensitized to dinitrochlorobenzene by skin application (Twomey *et al.*, 1969); leukocytes from another patient failed to proliferate when cultured with concanavalin A but responded normally to other mitogens (Cowling *et al.*, 1974).

5. The ages at which atrophic gastritis and increased susceptibility to infections were recognized in 21 PA-IgDef patients (Cowling *et al.*, 1974; Douglas *et al.*, 1970; Manigand *et al.*, 1974; Clinicopathological Conference, 1965; Larsson *et al.*, 1961; Twomey, 1975) did not indicate a sequence suggestive of a cause-and-effect relationship. Indeed, the two clinical components were diagnosed in nine of these patients within a 5-year age period. Gastrointestinal disorders which include atrophic gastritis, carcinoma of the stomach, small bowel dysfunction, and perhaps pancreatic insufficiency, together with immunoglobulin deficiency and nodular dysplasia of intestinal lymphoid tissues, may be independent manifestations of one or more occult disease states. This disease complex appears to identify with common variable immunoglobulin deficiency specifically and not with primary humoral immunodeficiency in general.

6. Serum from at least 21 patients with PA-IgDef has been tested for parietal cell and intrinsic factor antibodies (Cowling *et al.*, 1974; Douglas *et al.*, 1970; Manigand *et al.*, 1974; Clinicopathological Conference, 1965; Larsson *et al.*, 1961; Twomey, 1975). In contrast to the high rate of seropositivity with classical pernicious anemia (Table 1), all 21 patients were seronegative for both autoantibodies. In light of the severe general impairment of humoral immunity, it is not likely that significant amounts of autoantibody were present at the gastric mucosal level in these patients which was not appreciated by serological testing. Although evidence exists that gastric autoantibodies may contribute to the pathogenesis of atrophic gastritis (see Section 5), it is evident from the PA-IgDef syndrome that detectable levels of gastric autoantibodies are not essential for the presence of atrophic gastritis. Cell-mediated autoimmunity is an alternative immunological mechanism that could cause atrophic gastritis in immunoglobulin-deficient individuals. Cell-mediated immune responses to gastric antigens have been identified in at least five PA-IgDef patients (James *et al.*, 1974; Gelfand *et al.*, 1972). Conversely, humoral autoimmunity may contribute more prominently to the pathophysiology of atrophic gastritis in patients with chronic mucocutaneous candidiasis where cell-mediated immunity is likelier to be compromised (Quie and Chilgren, 1971; Olin and Poindexter, 1972; Twomey *et al.*, 1975).

Multiple myeloma is a plasmacytoid neoplasm with which humoral rather than cell-mediated immune competence is deficient (Heath *et al.*, 1964;

Twomey and Douglass, 1974). At least nine patients with coexistent pernicious anemia and multiple myeloma have been reported (Selroos and von Knorring, 1973; Larsson, 1962; Nordenson, 1966; Frazer, 1969; Hoffbrand *et al.*, 1967; Twomey *et al.*, 1971*a*). The ages when pernicious anemia was recognized in these patients was within the usual range for classical pernicious anemia and considerably older than the range for PA-IgDef. One patient also had carcinoma of the stomach (Twomey *et al.*, 1971*a*). Serum from one patient who probably had a relatively small tumor cell mass had parietal cell antibody but did not have intrinsic factor antibody (Selroos and von Knorring, 1973). Three other patients with multiple myeloma plus pernicious anemia were seronegative for both autoantibodies (Twomey *et al.*, 1971*a*). It is not known whether patients with multiple myeloma plus pernicious anemia manifest cellular autoimmunity to gastric antigens. Apart from the reduced frequency of gastric autoantibody, the pernicious anemia in patients with multiple myeloma does not have characteristics that distinguish it from classical pernicious anemia. The low incidence of gastric autoantibody in these patients is probably related to impaired humoral immunity. We have observed a progressive decline in capacity for intrinsic factor secretion during the clinical course of multiple myeloma (Twomey, 1975). This could represent a cumulative increase in the incidence of gastric disease during the course of multiple myeloma or, alternatively, it could be a nonspecific reflection of chronic debilitating illness (Twomey, 1971).

Atrophic gastritis, achlorhydria, and intrinsic factor secretory failure have been detected in four out of ten unselected patients with common variable immunoglobulin deficiency (Twomey *et al.*, 1970). James *et al.* (1974) found impaired gastric acid and intrinsic factor secretion and cell-mediated autoimmunity to gastric antigens in four out of nine hypogammaglobulinemic individuals. Five of 12 additional patients with severe immunoglobulin deficiency (Hughes *et al.*, 1972) were achlorhydric and demonstrated vitamin B_{12} malabsorption (which was improved with exogenous intrinsic factor in four instances); a sixth patient was achlorhydric. This relatively uniform epidemiological experience indicates that greater than 40% of adults with primary immunoglobulin deficiency have coexistent pernicious anemia. In addition, three (7.7%) of 39 immunoglobulin-deficient patients seen at the Mayo Clinic over a 10-year period had cancer of the stomach (Hermans and Huizenga, 1972). The literature suggests that 1.6–2.3% of patients with multiple myeloma have coexistent pernicious anemia (Twomey, 1975). Furthermore, diseases coincidentally related to pernicious anemia (e.g., thyroid disorders) occur with unusual frequency among relatives of patients with multiple myeloma (Twomey, 1975). Conversely, one out of a series of 33 patients with pernicious anemia also had multiple myeloma (Selroos and von Knorring, 1973). It is therefore apparent that the incidence of pernicious anemia is considerably higher in patients with primary immunoglobulin deficiency and, to a lesser degree, in patients with multiple myeloma than in general (<0.2%) or hospital in-patient (0.5%) populations (Kaplan and Regler, 1945; Bisgaard Pedersen and Mosbech, 1968; Scott, 1960). The risk of developing cancer of the stomach is also increased with immunoglobulin deficiency (Krain, 1973). The epidemiological significance of case reports of dysglobulinemia and pernicious anemia (Ginsberg and Mullinax, 1970) remains to be determined.

Extensive studies (Talal and Steinberg, 1974; Stutman, 1972; Dauphinee and Talal, 1975) have associated autoimmunity in inbred New Zealand mice with a deficit of thymus-derived lymphocytes and a loss of normal immunoregulatory control. Autoimmune responses to gastric antigens are usually evident with classical pernicious anemia and may have pathophysiological significance. These findings suggest that immune suppressor cell activity may also be inadequate in patients with pernicious anemia. However, the possibility that atrophic gastritis in patients with common variable immunoglobulin deficiency or multiple myeloma may be related to an immunoregulatory deficit is challenged by recent evidence that the suppressive component of immune regulatory mechanisms may be hyperactive rather than impaired with these disorders (Waldmann *et al.,* 1974; Broder *et al.,* 1975).

9. Classification

The etiology of atrophic gastritis has not yet been identified. Indeed, this gastric lesion may result from more than one pathogenetic mechanism. There is little opportunity to identify the evolution of different histopathological patterns from the advanced stage of atrophic gastritis that is present with pernicious anemia. Intrinsic factor deficiency due to atrophic gastritis, which is the basic disorder of pernicious anemia, must be distinguished from intrinsic factor deficiency resulting from gastric resection (Hines *et al.,* 1967) and from rare instances where absence of intrinsic factor secretion occurs as an isolated congenital deficiency (Miller *et al.,* 1966).

Pernicious anemia has been classified as hereditary or sporadic. Hippe and Jensen (1969) have observed a higher frequency of diabetes mellitus, thyroid disorders, and vitiligo, lower (but normal) serum immunoglobulin levels, and an earlier age at diagnosis when more than one family member has pernicious anemia. However, a genetic classification of pernicious anemia has, as yet, little practical application because of the poorly defined role of genetic factors that pertain to the disease.

There is potential merit to grouping atrophic gastritis by the presence or absence of antral gastritis. These subgroups may be distinguished by measuring serum gastrin levels, which are usually elevated when normal antral mucosa is preserved (Strickland and Mackay, 1973). Patients with antral gastritis may have a greater risk of developing cancer of the stomach; this observation may be related to the high percentage of gastric carcinomas that are located in the antrum of the stomach. This type of atrophic gastritis that involves antral mucosa may be particularly relevant to the PA-IgDef syndrome. Patients having atrophic gastritis with which normal antral mucosa is preserved may be most likely to secrete insufficient intrinsic factor to maintain vitamin B_{12} nutritional equilibrium from dietary sources (i.e., classical pernicious anemia) and manifest autoimmume responses to gastric antigens. The reason why a small minority of patients with classical pernicious anemia do not express detectable gastric autoimmunity remains to be determined.

Pernicious anemia can also be classified by immunological criteria. Patients who demonstrate autoimmunity to gastric antigens and others who do not may have basically distinct disorders. The presence or absence of coincidentally related diseases and related autoimmune phenomena involving other organs may eventually help identify different forms of pernicious anemia. PA-IgDef has distinguishing features that qualify it as a syndrome; the relationship (if any) between the gastric lesion with PA-IgDef and that of classical pernicious anemia remains to be determined. The grouping of pernicious anemia plus multiple myeloma and of pernicious anemia plus chronic mucocutaneous candidiasis is valid on an epidemiological basis. However, the gastric lesion or the immunological disorders that occur together in these patients lack features that distinguish them from those found when pernicious anemia, multiple myeloma, or chronic mucocutaneous candidiasis manifests as a single entity. It is not apparent why patients with either immunological disorder should be unduly susceptible to atrophic gastritis.

10. Concluding Comments

The high frequency of autoantibody and cell-mediated immune responses to gastric antigens in patients with classical pernicious anemia has been well documented. There is strong clinical inference, which is supported by experimental data, that autoimmune responses to gastric antigens contribute to the pathogenesis of atrophic gastritis. This does not necessarily imply that autoimmune responses initiate the gastric lesion. It remains to be proven that an intrinsic abnormality of gastric mucosa is not the primary cause of atrophic gastritis; gastric autoimmunity may be a secondary phenomenon that also contributes to the disease process.

The reason why patients with certain immunodeficiencies have an unusually high incidence of pernicious anemia remains to be explained. The increased incidence of atrophic gastritis among patients with common variable immunoglobulin deficiency, multiple myeloma, and, perhaps, chronic mucocutaneous candidiasis, on the surface, challenges the pathophysiological relevance of autoimmune responses to atrophic gastritis. However, patients with severe impairment of humoral immunity may still have immunologically induced atrophic gastritis effected by cellular mechanisms and *vice versa*. The relative pathophysiological importance of antibody and cell-mediated autoimmunity to gastric antigens has not been established. Additional information may be obtained on this subject from further studies on patients with atrophic gastritis and various immune deficiency diseases. A coincidental relationship may also be established between pernicious anemia and other immunodeficiency disorders.

Atrophic gastritis is the central lesion of pernicious anemia. Since many patients with cancer of the stomach also have atrophic gastritis, it is not surprising that this neoplasm and pernicious anemia are coincidentally related. However, the frequencies of circulating gastric autoantibodies with these two disease states are quite different, being high with pernicious anemia and low with cancer of the stomach. This difference suggests that atrophic gastritis may have more than one pathogenetic mechanism and that the risk of developing gastric carcinoma may be greatest when atrophic gastritis is not accompanied by circulating gastric autoantibody. The question of whether antral gastritis has a role in determining the prevalence of gastric autoantibody and the risk of developing carcinoma of the stomach is worthy of further investigation. The frequency of cell-mediated autoimmunity to gastric antigens with carcinoma of the stomach also needs documentation.

11. References

Ardeman, S., and Chanarin, I., 1965, Steroids and Addisonian pernicious anemia, *N. Eng. J. Med.* **273:**1352–1355.

Ardeman, S., Chanarin, I., Jacobs, A., and Griffiths, L., 1966, Family study in Addisonian pernicious anemia, *Blood* **27:**599–610.

Bar-Shany, S., and Herbert, V., 1967, Transplacentally acquired antibody to intrinsic factor with vitamin B_{12} deficiency, *Blood* **30:**777–784.

Baur, S., Roitt, I. M., and Doniach, D., 1965, Characterization of the human gastric parietal cell auto-antigen, *Immunology* **8:**62–68.

Baur, S., Fisher, J. M., Strickland, R. G., and Taylor, K. B., 1968, Autoantibody-containing cells in the gastric mucosa in pernicious anemia, *Lancet* **2:**887–890.

Bierfeld, J. L., Scheiner, M. I., Schultz, D. R., Moral, M. D., and Rogers, A. I., 1973, Alpha-fetoprotein and carcinoembryonic antigen in a case of gastric carcinoma metastatic to the liver, *Am. J. Digest. Dis.* **18:**517–520.

Bisgaard Pedersen, A., and Mosbech, J., 1968, The incidence of pernicious anemia in the population of Denmark, *Ugeskr Laeg.* **130:**1264–1278.

Blizzard, R. M., Chee, D., and Davis, W., 1966, The incidence of parathyroid and other antibodies in the sera of patients with idiopathic hypoparathyroidism, *Clin. Exp. Immunol.* **1:**119–128.

Blizzard, R. M., Chee, D., and Davis, W., 1967, The incidence of adrenal and other antibodies in the sera of patients with idiopathic adrenal insufficiency, *Clin. Exp. Immunol.* **2:**19–30.

Bor, S., Feiwel, M., and Chanarin, I., 1969, Viteligo and its aetiological relationship to organ-specific autoimmune disease, *Br. J. Dermatol.* **81:**83–88.

Broder, S., Humphrey, R., Durm, M., Blackman, M., Meade, B., Goldman, C., Strober, W., and Waldmann, T., 1975, Impaired synthesis of polyclonal immunoglobulins in myeloma—Role of suppressor cells, *N. Eng. J. Med.* **293:**887–892.

Brody, E. A., Estren, S., and Herbert, V., 1966, Coexistent pernicious anemia and malabsorption in four patients, *Ann. Intern. Med.* **64:**1246–1251.

Brunschwig, A., Van Prohaska, J., Clarke, T. H., and Kandel, E. V., 1939, Secretory depressant in gastric juice of patients with pernicious anemia, *J. Clin. Invest.* **18:**415–422.

Calder, E. A., McLeman, D., Barnes, E. W., and Irvine, W. J., 1972, The effect of thyroid antigens on the *in vitro* migration of leukocytes from patients with Hashimoto's thyroiditis, *Clin. Exp. Immunol.* **12:**429–438.

Castle, W. B., 1929, Observations on the etiological relationship of achylia gastrica and pernicious anemia, *Am. J. Med. Sci.* **178:**748–764.

Chanarin, I., 1972, Pernicious anemia as an autoimmune disease, *Br. J. Haematol. Suppl.* **23:**101–107.

Chanarin, I., and James, D., 1974, Humoral and cell-mediated intrinsic-factor antibody in pernicious anemia, *Lancet* **1**:1078–1080.

Charache, P., Hodkinson, B. A., Lambiotte, B., and McIntyre, P. A., 1968, Genetic and autoimmune features of pernicious anemia, *Johns Hopkins Med. J.* **122**:184–195.

Clinicopathological Conference, 1965, A case of primary acquired hypogammaglobulinemia with pernicious anemia and amyloidosis, *Br. Med. J.* **1**:35–38.

Coghill, N. F., 1960, The significance of gastritis, *Postgrad. Med. J.* **36**:733–742.

Cooper, M., and Lipkin, M., 1973, Growth and development of normal and diseased gastrointestinal cells, *Digestion* **8**:191–200.

Cowling, D. C., Strickland, R. G., Ungar, B., Whillingham, S., and Rose, W. McI., 1974, Pernicious anemia like syndrome with immunoglobulin deficiency, *Med. J. Aust.* **1**:15–17.

Cruze, K., Clarke, J. S., and Elfarra, S., 1961, Familial aspects of gastric adenocarcinoma: Report of 13 families, *Am. J. Digest. Dis.* **6**:7–10.

Dauphinee, M. J., and Talal, N., 1975, Reversible restoration by thymosin of antigen-induced depression of spleen DNA synthesis in NZB mice, *J. Immunol.* **114**:1713–1716.

David, J. R., 1966, Delayed hyposensitivity *in vitro:* Its mediation by cell free substances formed by lymphoid cell-antigen interaction, *Proc. Natl. Acad. Sci. USA* **56**:72–77.

Davidsohn, I., Kovarik, S., and Chang, L. L., 1966, A, B, and O substances in gastrointestinal carcinoma, *Arch. Pathol.* **81**:381–390.

Denk, H., Tappeiner, G., Davidovits, A., and Eckerstorfer Rand Holzner, J. H., 1974, Carcinoembryonic antigen and blood group substances in carcinoma of the stomach and colon, *J. Natl. Cancer Inst.* **53**:933–942.

Doniach, D., and Roitt, I. M., 1964, An evaluation of gastric and thyroid autoimmunity in relation to hematologic disorders, *Sem. Hematol.* **1**:313–343.

Douglas, S. D., Goldberg, L. S., Fudenberg, H. H., and Goldberg, S. B., 1970, Agammaglobulinemia and co-existent pernicious anemia, *Clin. Exp. Immunol.* **6**:181–187.

Fenwick, S., 1870, On atrophy of the stomach, *Lancet* **2**:78–80.

Finlayson, N. D. C., Fanconnet, M. H., and Krohn, K., 1972, *In vitro* demonstration of delayed hypersensitivity to gastric antigens in pernicious anemia, *Am. J. Digest. Dis.* **17**:631–638.

Fisher, J. M., and Taylor, K. B., 1965, Comparison of autoimmune phenomena in pernicious anemia and chronic atrophic gastritis, *N. Eng. J. Med.* **272**:499–503.

Fisher, J. M., Rees, C., and Taylor, K. B., 1965, Antibodies in gastric juice, *Science* **150**:1467–1469.

Fixa, B., and Thiele, H. G., 1969, Delayed hypersensitivity to intrinsic factor in patients with pernicious anemia, *Med. Exp.* **19**:231–239.

Fixa, B., Komarkova, O., Vejbora, O., Langr, F., and Brzek, V., 1970, Transfer of experimental gastric lesions in dogs by means of thoracic duct cells, *Sborn. ved. Praci lek. Fak. Hradci Kralove Suppl.* **13**:169–174.

Foroozan, P., and Trier, J. S., 1967, Mucosa of the small intestine in pernicious anemia, *N. Eng. J. Med.* **277**:553–557.

Forssman, O., and Homer, B., 1964, Acquired agammaglobulinemia and malabsorption, *Acta Med. Scand.* **176**:779–786.

Frazer, K. J., 1969, Multiple myeloma and pernicious anemia, *Med. J. Aust.* **1**:298–299.

Gefro, P. L., Krupey, J., and Hansen, H. H., 1971, Demonstration of an antigen common to several varieties of neoplasia, *N. Eng. J. Med.* **285**:138–141.

Geha, R. S., Schneeberger, E., Merler, E., and Rosen, F. S., 1974, Heterogenicity of "acquired" or common variable agammaglobulinemia, *N. Eng. J. Med.* **291**:1–6.

Gelfand, E. W., Berkel, A. L., Godwin, H. A., Rocklin, R. E., David, J. R., and Rosen, F. S., 1972, Pernicious anemia, hypogammaglobulinemia and altered lymphocyte reactivity, *Clin. Exp. Immunol.* **11**:187–199.

Ginsberg, A., and Mullinax, F., 1970, Pernicious anemia and monoclonal gammopathy in a patient with IgA deficiency, *Am. J. Med.* **48**:787–791.

Glass, G. B. J., 1963, Gastric intrinsic factor and its function in the metabolism of vitamin B_{12}, *Physiol. Rev.* **43**:529–849.

Glynn, L. E., Holborow, E. J., and Johnson, G. D., 1957, The distribution of blood-group substances in human gastric and duodenal mucosa, *Lancet* **2**:1083–1088.

Gold, P., and Freedman, S. O., 1965, Specific carcinoembryonic antigens of the human digestive system, *J. Exp. Med.* **122**:467–481.

Goldberg, L. S., and Bluestone, R., 1970, Hidden gastric autoantibodies to intrinsic factor in pernicious anemia, *J. Lab. Clin. Med.* **75**:449–456.

Goldberg, L. S., Barnett, E. V., and Desai, R., 1967, Effect of transplacental transfer of antibody to intrinsic factor, *Pediatrics* **40**:851–855.

Goldberg, L. S., Shuster, J., Stuckey, M., and Fudenberg, H. H., 1968, Secretory immunoglobulin A: Autoantibody activity in gastric juice, *Science* **160**:1240–1241.

Goldberg, L. S., Samloff, I. M., and Barnett, E. V., 1969, Studies on the antigenic structure of human and hog intrinsic factors, *Clin. Exp. Immunol.* **5**:371–379.

Goldberg, L. S., Cunningham, J. E., and Terasaki, P., 1972, Lymphocytotoxins and pernicious anemia, *Blood* **39**:862–873.

Goldstone, A. H., Calder, E. A., Barnes, E. W., and Irvine, W. J., 1973, The effect of gastric antigens on the *in vitro* migration of leukocytes from patients with atrophic gastritis and pernicious anemia, *Clin. Exp. Immunol.* **14**:501–508.

Hakkinen, I. P. T., 1974, Gastric fetal sulphoglycoprotein antigen (FSA) and blood group antigens A and B, *Int. Arch. Allergy* **47**:380–387.

Hauseman, T. U., Halcrow, D. A., and Taylor, K. B., 1969, Biological effects of gastrointestinal antibodies, *Gastroenterology* **56**:1062–1070.

Heath, R. B., Farley, G. H., and Malpas, J. S., 1964, Production of antibodies against viruses in leukemia and related diseases, *Br. J. Haematol.* **10**:365–370.

Hennes, A. R., Sevelins, H., Lewellyn, T., Walter, J., Wood, A. H., and Wolf, S., 1962, Atrophic gastritis in dogs, *Arch. Pathol.* **73**:281–287.

Herbert, V., 1967, Immunologic factors in pernicious anemia, *Postgrad. Med.* **42**:298–301.

Hermans, P. E., and Huizenga, K. A., 1972, Association of gastric carcinoma with idiopathic late-onset immunoglobulin deficiency *Ann. Intern. Med.* **76**:605–609.

Hermans, P. E., Huizenga, K. A., Hoffman, H. N., Brown, A. L., and Markowitz, H., 1966, Dysgammglobulinemia associated with nodular lymphoid hyperplasia of the small intestine, *Am. J. Med.* **40**:78–89.

Higgs, J. M., and Wells, R. S., 1972, Chronic mucocutaneous candidiasis: Associated abnormalities of iron metabolism, *Br. J. Dermatol.* **86**:88–102 (Suppl. 8).

Hines, J. D., Hoffbrand, A. V., and Mollin, D. L., 1967, The hematologic complications following partial gastrectomy, *Am. J. Med.* **43**:555–569.

Hippe, E., and Jensen, K. B., 1969, Hereditary factors in pernicious anemia and their relation to serum immunoglobulin levels, *Lancet* **2**:721–722.

Hoffbrand, A. V., Hobbs, J. R., and Kremenchusky, S., 1967, Incidence and pathogenesis of megaloblastic erythropoiesis in multiple myeloma, *J. Clin. Pathol.* **20**:699–705.

Hooper, B., Whittingham, S., Mathews, J. D., Mackray, I. R., and Curnow, D. H., 1972, Autoimmunity in a rural community, *Clin. Exp. Immunol.* **12**:79–87.

Hoskins, L. C., Winawer, S. J., Broitman, S. A., Gottlieb, L. S., and Zamcheck, N., 1967, Clinical giardiasis and intestinal malabsorption, *Gastroenterology* **53**:265–271.

Howitz, J., and Schwartz, M., 1971, Viteligo, achlorhydria and pernicious anemia, *Lancet* **1**:1331–1334.

Hughes, W. S., Cerda, J. J., Holtzapple, P., and Brooks, F. P., 1971, Primary hypogammglobulinemia and malabsorption, *Ann. Intern. Med.* **74**:903–910.

Hughes, W. S., Brooks, F. P., and Conn, H. O., 1972, Serum gastrin levels in primary hypogammaglobulinemia and pernicious anemia, *Ann. Intern. Med.* **77**:746–750.

Huizenga, K. A., Wollaeger, E. G., and Green, P. A., 1961, Serum globulin deficiencies in non-tropical sprue with report of two cases of acquired agammaglobulinemia, *Am. J. Med.* **31**:572–580.

Irvine, W. J., 1965, Immunologic aspects of pernicious anemia, *N. Eng. J. Med.* **273**:432–438.

Irvine, W. J., Davies, S. H., Delamore, I. W., and Williams, A. W., 1962, Immunological relationship between pernicious anemia and thyroid disease, *Br. Med. J.* **2**:454–456.

Irvine, W. J., Stewart, A. G., and Searth, L., 1967, A clinical and immunological study of adrenocortical insufficiency (Addison's disease), *Clin. Exp. Immunol.* **2**:31–69.

Irvine, W. J., Clarke, B. F., Scarth, L., Cullen, D. R., and Duncan, L. J. P., 1970, Thyroid and gastric autoimmunity in patients with diabetes mellitus, *Lancet* **2**:163–168.

James, D., Asherton, G., Chanarin, I., Coghill, N., Hamilton, S., Himsworth, R. L., and Webster, D., 1974, Cell-mediated immunity to intrinsic factor in autoimmune disorders, *Br. J. Med.* **4**:494–496.

Jeffries, G. H., 1965, Recovery of gastric mucosal structure and function in pernicious anemia during predisolone therapy, *Gastroenterology* **48:**371–378.

Jeffries, G. H., and Sleisenger, M. H., 1965, Studies of parietal cell antibody in pernicious anemia, *J. Clin. Invest.* **44:**2021–2028.

Kabat, E. A., Bendich, A., Bezer, A. E., and Beiser, M., 1947, Immunochemical studies on blood groups, *J. Exp. Med.* **85:**685–699.

Kaplan, H. S., and Regler, L. G., 1945, Pernicious anemia and carcinoma of the stomach—Autopsy studies concerning their interrelationship, *Am. J. Med. Sci.* **209:**339–348.

Kerby, G. R., 1968, Correlation of tuberculin skin reaction with *in vitro* lymphocyte transformation, *Am. Rev. Resp. Dis.* **97:**904–908.

Kirkpatrick, C. H., Rich, R. R., and Bennett, J. E., 1971, Chronic mucocutaneous candidiasis: Model-building in cellular immunity, *Ann. Intern. Med.* **74:**955–978.

Kopp, W. L., Trier, J. S., Stiehm, R., and Foroozan, P., 1968, "Acquired" agammaglobulinemia with defective delayed hypersensitivity, *Ann. Intern. Med.* **69:**309–317.

Krain, L. S., 1973, Why is pancreatic cancer incidence up; stomach cancer down? *Geriatrics* **28(4):**140.

Krolin, K. J. E., and Finlayson, N. D. C., 1973, Interrelations of humoral and cellular immune responses in experimental canine gastritis, *Clin. Exp. Immunol.* **14:**237–245.

Larsson, S. O., 1962, Myeloma and pernicious anemia, *Acta Med. Scand.* **172:**195–205.

Larsson, S. O., Hagelquist, E., and Coster, C., 1961, Hypogammaglobulinemia and pernicious anemia, *Acta Haematol.* **26:**50–62.

LeCompte, P. M., Steinke, J., Soeldner, J. S., and Renold, A. E., 1966, Changes in the islets of Langerhans in cows injected with heterologous homologous insulin, *Diabetes* **15**:586–596.

Lee, F. I., Jenkins, G. C., Hughes, D. T. D., and Kazentis, G., 1964, Pernicious anemia, myxedema and hypogammglobulinemia—A family study, *Br. Med. J.* **1**:598–602.

Lehner, T., Wilton, J. M. A., and Ivanyi, L., 1972, Immunodeficiencies in chronic mucocutaneous candidiasis, *Immunology* **22:**775–787.

Levine, S. A., and Ladd, W. S., 1921, Pernicious anemia: A clinical study of one hundred and fifty consecutive cases with special reference to gastric anacidity, *Bull. Johns Hopkins Hosp.* **32:**254–267.

Lipkin, M., 1973, Proliferation and differentiation of gastrointestinal cells, *Physiol. Rev.* **53:**891–915.

Luderitz, O., Staub, A. M., and Westphal, O., 1966, Immunochemistry of O and R antigens of *Salmonella* and related Enterobacteriaceae, *Bacteriol. Rev.* **30:**192–255.

Lupulescu, A., Pop, A., Merculiev, E., Neascu, C., and Heithmanek, C., 1965, Experimental iso-immune hypoparathyroidism in rats, *Nature (London)* **206:**415–418.

MacCuish, A. C., Urbaniak, S. J., Goldstone, A. H., and Irvine, W. J., 1974. PHA responsiveness and subpopulations of circulating lymphocytes in pernicious anemia, *Blood* **44:**849–855.

Mancini, A. M., Constanzi, G., and Zampa, G. A., 1964, Human insulin antibodies detected by immunofluorescent technique, *Lancet* **1**:726.

Manigand, G., Seligman, M., Foulon, D., Perrigot, M., Allard, C., and Deparis, M., 1974, Hypogammaglobulinemia primative et anemia de Biermer, *Nouv. Presse Med.* **3**:2087–2090.

McConnell, R. B., 1966, The stomach, in: *The Genetics of Gastrointestinal Disorders,* pp. 46–75, Oxford University Press, London.

McGuigan, J. E., and Trudeau, W. L., 1970, Serum gastrin concentrations in pernicious anemia, *N. Eng. J. Med.* **282:**358–361.

McIntyre, P. A., Hahn, R., Conley, C. L., and Glass, B., 1959, Genetic factors in predisposition to pernicious anemia, *Bull. Johns Hopkins Hosp.* **104:**130–142.

McMaster, P. R. B., and Lerner, E. M., 1967, The transfer of allergic thyroiditis in histocompatible guinea pigs by lymph node cells, *J. Immunol.* **99:**208–214.

Miller, D. R., Bloom, G. E., Streiff, R. R., LoBuglio, A. F., and Diamond, L. K., 1966, Juvenile "congenital" pernicious anemia, *N. Eng. J. Med.* **275:**978–983.

Montplasir, S., Rabin, B., Pelletier, M., Rose, N. R., and Alpert, E., 1973, Alpha$_1$-fetoprotein content of gastric carcinoma and hepatic metastases, *Am. J. Digest. Dis.* **18:**416–418.

Morgan, W. T. J., 1970, Molecular aspects of human blood-group specificity, *Ann. N.Y. Acad. Sci.* **169:**118–130.

Morse, W. I., Cochrane, W. A., and Landrigan, P. L., 1961, Familial hypoparathyroidism with pernicious anemia, steatorrhea, and adrenocortical insufficiency; a variant of mucoviscidosis, *N. Eng. J. Med.* **264:**1021–1024.

Munichoodappa, C., and Kozak, G. P., 1970, Diabetes mellitus and pernicious anemia, *Diabetes* **19:**719–723.

Nakamura, R. M., and Weigle, W. O., 1969, Transfer of experimental autoimmune thyroiditis by serum from thyroidectomized donors, *J. Exp. Med.* **130:**263–281.

Nerup, J., Anderson, V., and Bendixen, G., 1969, Antiadrenal cellular hypersensitivity in Addison's disease, *Clin. Exp. Immunol.* **5:**357–364.

Nerup, J., Anderson, O. O., Bendixen, G., Egeberg, J., and Poulsen, J. E., 1971, Antipancreatic cellular hypersensitivity in diabetes mellitus, *Diabetes* **20:**424–427.

Nordenson, N. G., 1966, Myelomatosis: A clinical review of 310 cases, *Acta Med. Scand.* **179:**178–186 (Suppl. 445).

Ochs, H. D., Ament, M. E., and Davis, S. D., 1975, Structure and function of the gastrointestinal tract in primary immunodeficiency syndromes and in granulocyte dysfunction, *Birth Defects: Orig. Art. Ser.* **11:**199–207.

Odgers, R. J., and Wangel, A. G., 1968, Abnormalities in IgA-containing mononuclear cells in the gastric lesion of pernicious anemia, *Lancet* **2:**846–849.

Olin, R., and Poindexter, M. H., 1972, Familial idiopathic hypoparathyroidism, *Minn. Med.* **55:**701–704.

Penhale, W. J., Farmer, A., and Irvine, W. J., 1975, Thyroiditis in T-cell depleted rats, *Clin. Exp. Immunol.* **21:**362–375.

Pirofsky, B., and Vaughn, M., 1968, Addisonian pernicious anemia with positive antiglobulin tests, *Am. J. Clin. Pathol.* **50:**459–466.

Quie, P. G., and Chilgren, R. A., 1971, Acute disseminated and chronic mucocutaneous candidiasis, *Sem. Hematol.* **8:**227–242.

Ramsey, C., and Herbert, V., 1965, Dialysis assay for intrinsic factor: Demonstration of species specificity of antibodies to human and hog intrinsic factor, *J. Lab. Clin. Med.* **65:**143–152.

Richens, E. R., Irvine, W. J., Williams, M. J., Hartog, M., and Ancill, R. J., 1974, Cellular hypersensitivity to mitochondrial antigens in diabetes mellitus and its relationship to the presence of circulating autoantibodies, *Clin. Exp. Immunol.* **17:**71–75.

Roitt, I. M., Ling, N. G., Doniach, D., and Conchman, K. G., 1964, The cytoplasmic autoantigen of the human thyroid: Immunological and biochemical characterization, *Immunology* **7:**375–393.

Rose, M. S., and Chanarin, I., 1969, Dissociation of intrinsic factor from its antibody: Application to study pernicious anemia gastric juice specimens, *Br. Med. J.* **1:**468–470.

Rose, M. S., and Chanarin, I., 1971, Intrinsic-factor antibody and absorption of vitamin B_{12} in pernicious anemia, *Br. Med. J.* **1:**25–26.

Salupere, V., Nutt, H., and Jarve, E., 1972, Lymphocyte blast-transformation test *in vitro* in cases of chronic gastritis, *Scand. J. Gastroenterol.* **7:**215–218.

Schade, S. G., Feick, P., Muckerliede, M., and Schilling, R. F., 1966, Occurrence in gastric juice of antibody to a complex of intrinsic factor and vitamin B_{12}, *N. Eng. J. Med.* **275:**528–531.

Schiff, F., and Sasaki, H., 1932, Ueber die Vererbung das serologischen Ausscheidungstypus, *Ztschr. Immunitatsforsch.* **77:**129–139.

Schwartz, M., 1958, Intrinsic factor inhibiting substance in serum of orally treated patients with pernicious anemia, *Lancet* **2:**61–62.

Scott, E., 1960, Prevalence of pernicious anemia in Great Britain, *J. Coll. Gen. Pract.* **3:**80–84.

Selroos, O., and von Knorring, J., 1973, Immunoglobulins in pernicious anemia, *Acta Med. Scand.* **194:**571–574.

Sheahan, D. G., Horowitz, S. A., and Zamchek, N., 1971, Deletion of epithelial ABH isoantigens in primary gastric neoplasms and in metastatic cancer, *Am. J. Digest. Dis.* **16:**961–969.

Shulman, S., Centeno, E., Milgrom, F., and Witebsky, E., 1965, Immunological studies on adrenal glands, *Immunology* **8:**531–588.

Simons, D. A. R., 1971, Immunochemistry of *Shigella flexneri* O antigens, *Bacteriol. Rev.* **35:**117–148.

Simons, D. A. R., and Perlmann, P., 1973, Carcinoembryonic antigen and blood group substances, *Cancer Res.* **33:**313–322.

Siurala, M., Varis, K., and Wiljasalo, M., 1966, Studies on patients with atrophic gastritis: A 10–15 year follow-up, *Scand. J. Gastroenterol.* **1:**40–48.

Siurala, M., Isokoski, M., Varis, K., and Kekki, M., 1968, Prevalence of gastritis in a rural population, *Scand. J. Gastroenterol.* **3:**211–223.

Strickland, R. G., and Mackay, I. R., 1973, A reappraisal of the nature and significance of chronic atrophic gastritis, *Am. J. Digest. Dis.* **18:**426–440.

Strickland, R. G., Baur, S., Ashworth, A. E., and Taylor, K. B., 1971, A correlative study of immunological phenomena in pernicious anemia, *Clin. Exp. Immunol.* **8:**25–36.

Stutman, O., 1972, Lymphocyte subpopulations in NZB mice: Deficit of thymus dependent lymphocytes, *J. Immunol.* **109:**602–611.

Szulman, A. E., 1960, The histological distribution of blood group substances A and B in man, *J. Exp. Med.* **111:**785–800.

Tai, C., and McGuigan, J. E., 1969, Immunologic studies in pernicious anemia, *Blood* **34:**63–71.

Talal, N. J., and Steinberg, A. D., 1974, The pathogenesis of autoimmunity in New Zealand black mice, *Current Topics Microbiol. Immunol.* **64:**79–103.

Tanaka, N., and Jerzy Glass, G. B., 1970, Effect of prolonged administration of parietal cell antibodies from patients with atrophic gastritis and pernicious anemia on the parietal cell mass and hydrochloric acid output in rats, *Gastroenterology* **58:**482–494.

Taylor, K. B., 1959, Inhibition of intrinsic factor by pernicious anemia serum, *Lancet* **2:**106–108.

Taylor, K. B., Roitt, I. M., Doniach, D., Conchman, K. G., and Shapland, C., 1962, Autoimmune phenomena in pernicious anemia: Gastric autoantibodies, *Br. Med. J.* **2:**1347–1352.

TeVelde, K., Abels, J., Anders, G. J., Arends, P. A., Hoedemaeker, P. J., and Nieweg, H. O., 1964, A family study of pernicious anemia by an immunologic method, *J. Lab. Clin. Med.* **64:**177–187.

Tormey, D. C., Kamin, R., and Fudenberg, H. H., 1967, Quantiative studies to phytohemagglutinin-induced DNA and RNA synthesis in normal and agammaglobulinemic leukocytes, *J. Exp. Med.* **125:**863–872.

Twomey, J. J., 1971, Gastric secretory and serologic studies on patients with neoplastic and immunologic disorders, *Arch. Intern. Med.* **128:**746–749.

Twomey, J. J., 1975, An immunologic classification of pernicious anemia, *Birth Defects: Orig. Art. Ser.* **11:**215–218.

Twomey, J. J., and Douglass, C. C., 1974, An *in vitro* study of lymphocyte and macrophage function with lymphoproliferative neoplasms, *Cancer* **33:**1034–1038.

Twomey, J. J., Jordan, P. H., Jarrold, T., Ritz, N. D., and Conn, H. O., 1969, The syndrome of immunoglobulin deficiency and pernicious anemia, *Am. J. Med.* **47:**340–350

Twomey, J. J., Jordan, P. H., Laughter, A. H., Neuwissen, H. J., and Good, R. A., 1970, The gastric disorder in immunoglobulin deficient patients, *Ann. Intern. Med.* **72:**499–504.

Twomey, J. J., Laughter, A. H., Villanueva, N. D., Kao, Y. S., Lidsky, M. D., and Jordan, P. H., 1971*a,* Gastric secretory and serologic studies on patients with neoplastic and immunologic disorders, *Arch. Intern. Med.* **128:**746–749.

Twomey, J. J., Laughter, A. H., and Jordan, P. H., 1971*b,* Studies into human IF secretion, *Am. J. Digest. Dis.* **16:**1075–1081.

Twomey, J. J., Villanueva, N. D., Laughter, A. H., Danna, S. T., Hyanie, T. P., and Jahns, M. F., 1972, Daily requirements and physiological efficiency of intrinsic factor in man, *Acta Haematol.* **48:**65–71.

Twomey, J. J., Waddell, C. C., Krantz, S., O'Reilly, R., L'Esperance, P., and Good, R. A., 1975, Chronic mucocutaneous candidiasis with macrophage dysfunction, a plasma inhibitor and coexistent pernicious anemia, *J. Lab. Clin. Med.* **85:**968–977.

Ungar, B., Stocks, A. E., Martin, F. I. R., Whittingham, S., and Mackay, I. R., 1968, Intrinsic factor antibody, parietal cell antibody and latent pernicious anemia in diabetes mellitus, *Lancet* **2:**415–418.

Ungar, B., Strickland, R. G., and Francis, C. M., 1971, The prevalence and significance of circulating antibodies to gastric intrinsic factor and parietal cell in gastric carcinoma, *Gut* **12:**903–905.

Walder, A. I., 1968, Experimental achlorhydria: Techniques of production with parietal cell antibody, *Surgery* **64:**175–184.

Waldmann, T. A., Durm, M., Broder, S., Blackman, M., Blaese, R. M., and Strober, W., 1974, Role of suppressor T cells in pathogenesis of common variable hypogammaglobulinemia, *Lancet* **2:**609–613.

Wall, J. R., Good, B. F., Forbes, I. J., and Hetzel, B. S., 1973, Demonstration of the production of the long acting thyroid activator (LATS) by peripheral lymphocytes cultured *in vitro, Clin. Exp. Immunol.* **14:**555-561.

Weisbart, R. H., Cunningham, J. E., Bluestone, R., and Goldberg, L. E., 1973, A modified agarose method for detection of migration inhibitory factor and delineation of its antigenic dependency, *Int. Arch. Allergy Appl. Immunol.* **45:**612–619.

Weisbart, R. H., Bluestone, R., and Goldberg, L. S., 1975, Cellular immunity to intrinsic factor in pernicious anemia, *J. Lab. Clin. Med.* **85:**87–92.

Wick, G., Kite, J. H., and Witebsky, E., 1970, Spontaneous thyroiditis in the obese strain of chickens, *J. Immunol.* **104:**54–62.

Winawer, S. J., and Lipkin, M., 1969, Cell prlliferation kinetics in the gastrointestinal tract of man. IV. Cell renewal in the intestinalized gastric mucosa, *J. Natl. Cancer Inst.* **42:**9–17.

Wintrobe, M. M., 1961, in: *Clinical Hematology,* p. 468, Lea and Febiger, Philadelphia.

Witebsky, E., and Milgrom, F., 1962, Immunological studies on adrenal glands, *Immunology* **5:**67–78.

Witebsky, E., and Rose, N. R., 1956, Studies on organ specificity. IV. Production of rabbit thyroid antibodies in the rabbit, *J. Immunol.* **74:**408.

Wood, I. J., Ralston, M., Ungar, B., and Cowling, D. C., 1964, Vitamin B_{12} deficiency in chronic gastritis, *Gut* **5:**27–37.

Wuepper, K. D., and Fudenberg, H. H., 1967, Moniliasis, "autoimmune" polyenocrinopathy and immunologic family study, *Clin. Exp. Immunol.* **2:**71–82.

Zamcheck, N., Grable, E., Ley, A., and Norman, L., 1955, Occurrence of gastrointestinal cancer among patients with pernicious anemia at the Boston City Hospital, *N. Eng. J. Med.* **252:**1103–1110.

Zittoun, R., Zittoun, J., Seignalet, J., and Dausset, J., 1975, HL-A and pernicious anemia, *N. Eng. J. Med.* **293:**1324.

6

The Digestive Form of α-Chain Disease

Maxime Seligmann and Jean-Claude Rambaud

1. Introduction

Alpha-chain disease (α-CD) is a proliferative disorder of B-lymphoid cells involving primarily the IgA secretory system, in which plasma cells produce a presumably homogeneous population of immunoglobulin molecules consisting of incomplete α chains devoid of light chains. Since the first description of this new immunoglobulin abnormality (Seligmann *et al.*, 1968) in a young Syrian patient affected with malabsorption and diffuse plasmacytic infiltration of the small intestine (Rambaud *et al.*, 1968), more than 100 cases have been recognized to our knowledge. Alpha-chain disease is thus the most frequent of the heavy-chain diseases. In three of these patients α-CD was apparently confined to the respiratory tract (Stoop *et al.*, 1971; Faux *et al.*, 1973; Florin-Christensen *et al.*, 1974). All the other patients were affected with the digestive form of α-CD, which is mainly localized in the small intestine and the mesenteric lymph nodes.

There appears to be an early "premalignant" stage of the digestive form of α-chain disease which progresses to a fatal malignancy. The frequency of this disease among populations exposed to conditions of poor hygiene and the evidence for complete remissions induced in early stage by oral antibiotic therapy implicate environmental factors in the pathogenesis of the disorder, which may serve as a model offering unique opportunities for research into the oncogenesis of human lymphomas.

Maxime Seligmann • Laboratory of Immunochemistry and Immunopathology (INSERM U 108), Research Institute on Blood Diseases, Hôpital Saint-Louis, Paris 10, France. ***Jean-Claude Rambaud*** • Department of Gastroenterology and Research Unit on Physiopathology of Digestion (INSERM U 54), Hôpital Saint-Lazare, Paris, 10, France.

Table 1. Geographical Origin of 97 Patients with α-Chain Disease

Africa		South and Central America	
Tunisia	19	Colombia	1
Algeria	18	North Argentina	1
South Africa	2	Mexico	1
Morocco	1	Europe	
Middle East		Spain	8
Iran	10	South Italy	5
Israel	8	Turkey	5
Lebanon	2	Yugoslavia	2
Syria	1	Greece	2
Libya	1	Portugal	1
Iraq	1	Finland	1
Far East		Netherlands	1[a]
Pakistan	2	Great Britain	1[a]
Cambodia	1	North America	
India	1	United States	1[a]

[a]Respiratory form.

2. Epidemiology

The age distribution of α-CD is in sharp contrast to that of multiple myeloma and of intestinal lymphoma occurring in Western Europe, since the great majority of patients affected with α-CD are between 10 and 30 years old (Seligmann, 1975*a*). The sex distribution shows a moderate prevalence of males, with a 3:2 ratio (Seligmann, 1975*a*).

The geographical origins of 97 patients affected with α-CD, diagnosed or confirmed in our laboratory in the vast majority of cases, are listed in Table 1. Although early reports of α-CD concerned mainly patients living in the Mediterranean region, there now appears to be a wide spectrum of racial and ethnic origins and cases have now been described in many parts of the world. Two cases have recently been recognized in Central Africa. It should be emphasized that the three patients from the Netherlands, Great Britain, and the United States were those with a respiratory form of the disease and without detectable intestinal involvement. The digestive form of the disease appears to be extremely rare in Western "developed" nations. Most patients originated from and had been living in areas with a high degree of infestation by intestinal microorganisms and were exposed to conditions of poor hygiene in low socioeconomic circumstances.

There appears to be no strong predilection for cases to cluster in families. No clear immunoglobulin abnormalities have been found in a limited number of sera from close relatives of patients (Seligmann *et al.*, 1971; Ramot and Hulu, 1975; Lewin *et al.*, 1976).

3. *Clinical Features*

The clinical features of intestinal α-chain disease are markedly uniform (Tables 2 and 3). The disease is usually revealed by severe malabsorption syndrome. Its onset may be either progressive or abrupt. In most cases, the first and main symptom all along the course of the disease is chronic diarrhea. Steatorrhea is usually obvious, but stools not rarely appear watery and sometimes are very copious. Patients complain of abdominal pains of variable intensity and localization, and vomiting is frequent. Several patients first experienced localized, acute pains and vomiting, and some were operated on with the diagnosis of appendicitis or acute pancreatitis. Time elapsed between the first symptom and diagnosis ranged from 1 month to 6 years. In some cases (Bognel *et al.*, 1972; Bonomo *et al.*, 1972) the usual clinical patient of α-CD was preceded by a protracted prodromic period with symptoms simulating the irritable colon syndrome.

The abdomen is usually distended and tender, and some ascitic fluid may be present. Hypertrophied mesenteric lymph nodes may be palpated as abdominal masses. Signs of chronic small bowel obstruction with or without palpable abdominal mass(es), and/or surgical emergencies such as intestinal intussusception or perforation or epiploic infarction, may reveal the disease (Bonomo *et al.*, 1972; unpublished data, 1975), but these "tumoral" symptoms are more often observed in the later stages of evolution. It should be em-

Table 2. Main Clinical Findings in 34 Cases of α-CD[a]

Chronic diarrhea		100%
With overt steatorrhea	47%	
Watery appearance	24%	
Type not determined	29%	
Abdominal pains		93%
Diffuse	38%	
Epigastric	16%	
Periumbilical	6%	
Right sided	6%	
Site unknown	34%	
Vomiting		41%
Fever		21%
Loss of weight		97%
Edema		24%
Tetany		38%
Finger clubbing		47%
Abdominal mass(es)		24%
Ascites		12%

[a]Including cases referenced in the text and cases reported by Irunberry *et al.* (1970), Zlotnick and Levy (1971), Bernadou *et al.* (1972), Guardia *et al.* (1972), Henry *et al.* (1974), Metrass *et al.* (1974), Pittman *et al.* (1975), Shahid *et al.* (1975), and personal unpublished cases.

Table 3. Main Laboratory and Radiological Findings Related to the Intestinal Involvement in 34 Cases of α-CD[a]

Biology	
Hemoglobin	
10–13 g/100 ml	54% (28)
<10 g/100 ml	14% (28)
Serum potassium <3.5 mEq/liter	55% (20)
Serum albumin	
25–35 g/liter	46% (28)
<25 g/liter	46% (28)
Serum cholesterol <0.15 g/100 ml	89% (19)
Serum calcium <9.0 mg/100 ml	71% (28)
Raised serum alkaline phosphatase	81% (21)
Fecal fats (24-hr output)	
<6 g	5% (22)
6–15 g	45% (22)
>15 g	50% (22)
Abnormal D-xylose test	83% (18)
Abnormal oral glucose tolerance test	93% (13)
Abnormal Schilling test	56% (9)
Protein-losing enteropathy	71% (7)
Small intestinal X-rays	
Hypertrophic folds ("pseudopolypoid" pattern)	86% (28)
Strictures and/or defects	43% (28)
Intestinal bacteriology and parasitology	
Jejunal fluid bacteria overgrowth	80% (5)
Stool and/or jejunal fluid parasites	
Giardia lamblia	24% (34)
Ascaris	3% (34)
Hookworm	3% (34)
Trichuris trichuria	3% (34)
Coccidia	3% (34)
Schistosoma mansoni	3% (34)

[a]Numbers in parentheses indicate the number of cases where data are available.

phasized that hepatosplenomegaly is usually not observed and that peripheral lymphadenopathy is a very rare sign at presentation. Nasopharyngeal, gastric, and rectal localizations of the lymphoid proliferation have occasionally been described.

Finger clubbing appears more frequent than in any other intestinal disease. Fever is uncommon. Asthenia and loss of weight, often rapid and massive, are consistently observed. Severe protein malnutrition may be evidenced by edema, alopecia, and amenorrhea.

Low serum albumin level and creatorrhea are nearly constant features, and search for protein-losing enteropathy is usually positive. Dehydration and electrolyte imbalance may require emergency intravenous fluid replacement. The severity of diarrhea has on occasions led to hypokalemic nephropathy with polyuria. Tetany is frequently observed and may be the major presenting symptom. Hypocalcemia, often deep, is secondary to magnesium deficiency rather than to vitamin D deficiency (Dent *et al.*, 1968; Rambaud *et al.*, 1976). Hemorrhagic syndrome and overt osteomalacia are absent. The frequent high level of serum alkaline phosphatase is usually accounted for by the increase in intestinal isoenzyme (Doe *et al.*, 1972). Anemia of variable type, with low iron, folate, and/or B12 serum level, remains mild or moderate. Total serum lipids and cholesterol are low, even in the frequent eventuality of mild steatorrhea. Xylose, glucose, and folic acid oral tests are usually but not always

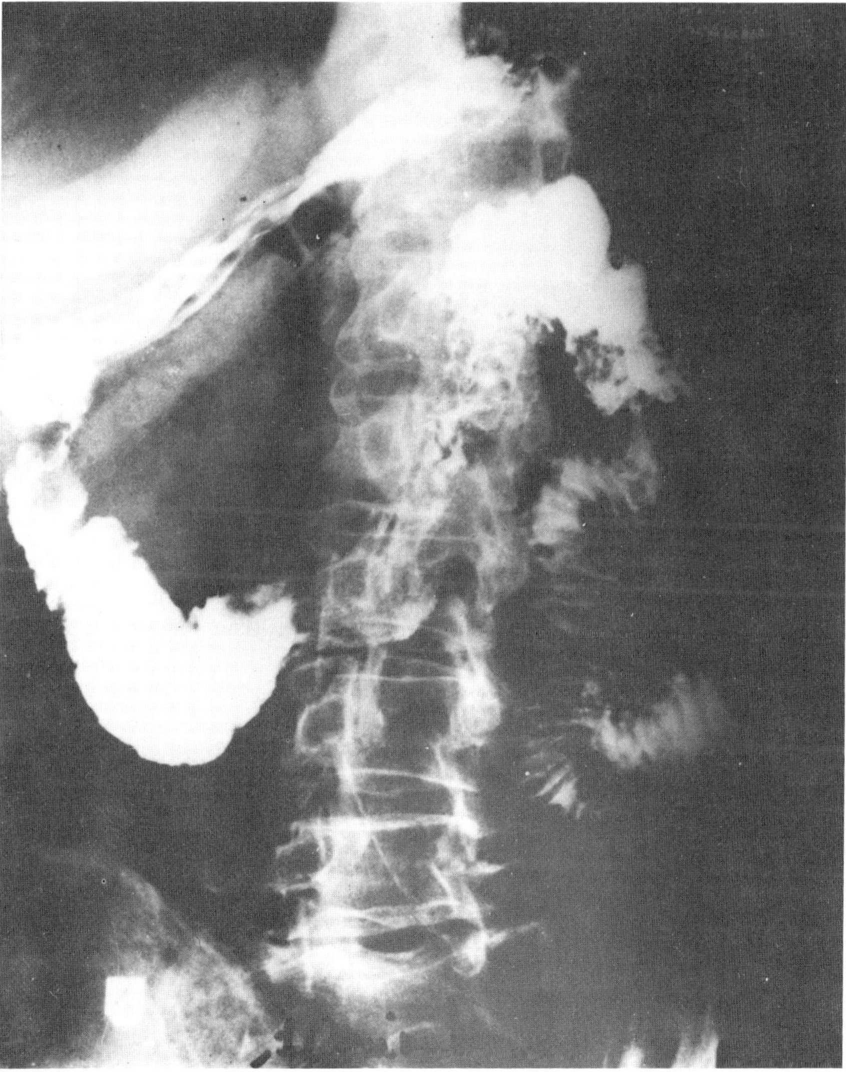

Fig. 1. Barium meal in a patient with α-CD. Note the enlarging of the duodenal loop, the narrowing of D2, and the hypertrophy of duodenal and proximal jejunal folds.

abnormal, and Schilling test with intrinsic factor is low in nearly two-thirds of cases.

Small intestine X rays, with a thin and nonflocculable barium, show very hypertrophic and pseudopolypoid mucosal folds in duodenum and jejunum sometimes associated with stricture or defect areas, suggesting extrinsic compression by hypertrophic peripancreatic and/or mesenteric lymph nodes (Fig. 1). Mediastinal adenopathy is usually not observed. Abdominal lymphangiography may reveal an involvement of the retroperitoneal lymph nodes. Radiological features of osteomalacia are absent, and skeletal surveys do not show any evidence of osteolytic lesions.

Limited bacteriological studies of stools have not revealed any consistent pathogens. In several patients overgrowth of aerobes and anaerobes has been demonstrated in jejunal fluid, often associated with bile salt deconjugation and high indicanuria. Evidence of parasitic infestation is common but not constant. A variety of parasites have been found, giardiasis being the most frequent (Table 3).

4. *Pathology*

The intestinal lesions of α-chain disease usually predominate in duodenum and jejunum, in contrast to the common lymphomas of the digestive tract which have a predilection for the stomach, terminal ileum, and colorectal areas. The whole length of the small intestine is most often involved. During the first stage of the disease, its serosal surface, apart from possible lymphatic dilation, appears normal without nodular formation. Its wall is mildly thickened at palpation. Intestinal ulcerations are rare. The mesenteric nodes are often greatly enlarged. Multiple biopsies taken during laparotomy or with a peroral capsule show a massive infiltration of the lamina propria by round cells (Fig. 2). Occasionally these infiltrates penetrate into the submucosa. Most cells in this infiltrate belong to the plasma cell series (Fig. 3A), as confirmed by electron microscopy (Scotto *et al.*, 1970; Doe *et al.*, 1972). These plasma cells do not usually show cellular atypia. In some instances, small lymphocytes and transitional forms are found in addition to the plasma cells. The plasma cell infiltration is usually massive, causing wide separation and sparsity of the crypts and obliteration of the villous architecture without significant impairment of the integrity of the surface epithelium (Fig. 2). The villous atrophy may be incomplete, and focal areas remain in which the villous architecture is preserved with heavy infiltration of the villous stroma by plasma cells and/or lymphocytes.

In some instances, the infiltrate extends to deep submucosa and even muscularis propria. In these areas, plasma cells are often atypical and large pyroninophilic immunoblastlike cells are scattered within the plasmacytic infiltrate, either isolated or gathered in small islets or even large nodules (Galian *et al.*, 1977).

Mesenteric lymph nodes very often show the same cellular infiltrate as

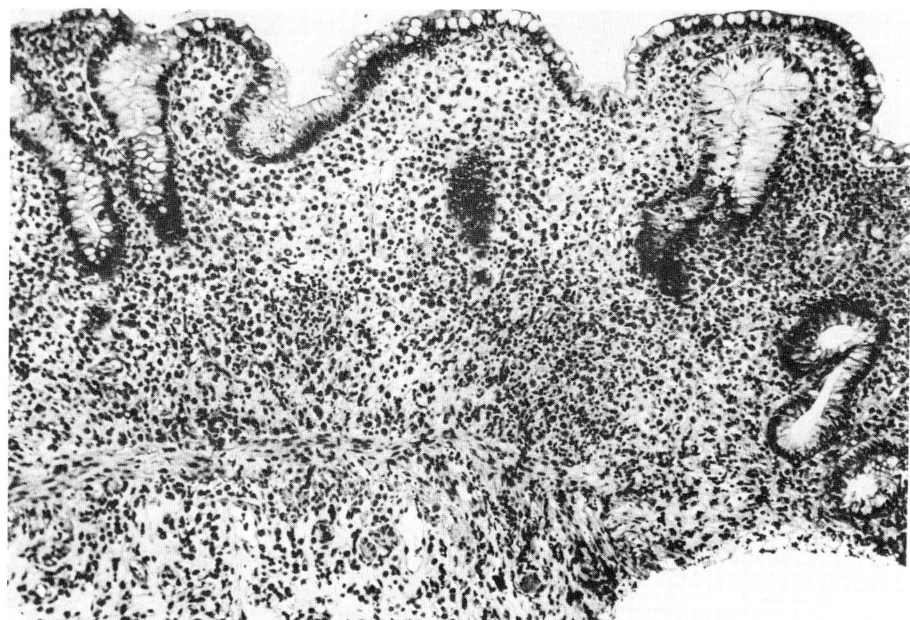

Fig. 2. Jejunal peroral biopsy. Note the subtotal villous atrophy, the increased number of goblet cells, and the sparsity and destruction of the crypts by the massive lamina propria infiltrate, which extends slightly to submucosa. Hematoxylin and eosin; ×125, reproduced at 70%. (From Rambaud *et al.* (1972), with permission of the *Annales de Gastroentérologie et d'Hépatologie.*

small intestinal lamina propria, often leading to an obliteration of the normal architecture, especially when immunoblastic cells are present.

In some cases (Bognel *et al.*, 1972; Bonomo *et al.*, 1972), a first biopsy of jejunum and/or mesenteric lymph nodes merely showed a nonspecific hyperplastic lymphoid infiltration. Subsequently, the typical plasma cell infiltration became apparent. In the absence of appropriate immunological studies, one cannot determine whether these initial findings were truly related to an early stage of the disease.

In some patients, frequently those who present with the "tumoral" symptoms mentioned above, pathological evidence of a truly malignant lymphoma is found in the gut (Fig. 3B) and/or the mesenteric nodes. In the small intestine, the lymphoma cells may form single (Novis *et al.*, 1973) or multiple (Rappaport *et al.*, 1972; Bonomo *et al.*, 1972; Montoro-Marin *et al.*, 1974; Manousos *et al.*, 1974; Teulieres, 1975) circumscribed tumors. In some of these cases, the characteristic plasma cell infiltration of α-chain disease may not be recognized if intestinal biopsies are not performed at a site distant from the tumoral formation(s). In other cases, the malignant lymphoma cells are intermixed with the plasma cell proliferation and invade the deeper layers of the gut wall (Bognel *et al.*, 1972; Bonomo *et al.*, 1972; Chadli *et al.*, 1973; Galian *et al.*, 1977). At this stage, the malignant process may spread out of the enteromesenteric area. Histologically, the malignant lymphoma is composed of

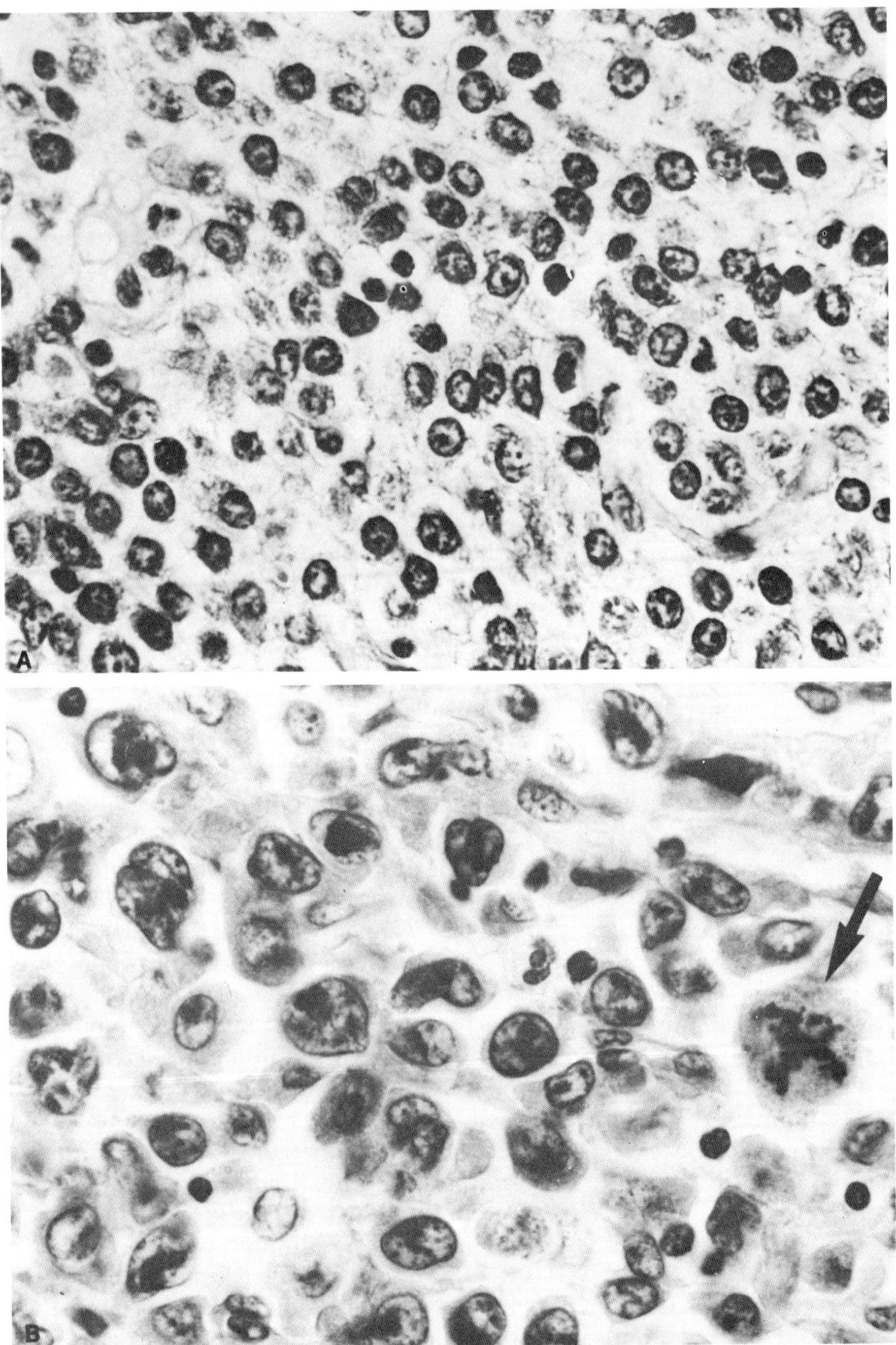

Fig. 3. Details of the lamina propria infiltrate. Hematoxylin and eosin; ×1200, reproduced at 80%. A: At the time of diagnosis, most cells are plasma cells, sometimes mature, often young, but not dystrophic. B: At a later stage of the disease (immunoblastic lymphoma), all cells appear dystrophic and some of these are large, with a polysegmented nucleus containing multiple nucleoli and with occasional mitoses (arrow). From Rambaud *et al.* (1972), with permission of the *Annales de Gastroentérologie et d'Hépatologie.*

large neoplastic cells. These tumors have been called reticulum cell sarcomas or histiocytic lymphomas according to the older classifications. However, the features of these cells strongly suggest that we are dealing with the so-called immunoblastic lymphoma. Cells resembling Reed–Sternberg cells may be part of the infiltrate of the tumor, but they usually have a pyroninophilic cytoplasm.

Extensive histological studies have failed to reveal evidence of amyloid deposition.

5. *Immunochemical Diagnosis*

The diagnosis of α-CD relies entirely on laboratory studies including immunochemical analysis of the serum proteins and, as previously emphasized (Seligmann *et al.,* 1969, 1971), may be difficult in the average laboratory. The abnormality can easily be missed on the serum protein electrophorogram, and the pathological protein was not noticeable in half of the

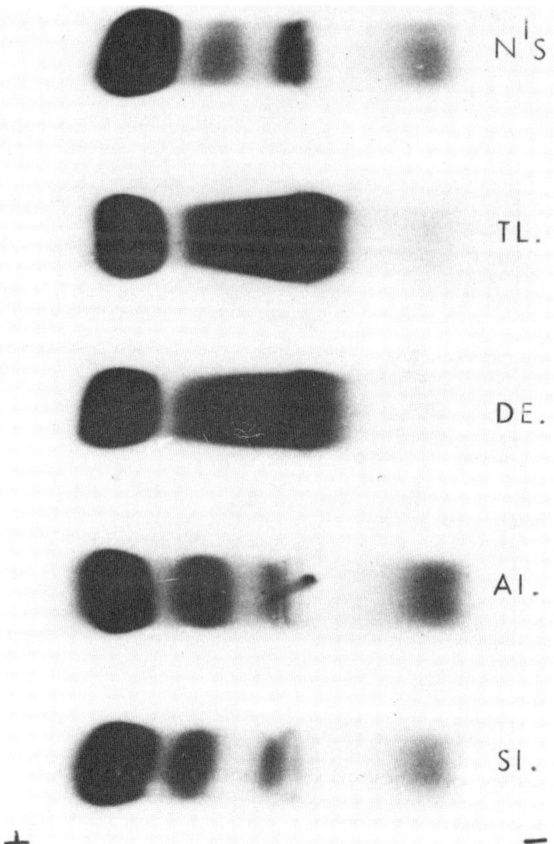

Fig. 4. Agar gel electrophoretic pattern of the serum of our patients with α-CD, compared with normal serum (N'S.). In patients TL. and DE. an abnormal, very broad band is observed. In patient AI. there is only an increase in α_2-globulins. In patient SI. the pathological protein is not noticeable. From Seligmann *et al.* (1969), with permission of the *Journal of Clinical Investigation*.

80 cases studied in our laboratory. When detectable by electrophoresis, the pathological α-CD protein shows an abnormal broad band, usually in the α_2 or β region (Fig. 4). The characteristic narrow band, which is suggestive of a monoclonal Ig abnormality, is always lacking. In most of the cases where the pathological protein was not noticeable, serum electrophoresis showed only a decrease in serum albumin and a moderate to severe hypogammaglobulinemia (Fig. 4).

The diagnosis is usually suspected or established by immunoelectrophoretic analysis of the serum of these patients (Fig. 5). In many cases the protein abnormality has escaped detection by routine immunoelectrophoresis using polyvalent antiserum to human normal serum, and analysis with monospecific antisera to IgA is essential. The abnormal component usually gives an abnormal precipitin line either extending from the α_1-globulins to the slow β_2 region or showing a faster electrophoretic mobility than normal IgA. However, in a few patients the α-CD protein has a slow electrophoretic

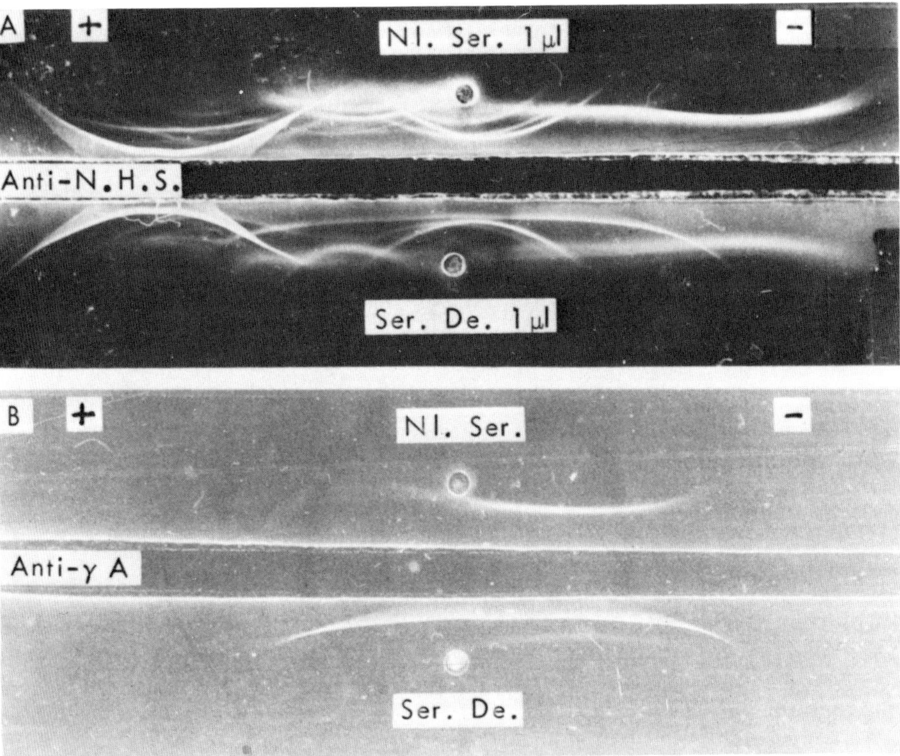

Fig. 5. Immunoelectrophoretic analysis of the serum of a patient with a α-CD (De.) compared with normal serum (Nl. Ser.) developed with (A) a polyvalent antiserum to whole normal human serum (Anti-N.H.S.) and (B) an antiserum to α chains (Anti-γA). Note the abnormal broad precipitin line. The line given by this abnormal component was not revealed by antisera to κ or λ light chains. From Seligmann *et al.* (1971), reproduced with permission of the *Annals of the New York Academy of Science.*

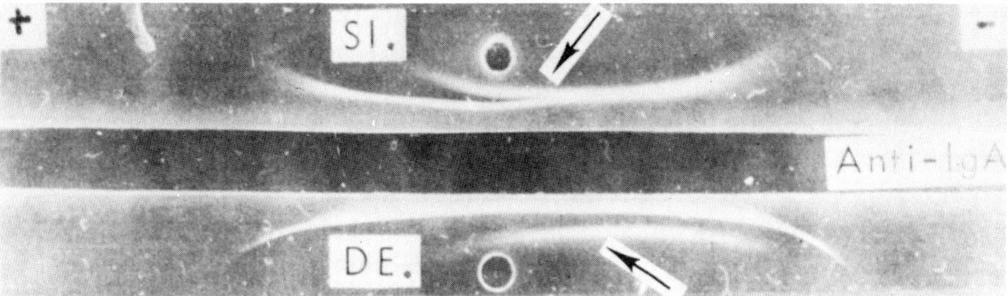

Fig. 6. Immunoelectrophoretic analysis of two α-CD sera using a specific antiserum to IgA which contains, after adsorption with light chains, precipitating antibodies reacting with the light-heavy chain combination. The precipitin line corresponding to normal IgA is shown by the arrows. This line spurs over the α-CD protein line of serum SI., whereas it is inside the α-CD protein line in serum DE. From Seligmann *et al.* (1971), reproduced with permission of the *Annals of the New York Academy of Sciences.*

mobility. The anomalous component does not of course precipitate with antisera to light chains. It should, however, be emphasized that this lack of precipitation with anti-κ and anti-λ antisera is not a sufficient criterion for the diagnosis of α-CD since many IgA myeloma proteins, even though they contain light chains (mainly λ chains), fail to precipitate with such antisera.

Selected antisera to IgA that contain antibodies related to the conformational specificity of the Fab region, which precipitate only with α and light chains combined, have been found to be very useful for the diagnosis of α-CD by immunoelectrophoresis (Fig. 6) or the Ouchterlony technique (Fig. 7) (Seligmann *et al.,* 1969), as is the immunoselection plate method of Radl (Doe *et al.,* 1972). In all doubtful cases the pathological protein should be purified, reduced, and alkylated, and the lack of light chains should be demonstrated directly by starch or polyacrylamide gel electrophoresis or by gel filtration after dissociation of the molecule.

The striking and unexpected electrophoretic heterogeneity of these presumably monoclonal α-CD proteins is certainly due in part to the heterogeneity of their *N*-terminal sequences, as discussed below. It may also

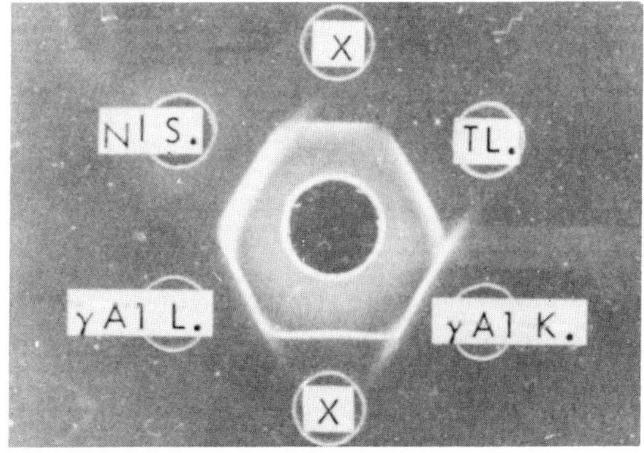

Fig. 7. Ouchterlony test useful for identification of α-CD protein. The selected antiserum to IgA in the center well is that used in Fig. 6. It shows that the serum under study (X) contains an α-CD protein since the precipitin line is deficient when compared to normal IgA and to IgA_1 myeloma proteins of both light-chain types but in identity with the reference α-CD protein TL. From Seligmann *et al.* (1969), reproduced by permission of the *Journal of Clinical Investigation.*

be related to two other features, the high carbohydrate content of most α-CD proteins (Seligmann *et al.*, 1971) and their high tendency to polymerize. Indeed, on ultracentrifugation α-CD proteins appear to consist of dimers with a 3–4 S sedimentation constant and, in most instances, of larger polymers of various sizes (Seligmann *et al.*, 1969). J chain has been found in all α-CD proteins so far studied (Seligmann, 1975*a*).

The serum levels of normal IgA, IgG, and IgM molecules are usually depressed. These decreases are not solely due to a protein-losing enteropathy, as shown by the disproportionate depression of serum Ig levels relative to the serum albumin concentration. Deficiencies of humoral immunity as well as cellular immunity have been demonstrated in a few patients (Rambaud *et al.*, 1970; Manousos *et al.*, 1974). No functional tests of the secretory immune system have been performed in these patients, to our knowledge.

The diagnosis of α-CD is made more difficult by the very low concentration of pathological protein in the urine. In most patients, however, it can be detected in concentrated urine and has the same electrophoretic and immunochemical characteristics as that in the serum. Bence Jones proteinuria has never been found. The pathological protein is also found in significant amounts in jejunal fluid, as expected from the involvement of the intestine, whereas the IgA in the parotid saliva is normal (Seligmann *et al.*, 1969).

In order to establish a true incidence of α-CD, it will be necessary to study systematically the immunoglobulins of the intestinal fluid in those patients with similar clinicopathological features but without detectable α-CD protein in the serum. In those patients without detectable α-CD protein in the serum and intestinal fluid, demonstration of the production of the α-CD protein by the proliferating cells, using immunofluorescence or biosynthetic studies (Seligmann *et al.*, 1969; Buxbaum and Preud'homme, 1972), may lead to the discovery of nonsecreting forms of α-CD.

Interesting exceptions to the usual immunoglobulin findings in α-CD have been reported. A small homogeneous IgG component has been found in addition to α-CD protein in serum in two cases (Seligmann, 1975*a*). In the serum from two patients presenting with the typical clinicopathological features of the intestinal form of α-CD, an entire IgA myeloma globulin was found, and Bence-Jones protein was present in the urine of one of these patients (Chantar *et al.*, 1974; Tangun *et al.*, 1975). In another young girl presenting with the typical clinicopathological features of intestinal α-CD, a γ-chain disease protein was demonstrated in the serum and in the intestinal biopsy (Seligmann, 1975*b*).

6. *Structural and Cellular Studies of the Immunoglobulin Abnormality*

Alpha-chain disease is defined as the production of a presumably homogeneous population of molecules consisting of incomplete heavy α chains devoid of light chains.

The molecular weight of the monomeric polypeptide subunit was found to vary between 29,000 and 34,000 (Dorrington *et al.*, 1970; Seligmann *et al.*, 1971). The length of these chains was thus greater than half but smaller than three-quarters of the length of normal α_1 heavy chains. Antigenic analysis (Seligmann *et al.*, 1969) and chemical studies (Seligmann *et al.*, 1971) indicated that the entire Fc fragment was present in α-CD proteins, that their *C*-terminus was identical to that of normal α_1 chains, and that the heavy–light peptide was missing. The hinge region has been shown by chemical methods to be present in all eight proteins so far studied. All attempts to raise individually specific antibodies to α-CD proteins have failed, indicating the paucity of antigenic determinants in the variable portion of the chain. In view of these results and of the molecular weight data, the missing portion of the chain is located in the Fd segment and involves both the V_H and C1 regions.

The *N*-terminal sequences of several α-CD proteins were shown to be heterogeneous (Seligmann *et al.*, 1971). Even for those proteins with the same *N*-terminal amino acid, marked heterogeneity became apparent after two steps in degradation. Attempts to obtain the *N*-terminal sequence on an automated sequencer were unsuccessful. The *N*-terminal residues were different from those found in any of the subgroups of the variable regions of normal heavy chains. The most likely explanation of this heterogeneity is that it is the consequence of intracellular proteolysis occurring after synthesis. The fact that the *N*-terminal residues found in the seven proteins studied were valine and/or isoleucine suggests that the degradation stops at this level for some reason, which could possibly be enzyme specificity, steric hindrance, or the presence of a carbohydrate moiety. An analogous limited intracellular postsynthetic proteolysis of the *N*-terminus of an incomplete protein has been described for a nonsense mutant of alkaline phosphatase produced by *Escherichia coli* (Natori and Garen, 1970). Alternatively, postsynthetic cleavage may occur extracellularly. In one case of γ-CD, the nascent abnormal chain in the cytoplasm and in the culture fluid during biosynthetic studies had a molecular weight of 36,000, in contrast to the molecular weight of the serum α-CD protein, which was 28,000 (Buxbaum and Preud'homme, 1972).

The demonstration of a large internal deletion in a γ-heavy-chain disease protein (Frangione and Milstein, 1969) led us to postulate that in α-CD we were dealing with a similar primary deletion followed and obscured by a secondary limited proteolysis (Seligmann *et al.*, 1971). This hypothesis has been supported to some extent by biosynthetic and structural studies. Cellular biosynthetic studies in a case of α-CD excluded the possibility of the synthesis of a normal α chain with subsequent degradation to a smaller fragment after its release from the ribosomes (Buxbaum and Preud'homme, 1972). Comparison of the amino acid sequence of the hinge region of this protein (Def) with that of a normal IgA1 showed that, after a short segment thought to correspond to the variable region, protein Def displays a gap which comprises almost the whole Fd segment including C_H1 domain (Wolfenstein-Todel *et al.*, 1974). It is, however, not excluded that the *N*-terminal sequence of this protein is not a portion of the V region but rather a noncleaved polypeptide (?precursor ?viral genome). Normal synthesis resumes in protein Def at a valine residue in the hinge region just preceding a segment which contains a partially duplicated fragment and the inter-heavy-chain disulfide bonds. From there on, the molecule is apparently normal, with the exception of a substitution of threonine for serine in position 12. It is of interest that valine at position 9 of the hinge peptide, where the identity with a normal α_1 chain starts, could be the equivalent of glutamine at position 216 of γ chains, the site where normal synthesis resumes in several γ-CD proteins with internal deletions (Frangione and Franklin, 1973). Similar conclusions were reached from the structural study of another α-CD protein (Wolfenstein-Todel *et al.,* 1975). Thus the primary defect in α-CD proteins appears to be a deletion affecting the variable and first constant regions of the heavy chains, which are under independent genetic control.

Cultures of jejunal biopsy specimens from α-CD patients in medium containing ^{14}C-labeled amino acids have established that the α-CD protein is synthesized *in vitro* by the proliferating cells (Seligmann *et al.,* 1968). Radioimmunoelectrophoretic analysis of protein synthesized *in vitro* by cells teased from mesenteric nodes also demonstrated the production of labeled α-CD proteins (Seligmann *et al.,* 1969). Immunofluorescent studies of intestinal mucosa and mesenteric nodes revealed variable and sometimes weak staining in the cytoplasm of cells composing the cellular infiltrate (Seligmann *et al.,* 1969). No membrane-bound immunoglobulin was detectable on the surface of α-CD protein-synthesizing cells in several patients (Preud'homme and Seligmann, 1972), whereas in other patients the cells bore α chains and no light chains (unpublished results from our laboratory).

Immunofluorescent studies failed in most cases to detect any light-chain production in the cells which secrete α-CD proteins (Seligmann *et al.,* 1969). No free labeled light chains were found upon radioimmunoelectrophoretic analysis of proteins synthesized *in vitro* by intestinal or mesenteric node proliferating cells (Seligmann *et al.,* 1969). This failure of light-chain synthesis has been confirmed by biosynthetic studies of nascent Ig subunits in such patients (Buxbaum and Preud'homme, 1972). Since light and heavy chains are under the control of unlinked genes, this peculiar situation raises a puzzling problem for the cellular geneticist. The possibility remains that the light chain is transcribed but not translated. Studies looking for the presence or absence of its messenger are warranted since Cowan *et al.* (1974) have detected an inactive light-chain messenger RNA in a nonsecreting variant of a mouse myeloma which contained an abnormally short heavy chain and failed to synthesize light chain. In one patient whose cells were recently studied in our laboratory, monotypic light chains were synthesized but not secreted, as shown by immunofluorescence and biosynthesis experiments.

All 50 α-CD proteins which have been typed to date in our laboratory belong to the α_1 subclass. The absence of a single case of α_2-heavy-chain disease in this series is probably not accidental since 30% of the normal secretory IgA molecules belong to the α_2 subclass (Grey *et al.,* 1968). This finding that all the molecules of α-CD protein in a given patient belong to only one IgA subclass, together with the amino acid substitution in position 12 of protein Def, suggests that α-CD proteins are monoclonal. However, this assumption cannot be confirmed because the other essential criteria for monoclonality; i.e., homogeneity of the V regions of light and heavy chains leading to shared idiotypic specificity and antibody activity, cannot be tested.

Whether α-CD proteins should be considered as "abnormal" is still an open question. Polypeptides analogous to the proteins of γ-chain disease have been reported to be present in very small amount in normal plasma (Lam and Stevenson, 1973). However, if heavy-chain diseases arises from proliferation of a clone of cells producing such polypeptides, it is necessary to postulate a wide variety of cells carrying such deletions in normal individuals since the site and length of the deletion appear to vary from one α-CD protein to another.

7. *Course of the Disease*

The natural history of α-CD is probably of utmost importance, but is not yet fully elucidated.

The spontaneous course of α-CD may be continuous, but often proceeds as exacerbations separated by more or less complete and prolonged improvements. The disease appears to proceed in two stages. The early "premalignant" stage is characterized by diffuse and extensive plasma cell infiltration which remains confined to the enteromesenteric area. In the absence of therapy there is progressive deterioration, usually culminating in frank malignancy with immunoblastic tumours which may lead to obstruction, intussuception, or perforation of the small intestine. Death is usually due either to cachexia and infection or to complications of the localized tumors. Dissemination of the immunoblastic tumor outside the abdomen is rare and a late event of the disease. Patients with well-documented initial status and adequate long-term follow-up are still scarce. However, in two patients who were regularly followed until death, it was possible to observe the progressive passage from the mature plasmacytic proliferation of α-CD to these overt malignant lymphomas (Bognel *et al.,* 1972; Galian *et al.,* 1977). In the gut, foci of large malignant cells first appeared in the deep mucosa and in submucosa, and all transitional forms between these cells and the plasma cells were observed. Noticeably, at any stage of the lymphoma growth, mesenteric lymph nodes showed a higher degree of malignancy than intestinal wall.

Several lines of evidence strongly suggest that the overt malignant lymphomas, first classified as reticulum cell sarcoma or Hodgkin's disease, which arise in the late course of α-CD, are in fact "immunoblastic" sarcomas derived from the same B-cell clone as the initial plasma cell proliferation. Both proliferations can be topographically intricated in the lymph nodes and in the gut (Bognel *et al.,* 1972). Rough endoplasmic reticulum may be found by electron microscopy in the apparently poorly differentiated malignant cells (Doe, 1975). All transitional forms between the large undifferentiated malignant cells and the mature plasma cells may be found in some patients. Intracytoplasmic α-CD protein may be undetectable by immunofluorescence in the most malignant and undifferentiated cells (Bognel *et al.,* 1972; Teulières, 1975), and it must be emphasized that the α-CD protein may be no more detectable in the serum as the lymphoma develops (Teulières, 1975). However, α-CD protein has been identified in one patient in the perinuclear cisternae of the large lymphomatous cells found in the bone marrow (Reyes, personal communication). Furthermore, the study of membrane-bound immunoglobulins has provided conclusive evidence that the sarcomatous cells of morphologically similar lymphomas arising in two other immunoproliferative disorders, i.e., chronic lymphocytic leukemia and Waldenström macroglobulinemia, originate from the same clone as the previous lymphoid proliferation (Brouet *et al.,* 1975). Recently, α chains were found on the surface of the large lymphomatous cells in one patient with α-CD (Brouet *et al.,* 1977), and very recent studies of immunoglobulin biosynthesis provide evidence that these lymphomatous cells do indeed derive from the same clone as the plasma cell proliferation (Ramot *et al.,* 1977, and unpublished results from our laboratory).

Whether the plasmacytic phase of α-CD is truly benign is open to question. The hypothesis of a benign process seems unlikely in those patients with high and rising serum levels of the pathological protein if its monoclonal nature is confirmed. This hypothesis is also unlikely when the plasma cell proliferation penetrates deeply into the submucosa and possibly muscularis propria, or disorganizes completely the architecture of the mesenteric nodes and shows atypical forms with an admixture of large "immunoblastic" cells. This pleomorphic invasive proliferation probably represents the early stage of the malignant lymphoma.

However, in most cases, the plasma cells of the infiltrate appear to be mature and well-differentiated with scarce mitoses. This does not necessarily militate against malignancy since in other malignant lymphoproliferative disorders such as chronic lymphocytic leukemia and Waldenström's macroglobulinemia the proliferating cells are normal in appearance. Karyotypic studies of plasma cells taken from the intestinal infiltrate during the "benign" phase may help to resolve this question. The truly benign nature of α-CD at its initial stage is a real possibility since apparently complete remission of the disease was achieved in several patients treated only with oral antibiotics (Rogé *et al.* 1970; Monges *et al.,* 1975; Rambaud *et al.,* 1978; Ramot, personal communication). Disappearance of the α-CD protein from the serum and intestinal fluid was noted in these patients together with a normal histological appearance and negative immunofluorescent studies. It should be emphasized that in one of these patients (Rogé *et al.,* 1970) the complete remission has lasted since 5 years after withdrawal of the antibiotherapy. It is also noteworthy that, in the three published cases, the initial serum level of α-CD protein was relatively low.

8. Treatment

Since relatively few data are available to date, we can give only our present and provisional opinion on the main therapeutic guidelines.

All patients in whom α-CD has been diagnosed and in whom signs of overt malignancy are not found on peroral biopsies should be submitted to laparotomy if there is no major contraindication, in order to perform multiple transmural and large biopsies of the small intestine and biopsies of several mesenteric lymph nodes and of the liver.

Patients without any evidence of a sarcomatous process should first be treated with oral antibiotics alone. The same could perhaps apply to patients with suspected but not documented malignancy (i.e., patients with submucosal infiltration, complete obliteration of nodal architecture, or the presence of scattered immunoblastlike cells). Unless the antibiotic choice can be directed by repeated quantitative bacteriological studies of jejunal fluid and antibiograms, tetracycline should be given at a dosage of 2 g per day. As a dramatic improvement in clinical and biological symptoms of malabsorption may occur with such a treatment without any significant changes in intestinal lesions (Teulières, 1975; Galian *et al.,* 1977) or without disappearance of the α-CD protein (Seligmann and Danon, unpublished results), the survey should be mainly based on intestinal biopsies (with immunofluorescence studies whenever possible) and on repeated search for α-CD protein in blood and, if negative, in jejunal fluid. If no marked improvement is observed after a 3-month treatment or if complete remission is not achieved after 9–12 months, cyclophosphamide should be administered at a dose of 200 mg/m^2 intramuscularly or intravenously weekly. In those patients where the disease remains stable or progressive or in whom a recurrence occurs, multiple intestinal biopsies should be performed and a second laparotomy may be advisable.

In patients with overt malignant lymphoma diagnosed at onset or later in the course of the disease and localized to the enteromesenteric area, total abdominal irradiation should be performed after a short course of tetracycline, prednisone, and possibly chemotherapy. A maximum dosage of 3500 rads over the entire abdominal cavity seems to be required. Liver and kidneys should be protected as usual, and the weekly dosage should not exceed 750 rads. After a 1-month rest, irradiation should be followed by polychemotherapy for residual disease. Polychemotherapy should be given first to patients with malignant lymphomas involving the liver and/or extraabdominal nodes or viscera. A subsequent abdominal irradiation may be indicated in these patients for focal residual tumor. The most advisable polychemotherapy seems to be the classical CHOP protocol: a combination of cyclophosphamide, adriamycin, vincristine, and prednisone administered in cycles at monthly intervals for 6 months at least.

At all stages of the disease, supportive therapy is essential and should include fluid and electrolyte intravenous replacement, blood or serum albumin infusions, vitamins and iron, and an appropriate diet.

9. Relationship to So-Called Mediterranean Lymphoma

The so-called Mediterranean lymphoma, i.e., diffuse primary intestinal lymphoma associated with malabsorption, was first reported in Israel (Ramot *et al.,* 1965; Eidelman *et al.,* 1966). This syndrome, which affects underprivileged young adults, has since been described in Iran (Nasr *et al.,* 1970), Iraq (Al-Bahrani and Bakir, 1971), and South Africa (Novis *et al.,* 1971). In Israel these lymphomas are found relatively frequently among Arabs and first- and second-generation Jewish immigrants from Mideastern and North African countries but almost never affect Israeli Jews of Ashkenazi origin. A variety of histological types have been described, and there is much confusion in the literature about the pathology of these lymphomas. In fact, it is likely that most cases could be described under the heading of immunoblastic lymphoma. Initial reports of these so-called Mediterranean lymphomas did not include immunoglobulin studies. Recent evidence suggests that the majority of these primary diffuse intestinal lymphomas causing malabsorption in underprivileged populations begin as an apparently benign infiltration of the small intestine by plasma cells. As mentioned above, α-CD patients have been observed over several years to progress from an apparently benign plasmacytic stage to a malignant intestinal lymphoma identical to the so-called Mediterranean lymphoma. A retrospective pathological study from a group of 20 patients suffering from so-called Mediterranean lymphoma revealed that in 16 cases a diffuse plasma cell infiltrate was present in association with the malignant lymphoma (Rappaport *et al.,* 1972). The remaining four patients showed a purely plasmacytic proliferation in the small intestine without histological evidence of malignancy. The true incidence of α-CD among the so-called Mediterranean lymphomas is still open to discussion. Our hypothesis (Seligmann and Rambaud, 1969) that many of these lymphomas are in fact α-CD, provided that their definition is restricted to cases showing a diffuse plasma cell proliferation with or without superimposed sarcoma, has been confirmed by the study of serum immunoglobulins in numerous such patients. Serum α-CD protein has been found in several cases classified histologically as reticulum cell sarcoma (Ramot and Hulu, 1975). However, we and others have been unable to detect the α-CD protein in the serum of some such patients. Such a failure may reflect the insensitivity of techniques used or the advanced undifferentiated stage of the malignancy. Careful prospective studies should include a systematic search for the abnormal protein in jejunal fluid and, in negative cases, at the intracellular level by immunofluorescence and biosynthetic studies since nonsecretory forms of α-CD may exist. Current findings suggest that the majority, if not all, cases of diffuse "Mediterranean lymphoma" represent the late malignant phase of α-CD.

10. Pathogenesis

The very peculiar geographical distribution of α-CD patients and the clear predilection of α-CD for underprivileged populations suggest that environmental factors providing a local and protracted antigenic stimulation may play an important role in its pathogenesis (Seligmann *et al.,* 1971). One common factor among susceptible populations of various ethnic origins is their exposure to an environment of poor hygiene in areas with high degree of infestation by intestinal pathogens. Studies conducted in affected populations have shown that chronic gastrointestinal infection and diarrhea are common, and serial intestinal biopsies in healthy people have shown an increased lymphocytic and plasma cell infiltration within the lamina propria of the small bowel. Since orally ingested microorganisms are known to be a powerful proliferative stimulus to the secretory IgA system, the early phase of α-CD could represent an aberrant humoral immune response following sustained topical antigenic stimulation of the intestinal mucosa. The specific or nonspecific nature of the postulated stimulating microorganisms is open to question. Investigation of possible specific environmental agents has been unrewarding. Limited bacteriological parasitic and virological studies have not revealed evidence for a specific agent associated with α-CD. However, the postulated antigenic stimulation may have occurred many years before α-CD became clinically manifest. The clinical onset of the disease has occurred in some patients more than 10 years after withdrawal from the environmental factors. Microorganisms involved in the pathogenesis of α-CD may be present only during infancy or childhood and absent in identifiable form years later at the time of diagnosis. Unfortunately, the absence of Fab in α-CD protein precludes its use for identifying putative antigenic stimuli. These environmental factors could trigger the clonal proliferation directly. Alternatively, they may only be predisposing factors causing a nonspecific stimulation of immunocytes which could potentiate the oncogenic effect of a virus interfering with genes controlling IgA synthesis (Rambaud and Matuchansky, 1973).

In either case, it is remarkable that the plasma cell proliferation resulting from the postulated antigenic stimulation appears to lead to heavy-chain disease rather than to myeloma. This could be explained by two main possibilities, (WHO, 1976). An abnormal B-cell clone synthesizing the α-CD protein could be produced in the gut through a series of recombinant events during embryogenesis. Another possibility which is not excluded is that a somatic mutation event gives rise to a cell producing the α-CD protein, permitting it to enter into the gut-associated lymphoid system and to home into the lamina propria. In either case, the abnormal clone would overgrow in abnormal microenvironmental situations and could, for instance, be susceptible to the proliferation stimulus of bacterial lipopolysaccharide in the intestinal lumen. In addition, the abnormal clone could have a selective advantage for proliferation because of the lack of antibody activity of its immunoglobulin product, possibly resulting in the suppression of a feedback mechanism (Rambaud and Matuchansky, 1973).

The postulated environmental antigenic stimulus might be associated with an underlying immunodeficiency. This could be a defect rendering the host more susceptible to infection with oncogenic organisms or a basic defect of the feedback mechanisms controlling the cellular proliferative response to stimulation. Immunodeficiency could be due to malnutrition, especially in early infancy, or to genetic factors.

In fact, the role of environmental factors, either specific or nonspecific, does not exclude the possibility of predisposing genetic factors. Although limited family studies have failed to reveal evidence of a heritable trait for α-CD, a search for genetic markers may help to identify predisposed subjects. Raised serum levels of the intestinal isoenzyme of alkaline phosphatase were reported in patients with α-CD and Mediterranean lymphoma and in their healthy relatives (Ramot and Streifler, 1968; Doe *et al.*, 1972; Lewin *et al.*, 1976). The histocompatibility antigens (both HLA and LD) of the patients and other relatives should be determined, in view of their implication in susceptibility to some diseases.

Alpha-chain disease probably represents a model of a lymphoma characterized by a continuous sequence of events ranging from an apparently benign hyperplastic process reversible by the administration of antibiotics to an overt neoplastic proliferation. The elucidation of this sequence of events may offer a revealing insight into the development of lymphomas in man.

11. References

Al-Bahrani, Z. R., and Bakir, F., 1971, Primary intestinal lymphoma, *Ann. R. Coll. Surg. England* **48:**103–113.

Bernadou, A., Segond, P., Bilski-Pasquier, G., Mihaesco, E., Preud'homme, J. L., and Bousser, J., 1972, La maladie des chaines alpha: A propos d'une observation, *Nouv. Rev. Fr. Hematol.* **12:**333–350.

Bognel, J. C., Rambaud, J. C., Modigliani, R., Matuchansky, C., Bognel, C., Bernier, J. J., Scotto, J., Hautefeuille, P., Mihaesco, E., Hurez, D., Preud'homme, J. L., and Seligmann, M., 1972, Etude clinique, anatomo-pathologique et immunochimique d'un nouveau cas de maladie des chaines alpha suivi pendant cinq ans, *Rev. Eur. Etud. Clin. Biol.* **17:**362–374.

Bonomo, L., Dammacco, F., Marano, R., and Bonomo, G. M., 1972, Abdominal lymphoma and alpha chain disease, *Am. J. Med.* **52:**73–86.

Brouet, J. C., Labaume, S., and Seligmann, M. 1975, Evaluation of T and B lymphocyte membrane markers in human non Hodgkin malignant lymphomas, *Br. J. Cancer* **31:**121–127 (Suppl. 2).

Brouet, J. C., Mason, D. Y., Danon, F., Preud'homme, J. L., Seligmann, M., Reyes, F., Navab, F., Galian, A., René, E., and Rambaud, J. C., 1977, Alpha chain disease: Evidence for a common clonal origin of intestinal immunoblastic lymphoma and plasmacytic proliferation, *Lancet* **1:**861.

Buxbaum, J. N., and Preud'homme, J. L., 1972, Alpha and gamma heavy chain diseases in man: Intracellular origin of the aberrant polypeptides, *J. Immunol.* **109:**1131–1137.

Chadli, A., Hafsia, M., Maamouri, M. T., Haddad, N., and Ayed, K., 1973, Lymphome méditerranéen avec maladie des chaines alpha: Etude anatomo-pathologique à propos du premier cas tunisien, *Arch. Anat. Pathol.* **21:**199–210.

Chantar, C., Escartin, P., Plaza, A. G., Corugedo, A. F., Arenas, J. I., Sanz, E., Anaya, A., Bootello, A., and Segovia, J. M., 1974, Diffuse plasma cell infiltration of the small intestine with malabsorption associated to IgA monoclonal gammapathy, *Cancer* **34:**1620–1630.

Cowan, N. J., Secher, D. S., and Milstein, C., 1974, Intracellular immunoglobulin chain synthesis in non-secreting variants of a mouse myeloma: Detection of inactive light-chain messenger RNA, *J. Mol. Biol.* **90:**691–701.

Dent, C. E., Norris, T. St. M., Smith, R., Sutton, R. A. L., and Temperley, J. M., 1968, Steatorrhoea with striking increase of plasma alkaline-phosphatase of intestinal origin, *Lancet* **1:**1333–1336.

Doe, W. F., 1975, Alpha chain disease: Clinicopathological features and relationship to so-called Mediterranean lymphoma, *Br. J. Cancer* **31:**350–355 (Suppl. 2).

Doe, W. F., Henry, K., Hobbs, J. R., Avery Jones, E., Dent, C. E., and Booth, C. C., 1972, Five cases of alpha-chain disease, *Gut* **13**:947–957.

Dorrington, K. J., Mihaesco, E., and Seligmann, M. 1970, The molecular size of three α-chain disease proteins, *Biochim. Biophys. Acta* **221**:647–649.

Eidelman, S., Parkins, A., and Rubin, C., 1966, Abdominal lymphoma presenting as malabsorption: A clinicopathologic study of 9 cases in Israel and a review of the literature, *Medicine* **45**:111–137.

Faux, J. A., Crain, J. D., Rosen, F. S., and Merler, E., 1973, An alpha heavy chain abnormality in a child with hypogammaglobulinemia, *Clin. Immunol. Immunopathol.* **1**:282–290.

Florin-Christensen, A., Doniach, D., and Newcomb, P. B., 1974, Alpha chain disease with pulmonary manifestations, *Br. Med. J.* **2**:413–415.

Frangione, B., and Franklin, E. C., 1973, Heavy chain diseases: Clinical features and molecular significance of the disordered immunoglobulin structure, *Sem. Hematol.* **10**:53–64.

Frangione, B., and Milstein, 1969; Partial deletion in the heavy chain disease protein ZUC, *Nature (London)* **224**:597–599.

Galian, A., Lecestre, M. J., Scotto, J., Bognel, C., Matuchansky, C., and Rambaud, J. C., 1977, Pathological study of alpha-chain disease, with special emphasis on evolution, *Cancer* **39**:2081–2101.

Guardia, J., Moragas, A., Pedreira, J. D., Ferragut, A., Gomez-Perez, J., Martinez-Vasquez, J. M., and Llorens, V., 1972, Enfermedad de las cadenas pesadas alfa (Enfermedad de Seligmann), *Rev. Clin. Esp.* **127**:923–926.

Grey, H. M., Abel, C. A., Yount, W. J., and Kunkel, H. G., 1968, A subclass of human γA-globulins(γA2) which lacks the disulfide bonds linking heavy and light chains, *J. Exp. Med.* **128**:1223–1236.

Henry, K., Bird, R. G., and Doe, W. F., 1974, Intestinal coccidiosis in a patient with alpha-chain disease, *Br. Med. J.* **1**:542–543.

Irunberry, J., Benallegue, A., Illoul, G., Timsit, G., Abbadi, M., Benabdallah, S., Boucekkine, T., Ould-Aoudia, J. P., and Colonna, P., 1970, Trois cas de maladie des chaines alpha observés en Algérie, *Nouv. Rev. Fr. Hematol.* **10**:609–616.

Lam, C. W. K., and Stevenson, G. T., 1973, Detection in normal plasma of immunoglobulin resembling the protein of γ-chain disease, *Nature (London)* **246**:419–421.

Lewin, K. J., Kahn, L. B., and Novis, B. H., 1976, Primary intestinal lymphoma of "Western" and "Mediterranean" type, alpha chain disease and massive plasma cell infiltration. A comparative study of 37 cases, *Cancer* **38**:2511–2528.

Manousos, O. N., Economidou, J. C., Georgiadou, D. E., Pratsika-Ougourloglou, K. G., Hadziyannis, S. J., Merikas, G. E., Henry, K., and Doe, W. F., 1974, Alpha chain disease with clinical, immunological and histological recovery, *Br. Med. J.* **2**:409–412.

Metrass, M. J., Virella, G., Baptista-Cunha, M. A., and Alfonso, G., 1974, Linfoma intestinal productor de cadenas alfa, *Sangre* **19**:418–434.

Monges, H., Aubert, L., Chamlian, A., Remacle, J. P., Mathieu, B., Cougard, A., and Arroyo, H., 1975, Maladie des chaines alpha à forme intestinale: Présentation d'un cas traité par antibiothérapie avec rémission clinique, histologique et immunologique, *Arch. Fr. Mal. App. Dig.* **64**:223–231.

Montoro-Marin, F., Bermejo, M. R., Monzonis Torres, M. C., and Perez Pena, F., 1974, Aspectos evolutivos y necropsicos de un caso de linfoma mediterraneo con enfermedad de cadenas alfa, *Med. Clin.* **62**:158–161.

Nasr, K., Haghighi, P., Bakhshandeh, K., and Haghshenas, M., 1970, Primary lymphoma of the upper small intestine, *Gut* **11**:673–678.

Natori, S., and Garen, A., 1970, Molecular heterogeneity in the amino-terminal region of alkaline-phosphatase *J. Mol. Biol.* **49**:577–588.

Novis, B. H., Bank, S., Marks, I. N., Selzer, G., Kahn, L., and Sealy, R., 1971, Abdominal lymphoma presenting with malabsorption, *Q. J. Med.* **40**:521 540.

Novis, B. H., Kahn, L. B., and Bank, S. 1973, Alpha-chain disease in sub-Saharan Africa, *Am. J. Digest. Dis.* **18**:679–688.

Pittman, F. E., Tripathy, K., Isobe, T., Bolanos, O. M., Osserman, E. F., Pittman, J. C., and

Lotero, H. R., 1975, IgA heavy chain disease: A case detected in the western hemisphere, *Am. J. Med.* **58**:424–430.

Preud'homme, J. L., and Seligmann, M., 1972, Surface-bound immunoglobulins as a cell marker in human lymphoproliferative diseases, *Blood* **40**:777–794.

Rambaud, J. C., and Matuchansky, C., 1973, Alpha-chain disease: Pathogenesis and relation to Mediterranean lymphoma, *Lancet* **1**:1430–1432.

Rambaud, J. C., Bognel, C., Prost, A., Bernier, J. J., Le Quintrec, Y., Lambling, A., Danon, F., Hurez, D., and Seligmann , M., 1968, Clinico-pathological study of a patient with "Mediterranean" type of abdominal lymphoma and a new type of IgA abnormality ("alpha chain disease"), *Digestion* **1**:321–336.

Rambaud, J. C., Matuchansky, C., Bognel, J. C., Bognel, C., Bernier, J. J., Scotto, J., Perol, C., Ferrier, J. P., Mihaesco, E., Hurez, D., and Seligmann, M., 1970, Nouveau cas de maladie des chaines alpha chez un eurasien, *Ann. Med. Int.* **121**:135–148.

Rambaud, J. C., Matuchansky, C., Bognel, C., Galian, A., Le Quintrec, Y., and Bernier, J. J., 1972, La maladie des chaines alpha: Rapport avec le "lymphome méditerranéen"; diagnostic et orientations thérapeutiques actuelles, *Ann. Gastro-enterol. Hepatol.* **8**:481–494.

Rambaud, J. C., Piel, J. L., Galian, A., Leclerc J. P., Danon, F., Girard-Pipeau, F., Modigliani, R., and Illoul, G., 1978, Rémission complète clinique, histologique et immunologique d'un cas de maladie des chaines alpha traité par antibiothérapie orale, *Gastroenterol. Clin. Biol.* **2**:49–61.

Ramot, B., and Hulu, N., 1975, Primary intestinal lymphoma and its relation to alpha heavy chain disease, *Br. J. Cancer* **31**:343–349 (Suppl. 2).

Ramot, B., and Streifler, C., 1968, Raised serum-alkaline phosphatase, *Lancet* **2**:587.

Ramot, B., Shanin, N., and Bubis, J. J., 1965, Malabsorption syndrome in lymphoma of small intestine, *Israel J. Med. Sci.* **1**:221–226.

Rappaport, H., Ramot, B., Hulu, N., and Park, J. K., 1972, The pathology of so-called Mediterranean abdominal lymphoma with malabsorption, *Cancer (Philadelphia)* **20**:1502–1511.

Ramot, B., Levanon, M., Hahn, Y., Lahat, N., and Moroz, C., 1977, The mutual clonal origin of the lymphoplasmocytic and lymphoma cell in alpha-heavy chain disease, *Clin. Exp. Med.* **27**:440–445.

Rogé, J., Druet, P., and Marche, C., 1970, Lymphome méditerranéen avec maladie des chaines alpha: Triple rémission clinique, anatomique et immunologique, *Pathol. Biol.* **18**:851–858.

Scotto, J., Stralin, H., and Caroli, J., 1970, Ultrastructural study of two cases of α-chain disease, *Gut* **11**:782–788.

Seligmann, M., 1975*a*, Immunochemical, clinical and pathological features of α-chain disease, *Arch. Intern. Med.* **135**:78–82.

Seligmann, M., 1975*b*, Alpha chain disease, *J. Clin. Pathol.* **28**:72–76. (Suppl. Assoc. Clin. Pathol. 6).

Seligmann, M., and Rambaud, J. C., 1969, IgA abnormalities in abdominal lymphoma (α-chain disease), *Israel J. Med. Sci.* **5**:151–157.

Seligmann, M., Danon, F., Hurez, D., Mihaesco, E., and Preud'homme, J. L., 1968, Alpha-chain disease: A new immunoglobulin abnormality, *Science* **162**:1396–1397.

Seligmann, M., Mihaesco, E., Hurez, D., Mihaesco, C., Preud'homme, J. L., and Rambaud, J. C., 1969, Immunochemical studies in four cases of alpha chain disease, *J. Clin. Invest.* **48**:2374–2389.

Seligmann, M., Mihaesco, E., and Frangione, B., 1971, Studies on alpha chain disease, *Ann. N.Y. Acad. Sci.* **190**:487–500.

Shahid, M. J., Alami, S. Y., Nassar, V. H., Balikian, J. B., and Salem, A. A., 1975, Primary intestinal lymphoma with paraproteinemia, *Cancer* **35**:848–858.

Stoop, J. W., Ballieux, R. E., Hijmans, W., and Zegers, B. J. M., 1971, Alpha chain disease with involvement of the respiratory tract in a Dutch child, *Clin. Exp. Immunol.* **9**:625–635.

Tangun, Y., Saracbasi, Z., Inceman, S., Danon, F., and Seligmann, M., 1975, IgA myeloma globulin and Bence-Jones proteinuria in a diffuse plasmacytoma of small intestine, *Ann. Intern. Med.* **83**:673.

Teulières, J. P., 1975, La maladie des chaines lourdes alpha, M. D. thesis, Claude Bernard University, Lyon, France.

WHO Meeting Report, 1976, Alpha-chain disease and related small intestinal lymphoma, *Arch. Fr. Mal. App. Dig.* **65**:591–607.

Wolfenstein-Todel, C., Mihaesco, E., and Frangione, B., 1974, "Alpha chain disease" protein Def: Internal deletion of a human immunoglobulin A_1 heavy chain, *Proc. Natl. Acad. Sci. USA* **71**:974–978.

Wolfenstein-Todel, C., Mihaesco, E., and Frangione, B., 1975, Variant of a human immunoglobulin: α chain disease protein AIT, *Biochem. Biophys. Res. Commun.* **65**:47–53.

Zlotnick, A., and Levy, M., 1971, α Heavy chain disease: A varient of Mediterranean lymphoma, *Arch. Intern. Med.* **128**:432–436.

IIB

Individual and Familial Susceptibility to Gastrointestinal Malignancy: Environmental and Hereditary Factors

7

Epidemiology of Esophageal Cancer

Joanna F. Haas and David Schottenfeld

1. Introduction

Dramatically different patterns of occurrence are observed for esophageal cancers in different parts of the world, among different ethnic groups, and between males and females. While the clues to the origin of this neoplasm are myriad, they defy explanation within a unifying etiological framework. Clinically, esophageal cancer presents a distinctive picture, which facilitates its diagnosis even in the face of limited diagnostic technology. The commonest presenting feature, dysphagia, occurs in virtually all cases. Often the patient is able to identify the site of the tumor by localizing the dysphagia. Obstruction progresses with increasing dysphagia, regurgitation, and aspiration. This sequence, followed by a rapid downhill course, is so characteristic that in areas where cancer of the esophagus is hyperendemic, the symptoms and outcome are well known to the population.

X-ray findings of an obstructing or constricting lesion are often diagnostic. Histological confirmation is readily obtained through endoscopic examination and biopsy. In the United States, the diagnosis is confirmed microscopically in 88% of cases (Cutler and Young, 1975). In medically isolated regions, more reliance must be placed on the clinical and radiological features of the disease. The specificity of the clinical and radiological findings permits reasonable confidence in the diagnosis even in the absence of confirmatory tissue. Fruitful epidemiological study of cancer of the esophagus has thus been possible in areas with limited medical resources.

Joanna F. Haas • Assistant Professor of Public Health, Cornell University Medical College, New York, New York 10021. ***David Schottenfeld*** • Chief, Epidemiology and Preventive Medicine, Memorial Sloan-Kettering Cancer Center, New York, New York 10021, and Professor of Public Health, Cornell University Medical College, New York, New York 10021.

The tumor is generally described both by its cell type and by its anatomical location along the length of the esophagus. Most esophageal cancers are epidermoid. Of 1918 patients with cancer of the esophagus seen at Memorial Hospital from 1926 to 1968, only 66 (3.4%) showed other cellular patterns. Of these cancers, 44 were adenocarcinomas and ten were atypical epidermoid carcinomas with glandular or spindle cell features (Turnbull *et al.,* 1973). In other areas of the world, too, epidermoid carcinomas predominate, although some reports include up to 20% adenocarcinomas (Schonland and Bradshaw, 1969; Mohan Kumar *et al.,* 1971; Krain, 1973; Cutler and Young, 1975). In the case of adenocarcinoma of the lower third of the esophagus, care must be taken to exclude stomach primaries. Benign tumors of the esophagus such as the leiomyoma or granular cell myoblastoma are rare (Farrell *et al.,* 1973).

The majority of esophageal cancers are located in the middle and lower thirds of the esophagus (Cutler and Young, 1975; Waterhouse, 1974; Martinez, 1969; Schonland and Bradshaw, 1969). Some 5.9–17.3% of esophageal cancers occur in the upper third of the esophagus. In Sweden and southeast Scotland, a higher proportion of esophageal neoplasms in females have been in the upper third. Pearson (1966) reports that 32% of esophageal cancers in female patients from southeast Scotland (1931–1964) were in the upper third. For males the comparable figure was 6%. The female predominance and the geographical distribution of this unusual anatomic pattern suggest a role for Plummer-Vinson syndrome in these areas.

2. *Geographical Pathology*

2.1. *United States*

In the United States, esophageal cancer accounts for 1.1% of all cancers in both sexes (excluding skin and *in situ* tumors); in males 1.7%, in females 0.6%. It is the cause of a higher proportion of all cancers among blacks, and its importance among black males is noteworthy (Table 1). Some 7400 cases and

Table 1. Esophageal Cancer Incidence[a] *and Esophageal Cancer as Percent of All Cancer Cases*[b] *in the United States, 1969–1971*[c]

	All races		White		Black	
	Incidence	Percent of cancer	Incidence	Percent of cancer	Incidence	Percent of cancer
Males	5.7	1.7	4.7	1.4	16.7	4.5
Females	1.6	0.6	1.3	0.5	3.7	1.5
Total	3.4	1.1	2.8	0.9	9.7	3.1

[a]Incidence rates are given per 100,000 population per annum and adjusted to the 1970 U.S. population.
[b]Excluding skin and *in situ* malignancies.
[c]Source: Third National Cancer Survey (Cutler and Young, 1975).

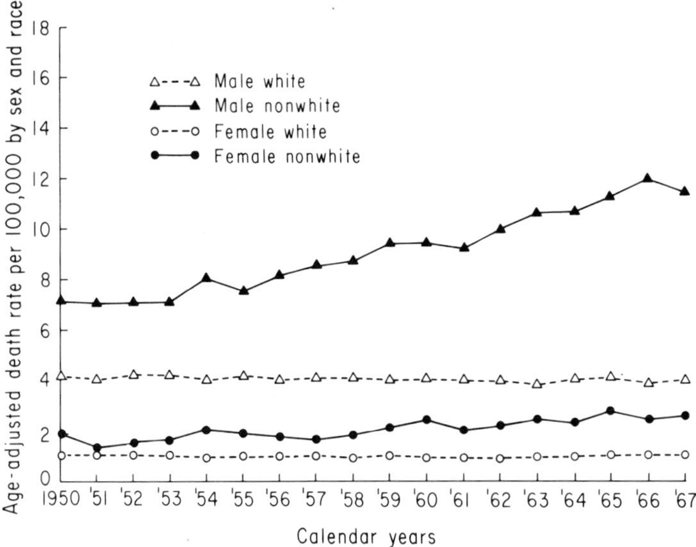

Fig. 1. Trends in esophageal cancer mortality, United States, average annual rates 1950–1967. Source: Burbank (1971).

6300 esophageal cancer deaths occur annually in the United States (Silverberg and Holleb, 1975). The average age-adjusted incidence rate for esophageal cancer determined by the Third National Cancer Survey was 3.4 cases per 100,000 (adjusted to the U.S. 1970 population). The rate for black males, 16.7 per 100,000, is 3.6 times that of white males.

Because of low survivorship, esophageal cancer mortality closely reflects incidence rates. In the United States, mortality rates in whites have been quite stable, but for black males the mortality rate has been rising since 1940 (Fig. 1). From 1950 to 1966, age-adjusted mortality in black men rose from 7.29 to 11.49. The average 1969–1971 incidence rate among black males, 16.7 per 100,000, suggests that the increase has continued. The age-adjusted mortality rates for white males ranged between 3.88 and 3.69 per 100,000 during 1950–1966. While rates for Chinese and Japanese males (7.24 and 5.18, respectively, in 1965–1966) have been intermediate between those of whites and blacks in the United States, they have not shown an upward trend. In an effort to clarify the increase among blacks, age-specific mortality rates for cancer of the esophagus were examined in successive cohorts of nonwhite males. Age-specific risk of death from esophageal cancer has risen in recent cohorts of black males, although there is some suggestion that this trend might have plateaued (Schoenberg *et al.*, 1971; Burbank, 1971).

Geographical patterns of esophageal cancer in the United States differ for males and females. Mortality data for white males for 1950–1969 have been mapped by state–economic area (Mason *et al.*, 1975). Age-adjusted mortality rates are significantly elevated in Chicago, San Francisco, and areas of the northeastern United States, including New York City, Long Island,

Connecticut, northern New Jersey, and Massachusetts. For white females, areas with high rates are found in North Carolina, Georgia, Mississippi, northern Florida, and Texas, as well as New York City, Long Island, Washington, D.C., San Francisco, and Seattle. By contrast, large areas of the Mid-, North-, and Southwest have significantly low death rates for white males and females for the same period. Since these figures are for whites only, they cannot be explained by the geographical distribution of the black population with its high esophageal cancer mortality. On the other hand, for males particularly, the disease seems concentrated in urban industrial areas. Average annual mortality rates for 1950–1969 for white males ranged from 0.23 to 8.54 per 100,000 and for white females from 0.11 to 2.32 per 100,000. The upper decile for males included areas with mortality rates of more than 5.09 and for females included areas with more than 1.34 deaths from esophageal cancer per 100,000.

2.2. *International Variation*

One of the most intriguing features of esophageal cancer is its geographical variability. Data from around the world present a mosaic of changing incidence rates and changing sex ratios (Mason *et al.*, 1964; Dunham and Bailar, 1968; Logan, 1976). For purposes of cross-cultural comparison, incidence rates for a selected age range are more useful than pooled rates for all age groups. Specifically, for neoplasms which primarily affect adults, truncated incidence rates for the ages 35–64 may be compared. Age-specific cancer incidence rates tend to decline after age 65 or 75. This can reflect a cohort effect wherein older groups with limited exposure to a newly introduced carcinogen may never experience increased mortality. More commonly, the falloff for rates in the advanced age groups reflects failure of the elderly to seek medical care or to receive the same diagnostic attention as the younger groups. Truncated rates utilize information from middle life and are most likely to provide relevant comparisons (Doll and Cook, 1967). Since in some circumstances only mortality information is available, factors for converting mortality data to incidence estimates have been calculated for several tumor sites. Using these factors, incidence rates may be estimated from mortality data (Table 2). In general the lower the survivorship the closer the conversion factor is to 1. For esophagus the incidence rate for ages 35–64 years is estimated at 1.19 times the mortality rate (Doll, 1969).

2.3. *Western Hemisphere*

In Canada, low rates of esophageal cancer prevail, and truncated incidence rates for males (ages 35–64) range from 2.1 in Manitoba to 5.3 per 100,000 in Newfoundland. Elsewhere in the Western Hemisphere rates vary considerably, and there are several foci of rather high incidence, albeit none which approaches levels found in parts of Africa and Asia. In Puerto Rico, the

Table 2. Truncated[a] Incidence Rates in Males for Esophageal Cancer, Selected Countries

Population	Rate
Africa	
Mozambique, Lourenco Marques	11.8
Nigeria, Ibadan	2.6
South Africa (colored)	28.0
South Africa (white)	6.1
South Africa, Durban (African)	98.9
South Africa, Durban (Indian)	14.7
South Africa, Johannesburg (African)	21.8
Uganda, Kyadondo	5.5
America	
Canada	2.2
United States (white)	5.8
United States (nonwhite)	20.5
Puerto Rico	35.2
Chile	18.9
Venezuela	4.8
Asia	
Singapore (Chinese)	24.6
Japan	20.7
Israel	4.2
Iran, Gonbad[b]	206.4
USSR (Turkmenistan)	110.5
USSR (Uzbekistan)	48.5
USSR (Georgia)	7.9
Northern China[c]	109.0
Europe	
Austria	4.9
Belgium	6.2
Denmark	3.9
France	25.5
Germany (Federal Republic)	4.8
Italy	6.5
Portugal	11.5
Switzerland	15.1
Sweden	3.4

[a]Incidence rates are given as average annual rates per 100,000 persons aged 35–64 years. Source: Doll (1969), except as indicated.
[b]From Mahboubi *et al.* (1973).
[c]From Dunham and Bailar (1968).

annual incidence for males ages 35–64 has averaged 35.2 per 100,000 population. In Kingston, Jamaica, it is also high, 26.6 per 100,000.

For Cali, Colombia, and for Chile, truncated rates for males are 8.2 and 18.9, respectively. In Chile, rates are higher in the north and lower in the south. The overall age-adjusted death rate for esophageal cancer in the more northern Chilean province of Aconagua was 11.1, whereas for the southern province of Bio-Bio it was 0.5 per 100,000 (Zaldivar, 1970). Esophageal cancer rates are negatively correlated with rainfall in Chile. Regions of low rainfall and high esophageal cancer also have highly alkaline soil conditions (Zaldivar and Robinson, 1971). An analogous geographical relationship has been noted for areas of eastern Iran. In Curaçao, the crude incidence of esophageal cancer for both males and females is about 21 per 100,000 (Morton, 1968). The high esophageal cancer rate reported in some areas of Brazil may be related to megaesophagus secondary to endemic Chagas' disease (Kruel de Almeida and Meinhardt, 1976).

2.4 Europe

For most of Europe low rates of esophageal cancer are the rule and are comparable to those of North American whites. France, Switzerland, and Portugal, with truncated incidence rates for males of 25.5, 15.1, and 11.5, respectively, are exceptions. In France, esophageal cancer is a major problem among males, particularly in Normandy and Brittany. In Ille-et-Vilaine, France, from 1968 to 1973 the truncated incidence rate for males was 56.1 per 100,000. The ratio of male to female cases in this area, 23.1:1, is severalfold that observed elsewhere in the world. While lower than rates in parts of Africa and Asia, the incidence of esophageal malignancy in Ille-et-Vilaine is not paralleled elsewhere in Europe or the Americas (Tuyns and Massé, 1975). The majority of the European areas of the USSR have moderate to high rates of death from esophageal cancer compared to other European countries. Truncated rates for males range from a low of 5.2 in Lithuania to 15.0 in Estonia and 24.1 in RSFSR. Areas of Soviet Central Asia experience exceptionally high rates of esophageal cancer.

2.5. Africa

Esophageal cancer in Africa has been the subject of intense interest for some years. The disease, while virtually unknown in West Africa, is common in circumscribed regions of South and East Africa with variation in rates as high as twentyfold between contiguous communities. In parts of Africa, the incidence of esophageal cancer appears to have been rapidly rising for the last three decades (Cook, 1971; Ahmed, 1966; Ahmed and Cook, 1969; Burrell, 1969; Schonland and Bradshaw, 1969; Wapnick *et al.*, 1972).

Reports from West Africa suggest that esophageal cancer is quite rare. Only 0.4% of 1920 tumors reported by the Ibadan Cancer Registry were of esophageal origin. Low rates of esophageal cancer appear to prevail in Ghana, Gabon, and the Cameroons as well as Zaire and the Congo (Brazzaville), although the data from these areas are rather sparse (Edington and Easmon, 1967; Solanke, 1969). In parts of South Africa, Rhodesia, Malawi, and Kenya, esophageal neoplasms represent 16–30% of all tumors and alternate with liver cancer as the most common neoplasm. Hyperendemic foci of esophageal cancer contrast with adjacent areas of low frequency. Liver cancer is widespread in these endemic areas, but more uniformly distributed. Where there is no systematic cancer registration system, the ratios of esophageal cancer cases to liver cancer cases have been compared among various hospitals to map out high-risk esophageal cancer regions (Cook, 1971). Incidence rates of esophageal cancer are available for some parts of Africa. Truncated incidence rates in males range from 98 per 100,000 in parts of South Africa to 39 in West Kenya. Sharp contrasts occur across political borders. In parts of Uganda, esophageal cancer is a rarity, while contiguous regions of western Kenya are high-incidence areas. In Lourenço Marques, Mozambique, the truncated incidence rate in males of 12 cases per 100,000 contrasts with high rates in Africans in adjacent Transvaal (Warwick and Harington, 1973). Regional differences are further illustrated in a study of African gold miners in the Transkei (Robertson *et al.,* 1971). Only six of 120 esophageal cancers in these miners were in workers from Mozambique. Sixty-eight percent (82) of the 120 esophageal cancers were among Cape Africans (mostly Xhosa) despite the fact that the number of individuals employed from the two areas was similar. The ratio of male to female cases varies in different areas of sub-Saharan Africa. Such ratios must be adjusted to reflect the sex ratio of the population at risk, since extensive migration of males occurs out of rural areas to areas where jobs are available.

While the evidence is fragmentary, it appears as though the frequency of esophageal cancer has risen dramatically over the past decade. A multifold increase in number of cases was noted among African patients attending hospitals in Cape Province. Moreover, while esophageal cancer is familiar to tribesmen as *umntaza wombiza* ("defilement of the gullet"), it was previously unknown, and "the old folks are emphatic that it was unheard of in their younger days" (Burrell, 1962). Registration of esophageal cancer at the Glen Grey Mission Hospital for the Ciskei, Transkei, and Tembuland regions of South Africa has indicated a rise in incidence from 16.45 before 1970 to over 40 per 100,000 in later years (Von Zeynek, 1973). Doctors who have spent long periods in the area have made similar observations. In East Africa too, there appears to have been an increase of such magnitude that esophageal cancer, which was previously rare, is now a commonplace disease. Etiological speculation must account for the appearance of the malignancy in these regions during the last 30–40 years. In addition, it must explain a mosaic spatial distribution which follows no recognized geographical boundaries. McGlashan (1969) abandons any attempt to explain these patterns by geographical or geological factors, and looks instead to sociocultural differences. Curdled milk, for example, is extensively consumed by children of the Transkeian Bantu. The agent used to curdle the milk, the juice of the fruit of the solanaceous bush (*Solanum incanum*), has been found to contain dimethylnitrosamine (DePlessis *et al.,* 1969).

2.6. *Asia*

Geographical pathology has provided intriguing insights into the etiology of esophageal cancer in Iran. Initial reports of a belt of hyperendemic disease have been supported by findings of the Caspian Cancer Registry, operating in the Caspian littoral of Iran. Five hundred doctors were distributed fairly evenly over the area covered by the Caspian Cancer Registry, giving a ratio of one physician per 8000 inhabitants. Results from that registry suggest a thirtyfold variation in the incidence of the disease in females across the region, and a tenfold variation for males. In the northeastern area of Gonbad, truncated incidence rates reach 262.9 for females and 206.4 for males. In the administrative units (shahrestans) with the highest rates, the male-to-female ratio is reversed. In shahrestans with slightly lower rates there is a slight male predominance. In parts of the northeast of Iran, the actuarial risk of developing esophageal cancer before age 65 is approximately 1 in 6. No such geographical shift is discernible for other cancers in the Caspian littoral. Most of the esophageal cancers are in the middle and lower thirds of the esophagus, with no hint of any excess of upper esophageal lesions. In addition to providing valuable information on esophageal cancer, these studies have demonstrated the possibility of conducting sophisticated cancer registration studies in isolated and underdeveloped regions, at least for readily diagnosable tumors (Mahboubi *et al.,* 1973).

Geographically, the Caspian littoral has striking variations in climate and landscape which parallel shifts in esophageal cancer frequency. The regions of very high incidence in the northeast are characterized by arid climate and saline, alkaline soil. Nearby, in areas of low risk such as the piedmont of the Elburz Mountains, precipitation is abundant and soils are not saline. Cases of cancer of the esophagus become less frequent and occur mostly in males as one moves west into the almost subtropical Caspian rainbelt, where "changes in the natural vegetation and in the agricultural practices parallel the changing features of the climate" (Kmet and Mahboubi, 1972; Mahboubi *et al.,* 1973; Mahboubi, 1971).

A study of esophageal cancer patients from the Caspian littoral matched by age and sex with healthy controls from the same or nearest village confirmed that neither alcohol nor tobacco use contributes to the high incidence rates noted. Use of both substances is minimal in males and essentially nonexistent among females. Opium use exists but is difficult to evaluate, since healthy persons are reluctant to admit to its use. It is used as an analgesic in the sick, making it difficult to sift out premorbid from therapeutic drug use. Nass, a mixture of ash, lime, and tobacco, is used in the area and may play a role in the Persian-speaking group, but does not seem to be a factor in the Turkoman population, which is at high risk for esophageal cancer (Mahboubi *et al.,* 1976).

Long-term nutritional deficiencies may be involved in esophageal cancer in Iran, and rather detailed studies of food preparation and consumption have been undertaken in 38 villages representing a range of ecological conditions and esophageal cancer experience. More bread and less rice are consumed in the high-incidence areas compared to the low-incidence areas. Deficiencies of vitamin A, riboflavin, and vitamin C are more serious in the high-incidence areas. Iron deficiency anemia is more prevalent in low-incidence regions. Cooking with spices and constant sipping of hot tea are practices rather uniformly distributed through high- and low-incidence areas. Foodstuffs consumed in high-incidence regions have been studied for the presence of nitrosamines, aflatoxin, and other known carcinogens. To date, none of these investigations has yielded positive results (Hormozdiari *et al.*, 1975). Even in the highest esophageal cancer areas of the Caspian littoral there is said to be a marked social gradient. Esophageal cancer affects the poorest families. Those of slightly higher means, owners of livestock, for example, are rather less likely to be afflicted. Considerable modernization has affected the way of life of these formerly nomadic peoples, and it has been suggested that, with socioeconomic evolution alone and without specific intervention, rates of esophageal cancer may decline (Mahboubi *et al.*, 1976).

The situation in Iran does not stop at the border. Turkoman and Kazakh tribesmen inhabiting Turkmenistan, USSR, have exceedingly high rates of esophageal cancer, 111 per 100,000 for males ages 35–64. It is reported, however, that ethnic Russians living in the same areas do not suffer high incidence rates. Localized pockets of esophageal cancer occur in Kazakhastan and Uzbekistan. As in Iran, the contiguous low-incidence areas are distinguished by abundant rainfall. The intermediate events by which geographical factors are expressed have yet to be characterized, although the interaction of soil, crops, and diet may play a role (*Lancet* editorial, 1973). In Iran these sparsely inhabited areas have been settled largely by Turkomans, and while these people have the highest incidence rate, this probably reflects environmental more than ethnic characteristics. In high-incidence areas around the Caspian Sea in the USSR, other ethnic groups are involved.

The high-incidence belt for esophageal cancer extends into northern China, where the truncated incidence rate for males is estimated to be 109 per 100,000 (Dunham and Bailar, 1968). The high incidence of esophageal cancer in this area was noted as early as 1924 by a missionary who reported that esophageal cancer was the third most frequently seen neoplasm following breast and cervix cancer (Davies, 1924).

Outside the Central Asian belt, rates of esophageal cancer are much lower but the disease is far from uncommon. The Bombay Cancer Registry reports high rates of esophageal cancer and cancers of the buccal cavity, pharynx, and larynx. The registry, functioning since 1963, covers a heterogeneous population of some 5,500,000 persons (Jussawalla and Deshpande, 1971). Esophageal cancer is the third commonest tumor. The age-adjusted incidence rate is established at 14.4 per 100,000 for males and 11 per 100,000 for females (Desai *et al.*, 1969). The truncated incidence rate for males aged 35–64 in Bombay is about 21.3 per 100,000. There is evidence from studies of railroad workers that the disease may be more common in western and southern India than in the northern, central, and eastern regions (Malhotra, 1967).

In Ceylon, esophageal cancer is the most commonly seen cancer of the gastrointestinal tract, and the most common tumor of patients admitted to thoracic units. In one series of 237 cases, not only were 58.6% of cases in females, but also, of 138 female patients, 23.2% (32) were under age 40. Ten of 99 male patients in the same series were under 40 years old. In both India and Ceylon the practice of betel chewing has been implicated in the etiology of esophageal cancer (Stephen and Uragoda, 1970).

2.7. Animals

Several foci of upper gastrointestinal neoplasms have been identified in animals. A "remarkable parallel" between high rates of squamous cell carcinoma of the esophagus in humans and in chickens in Linhsien County of the People's Republic of China has recently been highlighted. In nearby Fanhsien province, rates are low for both species (Miller, 1975). An epidemic of squamous cell cancer of the rumen, involving as many as 2.5% of cattle, has been reported in Kenya Masailand (Plowright *et al.,* 1971). All affected animals appear to have grazed in the Nasampolai Valley. The disease, locally known as *embonget,* has been recognized by the Masai since 1935. Other animals found to be affected have been forest hogs in the same area. The human population of the region does not appear to suffer high rates of esophageal cancer.

Esophageal tumors developed in 8% of sheep on one large South African farm in Cape Province during a 10-year period. The tumors began to occur after the introduction of a mass treatment program for intestinal parasites with oral instillation of nicotine sulfate and copper sulfate in lambs. The disease disappeared after the lamb-drenching solution was replaced by one containing 98% tetrachloroethylene. Animals were first affected at about 3 years of age. Tumors developed only in treated sheep grazing in plateau grasslands; animals in other grazing areas, although exposed to identical methods of animal husbandry, did not develop these tumors. The fact that esophageal tumors developed only in those treated animals which had also grazed in certain geographical areas is of special interest in light of evidence showing distinctive soil and geological characteristics in some high esophageal cancer incidence areas of Africa (Schütte, 1968).

2.8. Urban–Rural Differences

In the United States and Western Europe, esophageal cancer tends to be a disease of urban communities, with significantly higher rates among U.S. white males in the Northeast and in major population centers (Mason *et al.,* 1975). Age-, sex-, and race-adjusted esophageal cancer mortality rates for each state were significantly correlated with urbanization ($r = +0.63$) as well as alcohol ($r = +0.62$) and cigarette ($r = +0.64$) sales. When partial correlation coefficients were calculated, only degree of urbanization remained significantly correlated with esophageal cancer rates ($r = +0.51, P < 0.001$), suggesting that factors other than high alcohol and tobacco sales in urban environments were involved (Schoenberg *et al.,* 1971). In the state of Connecticut, incidence rates for cancer of the esophagus were highest in towns of highest population density. Within areas of comparable density, no correlation with degree or nature of industrialization was found. Survival did not vary with population density (Mason *et al.,* 1964). Urban counties in California had higher rates of esophageal cancer than rural counties (Krain, 1973), but the concentration of the high-risk black population in urban areas must be taken into account. Patients with esophageal cancer in Puerto Rico are most often from rural areas (Martinez, 1969). Rural predominance of cancer of the esophagus has been reported in France for the years 1961–1963 and 1966–1967 (Garbe and Brunet, 1970). In Iran, highest-incidence regions are rural and sparsely settled. The majority of high-risk African areas are also rural, but high rates are also noted for Johannesburg. In Japan, the relative risk of developing esophageal carcinoma is said to be higher among rural residents than urban dwellers. This has been attributed to a poor diet consisting largely of soy soup, rice, and noodles (Takano *et al.,* 1968). Cases of upper-third esophageal cancer in Swedish women are also most frequently encountered among residents of rural areas; again a nutritional factor is in question (Wynder *et al.,* 1957).

3. Demographic Characteristics

3.1. Age

Esophageal cancer is essentially unknown in childhood. A 5-year survey in the United States found a total of three deaths from esophageal cancer in this age group (Pickett and Briggs, 1967). The Third National Cancer Survey, which covered a total population of 21,003,451 persons throughout the

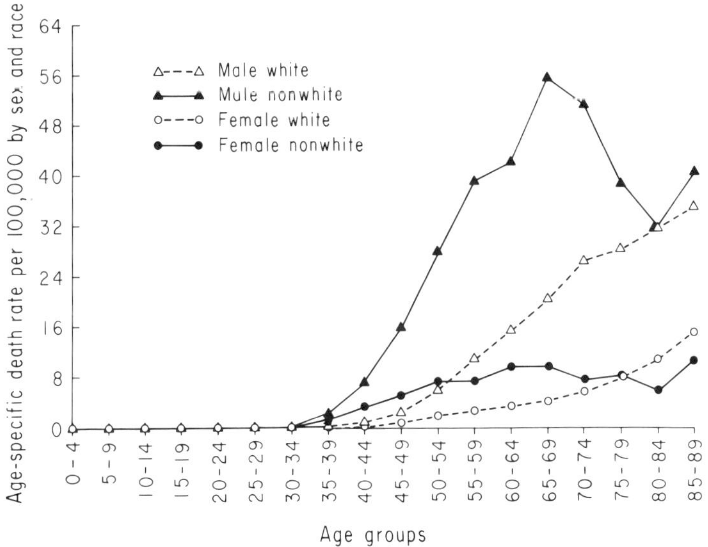

Fig. 2. Age-specific mortality rates from esophageal cancer, United States, average annual rates 1950–1967. Source: Burbank (1971).

United States, identified three new cases of esophageal cancer in persons under 30 during 1969–1971, two of whom were in the 15–19 year group. Figure 2 shows the average annual age-specific mortality rates for esophageal cancer in the United States for the period 1950–1967. Age-specific mortality rates rise steeply for males until about age 60, at which time the rate of increase slows for whites and rates actually decline for blacks (Burbank, 1971). Similar patterns are noted in England. In England there were no deaths from this neoplasm in the age group 0–14 years from 1952 to 1956. The median age for cases of esophageal cancer reported to the Birmingham Cancer Registry (U.K.) was 67.9 years for males, 68.2 for females. Ninety-five percent of cases in males were in persons between ages 45 and 88. For both males and females, increasing rates of esophageal cancer have occurred in the last decade (Waterhouse, 1974). In South Africa among Transkeian blacks, Burrell (1969) noted that mortality peaked for females at about 50 years of age, whereas for males the age-specific mortality continued to rise steeply after 60.

3.2. Sex

Considerable attention has been paid to variation in the sex ratio between regions with varying rates of esophageal cancer. In general, the ratio of male to female cases is greater than 1. The ratio may vary dramatically between adjacent regions. In the United States the male–female ratio of incidence rates is 3.6:1 for whites and 4.5:1 for blacks. In Western countries the ratio varies from about 8:1 in Switzerland and 9:1 in France to 1.3:1 in Ireland (Wynder and Bross, 1961). Switzerland and France have high esophageal cancer rates compared to most of Western Europe. In areas of Iran with exceedingly high rates of esophageal cancer there is little male predominance. In the Iranian shahrestan Gonbad, which has the highest rate of esophageal cancer, the male–female ratio was reversed, 0.85. In Africa, ratios of estimated incidence rates of cancer of the esophagus for males to females vary from 11.8:1 in West Kenya to 1.5:1 in the Transkei. No association seems to exist here between absolute rates and the sex ratio. There is evidence that the relative frequency between the sexes is changing in some areas. Reports for 1953–1955 in Johannesburg indicated that the sex ratio was 11.0:1. A later study in Johannesburg, 1962–1964, found a ratio of 5.3:1 (Cook, 1971). Variation in the sex ratio in esophageal neoplasms must be accounted for by proposed etiological mechanisms. Presumably in some areas consumption of alcohol and tobacco or other habits may contribute to a male excess. Flamant *et al.* (1964) have pointed out that the higher the correlation between a neoplasm and the consumption of tobacco or alcohol, the higher the sex ratio. In areas where male and female rates are close, a geophysical factor or dietary factor may be most important. In the high-incidence regions of the Caspian littoral, males and females presumably are comparably exposed to unknown environmental carcinogenic factors.

3.3. Race, Ethnicity, and Religion

In the United States, black, Japanese, and Chinese males have higher rates of esophageal cancer than white males. Age-specific rates among black males have been rising in successive cohorts. Genetic susceptibility among blacks might be suspected in view of high rates of esophageal cancer in Africa. However, the forefathers of most American blacks were from West Africa, an area of low esophageal cancer incidence (Kovi and Heshmat, 1973). The Bantu-speaking peoples of southern Africa, who experience high esophageal cancer rates, have contributed little to the genetic makeup of the American black. Studies of Alaskan Yupik Eskimos have demonstrated a striking excess of esophageal cancer in men and women, in the face of a generally low incidence of malignant disease. Esophageal cancer may be the most frequent malignancy encountered in this group (Fortuine, 1969).

It is difficult to separate ethnic factors from physical factors in Iran, where one population group with high esophageal cancer rates, the Turkomans, inhabits areas of the country with distinctive geographical and climatic features. In nearby regions of the USSR, Kazakhs and Uzbeks as well as Turkomans have high rates of esophageal cancer. Shaposhnikov (1964) reported that while the incidence of carcinoma of the esophagus in the Kzyl-Orda district of Soviet Central Asia was 13 per 100,000 overall, it was 35 for the Kazakhs and only 2.8 per 100,000 for other nationalities living in the same area. This elevated risk may arise from the interaction of environmental, cultural, and genetic factors.

Esophageal cancer is relatively common in Singapore. The overall incidence among Chinese males is 19.3 per 100,000 per annum. In the Teochew- and the Hokkien-speaking populations, the largest dialect groups, comparable rates are 30.8 and 26.3, respectively. Among Cantonese-speaking residents of Singapore the incidence in men is 4.1 per 100,000. Specific differences in diet, habits, and degree of adherence to traditional practice distinguish esophageal cancer patients from hospitalized controls. These factors no doubt vary in turn among language groups (DeJong *et al.,* 1974).

Religious practices may modify the behavior of adherents and thus influence health status. Ethnic and genetic factors may be confounded with religious affiliation. Certain religious groups have conspicuously different rates of esophageal cancer from those of surrounding populations. In India, the Bombay Cancer Registry showed that esophageal incidence rates were lower for the Parsi community than for the Greater Bombay population as a whole. This group is distinguished by its high socioeconomic status and by prohibition of tobacco smoking (Jussawalla *et al.,* 1970).

In the United States, the state of Utah had 22% less cancer mortality than the United States as a whole from 1950 to 1969. This was largely attributed to very low cancer rates among Mormons, who make up 72% of the state's population. Use of tobacco, alcohol, tea, and coffee is proscribed by the Mormon faith. Standardized incidence ratios for Mormons, compared to ex-

Table 3. Esophageal Cancer Incidence in the Israeli Jewish Population, 1960–1966, by Country of Origin[a]

	Males		Females	
	Rate[b]	Number	Rate[b]	Number
Total Jews	6.09	127	4.96	98
Yemen	8.11	7	11.70	9
Iran	12.32	7	26.58	9

[a]Source: Steinitz and Costin (1971).
[b]Average annual age-standardized incidence rate per 100,000 population, ages 44–74.

pected figures derived from the Third National Cancer Survey, were extremely low. Mormon males experienced 33.7% of the expected incidence of esophageal cancer and Mormon females only 10.6%. Esophageal cancer rates for the non-Mormon population of Utah were only slightly lower than the national norms (Lyon *et al.,* 1976).

3.4. Migration Studies

Mortality rates from cancer at all sites and for most specific sites in the digestive tract are higher for foreign-born than native-born U.S. whites. For esophageal cancer, the standardized mortality rate (SMR) for foreign-born males was 214; for females it was 211. The SMRs for males among the foreign-born originating in nine European countries as well as Canada and Australia were significantly higher than those of the native-born. The excess among males was especially noteworthy for persons born in Poland, Czechoslovakia, and Ireland. For females, a similar situation prevailed, with significant elevations of the SMR for persons born in England and Wales, Ireland, Sweden, Germany, Czechoslovakia, USSR, and Canada. For females originating in the USSR, the SMR, based on 42 cases, was 442, perhaps reflecting immigration from parts of the USSR with extremely high esophageal cancer rates. Age-specific mortality rates from esophageal cancer in the foreign-born rose more steeply and to much higher levels with advancing age. For foreign-born whites at 80 years of age, the mortality rate for esophageal cancer was 60 per 100,000, compared with about 20 per 100,000 among native-born U.S. whites. Since all deaths occurred in the United States, this variation could not be accounted for by classification differences (Haenszel, 1961; Kmet, 1970).

The sex ratio for esophageal cancers varied among immigrant groups from different countries. Among Polish immigrants, a high proportion of esophageal cancer deaths were in males, with 131 male and 12 female deaths in this group in the United States in 1950. Forty-nine percent of the Polish-born population over age 35 in the United States in that year was female (Staszewski and Haenszel, 1965). The low sex ratio of esophageal cancer rates in immigrants from the USSR may reflect the fairly large proportion of

Jewish immigrants in that group. The ratio of sex-specific death rates from esophageal cancer for Israeli Jews, 1.2:1, is consistent with that explanation.

Data from the Israel Cancer Register have permitted the evaluation of differences in cancer rates among Jews immigrating to Israel from different parts of the world. Esophageal cancer rates in Yemenite Jews and Iranian Jews are quite high, among both males and females. Age-standardized incidence rates for the two groups are shown in Table 3. The high esophageal cancer rates for Yemenite Jews are particularly noteworthy, since this group experienced low death rates from malignant neoplasms compared to the rest of the Israeli Jewish population (Steinitz and Costin, 1971).

3.5. Social Class

Esophageal cancer tends to be a disease of lower socioeconomic groups (Table 4). In data from the United States Second National Cancer Survey (1947), a gradient in standardized incidence rates is apparent, with class I (highest) having 55% of expected incidence compared to 137% in class V (lowest). For females, the gradient is less marked, but an excess is apparent in the lowest socioeconomic group. From the U.S. figures it is not possible to separate out the effect of race from low socioeconomic status, since nonwhites are concentrated in the lower strata. Excess deaths from esophageal cancer occur in class V males in Denmark and in England and Wales. Married females of class V in England and Wales have a Standardized Mortality Ratio (SMR) of 126. For unmarried females of class V in England and Wales, the SMR for esophageal cancer is 46 (Levin *et al.,* 1974). In Puerto Rico, about one-third of esophageal cancer patients were illiterates, in contrast to 12.8% of the island population over age 10. Approximately one-fourth had less than a grade 4 education. Some 35% were agricultural workers compared with 19.4% of the total labor force. Most patients were in the lowest-salary occupations. Not surprisingly, poor diets and poor dentition were also common (Martinez, 1969). Eighty-five percent of the group were described by interviewers as being white. The extent to which differences in smoking and drink-

Table 4. Standardized Incidence and Mortality Ratio for Cancer of the Esophagus by Socioeconomic Class in Males: United States, Denmark, and England and Wales[a]

Class	U.S., white, 10 cities, 1947, incidence	Denmark, 1943–1947, incidence	England and Wales, 20–64 years of age, 1949–1953, mortality
I (highest)	55	104	132
II	88	103	92
III	105	67	91
IV	102	80	98
V (lowest)	137	122	130

[a]Source: Levin *et al.* (1974).

ing habits can explain observed social class differences is not known. Poor diet and consumption of home-brewed beverages are also related to social class.

3.6. Occupation

Few specific occupational factors have been implicated in esophageal cancer. The SMR for esophageal cancer by broad occupational category suggests excesses among "Laborers, except farm and mine" (182), "Service workers except private household" (149), "Operatives and kindred workers" (122), and "Draftsmen, foremen and kindred workers" (117) (Levin, 1974). These differences may reflect racial, socioeconomic, and urban–rural factors more than specific occupational risks. The prevalence of smoking varies by occupational group. It is highest among blue-collar workers and lowest among professionals, managers, and proprietors (Sterling and Weinkam, 1976). In Puerto Rico the age-adjusted death rate for esophageal cancer in the professional and managerial group was less than half that for farm and service workers (Martinez, 1964).

The excess of esophageal cancer in males and its concentration in urban settings, however, are clues that occupational factors could play a role. One study has suggested that chromium ferroalloys might be such agents (Pokrovskaia and Shabynina, 1973). Among African workers in Natal, reported exposures to a number of occupational carcinogens (petrol and oil, tar, lead, asbestos, soot, and bagasse) were more common for both esophageal cancer patients and lung cancer patients than for controls. However, a large proportion of patients with these neoplasms had no history whatever of exposure to industrial carcinogens (Bradshaw and Schonland, 1969). Young and Russell (1926) described excesses of esophageal cancer among workers in the metal trades. They observed, as have others since, a predilection to the disease in groups such as "brewers, innkeepers, and publicans, whose work is said to facilitate consumption of alcohol." Wynder and Bross (1961) observed an excess of "alcohol-exposed" workers, including bartenders, brewery workers, waiters, and longshoremen among esophageal cancer patients. No other differences in occupational exposures were in evidence between study and control groups. Similar conclusions were suggested by a study of Danish male patients with esophageal cancer (Mosbech and Videbaek, 1955).

3.7. Heredofamilial Factors

Tylosis is the one heredofamilial disorder clearly associated with esophageal cancer. This disorder, marked by hyperkeratosis of the palms and soles, can be inherited as an autosomal dominant trait. Two Liverpool families with this form of tylosis have been followed from 1958 to 1970. Cancer has been occurring among them at a rate which will, if it continues, result in death before age 65 in 95% of family members with tylosis. All cases of esophageal cancer have developed in individuals with tylosis. Two deaths in persons with tylosis were due to other causes. No cases of esophageal cancer have occurred in family members without tylosis (Howel-Evans *et al.*, 1958; Harper *et al.*, 1970). This hereditary form of tylosis associated with esophageal cancer occurs about 10 years later than usual (Harper, 1971). The esophageal neoplasms occur at early ages in these individuals. Esophageal cancer occurred in a 30-year-old individual with hereditary tylosis who did not smoke or drink. The prospects of preventing the neoplasm or of diagnosing it in a curable stage are doubtful. Cytogenetic studies have not been revealing (Lynch, 1976).

4. *Etiological Considerations*

No single carcinogenic agent is involved in all areas in which excesses of esophageal cancer occur. Several factors have been incriminated which are no doubt part of complex sequences. Environmental carcinogens, nutritional deficiencies, chronic irritation, and mucosal damage all have been implicated in the etiology of esophageal cancer (Table 5).

4.1. Alcohol

Esophageal cancer has been induced in mice by the administration of ethanol containing benzo[α]pyrene and 4-nitroquinoline 1-oxide (Horie *et al.*, 1965). A variety of brands of bourbon, scotch, and whiskey have been shown by Japanese investigators to contain small amounts of polycyclic aromatic hydrocarbons (Masuda *et al.*, 1966).

In Europe and the Americas, alcohol appears to be a major etiological factor in esophageal cancer. Mortality rates for alcoholism and for esophageal cancer in males ages 45–64 were significantly correlated in data reported by administrative units in France for the years 1960–1963 (Tuyns, 1970), and the association with "occupational" exposure to alcohol has been alluded to. There is an excess of heavy drinkers among esophageal cancer patients. Wynder and Bross (1961) demonstrated that the average daily alcohol intake of male esophageal cancer patients from two New York City hospitals was significantly greater than that of male control patients with cancers at other sites. The proportion admitting to drinking greater than the equivalent of 3 oz of whiskey per day was higher in the esophageal cancer group (71% vs. 26%), while the proportion who denied drinking was smaller (3% vs. 15% in the control group). Binge drinkers and those drinking greater than the equivalent of 7 oz of whiskey daily made up 34% of the esophageal cancer group and only 13% of the controls. Differences in type or manner of alcohol consumption could not be demonstrated. Alcohol continued to be a factor when patients with similar smoking habits were compared. Among women patients with esophageal cancer there was a tendency to greater alcohol use than among controls, although the magnitude of the differences was more modest than in males, and might have occurred by chance. In a group of Puerto Rican patients with cancer of the esophagus there were significantly fewer nondrinkers and more heavy drinkers than in a group of neighborhood controls

Table 5. Proposed Etiological Factors in Esophageal Cancer

- Tobacco
  - Smoking cigarettes, pipes, and cigars and chewing tobacco all increase risk.
  - Epithelial changes in the esophagus are related to amount smoked.
  - Risk of esophageal cancer increases with number of cigarettes smoked.
  - Tobacco–alcohol synergism is a possibility.
- Quid chewing
  - Increased risk is present with or without tobacco in the quid.
  - Quid also contains slaked lime, betel nuts, liquified catechu, spices.
- Alcohol
  - Alcohol is especially important in Europe and North America.
  - Risk is increased among workers in "alcohol trades": bartenders, waiters etc.
  - Locally brewed beers may play a role in hyperendemic areas in Africa.
- Nutrition
  - Mice are more susceptible to some ingested carcinogens when diet is deficient in protein, vitamin A, and B complex
  - A role is possible in humans with riboflavin, and iron deficiencies, especially in rural areas.
- Carcinogenic contaminants in foods
  - Dimethylnitrosamine is present in fruit of solanaceous bush (used to curdle milk for children among Transkeian Bantu).
  - Contamination of home-brewed spirits in Africa with nitrosamines or other carcinogens is a possibility.
  - Use of highly spiced foods may play a role in parts of Asia.
- Carcinogenic fungal toxins
  - Soil factors could affect susceptibility of plants to toxic fungi.
  - Molybdenum deficiency in soil and plants may be a factor.
- Esophageal injury
  - Esophageal strictures from lye ingestion, but also congenital, very substantially increase risk of esophageal cancer in humans. Increased susceptibility to carcinogens in animals with experimental strictures has been shown.
  - Thermal injury occurs from ingestion of high-temperature beverages in Near and Far East.
  - Achalasia
    - There is a three- to tenfold increase of squamous cell carcinoma.
  - Barrett's esophagus
    - There is a clinical impression of increased risk, especially of adenocarcinoma of the esophagus.
- Other diseases associated with excess risk of esophageal cancer
  - Plummer-Vinson syndrome
    - The syndrome of iron deficiency anemia with esophageal webs and mucous membrane abnormalities is associated with carcinoma of the upper third of the esophagus or the hypopharynx, especially in women in rural Northern Europe. Possible roles for complex nutritional deficiencies.
  - Idiopathic steatorrhea or adult celiac disease
  - Tylosis
    - Tylosis was present in two kinships; hereditary pattern of autosomal dominance and complete penetrance; esophageal cancer occurrence in 95% of family members with tylosis.

matched by age and sex. When only pairs with similar tobacco use were considered, alcohol consumption continued to be greater in esophageal cancer patients, suggesting that the effect of alcohol was independent of tobacco consumption (Martinez, 1969).

In Africa, locally brewed alcoholic drinks have been under suspicion as a factor in esophageal cancer. Consumption of homemade beer is common in many places and it is primarily drunk by men. The techniques for preparing these beers reflect local ingenuity and the main ingredients vary from place to place. A number of mechanisms have been hypothesized which would be consistent with an association between consumption of local beers and esophageal cancer. It was suggested that nitrosaminelike compounds were present in native spirits (McGlashan *et al.,* 1968). This has not been confirmed by gas chromatographic or mass spectrometric analysis (Collis *et al.,* 1971). Nitrosamine contamination of local spirits does not appear to be widespread. An alternative explanation is offered by Cook (1971), who, after extensive evaluation of time trends and the geographical distribution of esophageal cancer in Africa, proposed that the introduction and spread of maize cultivation and its use as a major ingredient in alcoholic drinks could explain the observed patterns of esophageal cancer. Maize had spread widely as a food crop since the turn of the century, and had replaced sorghum as the basis for beer in parts of South Africa. Information on the extent and time of introduction is incomplete. More precise information about the content of beers in different areas would be needed to account for the sharp gradients of esophageal cancer in the Transkei. Esophageal cancer is not common in areas where millet is widely used. In Western Africa, with low rates of esophageal cancer, yams, cassava, bananas, rice, millet, and sorghum are staple foods and maize is not a traditional crop. Another fact nicely explained by the maize hypothesis is the abrupt disappearance of esophageal cancer at the Ugandan side of the Kenyan border. Since the 1930s Uganda discouraged the cultivation of maize while the Kenyan government actively encouraged its spread. There are no other geophysical or cultural factors which readily explain the concurrence of the esophageal cancer gradient with the political border. On the other hand, it is not evident why maize-based beer should be an etiological factor in esophageal cancer in Africa. One proposed mechanism is the contamination of maize beer with aflatoxin. Aflatoxin is known to be a cause of hepatoma in animals and may be responsible for a considerable amount of that disease in Africa. It is a widespread contaminant of food and is also found in fermented drinks. A number of facts may be marshaled against this suggestion. Liver cancer in Africa is more widespread and more uniformly distributed than esophageal cancer. It is common in West Africa and in parts of East Central and South Africa, where esophageal cancer is virtually not seen. Aflatoxin contaminates food and wine in West Africa and in other areas of low esophageal cancer incidence. At higher altitudes, stored grains are less frequently contaminated with aflatoxin. Esophageal cancer frequency does not change with altitude. Moreover, the fact that aflatoxins are more common contaminants of food than fermented drinks is inconsistent with the large male predominance of esophageal cancer in most areas (Cook and Collis, 1972).

In Iran, alcohol cannot be implicated in areas of high incidence of esophageal cancer. These areas are inhabited by Islamic peoples for whom both alcohol and tobacco are proscribed. Consumption of alcohol and tobacco smoking is exceedingly low among male patients with esophageal cancer as well as among controls. Females, who in much of this region are at the same risk for esophageal cancer as males, simply do not use tobacco or alcohol. For these areas, alternative explanations must be sought (Mahboubi *et al.*, 1976).

4.2. Tobacco

Habits of tobacco use differ from culture to culture, and, as one might expect, so does the pathology associated with its use. Tobacco may be smoked, chewed, and sniffed. It may be used alone or in combination with a variety of other substances. Tobacco smoking seems to play a role in the genesis of oral and upper gastrointestinal tract malignancies as well as those of the respiratory tract. Autopsy assessment of nuclear atypia in esophageal specimens from 1202 men showed a clear and strong association between smoking and the presence of atypical nuclei. The extent of atypia increased with the number of cigarettes smoked. The mucosa of nonsmokers showed few abnormal cells. In 15 of 779 "current cigarette smokers," lesions with the general appearance of carcinoma *in situ* were found in which cells with abnormal nuclei extended from the tunica propria to the surface. Thicker epithelium in the esophagus was found in smokers, reflecting basal cell hyperplasia. This too increased with the number of cigarettes smoked. "Histologic changes in the esophagus are strikingly similar to findings in previous studies of the trachea and bronchial tubes" (Auerbach *et al.*, 1965).

The association between tobacco usage and esophageal cancer has been shown retrospectively and prospectively. Wynder and Bross (1961) found that those who never smoked constituted 5% of a series of patients with cancer of the esophagus but 15% of controls with cancers of other sites (excluding cancers known to be associated with cigarette smoking). More persons smoking greater than 21 cigarettes per day and a higher percentage of cigar and pipe smokers and tobacco chewers were found among patients with esophageal cancer than controls. Smokers in the cancer of the esophagus group smoked to a shorter butt length than controls. After standardizing for heavy and light use of alcohol, the relative risk of developing esophageal cancer was estimated by level of tobacco use. Among those drinking greater than the equivalent of 3 oz of whiskey a day, the relative risk was 1.7 for nonsmokers and 6 for cigar/pipe smokers. Although the number of patients who consumed less than 3 oz of alcohol a day was small, this group had a relative risk of developing esophageal cancer close to 1, regardless of smoking habits. Thus in heavy drinkers the risk of esophageal cancer is related to the amount smoked. In light drinkers, increased risk with smoking was not convincingly demonstrated. In a group of Swedish male patients smoking was significantly related to cancer of the esophagus as well as to other upper alimentary tract cancers. It did not account for the relatively high occurrence of esophageal neoplasms in Swedish women (Wynder *et al.*, 1957). Patients with esophageal cancer in Puerto Rico were also more likely to be heavy smokers. When patients with esophageal, mouth, and pharyngeal cancer were matched with neighborhood controls by alcohol intake as well as age and sex, the relative risk of malignancy continued to be related to increasing amounts of tobacco smoked. Few patients or controls chewed tobacco (Martinez, 1969).

These findings are consistent with those of several prospective studies which have estimated the risk of esophageal cancer in smokers as 2–6 times that of nonsmokers, with risk increasing with amount smoked. Cigar and pipe smokers also experienced risks of 2–4 times those of nonsmokers (Wynder and Mabuchi, 1973). Prospective analysis of the mortality and smoking habits of 68,153 labor union members in California revealed a relative risk of 1.82 for esophageal cancer in men smoking more than 1½ packs of cigarettes daily compared to nonsmokers (Weir and Dunn, 1970). Among British physicians the rate for all smokers was 2.5 times that of nonsmokers. The rates of esophageal cancer increased with increasing amounts smoked (Doll and Hill, 1964). In Bombay, cases of esophageal cancer were matched from voter lists with individuals of the same age, sex, and religion, and both groups were questioned about smoking and quid-chewing habits. The estimated relative risks for quid chewers and tobacco smokers were 2–3 times the risk for those with neither habit. For individuals with combined habits, the relative risk of esophageal cancer was greater than for those with only one habit. Smoking of "bidis," Indian cigarettes consisting of a small amount of tobacco in a dried leaf, was not uncommon. The relative risk of esophageal cancer associated with their use was 2.9. Tobacco chewing alone was associated with some 3.5 the expected risk of esophageal cancer. The role of tobacco in cancers associated with quid chewing is not certain. A variety of ingredients including betel leaves and lime may be chewed in quid along with tobacco. Quid chewed without tobacco may be involved in cancer of the oropharynx and esophagus. Among those chewing quid made without tobacco, the risk of esophageal cancer was comparable to the risk for those who chewed quid with tobacco (Jussawalla and Deshpande, 1971).

4.3. Other Pathological States Associated with Increased Esophageal Cancer

Mucosal damage or irritation from a variety of conditions appears to predispose to the development of esophageal carcinoma. Esophageal cancer is more readily induced in hamsters via instillation of carcinogen (benzo[α]pyrene) in animals which have had the lower esophagus surgically constricted (Dunham and Sheets, 1974). Strictures can lead to mechanical irritation above the stenosis and esophagitis below. Many such strictures have resulted from lye ingestion, although mechanical or thermal trauma and congenital defects are infrequently their cause. The shortest reported interval between stricture formation and esophageal cancer occurred in a 15-year-old Korean boy who had ingested lye 12 years earlier (Kinnmann *et al.,* 1968). Fourteen cases of malignancies were seen from 1953 to 1967 among a group of patients with histories of chemical burns 16–41 years before (Sytnik and Petrov, 1968). In a group of some 200 patients in whom reconstructive surgery for esophageal cicatricial stricture was performed between 1937 and 1969, five developed esophageal cancer some 15–20 years after the original injury (Rogacheva *et al.,* 1971). Based on nine cancers of the esophagus observed in 381 persons with corrosions (90% of which were due to lye ingestion), Kirivanta (1952) estimated that for Finnish patients aged 25–64 years with corrosions at least 24 years earlier, the risk of developing esophageal cancer was about a hundredfold that for other people in the same age group. The latency period between corrosion and cancer ranged from 24 to 44 years. It should be noted that achlorhydria was present in 80% and anemia in 85% of patients in this group and hence other factors besides corrosion may have augmented the risk.

Esophageal cancer has also been associated with achalasia, most often in patients with a long history of recurrent treatment with bouginage. Just-Viera and Haight (1969) identified 167 cases of esophageal cancer in patients with achalasia in the American and Western European literature since 1872. The reported frequency of esophageal cancer in various series of patients with achalasia varied from none to 20%. It seemed to be greatest for males, and few such patients were black. Esophageal cancer occurred at an earlier age than expected; one patient was 14 years old. Symptoms of achalasia had been present for an average of 17 years before the diagnosis of esophageal cancer. At the Mayo Clinic, 1318 patients were treated for esophageal achalasia for an average of 13 years. Seven developed esophageal cancer, for an overall incidence rate of 41 cases per 100,000 per year with 95% confidence limits of 16–84 per 100,000. Six additional patients with esophageal cancer had a history of achalasia. In these patients achalasia had been present an average of 28 years prior to the diagnosis of esophageal malignancy (Wychulis *et al.,* 1971). Tobacco and alcohol use were not considered but probably could not account for an increase of this magnitude.

Conflicting reports have appeared about gastric surgery as an antecedent to esophageal cancer. Prior gastric surgery was noted in eight out of 92 consecutive patients with esophageal squamous cell carcinoma seen for radiotherapy in Edinburgh (Shearman *et al.,* 1970). Chance or selection bias could readily account for this apparent excess. Review of necropsy reports in Norway did not suggest that the prior gastric surgery for benign condition was more frequent in patients dying of esophageal cancer than in controls matched by age, sex, and year of necropsy (Stalsberg, 1972).

Peptic reflux esophagitis from several anatomical abnormalities has been linked with esophageal cancer. In many cases it is not clear which came first (Smithers, 1955). Barrett's esophagus (columnar epithelial lined esophagus) has been regarded both as a congenital variant and as an acquired abnormality developing following destruction of esophageal squamous epithelium by gastroesophageal reflux (Paull *et al.,* 1976). Experience with the lesion is limited. It has been the impression of several observers that these patients have a high incidence of associated esophageal malignancy, particularly adenocarcinoma. In such a setting, special care must be taken to avoid confusion of gastric lesions with lower-third esophageal cancers (Burgess *et al.,* 1971; Jernstrom and Brewer, 1970).

Carcinomas of the digestive tract and particularly of the esophagus may complicate adult celiac disease and idiopathic steatorrhea. In 202 patients with these two disorders followed between 1941 and 1965, six cases of esophageal cancer occurred. A total of 31 malignant neoplasms occurred in 29 patients in this series. Five of the six cases of esophageal cancer were in males. The mean duration of celiac disease prior to diagnosis of esophageal carcinoma was 58.1 years (Harris *et al.,* 1967).

The association of esophageal cancers involving the upper third of the esophagus or the lower hypopharynx with the presence of Plummer-Vinson syndrome (Kelly-Paterson syndrome) has long been appreciated. In Sweden, the geographical distributions of the two diseases coincide. Both occur in northern rural areas and both are especially common in females. Iron deficiency anemia and vitamin B deficiencies are endemic in these outlying regions. Detailed interviews of Swedish female patients with cancer of the hypopharynx elicited a history of unexplained dysphagia preceding the tumor by more than 2 years in 70%. A variety of other signs and symptoms were compatible with Plummer-Vinson syndrome. Diets of these patients were high in carbohydrates, low in vitamins (especially vitamin C), and nearly devoid of fresh foods, whether fruits, vegetables, meat, or fish. Mucosal signs of Plummer-Vinson disease cleared with improved diets, and iron and riboflavin supplementation (Wynder *et al.,* 1957). Widespread recognition and treatment of the Plummer-Vinson syndrome have made elucidation of its role as a premalignant state difficult.

Others have drawn attention to the overlap of areas of molybdenum-deficient soil and esophageal cancer occurrence in the Transkei, South Africa. The mineral deficiency in the soil predisposes plants to fungal diseases as well as to the accumulation of nitrates as a result of impaired nitrogen metabolism. Dimethylnitrosamines have been isolated in this area from the fruit of the solanaceous bush. Curdled milk, a nutritional mainstay for boys up to age 20, is produced by the addition of juice from the solanaceous fruit. Females ingest little of this drink, however, and any proposed etiological agent must account for the checkered pattern of high-incidence esophageal cancer among females in the Transkei (Burrell *et al.,* 1966; DuPlessis *et al.,* 1969).

The risk of esophageal cancer is increased in individuals with previously diagnosed epidermoid malignancies of the upper digestive system, larynx, or lung. A tenfold increase of esophageal cancer has been observed in longitudinal studies and presumably reflects a common role for excessive tobacco and alcohol use (Schottenfeld *et al.,* 1974).

5. Conclusions

No unifying hypothesis explains the varied epidemiological picture presented by esophageal cancer in different regions of the world. No single factor among the many with which it has been associated accounts for its diversity in geographical distribution and sex ratio or its changing frequency. The epidemiological picture suggests more than one environmental determinant. These clues must be pursued since the only prospects for reducing the mortality from esophageal cancer lie in its prevention.

Alcohol plays a role, particularly in North America and Europe, in the genesis of esophageal cancer. Since there is no evidence that it acts directly as a carcinogen, alternative explanations must be sought. Ethanol may be consumed simultaneously with carcinogen-containing foodstuffs, or it may be a vehicle for them. It may serve as a promoting or cocarcinogenic agent. Alcohol consumption may be associated with nutritional deficiency and with chronic esophageal irritation. Both these factors have been independently correlated with esophageal cancer. Tobacco smoking, closely tied with alcohol consumption, seems to make an independent contribution to esophageal cancer. Smoking induces dose-related histological changes in the esophageal squamous epithelium strongly reminiscent of those preceding bronchogenic carcinoma. Other forms of tobacco use alone or in combination with a variety of substances are involved in esophageal cancer in parts of Asia. In areas such as the Caspian littoral where esophageal cancer is not tobacco or alcohol related, dietary factors are of special concern. Geophysical environment may be reflected in the effect of local soil characteristics on diet. Molds productive of carcinogens could be geographically limited food contaminants. Mucosa conditioned by chronic specific nutritional deficiency may be especially vulnerable to the action of carcinogens.

Enormous effort has gone into defining the worldwide patterns of this neoplasm. The mosaic of esophageal cancer is almost visible. The task which remains is to interpret what has been uncovered. Analytical studies designed to identify specific antecedents will be needed if strategies to control the disease are to be devised.

6. References

Ahmed, N., 1966, Geographical incidence of oesophageal cancer in West Kenya, *East Afr. Med. J.* **43**:235–248.

Ahmed, N., and Cook, P., 1969, The incidence of cancer of the oesophagus in West Kenya, *Br. J. Cancer* **23**:302–312.

Auerbach, O., Stout, A. P., Hammond, E. C., and Garfinkel, L., 1965, Histologic changes in esophagus in relation to smoking habits, *Arch. Environ. Health* **11**:4–15.

Bashirov, M.Sh., Nugmanov, S. N., and Kolycheva, N. I., 1968, Epidemiology of esophageal cancer in the Aktivbinsk region of Kazakh SSR, *Vopr. Onkol.* **14**:3–6 (in Goldsmith and Miller, 1975).

Bradshaw, E., and Schonland, M., 1969, Oesophageal and lung cancers in Natal African males in relation to certain socio-economic factors: An analysis of 484 interviews, *Br. J. Cancer* **23**:275–284.

Burbank, F., 1971, Patterns in cancer mortality in the United States: 1950–1967, *Natl. Cancer Inst. Monogr.*, No. 33.

Burgess, J. N., Payne, W. S., Andersen, H. A., Weiland, L. H., and Carlson, H. C., 1971, Barrett esophagus, the columnar epithelial-lined lower esophagus, *Mayo Clin. Proc.* **46**:728–734.

Burrell, R. J. W., 1962, Esophageal cancer among Bantu in the Transkei, *J. Natl. Cancer Inst.* **28**:495–514.

Burrell, R. J. W., 1969, Distribution maps of esophageal cancer among Bantu in the Transkei, *J. Natl. Cancer Inst.* **43**:877–889.

Burrell, R. J. W., Roach, W. A., and Shadwell, A., 1966, Esophageal cancer in the Bantu of the Transkei associated with mineral deficiency in garden plants, *J. Natl. Cancer Inst.* **36**:201–214.

Collis, C. H., Cook, P. J., Foreman, J. K., and Palframan, J. F., 1971, A search for nitrosamines in East African spirit samples from areas of varying oesophageal cancer frequency, *Gut* **12**:1015–1018.

Cook, P., 1971, Cancer of the oesophagus in Africa: A summary and evaluation of the evidence for the frequency of occurrence, and a preliminary indication of the possible association with the consumption of alcoholic drinks made from maize, *Br. J. Cancer* **25**:853–880.

Cook, P., and Collis, C. H., 1972, Cancer of the oesophagus and alcoholic drinks in East Africa (letter), *Lancet* **1**:1014.

Cutler, S. J., and Young, J. L., Jr., 1975, Third national cancer survey: Incidence data, *Natl. Cancer Inst. Monogr.*, No. 41.

Davies, S., 1924, Cancer in China (letter), *Br. Med. J.* (Jan. 19, 1924), p. 131.

DeJong, U. W., Breslow, N., Goh Ewe Hong, J., Sridharan, M., and Shanmugaratnam, K., 1974, Aetiological factors in oesophageal cancer in Singapore Chinese, *Int. J. Cancer* **13**:291–303.

Desai, P. B., Borges, E. J., Vohra, V. G., and Paymaster, J. C., 1969, Carcinoma of the esophagus in India, *Cancer* **23**:979–989.

Doll, R., 1969, The geographical distribution of cancer, *Br. J. Cancer* **23**:1–8.

Doll, R., and Cook, P., 1967, Summarizing indices for comparison of cancer incidence data, *Int. J. Cancer* **2**:269–279.

Doll, R., and Hill, A. B., 1964, Mortality in relation to smoking: Ten years' observations of British doctors, *Br. Med. J.* **1**:1399–1410.

Dunham, L. J., and Bailar, J. C., III, 1968, World maps of cancer mortality rates and frequency ratios, *J. Natl. Cancer Inst.* **41**:155–203.

Dunham, L. J., and Sheets, R. H., 1974, Effects of esophageal constriction on benzo[α]pyrene carcinogenesis in hamster esophagus and forestomach, *J. Natl. Cancer Inst.* **53**:875–881.

DuPlessis, L. S., Nunn, J. R., and Roach, W. A., 1969, Carcinogen in a Transkeian Bantu food additive, *Nature (London)* **222**:1198–1199.

Edington, G. M., and Easmon, C. O., 1967, Incidence of cancer of the alimentary tract in Accra, Ghana and Ibadan, Western Nigeria, in: *Tumors of the Alimentary Tract in Africans* (J. F. Murry, ed.), *Natl. Cancer Inst. Monogr.*, No. 25.

Editorial, 1973, Oesophageal cancer on the Caspian littoral, *Lancet* **2**:1365–1367.

Farrell, K. H., Devine, K. D., Harrison, E. G., and Olsen, A. M., 1973, Granular cell myoblastoma of the esophagus: Incidence and surgical treatment, *Ann. Otol.* **82**:784–789.

Flamant, R., Lasserre, O., Lazar, P., Leguerinais, J., Denoix, P., and Schwartz, D., 1964, Differences in sex ratio according to cancer site and possible relationship with use of tobacco and alcohol, *J. Natl. Cancer Inst.* **32**:1309–1314.

Fortuine, R., 1969, Characteristics of cancer in the Eskimos of southwestern Alaska, *Cancer* **23**:468–474.

Garbe, E., and Brunet, M., 1970, Cancer and air pollution: Aspects of geographical pathology, *Bull. Inst. Natl. Sante* **25(2)**:201–212.

Goldsmith, J. R., and Miller, G. L., 1975, *Abstracts and Indexes to Selected Literature on Occupational and Environmental Carcinogenic Hazards,* The Franklin Institute Research Laboratories, Philadelphia.

Haenszel, W., 1961, Cancer mortality among the foreign born in the United States, *J. Natl. Cancer Inst.* **26:**37–132.

Harper, P. S., 1971, Genetic heterogeneity in hyperkeratosis palmaris et plantaris, *Birth Defects: Orig. Art. Ser.*, VII(8), June.

Harper, P. S., Harper, R. M. J., and Howel-Evans, A. W., 1970, Carcinoma of the oesophagus with tylosis, *Q. J. Med.* **39:**317–333.

Harris, O. D., Cooke, W. T., Thompson, H., and Waterhouse, J. A. H., 1967, Malignancy in adult coeliac disease and idiopathic steatorrhoea, *Am. J. Med.* **42:**899–912.

Horie, A., Kohchi, S., and Kuratsune, M., 1965, Carcinogenesis in the esophagus. II. Experimental production of esophageal cancer by administration of ethanolic solution of carcinogens, *Gann* **56:**429–441.

Hormozdiari, H., Day, N. E., Aramesh, B., and Mahboubi, E., 1975, Dietary factors and esophageal cancer in the Caspian littoral of Iran, *Cancer Res.* **35:**3493–3498.

Howel-Evans, A. W., McConnell, R. B., Clarke, C. A., and Sheppard, P. M., 1958, Carcinoma of the oesophagus with keratosis palmaris et plantaris (tylosis): A study of two families, *Q. J. Med.* **27:**413–429.

Jernstrom, P., and Brewer, L. A., III, 1970, Primary adenocarcinoma of the midesophagus arising in ectopic gastric mucosa with associated hiatal hernia and reflux esophagitis (Dawson's syndrome), *Cancer* **26:**1343–1348.

Jussawalla, D. J., and Deshpande, V. A., 1971, Evaluation of cancer in tobacco chewers and smokers: An epidemiologic assessment, *Cancer* **28:**244–252.

Jussawalla, D. J., Deshpande, W., Haenszel, W., and Natekar, M. V., 1970, Differences observed in the site incidence of cancer between the Parsi community and the total population of Greater Bombay: A critical appraisal, *Br. J. Cancer* **24:**56–66.

Just-Viera, J. O., and Haight, C., 1969, Achalasia and carcinoma of the esophagus, *Surg. Gynecol. Obstet.* **128:**1081–1095.

Kinnman, J., Shin, H. I., and Wetteland, P., 1968, Carcinoma of the oesophagus after lye corrosion: Report of a case in a 15-year-old Korean male, *Acta Chir. Scand.* **134:**489–493.

Kiviranta, U. K., 1952, Corrosion carcinoma of the esophagus: 381 cases of corrosion and nine cases of corrosion carcinoma, *Acta Otolaryngol* **42:**89–15.

Kmet, J., 1970, The role of migrant population in studies of selected cancer sites: A review, *J. Chron. Dis.* **23:**305–324.

Kmet, J., and Mahboubi, E., 1972, Esophageal cancer in the Caspian littoral of Iran: Initial studies, *Science* **175:**846–853.

Kovi, J., and Heshmat, M. Y., 1973, Incidence of cancer in Negroes in Washington, D.C. and selected African cities, *Am. J. Epidemiol.* **96:**401–413.

Krain, L. S., 1973, Esophageal cancer in California 1942–1969: The California Tumor Registry experience, *J. Surg. Oncol.* **5:**267–275.

Kruel de Almeida, J., and Meinhardt, N. G., 1976, Esophagus carcinoma: Diagnostic and etiologic aspects, presented at the Third International Symposium on Detection and Prevention of Cancer, New York City.

Levin, D. L., Devesa, S. S., Godwin, J. D., II, and Silverman, D. T., 1974, *Cancer Rates and Risks*, DHEW Publ. No. (NIH) 76-691, U.S. Government Printing Office, Washington, D.C.

Logan, W. P. D., 1976, Cancers of the alimentary tract: International mortality trends, *WHO Chron.* **30:**413–419.

Lynch, H. T., 1976, Skin heredity and cancer, in: *Cancer Genetics* (H. T. Lynch, ed.), Thomas, Springfield, Ill.

Lyon, J. L., Klauber, M. R., Gardner, J. W., and Smart, C. R., 1976, Cancer incidence in Mormons and non-Mormons in Utah, 1966–1970, *N. Eng. J. Med.* **294:**129–133.

McGlashan, N. D., 1969, Oesophageal cancer and alcoholic spirits in central Africa, *Gut* **10:**643–650.

McGlashan, N. D., Walters, C. L., and McLean, A. E. M., 1968, Nitrosamines in African alcoholic spirits and oesophageal cancer, *Lancet* **2:**1017.

Mahboubi, E., 1971, Epidemiologic study of esophageal carcinoma in Iran, *Int. Surg.* **56:**68–71.

Mahboubi, E., Kmet, J., Cook, P. J., Day, N. E., Ghadirian, P., and Salmasizadeh, S., 1973,

Oesophageal cancer studies in the Caspian littoral of Iran: The Caspian Cancer Registry, *Br. J. Cancer* **28**:197–214.

Mahboubi, E., Day, N. E., Ghadirian, P., and Salmasizadeh, S., 1976, Negligible role of alcohol and tobacco in the etiology of esophageal cancer in Iran—A case control study, presented at the Third International Symposium on Detection and Prevention of Cancer, New York.

Malhotra, S. L., 1967, Geographical distribution of gastrointestinal cancers in India with special reference to causation, *Gut* **8**:361–372.

Martinez, I., 1964, Cancer of esophagus in Puerto Rico: Mortality and incidence analysis, 1950–1961, *Cancer* **17**:1279–1288.

Martinez, I., 1969, Factors associated with cancer of the esophagus, mouth, and pharynx in Puerto Rico, *J. Natl. Cancer Inst.* **42**:1069–1094.

Mason, M. J., Bailar, J. C., III, and Eisenberg, H., 1964, Geographic variation in the incidence of esophageal cancer, *J. Chron. Dis.* **17**:667–676.

Mason, T. J., McKay, F. W., Hoover, R., Blot, W. J., and Fraumeni, J. F., Jr., 1975, *Atlas of Cancer Mortality for U.S. Counties: 1950–1969,* DHEW Publ. No. (NIH) 75-780, Bethesda, Md.

Masuda, Y., Mori, K., Hirohata, T., and Kuratsune, M., 1966, Carcinogenesis in the esophagus. III. Polycyclic aromatic hydrocarbons and phenols in whiskey, *Gann* **57**:549–557.

Miller, R. W., 1975, High esophageal cancer rates in humans and chickens in North China (letter), *J. Natl. Cancer Inst.* **54**:535.

Mohan Kumar, K., Ramachandran, P., and Haridas, K. P., 1971, Carcinoma of the esophagus—A study of 103 cases (Part I: Clinico-pathologic features), *Indian J. Med. Sci.* **25**:705–711.

Morton, J. F., 1968, Plants associated with esophageal cancer cases in Curacao, *Cancer Res.* **28**:2268–2271.

Mosbech, J., and Videbaek, A., 1955, On the etiology of esophageal carcinoma, *J. Natl. Cancer Inst.* **15**:1665–1673.

Paull, A., Trier, J. S., Dalton, M. D., Camp, R. C., Loeb, P., and Goyal, R. K., 1976, The histologic spectrum of Barrett's esophagus, *N. Eng. J. Med.* **295**:476–480.

Pearson, J. G., 1966, The radiotherapy of carcinoma of the oesophagus and post cricoid region in south east Scotland, *Clin. Radiol.* **17**:242–257.

Pickett, L. K., and Briggs, H. C., 1967, Cancer of the gastrointestinal tract in childhood, *Pediatr. Clin. North Am.* **14**:223–234.

Plowright, W., Linsell, C. A., and Peers, F. G., 1971, A focus of rumenal cancer in Kenyan cattle, *Br. J. Cancer* **25**:72–80.

Pokrovskaia, L. V., and Shabynina, N. K., 1973, Carcinogenic hazards in the production of chromium ferroalloys, *Gig. Tr. Prof. Zabol.* **10**:23–26 (in Goldsmith and Miller, 1975).

Pour, P., and Ghadirian, P., 1974, Familial cancer of the esophagus in Iran, *Cancer* **33**:1649–1652.

Robertson, M. A., Harington, J. S., and Bradshaw, E., 1971, The cancer pattern in African gold miners, *Br. J. Cancer* **25**:395–402.

Rogacheva, V. A., Baidila, P. G., and Fomin, P. D., 1971, Malignant transformation of esophageal cicatrix strictures following chemical burning, *Khirurgiia (Moskva)* **47(8)**:23–25 (in Goldsmith and Miller, 1975).

Schoenberg, B. ., Bailar, J. C., III, and Fraumeni, J. F., Jr., 1971, Certain mortality patterns of esophageal cancer in the United States, 1930–67. *J. Natl. Cancer Inst.* **46**:63–73.

Schonland, M., and Bradshaw, E., 1969, Oesophageal cancer in Natal Bantu: A review of 516 cases, *South Afr. Med. J.* **16**:1028–1031.

Schottenfeld, D., Gantt, R. C., and Wynder, E. L., 1974, The role of alcohol and tobacco in multiple primary cancers of the upper digestive system, larynx and lung: A prospective study, *Prev. Med.* **3**:277–293.

Schütte, K. H., 1968, Esophageal tumors in sheep: Some ecological observations, *J. Natl. Cancer Inst.* **41**:821–824.

Shaposhnikov, V. I., 1964, Osobennosti zabolevaemosti rakom pishchevoda v Kzyl-Ordinskoĭ oblasti, *Vopr. Onkol.* **10**:72–73 (in Warwick and Harington, 1973, p. 94).

Shearman, D. J. C., Finlayson, N. D. C., Arnott, S. J., and Pearson, J. G., 1970, Carcinoma of the oesophagus after gastric surgery, *Lancet* **1**:581–582.

Silverberg, E., and Holleb, A. I., 1975, Major trends in cancer: 25 year survey, *Ca* **25**:2–20.

Smithers, D. W., 1955, The association of cancer of the stomach and oesophagus with herniation at the oesophageal hiatus of the diaphragm, *Br. J. Radiol.* **28**:554–564.

Solanke, T. F., 1969, Carcinoma of the esophagus in Ibadan, *Int. Surg.* **52**:204–209.

Stalsberg, H., 1972, Carcinoma of the oesophagus after gastric surgery (letter), *Lancet* **1**:381.

Staszewski, J., and Haenszel, W., 1965, Cancer mortality among the Polish-born in the United States, *J. Natl. Cancer Inst.* **35**:291–297.

Steinitz, R., and Costin, C., 1971, Cancer in Jewish immigrants, *Israel J. Med. Sci.* **7(12)**:1413–1436.

Stephen, S. J., and Uragoda, C. G., 1970, Some observations of oesophageal carcinoma in Ceylon, including its relationship to betel chewing, *Br. J. Cancer* **24**:11–15.

Sterling, T. D., and Weinkam, J. J., 1976, Smoking characteristics by type of employment, *J. Occup. Med.* **18**:743–754.

Sytnik, A. P., and Petrov, B. A., 1968, Cancer of the esophagus in post-burn scar stenosis, *Khirurgiia (Moskva)* **44(11)**:3–9 (in Goldsmith and Miller, 1975).

Takano, K., Osogoshi, K., Kamihura, N., Kanda, K., Kane, K., Kamiyama, R., Sakamoto, K., Sato, H., Shirai, Y., Sei, M., Tanabe, T., Horino, M., Minami, Y., Motoji, H., Morita, R., Orihata, H., and Hirayama, T., 1968, Epidemiology of cancer of the esophagus, Nippon Rinsho, *Jpn. J. Clin. Med.* **26(8)**:1823–1828 (in Goldsmith and Miller, 1975).

Turnbull, A. D., Rosen, P., Goodner, J. T., and Beattie, E. J., 1973, Primary malignant tumors of the esophagus other than typical epidermoid carcinoma, *Ann. Thorac. Surg.* **15**:463–473.

Tuyns, A. J., 1970, Cancer of the oesophagus: Further evidence of the relation to drinking habits in France, *Int. J. Cancer* **5**:152–156.

Tuyns, A. J., and Massé, G., 1975, Cancer of the oesophagus in Brittany: An incidence study in Ille-et-Vilaine, *Int. J. Epidemiol.* **4**:55–59.

Von Zeynek, E. R., 1973, Survey of cancer of the oesophagus in relation to other malignant neoplasms, *South Afr. Med. J.* **47**:325–331.

Wapnick, S., Zanamwe, L. N. D., Chitiyo, M., and Mynors, J. M., 1972, Cancer of the esophagus in central Africa, *Chest* **61**:649–654.

Warwick, G. P., and Harington, J. S., 1973, Some aspects of the epidemiology and etiology of esophageal cancer with particular emphasis on the Transkei, South Africa, *Adv. Cancer Res,* **17**:81–229.

Waterhouse, J. A. H., 1974, *Cancer Handbook of Epidemiology and Prognosis,* Churchill Livingstone, Edinburgh.

Weir, J. M., and Dunn, J. E., Jr., 1970, Smoking and mortality: A prospective study, *Cancer* **25**:105–112.

Wychulis, A. R., Woolam, G. L., Andersen, H. A., and Ellis, F. H., Jr., 1971, Achalasia and carcinoma of the esophagus, *J. Am. Med. Assoc.* **215**:1638–1641.

Wynder, E. L., and Bross, I. J., 1961, A study of etiological factors in cancer of the esophagus, *Cancer* **14**:389–413.

Wynder, E. L., Hultberg, S., Jacobsson, F., and Bross, E. J., 1957, Environmental factors in cancer of the upper alimentary tract: Swedish study with special reference to Plummer-Vinson (Paterson-Kelly) syndrome, *Cancer* **10**:470–487.

Wynder, E. L., and Mabuchi, K., 1973, Etiological and environmental factors, *J. Am. Med. Assoc.* **226**:1546–1548.

Young, M., and Russell, W. T., 1926, An investigation into the statistics of cancer in different trades and professions, Med. Res. Counc. (Gr. Brit.), Spec. Ref. Ser. SRS-99 (in Warwick and Harington, 1973).

Zaldivar, R., 1970, Geographic pathology of oral, esophageal, gastric and intestinal cancer in Chile. *Ztschr. Krebsforsch.* **75(1)**:1–13.

Zaldivar, R., and Robinson, H., 1971, Association between rainfall and esophageal cancer in Chile, *Beitr. Pathol.* **142(4)**:403–406.

8

Epidemiology of Gastric Cancer

Joanna F. Haas and David Schottenfeld

1. Introduction

Like esophageal neoplasms, gastric cancers are deadly but epidemiologically intriguing. A precipitous decline in death rates from gastric cancers has occurred at a time of slowly rising mortality from all cancers. The disappearance of gastric cancer as an important clinical entity has been divined, although clues to its etiology remain scant and contradictory.

Unlike esophageal cancer, gastric malignancies do not have a characteristic clinical, radiological, or even pathological appearance, and inconsistencies in diagnostic criteria plague the epidemiological investigator. Clinical onset is likely to be insidious, with anorexia, weight loss, early fullness, or vague epigastric discomfort as the first symptom. The pain may respond to routine medical measures and have ulcerlike characteristics. Signs of metastatic spread are often present at the time of the initial diagnosis. The majority of surgically resectable specimens show metastatic spread to lymph nodes (Hughes, 1966).

Radiological appearance can help separate malignancies from benign stomach disease, but the distinction is not definitive. Inadequate response to therapy, in a lesion which is radiologically benign, is reason for further diagnostic efforts. As many as 3–4% of patients treated medically for gastric ulcer disease which was diagnosed clinically or radiologically have ultimately been shown to have gastric cancer (Rønnov-Jessen *et al.,* 1965). Where the lesion

Joanna F. Haas • Assistant Professor of Public Health, Cornell University Medical College, New York, New York 10021. ***David Schottenfeld*** • Chief, Epidemiology and Preventive Medicine, Memorial Sloan-Kettering Cancer Center, New York, New York 10021, and Professor of Public Health, Cornell University Medical College, New York, New York 10021.

was radiologically classified as "indeterminant," the proportion ultimately diagnosed as malignant is higher, 9.4% in one series (Wenger *et al.*, 1971).

Fiberoptic gastroscopy has been employed for histological diagnosis and early detection of gastric cancer. Differential diagnosis between benign and malignant gastric ulcer can be made on the basis of gross endoscopic appearance of the lesion in up to 90% of cases. Diagnostic accuracy of 99% has been claimed for combined radiological and endoscopic findings (Colcher, 1974). If early diagnosis leads to resection with no regional node involvement, a 5-year survival of 60% can be hoped for, compared to dismal prospects in the presence of any tumor spread. In an effort to detect early, often presymptomatic gastric cancer, cytodiagnosis has been investigated as an adjunctive method. While some regard gastric cytology as an important diagnostic aid (Schade, 1974), others have pointed out that interest, skill, and available expertise are the overwhelming determinants of its successful application (Wenger *et al.*, 1971).

Gastric cancer is a leading cause of death in Japan. Efforts there at early detection through mass screening and combined use of cytological, roentgenological, and endoscopic approaches to diagnosis have uncovered comparatively large numbers of early gastric cancers, those confined to the gastric mucosa and submucosa. Follow-up of 222 such cases showed a 5-year survival of 98% (Kawashima, 1966). This rather astonishing figure does not take into account the distortions produced by lead time gained by early diagnosis through screening, or the bias introduced by the inherent weighting of cases detected through screening with cases of low biological aggressiveness.

The potential to over- or underdiagnose gastric malignancy has been considerable in the past, and diagnostic criteria have varied. The pathogenesis and malignant potential of stomach lesions may vary by site of origin and by gross and microscopic morphological features. These problems must be kept in mind when data from different regions and time periods are compared in an effort to describe the epidemiological features of the disease.

2. *Pathology*

Neoplasms of gastric origin are primarily carcinomas. Balfour and McCann (1930) reported 48 (1.2%) sarcomas among 4159 gastric malignancies. Other estimate the frequency of sarcomatous lesions as 3–6% of gastric neoplasms (Bazaz-Malik and Gupta, 1967). Among these are lymphoma, leiomyosarcoma, rhabdomyosarcoma, Kaposi's sarcoma, and neurofibrosarcoma. While the radiological appearance of noncarcinomatous tumors may be suggestive, diagnosis is generally first made at laparotomy. Of all smooth muscle tumors of the stomach occurring in Finland from 1953 to 1960, 17% were leiomyosarcomas. A total of 112 smooth muscle tumors of the stomach were registered during that time period, representing virtually all histologically confirmed cases in the country (Salmela, 1968). The Third National Cancer Survey has provided information about the frequency of various cell types among gastric neoplasms. Of 5041 microscopically confirmed stomach neoplasms, 365 (7.2%) were not carcinomas. Thirty-five were classified only as malignant neoplasms not otherwise specified, and 1207 other stomach cancer deaths had not been microscopically confirmed (Cutler and Young, 1975). In Table 1, the frequency of various histopathological diagnoses in microscopically examined specimens is recorded.

Pathologically gastric carcinomas are quite varied. Subclassification of gastric carcinomas into two main histological types has helped to clarify some of the controversy surrounding precursors of this neoplasm. Following review of clinical and histological material from 1344 patients treated between 1945

Table 1. Histological Diagnoses of Stomach Malignancies Reported to the Third National Cancer Survey (all races)[a]

Tumor	Total number	Males	Females
All microscopically confirmed	5041	3202	1839
Neoplasm, malignant, NOS[b]	35	20	15
Carcinoma, NOS	566	335	231
Giant and spindle cell carcinoma	3	2	1
Small cell carcinoma	17	7	10
Papillary carcinoma, NOS	3	2	1
Squamous cell carcinoma, NOS	6	4	2
Adenocarcinoma, NOS	3599	2354	1245
Adenocarcinoma in adenomatous polyp	8	5	3
Carcinoid tumor	12	6	6
Papillary adenocarcinoma	29	16	13
Clear cell adenocarcinoma	3	2	1
Papillary cystadenocarcinoma	1	1	—
Mucin-producing adenocarcinoma	334	211	123
Signet ring cell carcinoma	62	31	31
Medullary carcinoma, NOS	3	1	2
Adenosquamous cell carcinoma	2	1	1
Adenocarcinoma-squamous metaplasia	5	4	1
Sarcoma, NOS	1	—	1
Fibrosarcoma, NOS	1	—	1
Liposarcoma, NOS	1	1	—
Leimyosarcoma, NOS	96	56	40
Carcinosarcoma	1	1	—
Lymphoma, NOS	25	16	9
Stem cell lymphoma	1	—	1
Lymphosarcoma, NOS	50	28	22
Lymphocytic lymphosarcoma	22	10	12
Lymphoblastic lymphosarcoma	23	13	10
Reticulum cell sarcoma, NOS	132	75	57

[a]The Third National Cancer Survey conducted during 1969–1971 covered parts of the United States with about 10% of the total population. Source: Cutler and Young (1975).
[b]NOS, not otherwise specified.

and 1964 at the University of Turku, Finland, Lauren (1965) reaffirmed the existence of two histological types of stomach cancer: an intestinal type and a diffuse type. The intestinal variety, which accounted for 53% of the tumors in his series, typically formed prominent glandular lumina and had large distinct cells with variable shape. Extracellular secretion of mucus was noted in 78% of cases. Marked mucosal changes in the vicinity of the tumor were present in 90% of cases, frequently with prominent signs of chronic atrophic or hypertrophic gastritis. Grossly the tumors were most often polypoid or fungating. A quite different pathological picture is presented by diffuse-type carcinomas. This rubric would encompass such variants as linitis plastica and scirrhous carcinomas. Diffuse-type carcinomas are highly cellular tumors forming solid masses of relatively uniform and less distinct cells. Extracellular secretion of mucus was present in 37%. Adjacent gastric mucosa was less likely to show marked changes of chronic gastritis or intestinal metaplasia. Forty-three percent of diffuse-type gastric carcinomas were grossly infiltrating in the linitis plastica fashion. The differences in the mucosa surrounding the two types of lesions could not be accounted for by the age differences in the two groups of patients. In each age group, mucosal abnormalities in the tissue surrounding the tumor were more commonly associated with the intestinal type.

Lauren observed that the pathological distinctions were paralleled by clinical differences. A higher proportion of the intestinal variant was in males. The mean age of the patients was older (55.4 years for intestinal type compared with 47.7 for diffuse). Subsequent studies have substantiated differing epidemiological patterns for the two tumor types. These histological differences appear to have etiological and pathogenetic import (Muñoz *et al.*, 1968; Muñoz and Asvall, 1971; Muñoz and Connelly, 1971).

3. Gastric Polyps

Gastric polyposis is not a common lesion. It is in fact seen less frequently than gastric cancer. Invasive gastric cancer has been pathologically demonstrated to arise in villous or adenomatous polyps (Berg, 1958). It appears, however, that only polyps of epithelial origin have malignant potential. Hamartomatous gastric polyps, such as those which may occur in the Peutz-Jeghers syndrome, do not appear to precede gastric cancer (Ming, 1974). Epithelial polyps of the stomach may be classified into two groups: hyperplastic (regenerative) polyps and villous adenoma (adenomatous polyps). Ming and Goldman (1965) studied 49 patients with gastric polyps, of whom 79% had regenerative polyps and 21% had adenomatous polyps. The villous adenomas were solitary lesions, generally over 2 cm in size. All were in patients over 50. Focal malignant transformation was observed in four out of ten villous adenomas. In three of the remaining cases the patient had a separate coexisting carcinoma. Marked intestinal metaplasia was present in the mucosa adjacent to the villous adenoma. The remaining 39 patients had a total of 76 regenerative polyps,.which were smaller and often multiple. Although coexistent carcinomas occurred in three of the 39 patients, malignant transformation was not observed in any of the 76 polyps studied. Intestinal metaplasia was mild or absent in the adjacent mucosa. From evidence of this sort, the fact that gastric cancer may arise in villous adenomas seems clear. The exact nature of the relationship among villous adenomas, gastric carcinoma, and intestinal metaplasia is not resolved; a clear picture of the patterns of occurrence and frequency of gastric polyps is wanting. It is certain nonetheless that these lesions are not a major factor in the genesis of most gastric carcinomas.

3.1. Intestinal Metaplasia

Alteration of stomach mucosa to resemble small intestine, a process known as intestinal metaplasia, is frequently observed in patients with gastric cancer. There is evidence to suggest that these changes are closely related to the pathogenesis of gastric carcinoma. In experimental situations, gastric cancer may be preceded by mucosal atrophy and then atypical hyperplasia (Ming, 1974).

The terms "intestinal metaplasia," "mucosal atrophy," and "chronic atrophic gastritis" have been used interchangeably, although any one change may be present without the others. Such mucosal changes are increasingly prevalent with advancing age. When apparently healthy stomachs from autopsy specimens of Japanese in Japan and of whites in the United States were examined, intestinal metaplasia and gastric atrophy were found more often in the specimens from Japan (Imai *et al.*, 1971). This suggested that in high-risk gastric cancer areas like Japan the prevalence of intestinal metaplasia was increased. Studies in Colombia suggest that the prevalence of intestinal metaplasia is highest in natives of areas of high gastric cancer incidence (Correa *et al.*, 1970). Lauren's (1965) suggestion that intestinal metaplasia is most closely tied to the intestinal type of gastric cancer, independent of age, has received support from investigators studying other populations (Correa *et al.*, 1973).

Other lines of evidence suggest that while intestinal metaplasia may sometimes have been a precursor to gastric cancer, this is not invariably the case. The site of maximal intestinal metaplasia, as determined by stains for alkaline phosphatase activity, does not necessarily coincide with the site of a coexisting carcinoma (Stemmermann and Hayashi, 1968). Enzymes generally found only in the intestinal mucosa can be found both in carcinomas of the stomach and in intestinalized mucosa of the stomach. However, the histochemical characteristics of a tumor do not necessarily correlate with its degree of morphological differentiation. For these reasons, while intestinal-type gastric cancer is associated with intestinal metaplasia of the gastric mucosa, the causal sequence is not defined. It is possible that both intestinalization and carcinoma arise from common stimuli to undifferentiated cells of the gastric mucosa (Stemmermann, 1967). Alternatively, intestinalization of stomach mucosa with the associated rise in pH may increase the exposure and vulnerability of the gastric mucosa to other carcinogens.

3.2. Geographical Pathology

Frequency of stomach cancer has undergone striking change in some parts of the world over the last several decades. When comparing frequencies, it is essential that the time period be specified. Under these circumstances, comparison of trends may be more informative than absolute frequencies. By mapping mortality rates and relative frequency estimates of stomach cancer in males throughout the world as of about 1960–1961, Dunham and Bailar (1968) highlighted areas of high frequency in Japan, Central Europe, Finland, Iceland, West Germany, several Central Asian republics of the USSR, and eight major South American cities. The age-standardized mortality from gastric cancer among males in these areas was at least 40 per 100,000 per year. Worldwide reported age-standardized mortality rates for males from gastric cancer ranged from 112 per 100,000 in Russia to 10.7 in the southern U.S. white population. The percentage of all cancers in males attributed to stomach cancer ranged from a high of 38% in Costa Rica to a low of 0.6% in Ceylon. Age-standardized incidence rates which were available for a few areas through surveys and registries generally were consonant with mortality data. The highest reported age-standardized incidence rate for stomach cancer was in Iceland, with 109.3 cases per 100,000 males per year, and the lowest was 1.6 cases per 100,000 males in the Malay population of Singapore. While mortality rates for males are higher than those for females in each reporting country, the rank order of the countries is similar whether based on mortality rates for males or for females (Logan, 1976). Truncated (ages 35–64) incidence rates for males of selected countries are given in Table 2.

Regardless of reporting difficulties and discrepancies in diagnostic standards, there is no doubt that stomach cancer frequency varies dramatically throughout the world. Two highly industrialized societies, Japan and the United States, are near the top and bottom, respectively, of the rank order of gastric cancer mortality by country. Similarly, Chile and Mexico, while both only modestly industrialized, show a fivefold difference in gastric cancer mortality. Rates in Chile are comparable to those of Japan; those in Mexico resemble rates for the U.S. white population. Various climatic, geographical, environmental, hereditary, and dietary factors have been reported to be associated with high stomach cancer incidence. No single factor accounts for all of the observed international variation (Hammond and Seidman, 1974).

3.2.1. *Regional Differences within Countries*

Even within countries with uniform reporting and classification systems, gastric cancer mortality may show marked differences from area to area. Cancer of the stomach in Japan shows considerable regional variation. High-mortality areas are concentrated on the northeastern part of Honshu, along the coast of the Sea of Japan, and in the Nara prefecture. Relatively low rates are evident in the Kyushu and Shikoku districts in the south as well as

Table 2. Truncated Incidence Rates for Stomach Cancer, Males, Selected Countries[a]

Country	Rate[b]
Western Hemisphere	
Canada	24.5
Chile	85.2
Colombia, Cali	81.6
Jamaica, Kingston	40.2
Puerto Rico	42.8
United States (white)	14.8
United States (nonwhite)	35.6
Europe	
Austria	59.0
Belgium	42.1
Czechoslovakia	67.3
Denmark	37.4
England and Wales	45.5
Finland	72.0
France	33.0
Germany (Federal Republic)	51.3
Iceland	102.3
Ireland	38.8
Norway	38.6
Poland	74.8
Portugal	56.9
Sweden	32.5
Switzerland	34.4
Yugoslavia	38.6
Yugoslavia, Slovenia	74.6
USSR (towns, Europe)	
Latvia	76.2
RSFSR	172.3
Ukraine	104.3
USSR (towns, Asia)	
Georgia	48.7
Kazakhstan	149.5
Kirghizia	160.4
Asia	
India, Bombay	17.3
Japan, Miyagi	158.3
Singapore (Chinese)	29.5
Australia	22.7
Africa	
Nigeria, Ibadan	21.9
South Africa (colored)	79.0
South Africa (white)	36.2

[a]Source. Doll (1969).
[b]Per 100,000 males, ages 35–64; 1950 world population standard.

the Shizuoka and Iwate prefectures. These patterns hold true for males and females. They were observed when these regions were first studied, in 1949–1951, and then again in 1959–1961. The geographical distribution of gastric ulcer disease in Japan is quite different from that of gastric cancer (Hirohata and Kuratsune, 1969).

Similar variation has been noted between and within various Latin American countries. Zaldivar (1970) noted that stomach cancer rates for Chile are highest in the central province of Curico and lowest in Magallanes in the south. Highest death rates from cancer of the alimentary tract in Chile occur in agricultural provinces, suggesting an etiological role of nitrate fertilizers. In Colombia, the inland city of Cali had an age-adjusted incidence rate for gastric cancer in males of 50.1 per 100,000 per year compared to 12.2 in the coastal city of Cartagena (Muñoz *et al.,* 1968).

In Iceland, a country with high gastric cancer mortality, areas of excess frequency have been noted in the northwest of the country. This observation has led to efforts to reconstruct differences in diet, especially use of smoked food, in different regions of the country (Sigurjonsson, 1966). In Czechoslovakia, too, stomach cancer deaths for both males and females were higher in northern Moravia. The capital, Prague, had the lowest rates, 36% lower than northern Moravia. Differences could not be explained by reporting differences, nor did they correspond to known regional differences in consumption of fats, carbohydrates, or alcohol (Gregor *et al.,* 1969).

3.2.2. Gastric Cancer in the United States

Data from the Third National Cancer Survey (3rd NCS) provide information on the incidence of stomach cancer during the period 1969–1971 in representative regions of the United States covering approximately 10% of the population. This survey documented 6248 cases of stomach cancer in the 3-year period, of which 80.5% were microscopically confirmed (Cutler and Young, 1975). Based on 3rd NCS data, the American Cancer Society estimated that in 1974 some 23,100 new cases of gastric cancer occurred in the United States, 14,000 in males and 9100 in females. In that year an estimated 14,300 gastric cancer deaths occurred, of which 8400 were in males and 5900 in females (Silverberg and Holleb, 1975). Gastric cancer accounted for 13.8% of digestive system cancers and 3.5% of all new cases of cancer in the United States.

Mortality from cancer of the stomach in the United States, 1950–1969, was not uniformly distributed in the white population throughout the country. Counties in the highest decile had age-adjusted mortality rates of over 19.75 per 100,000 for males, 10.90 or greater for females. The average annual U.S. mortality rates for this period (1950–1969) were 15.22 and 7.70 per 100,000 for males and females, respectively (Mason *et al.,* 1975). Areas of significant elevation (in highest decile) of age-adjusted mortality rates for both men and women occur in the northern reaches of Michigan, Wisconsin, Minnesota, and North Dakota and Maine. By and large, the geographical pattern of gastric cancer within the United States is similar for both sexes. In Utah, coal-mining counties have had excess deaths from stomach cancer (Matolo *et al.*, 1972).

4. Time Trends in Gastric Cancer

A dramatic decline in stomach cancer incidence has occurred in the United States and many other countries (Fig. 1). The magnitude of the decline varies. In the United States the age-adjusted mortality rate for males dropped from 28 per 100,000 in 1930 to 9.7 per 100,000 in 1967. The rate of decline has been steepest among U.S. whites and in the older age groups of all race–sex categories. For white males over 80 years of age the decline in the mortality rate amounted to an average of 6.9 fewer deaths per 100,000 population each year between 1950 and 1967. The annual mortality rate in this age group dropped from 270 per 100,000 to 150 per 100,000 over this 17-year period (Burbank, 1971). An attempt was made to account for the decline in gastric cancer rates in Connecticut by attributing it to the decrease in the proportion of foreign-born individuals at high risk for gastric cancer. Based on age-, sex-, and nativity-specific mortality rates for stomach cancer from the Connecticut Cancer Registry, the decline in gastric cancer was found to be much too great to explain by this factor alone (Munõz and Connelly, 1971).

Declines in age-standardized mortality from stomach cancer between 1950–1951 and 1966–1967 have been noted in most developed countries, independent of the original rank or absolute level in 1950–1951. Males in

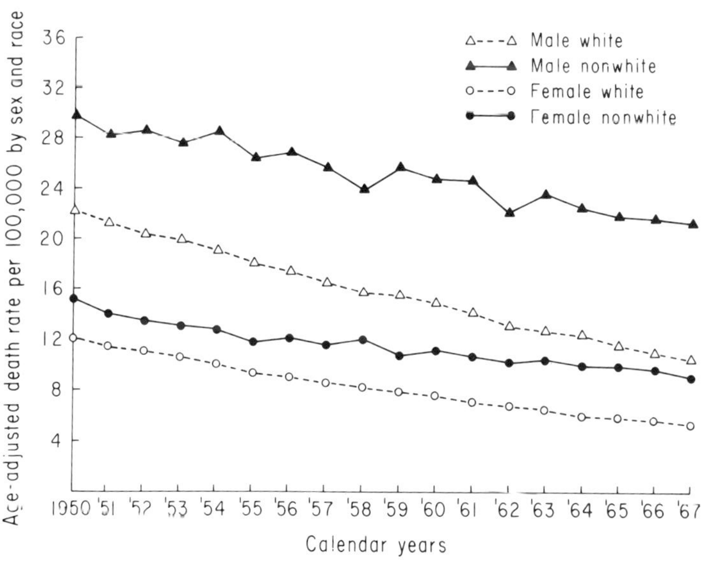

Fig. 1. Trends in gastric cancer mortality, United States, average annual rates, 1950–1967. Source: Burbank (1971).

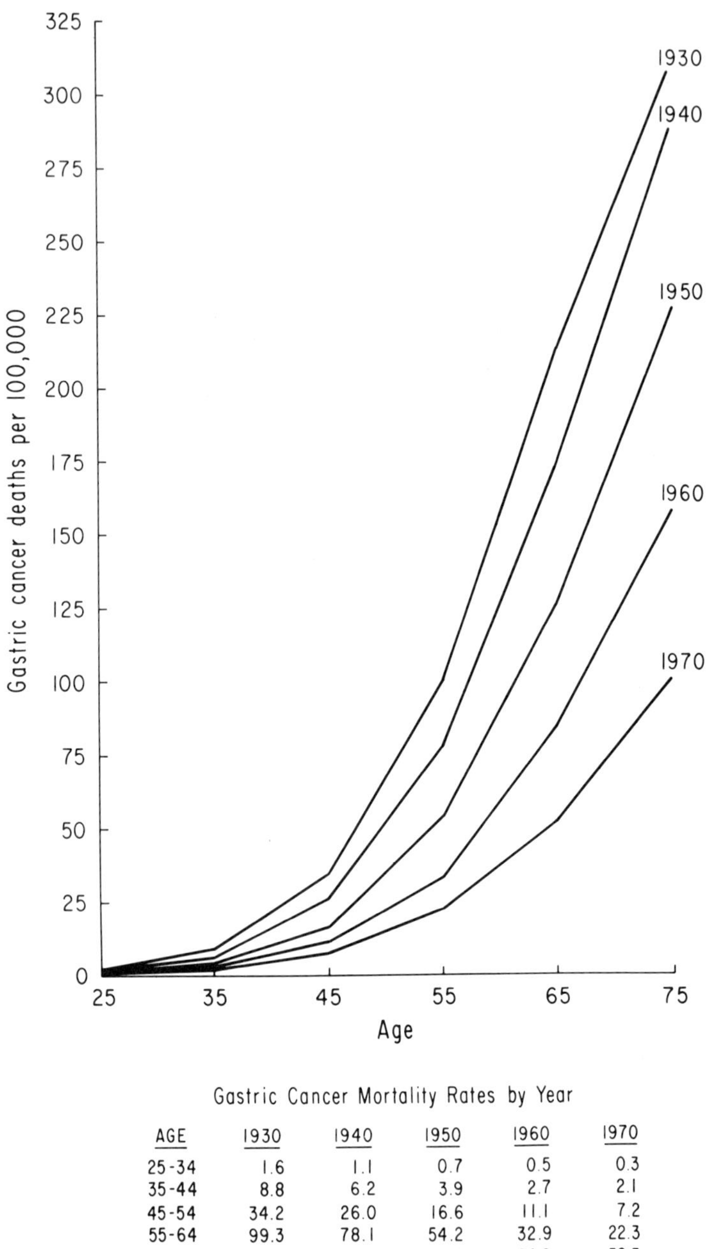

Gastric Cancer Mortality Rates by Year

AGE	1930	1940	1950	1960	1970
25-34	1.6	1.1	0.7	0.5	0.3
35-44	8.8	6.2	3.9	2.7	2.1
45-54	34.2	26.0	16.6	11.1	7.2
55-64	99.3	78.1	54.2	32.9	22.3
65-74	213.8	174.3	126.6	84.9	52.3
75-84	308.0	288.0	227.7	159.1	100.6

Fig. 2A. Gastric cancer mortality rates per 100,000 by age, United States, 1930–1970, white males.

Chile, Finland, and Austria had initial annual mortality rates of over 50 per 100,000, while those in the United States and New Zealand had initial rates less than 25 per 100,000. All experienced steep declines in stomach cancer mortality. Only among Japanese males and Portugese of both sexes was there an increase in stomach cancer mortality during this interval. Among men in

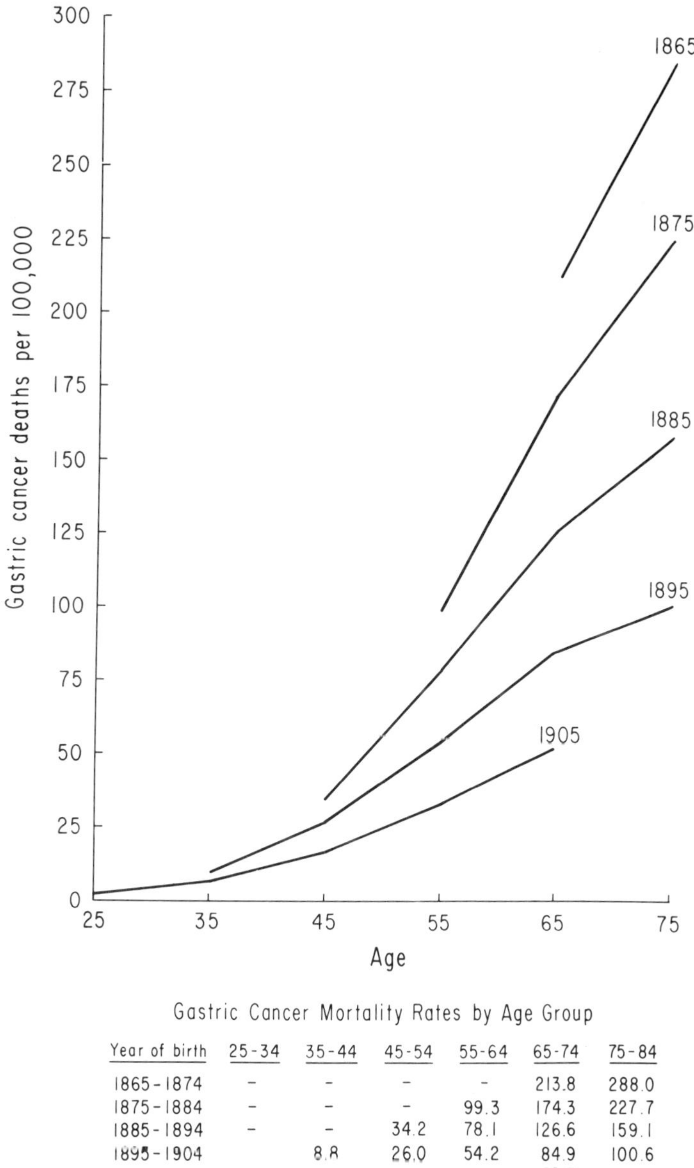

Gastric Cancer Mortality Rates by Age Group

Year of birth	25-34	35-44	45-54	55-64	65-74	75-84
1865-1874	-	-	-	-	213.8	288.0
1875-1884	-	-	-	99.3	174.3	227.7
1885-1894	-	-	34.2	78.1	126.6	159.1
1895-1904		8.8	26.0	54.2	84.9	100.6
1905-1914	1.6	6.2	16.6	32.9	52.3	-

Fig. 2B. Age-specific gastric cancer mortality rates per 100,000 by birth cohort, United States, white males. Source: Schottenfield (1975); Silverberg (1977).

Japan, annual mortality rose slightly from 67 per 100,000 in 1950–1951 to 70 per 100,000 in 1966–1967. In Portugal, the increase was from 27 to 33 per 100,000 (Hammond and Seidman, 1974).

Declining rates of stomach cancer suggest several possibilities. Recent environmental changes may have occurred which selectively decrease the risk of gastric cancer developing in persons over 70. Alternately, the decline could reflect the passing of earlier generations who carried an excess risk of stomach cancer with them throughout their lives. Studies on migrant populations suggest that some determinants of stomach cancer risk operate in the first few decades. It is also possible that both processes have occurred concurrently.

In Fig. 2A, the age-specific death rates are given for white males in the United States at 10-year intervals from 1930 to 1970. In Fig. 2B these data are differently displayed. For a group of individuals born in a given time interval, (termed "birth cohorts" and presented in 10-year intervals beginning with 1865), gastric cancer mortality rates are shown at successive ages. Thus men born in 1875–1884 had gastric cancer mortality rates at ages 55–64 of 99.3 per 100,000 and at ages 65–74 of 174.3 per 100,000. Men born during the next decade, 1885–1894, had lower mortality rates when they reached these ages: 78.1 per 100,000 at ages 55–64 and 126.6 per 100,000 at ages 65 to 74. Cohort analysis of gastric cancer mortality shows that age-specific gastric cancer mortality rates in the United States have declined with each successive birth cohort.

An analogous interpretation is suggested by data from the Finnish Cancer Registry. A decline in stomach cancer rates for successive cohorts is evident and is most pronounced in cohorts born around the turn of the century. For cohorts born in Finland in 1880, 1900, and 1920, the relative risk of stomach cancer declined with each successive group to about one-third of the risk of the preceding group. Stomach cancer mortality will probably continue to decline, but the rate of decline is expected to be more modest for subsequent cohorts (Hakama, 1972).

5. *Personal Risk Factors in Gastric Cancer*

Up to now, attention has focused primarily on differences in gastric cancer by geographical region and on trends in gastric cancer prevalence in the last decades. This section focuses on demographic characteristics associated with varying risks of gastric cancer.

5.1. *Age*

Stomach cancer incidence and mortality rates rise steeply with age (Fig. 3). Annual age-specific rates in the United States are nearly zero before age 20 but rise to over 110 cases per 100,000 after age 80. In 3 years only one case of stomach cancer occurred in an individual less than 15 years of age among

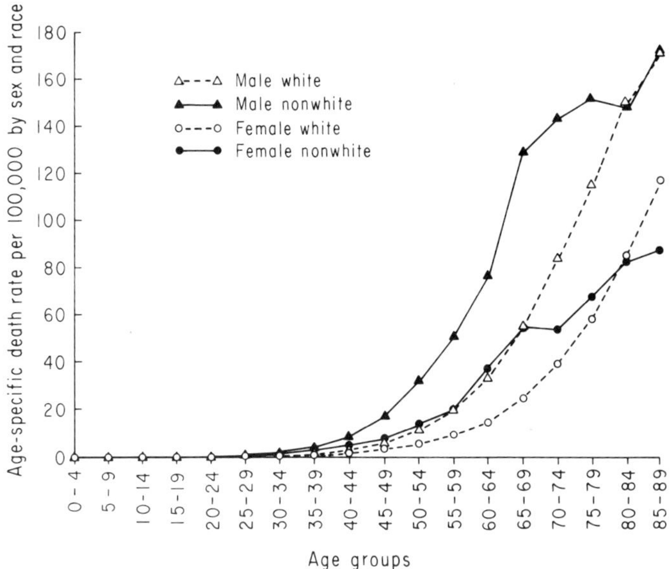

Fig. 3. Age-specific mortality rates from Gastric cancer, United States, average annual rates, 1950–1967. Source: Burbank (1971).

more than 20 million persons surveilled by the United States Third National Cancer Survey (Cutler and Young, 1975).

A rectilinear relationship has been observed between log stomach cancer mortality and log age in data from males in seven developed countries with markedly different levels of stomach cancer mortality. For females, a more complex relationship was noted which might be either curvilinear or two straight lines intersecting at about 50 years of age. The second possibility has been viewed as evidence for increased susceptibility at menopause to some histological variant of gastric cancer (Hems, 1968).

Review of material from several countries suggests that the intestinal type of gastric cancer is relatively more common among persons over 50 in both sexes. The diffuse type predominates before age 50. Such findings have been described in the United States, Finland, Japan, New Zealand, and Korea (Kubo, 1973).

5.2. *Sex*

Stomach cancer rates are higher among males than among females in virtually all settings. In the United States, age-adjusted incidence rates are 15.0 for males and 7.0 per 100,000 for females according to the 3rd NCS (U.S. 1970 population standard). Males rates are higher than female rates in both black and white populations at each level. The constancy of the overall sex ratio in different geographical settings and over time is a curious feature of the epidemiology of gastric cancer. It has been noted in numerous countries and in various geographical regions of the United States. Mortality rates of males and females are thus highly correlated (Logan, 1976). This is true within occupational groups as well as between geographical regions. The actual value of the sex ratio for stomach cancer mortality is not constant for each age group, however. Male predominance is greatest at ages 55–69, when the ratio of male to female death rates is greater than 2. At more advanced ages the ratio returns toward but does not reach unity. This pattern may be discerned in data from Japan, Germany, United States (whites), England, and Wales. No such pattern is noted when data for cancer of the large intestine and colon are similarly analyzed. The reproducibility of the sex ratio pattern by age suggests a biological phenomenon which needs to be accounted for (Griffith, 1968). When malignant tumors of the stomach are classified by location within the stomach, there is much more variation in the sex ratio. For gastric cancer occurring in the cardia of the stomach, the male–female ratio in a large series of Danish patients was 4, while for the cancers in the pylorus it was 1.5. The overall sex ratio, independent of site, was 2. The difference in the sex ratios of gastric cancer at the cardia and at the pylorus is statistically significant, and it persists when only adenocarcinomas are considered (Sterup and Mosbech, 1971).

High relative frequency of the diffuse-type histology among gastric cancer in females has been mentioned. Diffuse cancers constituted 37% of 827 gastric cancers in females from four different countries compared with 27% of 1724 male cases. The differences were most marked in the younger age groups and diminished thereafter. Above 80 years of age the proportion of males and females with diffuse histology was essentially the same (Kubo, 1973).

6. *Racial and Ethnic Differences in the United States*

Early in this century, gastric cancer incidence rates for U.S whites were higher than for blacks. For each age–sex group, during 1950–1967 gastric cancer rates declined more steeply in whites than in blacks so that by 1969 black rates were some 50% higher than those of whites (Levin *et al.*, 1974; Burbank, 1971). Average mortality rates from gastric cancer, 1950–1969, in black males are higher than those of whites within every state except Maine, Vermont, and New Mexico. This is true also for black females within every state except Connecticut, New Mexico, and North Dakota. Geographical distribution of gastric cancer in blacks is different from that in whites. In general, black rates for gastric cancer mortality are higher in the North than in the South for both males and females. The relatively high-risk area around the Great Lakes, described for whites, is not evident for blacks, although absolute mortality rates for blacks are high in those states (Burbank, 1971). In the African continent in diverse populations, the reported incidence rates are low. Operability and resectability rates for black patients are similar to those for whites, although survivorship among blacks is poorer regardless of stage of disease (Kovi *et al.,* 1974).

Among southwestern American Indians, annual gastric cancer mortality appears low. Based on cases referred to the major Indian referral center in Arizona, it has been estimated to be as low as 6.8 per 100,000. Tribal groups were not equally affected. Gastric cancer appeared to be more frequent among Hohakam (Pima–Papago) than among Apache–Navajo peoples (Sievers, 1973).

There is some evidence to suggest that the higher risk of gastric cancer which has been observed among Welsh in areas of Great Britain may not be entirely due to environmental factors. Northern seaboard counties of Wales have stomach cancer mortality up to 60% higher than that in the remainder of the British Isles. Standardized mortality rates by county are strongly correlated with the proportions of Welsh-speaking and Welsh-surnamed persons in the population. The risk of gastric cancer is estimated as 70% higher in Welsh than in non-Welsh residents of the same high-risk areas. Environmental conditions and dietary patterns are said to differ little between the two groups. The area is demographically rather isolated with little immigration from other areas, particularly for persons of marriageable age. The excess risk is not explained by differences in blood group patterns and prevalence of pernicious anemia is the same in the two groups (Maddock, 1966; Ashley and Davies, 1966; Ashley, 1969).

In general, considerable caution is advised before attributing racial differences in rates of gastric cancer to inherent biological differences in the populations. In most cases there are striking concurrent environmental, behavioral, and social class differences. Given the known importance of such factors in gastric cancer occurrence, it is difficult to separate the impact of differences in gene pool from environmental differences operating early in life. In the case of the Welsh in Great Britain, however, differences in life style are subtle at best. Moreover, there are heritable factors associated with differential susceptibility to gastric cancer. Racial differences in susceptibility to gastric cancer cannot be discounted, but their importance is not clear.

7. *Nativity and Migrant Studies*

Differences in stomach cancer mortality rates by place of birth are to be expected in light of the international variation in stomach cancer risk. In a study on mortality in New York City, 1953–1958, Newill (1961) observed that for all neoplasms average annual age-standardized death rates did not differ greatly between the native-born and foreign-born. For stomach cancer, however, there was a substantial excess among the foreign-born (21.0 compared to 14.1 per 100,000). When Jewish, Catholic, and Protestant populations were analyzed separately, the foreign-born in each religious group experienced excess stomach cancer (Hammond and Seidman, 1974). Subsequent declines in gastric cancer mortality in New York City were shown to have occurred among the native-born white, foreign-born white, and the black populations (Terris and Hall, 1963). The decline in stomach cancer mortality in the United States is thus not attributable only to the decreasing proportion of high-risk foreign-born population. High risk by virtue of nativity is not immutable; environmental factors later in life may modify the risk derived from place of birth or childhood residence.

In Manitoba, Canada, the average annual age-standardized death rate from stomach cancer was twice as high among the foreign-born as among the native-born. Among Scandinavian, Icelandic, Ukrainian, and Jewish ethnic groups, stomach cancer in Manitoba (1956–1965) was above that expected for the province. Within each ethnic group the risk for foreign-born was greater than that for the Canadian-born offspring. Only in the Jewish group was there no residual excess risk in the second generation (Choi *et al.,* 1971).

In Israeli Jews, a heterogeneous population, there is considerable variation in gastric cancer mortality by place of birth. European-born Jews have the highest gastric cancer rates, African-born the lowest, and Asians intermediate. The rates within these continental groupings vary when region of birth is defined more precisely. Within each continental grouping those persons who had lived in Israel for less than 10 years had significantly greater rates than those with longer residence (Tulchinsky and Modan, 1967).

Japanese residents of the United States experience a high risk of stomach cancer compared to the United States white population, but lower than that of Japanese in Japan. Differences in reporting standards or diagnostic criteria have been excluded as the explanation for differences in rates between the United States and Japan. Japanese migrants to the United States (referred to as Issei) experience stomach cancer rates lower than those of Japanese who remain in their native land, but much higher than those of the California white population. Among the first American-born generation of Japanese (Nisei), rates decline further in males but not in females. Rates for Nisei males are not as low as the rates of the California white population during the same time period (Buell and Dunn, 1965). Among Japanese living in Hawaii, Issei born in high-risk prefectures of Japan had a significantly higher relative risk of gastric cancer than Issei from low-risk prefectures. This difference did not carry through to the next generation. Among Nisei the birthplace of the parents did not alter the risk of gastric cancer (Haenszel *et al.,* 1972).

Chinese in the United States have standardized mortality rates (SMRs) for gastric cancer lower than those of the Chinese population in Taiwan, Hong Kong, and Singapore, but higher than those of U.S. whites. Gastric cancer occurs in excess among Chinese immigrants to the United States but not in their offspring (King and Haenszel, 1973).

Gastric cancer rates in Poland have been high in the past, although they have begun to decline. Poles migrating to the United States or Australia have gastric cancer rates lower than those in Poland. Immigrant Poles experience considerably higher rates of gastric cancer than do native-born Americans or Australians (Staszewski, 1971; Staszewski *et al.,* 1971). The reverse pattern prevails for lower intestinal tract cancer, where immigrant Poles have assumed the high incidence rates characterizing the host countries while rates in Poland remain low.

Migrant studies indicate that persons moving from high- to low-risk areas retain a considerable excess risk compared to natives of the low-risk areas. Offspring of migrants still have a small residual excess risk. Changes in intestinal-type gastric cancer frequency appear to account for much of the difference (Haenszel *et al.,* 1976). Early life factors appear to be important in determining subsequent gastric cancer risk. These disease patterns among migrant groups are consistent with an effect of dietary practices on gastric cancer risk.

8. Social Class and Occupation

Gastric cancer risk is greatest among the poor. Among U.S. whites there is an inverse gradient in both sexes in standardized incidence rates (SIRs) from the group with highest socioeconomic status (SIR 71, males) to the lowest (SIR 124, males). In New York City at least, this is independent of nativity and is thus not explained by a preponderance of high-risk foreign-born individuals in the lower socioeconomic strata (Hammond and Siedman, 1974). Gastric cancer excess among U.S. blacks may reflect low socioeconomic status. In England and Wales and in Denmark, excesses of gastric cancer are evident for males and females in the lowest socioeconomic strata. Gastric cancer mortality is low among professionals, sales workers, managers, and white-collar workers. It is increased in nonfarm laborers. These findings are, of course, consistent with the socioeconomic gradient described above (Levin *et al.,* 1974; Buell *et al.,* 1960).

As early as 1926, Young and Russell suggested that excesses of gastric cancer might prevail among iron, coal, and slate miners in Great Britain. Carbon and Emery counties, the only coal-mining regions in Utah, had age-adjusted incidence rates for gastric cancer during 1965–1969 that were 4 times those for the state of Utah as a whole. Risk was particularly high for males, and 59% of cases among males in these counties were in coal miners (Matolo *et al.,* 1972). Religious affiliation, which was not considered, is potentially important since in Utah members of the Church of Jesus Christ of Latter-Day Saints (Mormons) have stomach cancer incidence rates only about three-fourths as high as those of non-Mormons (Lyon *et al.,* 1976). In an effort to evaluate the association between coal mining and stomach cancer observed in Utah, the cancer mortality experience of 23 coal-mining counties in seven states of the United States was compared with that of non-coal-mining counties matched by educational level. The purpose of this matching was to distinguish effects of low socioeconomic status from factors specifically related to coal mining. A significant excess of stomach cancer was observed among persons in each coal-mining county, but other neoplasms related to low socioeconomic status (lung and cervix) were also present in excess. Rates for neoplasms (leukemia, breast, colon) associated with high SES were low in these same counties. The fact that the pattern of neoplasms in the coal-mining counties was that associated with low socioeconomic status suggests that low socioeconomic class remained a confounding factor despite matching of counties for education. Probably socioeconomic effects, rather than a specific coal-mining-related factor, account for the frequency of stomach cancer in these counties (Creagan *et al.,* 1974).

Analysis of detailed occupational histories taken from patients admitted to Roswell Park Memorial Institute, 1948–1951, suggested that a history of work in the metal products industry could be elicited significantly more frequently from patients with stomach cancer than from controls. In persons who had been employed in the metal products industry, iron dust and exposure to grain dust were the only specific exposures which were more common in stomach cancer patients than in controls (Kraus *et al.,* 1957). Among Russian workers in four nickel refineries in the Urals, stomach cancer rates were said to be significantly increased. Stomach cancers occurred primarily in persons with a 10–14 year history of employment in the industry (Saknyn' and Shabynina, 1973). Nickel is highly soluble in the acid environment of the stomach. In mice and rats the carcinogenic effects of nickel are local, but in man the target organs have generally been considered to be only lung and nasopharynx (Tomatis, 1976). Comparison of vital statistics and census data in Japan suggested that metal material workers (and farmers) were at high risk for stomach cancer (Hirayama, 1976). In Japan, stomach cancer mortality is said to be increased by more than 64% in miners, and excesses are reported among farmers and fishermen, and transportation and communication workers (Tsuchiga, 1967).

Review of death records for males dying in Washington state (USA) during 1950–1971 showed that the proportion of deaths due to stomach cancer was significantly elevated among loggers, plywood mill workers, sawmill and other mill workers, and carpenters (Milham, 1976). Asbestos workers may experience excess gastrointestinal cancer. The number of cases involved has been small, but the findings of several studies suggest that there may be an increase in gastric cancer risk in workers exposed to asbestos fibers, especially more than 20 years after first exposure (Selikoff *et al.,* 1968; Selikoff and Hammond, 1973; Enterline *et al.,* 1972).

Studies of rubber workers have shown excess stomach cancer mortality which appears to be widespread in the industry. Four plants, in which mortality experience from 1964 to 1973 was reviewed, each had elevated SMRs for gastric cancer among white male employees. The elevation was more marked in men aged 40–64 (SMR 183) than in those aged 65–84 (SMR 136). The overall SMR of 148 represented 80 deaths where 54 had been expected. It would be of interest to know the histological type of these cases. While specific exposures have not been defined, studies in one company with 42 of the stomach cancer cases showed that associated job categories included compounding and mixing, milling, tread extrusion and cementing, tube and flap building, and "green" tire preparation. Ingested carbon black (with absorbed carcinogens), asbestos, and nitrosamines are under consideration as agents which could be responsible for gastric cancer excesses in rubber workers (McMichael *et al.,* 1976).

Social class is an important confounding consideration when occupational hazards are explored. Workers who tolerate grossly unpleasant environments are likely to be of modest background and education. Nonetheless, for metal workers, miners, rubber workers, and those exposed to wood dusts and abestos, there is evidence that specific occupational hazards may exist for gastric malignancy.

9. Familial and Hereditary Influences

One must conclude that environmental factors play a leading role in gastric cancer. On the other hand, evidence exists to suggest that environmental factors may be superimposed on inherited susceptibility. Anecdotal accounts of gastric cancers in identical twins and of families with multiple cases arouse such suspicions. Two sibs with ataxia-telangiectasia, and their mother, an obligate heterozygote for that gene, developed gastric cancer (Lynch, 1972). In an isolated and inbred Virginia kinship, 12 stomach cancers were documented in four generations. The high frequency of antibody to gastric parietal cells and of cell-mediated immune defects was consistent with a genetic defect of T lymphocytes (Creagan and Fraumeni, 1973). Historically more eminent, if medically less well documented, was the experience of the Bonaparte family, in which cancer of the stomach caused the death of Napoleon in 1821 and also that of his grandfather, his father, and quite possibly his brother and three sisters (Sokoloff, 1938). Reports of such dramatic family concentrations of gastric cancer may be misleading. Some may represent chance occurrences, especially given the frequent occurrence of gastric cancer in previous years. Frequently, only a small portion of a kindred, that with the highest concentration of cases, may be the focus of the report, giving a misleading impression of the frequency of the disease in the family. Woolf and Isaacson (1961) pursued this question with five Mormon families in each of which three cases of gastric cancer had been identified in a family (parent–offspring) unit. Availing themselves of the extensive Mormon genealogical archives, they showed that high frequency of gastric cancer did not prevail in other parts of the kindred, and suggested that to the extent that a hereditary factor operated it must be polygenic. In a critique of Woolf's (1956) studies in Utah, Graham and Lilienfeld (1958) comment on the decision to limit the study to gastric cancer cases among members of the Mormon population in order to facilitate identification of kin of probands: "We cannot assume that the Mormon population is comparable to a probability sample of Utah population. The bias involved in the selection procedure used here could be very large." In fact, work published 18 years later supported just that concern by demonstrating substantially lower gastric cancer rates in Mormons than non-Mormons (Lyon *et al.,* 1976). A number of other studies suggest that gastric cancer is 2–3 times more frequent in the immediate relatives of gastric cancer patients (Woolf, 1961). Thoughtful criticism has been directed at the design of most published family and twin studies on gastric cancer (Graham and Lilienfeld, 1958; McConnell, 1966). Taken as a whole, however, various studies with different populations and with different flaws have been consistent in suggesting familial aggregation of gastric cancer. These observations are for the most part consistent with either genetic susceptibility to gastric cancer or an enduring impact of early home environmental factors. In rare families with immunological impairments, a major genetic factor may be operating.

10. *Epidemiological Investigations of the Pathogenesis and Etiology of Gastric Cancer*

10.1. *Gastric Cancer and Blood Group*

In 1953, Aird and his colleagues concluded from studies of patients in hospitals in England and Scotland that

> The frequency of blood group A is greater and the frequency of blood group O is less in patients suffering from cancer of the stomach than in the general population of the locality in which they live .... From this correlation of blood groups and cancer of the stomch, it follows that there is an inherited element in the susceptibility to or protection against cancer of the stomach.

Blood group A was also found to be unexpectedly frequent in gastric cancer patients in Denmark (Mosbech, 1960), Switzerland (Aird *et al.*, 1953), the United States (Hoskins *et al.*, 1965), the Netherlands (van Wayjen and Linschoten, 1973), and elsewhere (Roberts, 1959). Roberts (1959) showed that when data were pooled from a number of centers, including some which had failed to significantly demonstrate the posited relationship in their own data, the association of gastric cancer with blood group A was present and highly significant. The risk ratios among individual centers were not heterogeneous. The relative risk of gastric cancer in patients with blood type A compared to blood type O was estimated at 1.2 based on some 7858 cases from 13 centers throughout the world. Neither sampling error, given the numbers involved, nor systematic misclassification error, given the sophistication of the centers, is a plausible explanation for these differences.

The appropriateness of control groups used in these studies has been questioned. Considerable heterogeneity in blood group patterns may be present even in relatively isolated communities. Pooled areawide donor control series may thus not be representative of the populations from which the cases derive (Manuila, 1958). Control groups based on homogeneous patient groups may more accurately reflect the population in question than do those of transfusion centers, especially since inclusion of professional donors increases the frequency of blood group O (Buckwalter and Knowler, 1958). This last point is likely to be of special concern in the United States, where professionals constitute a higher proportion of blood donors. Findings of European series would be less influenced. Nonetheless, the weight of the now rather extensive evidence is that blood group A is significantly associated with an excess of gastric cancer. The increase in risk is modest, about 20%, and it needs to be further defined. Whether blood group A is associated with any given anatomical location is open to question (Glober *et al.,* 1971; van Wayjen and Linschoten, 1973). Similarly, whether the association is present in all age–sex groups has not been fully assessed. In a Japanese population, blood group A was associated only with the diffuse-type histology of gastric cancer (Haenszel *et al.,* 1976). This question needs further exploration. Further evaluation of the relationship between blood group A and gastric cancer may suggest that the association is greatest in some subgroup of gastric cancer cases. It has been suggested that the link between blood group and gastric cancer might reside in the nature of the mucopolysaccharide composition of gastric secretions and differential susceptibility to damage by environmental carcinogens (Lilienfeld *et al.,* 1976).

10.2. Pernicious Anemia and Gastric Cancer

Interest in a possible relationship between pernicious anemia and stomach cancer dates back to the turn of the century, as evidenced by numerous case reports of the coexistence of the two diseases. Interest in pernicious anemia was stimulated by the introduction of treatment with liver and stomach extracts. Several large autopsy series in the European and American literature suggested that the two diseases coincided in autopsy material about 3 times more frequently than expected, and moreover it seemed to constitute an unexpectedly high proportion, perhaps as much as 86% of all malignant neoplasms in these patients. Follow-up of pernicious anemia patients found variable frequencies of gastric cancer in such patients, although they generally were interpreted as representing an excess of gastric cancer and possibly of gastric polyps as well (Kaplan and Rigler, 1945). Among 181 patients with pernicious anemia, Jenner (1939) found eight cases of gastric cancer in Amsterdam; he estimated that this represented 12 times the expected number of cases. A total of 301 individuals with pernicious anemia (documented by typical blood findings, reticulocyte increase in response to therapy, and achlorhydria refractory to histamine) were followed in Copenhagen, 1928–1949. Surprisingly their mortality experience was exactly as expected, based on age- and sex-adjusted mortality rates of the population of Copenhagen in 1935–1939. Similarly, deaths from all types of malignant disease corresponded quite closely to the number expected based on figures from the Copenhagen population. Of the 21 deaths from malignant neoplasms, 14 (six of eight males and eight of 13 females) were attributed to carcinoma of the stomach. The authors indicated that the expected deaths from gastric cancer were 3.5 in females and 1.7 in males (Mosbech and Videbaek, 1950). The paucity of deaths from other causes is disturbing, since it would seem that death from other diseases, particularly other malignant neoplasms, might have been significantly underrepresented, suggesting the possibility of systematic diagnostic bias. Some 1222 patients with pernicious anemia were identified at Boston City Hospital during the years 1915–1951. Among these patients, some 28 cases of gastric cancer were identified. Analysis of a subgroup of these patients suggested that the incidence of gastric cancer was increased compared with estimates of the incidence in the Massachusetts general population. The excess seemed to be greatest in the age group 50–64 and only modestly elevated above age 65 (Zamcheck *et al.*, 1955). Given the uneven distribution of gastric cancer by social class, race, and nativity, the usefulness of the general population comparison must be questioned. The municipal hospital patient population may well have included an excess of high-risk persons so that the use of general population rates would then underestimate the expected number of cases. Later work originating in the same institution suggested an excess of type A blood group in pernicious anemia patients with gastric cancer (Hoskins *et al.* 1965). A recent study of some 138 patients with pernicious anemia followed from 1960 to 1968 found no cases of gastric cancer despite radiographic and gastroscopic follow-up specifically aimed at detecting early asymptomatic gastric cancer (Hoffman, 1970), The converse question was explored by Maddock (1966), who surveyed general practitioners in two areas of the British Isles about patients with pernicious anemia under their care to ascertain the degree to which differences in rates of pernicious anemia might explain the striking differences in gastric cancer rates between the two regions. No differences in pernicious anemia frequency were observed.

In summary, some of the evidence for a strong association between pernicious anemia and cancer of the stomach is less firm than generally appreciated and deserves a critical review and reassessment. In such review adequate emphasis must be given to methodological considerations such as duration of follow-up, adequacy of diagnostic criteria, the effect of treatment, and the appropriateness of comparison populations. It is possible that with the decline in gastric cancer, any association between stomach cancer and pernicious anemia has diminished.

10.3. Intestinal Metaplasia and Gastric Cancer

Various investigators have explored the possibility that variation in gastric cancer rates with place and time could be accounted for largely by changes in the frequency of intestinal-type gastric cancers. Clinicopathological correlation seemed to show that the intestinal variant predominated in higher-risk groups, males and persons over 50. Pathological evidence suggested that intestinal-type gastric cancer was related to intestinal metaplasia. If the epidemiological characteristics of intestinal metaplasia parallel those of intestinal-type gastric cancer, this would further support such a relationship.

Review of histological material from one high-risk city (Cali, Colombia) and three low-risk cities (Cartagena and Baranquilla, Colombia; Mexico City, Mexico) showed that the proportion of gastric cancers of intestinal type was highest in the high-risk city, Cali (Muñoz *et al.*, 1968). Subsequent study of gastric cancer deaths in Cali suggested that particularly high rates prevailed among individuals who had migrated to Cali from rural areas in the south of Colombia (Nariño, Cauca, and Upper Magdalena). Gastric cancer deaths among such migrants were in large part responsible for Cali's high gastric cancer rate. Specimens of gastric tissue from a general autopsy series were examined in an effort to correlate the prevalence of intestinal metaplasia with nativity. Intestinal metaplasia was found to be more widespread and more severe in the migrant group than among natives for Cali (Correa *et al.*, 1970).

This question has been explored in other settings. Review of material from all histologically confirmed gastric cancer cases from 1940–1944 and 1960–1964 in one Connecticut hospital led to the classification of 127 cases by age, sex, nativity, and histological type (Muñoz and Connelly, 1971). Cases were classified by nativity into high-risk and low-risk groups. Sixty-one of the cases had occurred in individuals born in high-risk countries; 66 were from low-risk countries. Intestinal-type tumors constituted a significantly higher proportion of gastric cancer cases in persons born in high-prevalence areas. In that group, 70.5% of tumors were intestinal type compared to 47.0% among persons born in low-prevalence areas. Gastric cancer rates in Connecticut had declined substantially between 1940–1944 and 1960–1964. The percentage of gastric cancers with intestinal-type histology was higher in the earlier time period (69.2% vs. 53.4%). The same trend was evident in each sex and nativity group, except among females born in low-prevalence areas, suggesting that a decrease in gastric cancers of the intestinal type explained much of the decline in gastric cancer which had occurred between 1940–1944 and 1960–1964.

The question of whether different time trends can be distinguished for diffuse and intestinal types of gastric carcinoma has also been investigated in a sample of histological material from one Norwegian cancer center. A decline in gastric cancer rates in Norway had been under way since the early 1930s, although rates plateaued from 1949 to 1951. Review of histological materials from 1940–1944, 1952–1953, and 1964–1966 suggested that this decline was due to decline in intestinal-type gastric cancer. The decline in intestinal-type cancer was most marked in females and persons under 50, groups that were initially at lower overall gastric cancer risk. During 1952–1953, the proportion of intestinal-type carcinomas remained stable in males, albeit a modest decline occurred among females. The authors point out that major dietary modifications prevailed during the 1940–1945 wartime period. They speculate that the plateau in the gastric cancer rates and in the proportion of intestinal-type gastric cancers during the postwar years may reflect these events, perhaps through a cocarcinogenic process acting in the presence of atrophic gastric mucosa (Muñoz and Asvall, 1971).

In England, gastric cancer rates have also declined in all age groups, 1940–1971. Using pathological material for 1940–1946 from the Radcliffe Infirmary (101 cases) and prospectively reviewed material for 1971–1973 (22 cases), British investigators determined that the proportion of gastric cancer due to the diffuse type rose from 24% to 38%. While this difference could still be attributable to chance (Whitehead *et al.*, 1974), the likelihood of having failed to prove a real difference is substantial with groups of this size (Fleiss, 1973).

Correa *et al.* (1973) pursued a related line of investigation, examining histology of gastric carcinomas in Japanese populations in Hawaii and in the Miyagi prefecture in Japan. The incidence of gastric carcinoma in the Japanese population of Hawaii is much lower than that of Japanese living in Japan. It was proposed that the difference might be accounted for by a lower incidence of intestinal-type gastric cancers among the Hawaiian Japanese. Surgically excised specimens were reviewed and classified histologically. Interobserver reliability in the classification system was confirmed. Specimens were typed into four groups: intestinal, mixed intestinal-diffuse, other, and diffuse. In analysis, however, the first three categories were pooled (IMO) since the histological groups "intestinal," "mixed," and "other" shared many clinical and epidemiological features. Age-, sex-, and histological-type-specific rates were estimated for both populations using gastric cancer rates recorded by Miyagi and Hawaiian cancer registries. Since histological typing had been done for each major age–sex group, comparisons could be made between the Miyagi and Hawaiian groups within each stratum without concern for selection bias in histological material, assuming that within each stratum the material reviewed was representative of gastric cancer in that age–sex group. It should be noted that the age strata employed (under 50, 50–59, over 60) were rather broad and that the Hawaiian Japanese population under 60 were probably born in Hawaii, whereas those over 60 were mainly immigrants. The proportion of IMO-type cancers increased with age in both populations. Within each age–sex group the proportion of IMO tumors in the Miyagi Japanese population was much greater than that among the Hawaiian Japanese. Estimated age–sex specific rates for IMO-type gastric cancer are higher among Japanese in Miyagi than Hawaii. Age–sex specific incidence rates for the diffuse histological variant are similar for the two groups. These findings support the suggestion that variation in the proportion of intestinal gastric cancer between these populations accounts for much of the variation in gastric cancer rates in these two populations.

Kubo (1971, 1973) evaluated pathological materials from Minnesota (USA), Kyushu (Japan), Korea, and New Zealand and did not find the kind of variation in tumor histology between high- and low-prevalence regions observed by Correa *et al.* (1973) after age and sex had been taken into account. Using a classification system similar to that of Lauren (1965) and other investigators, Kubo confirmed that the proportion of intestinal cancer is highest in males and the older age groups. However, when the percentages of diffuse carcinoma were compared within age–sex strata in specimens from New Zealand, the United States, Japan, and Korea, there was no significant variation among the four countries, despite large differences in their gastric cancer rates. This led Kubo to conclude that age–sex specific proportions of diffuse gastric carcinoma do not vary with overall gastric cancer incidence rates and that reports to the contrary have failed to take into full account the impact of selection factors for histological confirmation of cases, particularly age.

There is thus conflicting evidence on the question of how much international variation in gastric cancer rates reflects variation in rates of tumors with intestinal-type histology. Higher rates in gastric cancer in Miyagi compared to

Hawaiian Japanese are largely due to the higher rates of intestinal-type gastric tumors. In other settings this may not be the case. Among specimens from four other areas, the proportion of diffuse-type gastric cancer remains quite constant in each age–sex group.

There is thus a considerable body of evidence that differences in gastric cancer rates from place to place, over time, and between high-risk and low-risk populations in the same region may reflect variation in the rates of intestinal type and related histological variants. There are, however, several methodological questions which must be kept in mind. Uniformity in criteria for classification is essential, particularly if several observers are involved. Inter- and intraobserver reliability must be confirmed. The quality of specimens should uniformly reach a minimally acceptable standard. (Kubo, 1971, compared the results of classifying material from histological blocks of different sizes and found that there was no difference in histological diagnosis.) Perhaps the most serious problems have to do with the representativeness in histological materials examined. Criteria for selecting patients for biopsy, surgery, and autopsy vary over time, between places, and for different populations living in the same place. To the extent that pathological material is unrepresentative of all cases of gastric cancer, biased conclusions will be derived. This problem can be circumvented if all comparisons between groups are confined to defined strata, assuming that specimens studied are representative of the strata from which they are drawn.

10.4. Diet and Gastric Cancer

Considerable effort has gone into studies of diet to define food-borne carcinogens and other dietary factors which might explain the peculiarities of gastric cancer distribution. Food and eating habits were directly related to culture and socioeconomic status. Dietary factors could explain socioeconomic gradients amid striking intercultural variation. Modification of diet habits takes two or three generations and could account for the decline in rates in the children and grandchildren of immigrants. Diet is difficult to study accurately, for many reasons. In gastric cancer, the dietary patterns which are most important may have been those of decades before. To attempt to reconstruct those patterns in the face of secular changes and alterations in personal behavior is perilous and difficult. Not surprisingly, the results of diet studies have been confusing, the conclusions uncertain. Among the factors which have been associated with gastric cancer have been higher intake of starches, lower intake of fresh produce, the presence of large amounts of polycyclic hydrocarbons in the diet, and exposure to carcinogenic nitrosamines (Graham *et al.*, 1972).

10.4.1. Starch Intake

Low-socioeconomic-status groups take a larger proportion of their calories in starch. This may be especially the case with working males in these groups who meet their additional calorie requirements with inexpensive high-carbohydrate staples. Per capita consumption of potatoes and of flour and cereal products declined dramatically in the United States between 1909 and 1960, while consumption of all other major food groups increased (Wynder *et al.*, 1963). These facts are consistent with the socioeconomic gradient, the male preponderance, and the secular trends in gastric cancer.

Several retrospective studies suggest that gastric cancer patients eat more starchy foods than do comparison groups. Review of intake questionnaires recording social and dietary traits of patients admitted to Roswell Park Memorial Institute from 1957 to 1966 confirmed an earlier observation that male gastric cancer patients ate potatoes more frequently than male control patients. Control patients without cancer or gastrointestinal disease were matched by age, birthplace (U.S. or foreign), and "ethnic background" (determined by birthplace of parents or grandparents). There was, however, no difference in potato consumption between female gastric cancer cases and controls (Graham *et al.*, 1967, 1972). Another case-control study bearing on level of starch intake in gastric cancer was based on interviews with patients in six Tel Aviv hospitals, November 1967 to December 1969 (Modan *et al.*, 1974). Higher frequency of consumption of starchy foods was reported among gastric cancer patients than in three matched control groups. No single type of high-starch food was responsible for the difference, and the finding was independent of socioeconomic status. The study was conducted with particular care to avoid common pitfalls in investigation of dietary habits, and on that basis alone deserves special emphasis. Only histologically confirmed cancer patients were included. As a precaution against interviewer bias, the interviewers were not informed about the patient's diagnosed disease. There were three controls for each of the 166 gastric cancer patients. One was a neighborhood control, one a patient with a newly diagnosed colorectal cancer, and one a surgical patient who had neither malignancy nor gastrointestinal disorder. Each control had been matched by age, sex, ethnic origin, and length of residence in Israel. Selection of colorectal cancer patients helped protect against recall bias in patients with gastrointestinal disease. Use of a neighborhood control limited differences in socioeconomic factors. A reliability check was accomplished by reinterviewing a majority of neighborhood controls. A high degree of reproducibility of responses was demonstrated. In the analysis of data obtained from the interviews, an effort was made to avoid spurious associations which might result from multiple intergroup comparisons. The concept of "meaningful significance" was introduced in an effort to avoid artifactual associations where a large number of items were being cross-tabulated. A statistical association was termed meaningful only for items in which there were statistically significant differences in one direction between the gastric cancer case and two of the three control groups, and where differences in the third control group were in the same direction and of borderline significance. Finally, differences among the three control groups themselves must not have been significant. This rigorous definition served to exclude spurious associations. Food items were tabulated both as independent items and as food groups. The high-starch group consisted of items with starch content of 15% or more, and it contained 50 items. Gastric cancer patients had significantly higher consumption of food in this group, and the difference met the investigator's criteria for meaningful significance. The differences were due to an overall trend and not to excess consumption of any single item or subgroup. This finding was true of European- and non-European-born groups. Given the precautions taken in this investigation, the findings suggest a meaningful difference in the past dietary practices of Israelis who have developed gastric cancer.

In Japan, attention has been called to the fact that high-rice-consumption areas are those with the highest incidence of gastric cancer. It has also been shown that rice intake is higher for males than for females. However, other areas in the world in which rice is a staple food do not have unduly high gastric cancer incidence. It has been suggested that the Japanese preference for talc- and glucose-treated rice may be involved (Merliss, 1971; Matsudo *et al.*, 1974).

10.4.2. Nitrosamines

Discovery of the carcinogenicity of dimethylnitrosamine in animals followed upon observation of its hepatotoxicity in man (Weisburger and Raineri, 1975). Experimentally, nitrosamines and nitrosamides are carcinogens in at least ten animals species (Sander *et al.,* 1972). Ingestion, inhalation, injection, or transplacental passage of these agents may produce tumors. The stomach is among the organs affected in such models. The minimum dose for tumor induction in mice may be a single dose of less than 10 mg/kg. Nitrite-forming microorganisms are widespread in the environment and also can be found in the human nasal and oral cavities and under some circumstances in the upper gastrointestinal and urinary tracts. Since nitrites and nitrosatable amines and amides are widespread in the diet and environment (as drugs, for example), the potential exists for the formation *in vivo* of carcinogenic nitrosamines. The circumstances under which foods or water are stored affect the amount of nitrate produced. Brines used for preservation of a variety of foods are a deliberate mixture of sodium chloride and nitrate (Weisberger and Raineri, 1975). These observations have led to the suggestion that the introduction of modern storage methods, particularly refrigeration, has been responsible for the reduction of gastric cancer rates. With the adoption of lower storage temperatures come lower production of nitrites and less exposure to carcinogenic nitrosamines. The abandonment of other storage and preservation methods associated with considerable nitrate production in favor of refrigeration would concomitantly lead to the same result. Observed time trends and socioeconomic gradients are broadly compatible with this suggestion. Some more specific epidemiological support is based on observation of stomach cancer mortality in the town of Worksop in the United Kingdom, 1963–1971. Until 1953, the drinking water of this area had a nitrate concentration of 90 mg/liter compared to less than 10 mg/liter for neighboring control towns of similar social class structure. While deaths from all malignant neoplasms in Worksop were somewhat less than expected, those from stomach cancer were increased. The excess of stomach cancer was largely accounted for by deaths in the over 75-year age group, where the observed deaths were twice the number expected (Hill *et al.,* 1973). Other support for a role for nitrites in gastric cancer comes from study of gastric juice concentration of hydrogen ion, nitrites, and bacteria in 69 patients undergoing gastroscopy. Six patients with gastric carcinomas had higher nitrite concentrations and lower hydrogen ion concentrations than gastric ulcer patients or patients in whom no specific gastrointestinal pathology was detected. In patients with low levels of hydrogen ion concentration, higher counts of nitrate-reducing bacteria was detected. In the absence of bacteria the nitrosation reaction proceeds in an acid pH. In the presence of gastrointestinal bacteria, however, the process is facilitated by a neutral pH. These observations do not provide information on the premorbid status of gastric juice in gastric cancer patients, so it is possible that these changes were secondary to the disease process. There is no indication of the degree of intestinal metaplasia present in the 25% of "normals" in whom hypochlorhydria and high levels of nitrite were found (Ruddell *et al.,* 1976).

10.4.3. Polycyclic Hydrocarbons

Polycyclic hydrocarbons are another important group of potential carcinogens which are widely distributed in foodstuffs and the environment. Heated fats containing these compounds have produced papillomas in rat forestomach, although early reports of malignant tumors of the glandular stomach have not been confirmed O'Gara *et al.,* 1969). Smoked mutton and smoked trout have produced malignant tumor in rats (Dungal, 1961). Home-smoked food in Iceland, a country of high gastric cancer incidence, has been shown to contain particularly large amounts of benzopyrene (Thorsteinsson, 1969). Singed sheep heads and seabirds, similarly prepared and both with high concentrations of polycyclic hydrocarbons, are widely eaten in the high gastric cancer incidence Skagafjardarsýsla district of northern Iceland (Thorsteinsson and Thordarson, 1968). Dungal (1961) describes the importance of smoked food in the diet of some communities with high rates of gastric cancer:

> In a small community surrounding a little lake (Hofoavatn in Skagafjardarsýsla), sixty-three men died in the last 30 years. Discounting 7 who were drowned we find that of the remaining 56 there were 25 who died of stomach cancer, or 45% of the total deaths of disease in the men in the community .... The farmers go on special expeditions for weeks every spring to catch birds on an offshore island. On these expeditions they used to consume quantities of smoked trout and smoked meat. The fat breasts of the birds were also smoked and as they might catch up to 100,000 birds a year and live around a trout lake far from all markets, most of the trout was also smoked. Consequently, the consumption of smoked food was unusually high, especially among the men.

Among Icelanders who migrated to Manitoba, Canada, continued gastric cancer rates are more than double those of native-born Canadians in that province. Diet studies suggest that consumption of singed and smoked foods is higher for the migrant group than for native controls. The offspring of migrant Icelanders, with intermediate rates of gastric cancer, have rather lower consumption of such foods (Choi *et al.*, 1971). Other studies either have not addressed the question of smoked foods or have elected not to pursue it when it became apparent that such foods were not important in the diets of the groups studied (Graham *et al.*, 1967).

11. Models of Gastric Cancer Etiology

Recent efforts to consolidate information on gastric cancer into a plausible etiological model have concentrated on mechanisms by which the mucous barrier of the stomach might be damaged, exposing the gastric epithelium to carcinogens. It has been suggested that ingested abrasives and irritants (hard grains, foods of high salt content, surfactants) might overcome the barrier. Such damage might precede an initial mutation which would lead to intestinalization of the mucosa and a rise in pH. This environment would favor formation of carcinogenic nitroso compounds. A second mutation would lead to frank carcinogenic transformation and intestinal-type gastric cancer (Correa *et al.*, 1975). This model has been modified by Lilienfeld *et al.* (1976), who focus on the ability of some polysaccharides to breach the stomach's protective barrier. Covalent bonds might under some circumstances be formed between mucopolysaccharide and mucoprotein chains in stomach mucus and some ingested polysaccharides, especially in the presence of large amounts of starch. Biochemical damage to the gastric mucosa would occur. Cells would be damaged, leading to decline in hydrochloric acid production and development of intestinal-type mucosa. In this environment, the growth of bacteria producing carcinogenic nitrosamines is favored. Polysaccharide structures in the mucosa of persons with blood group A might be more vulnerable to damage than those of persons with other blood groups. The authors suggest that this might account for the association of blood group A with stomach cancer. Vitamin C, as a saccharide derivative similar in structure to blood group polysaccharide derivatives, might act protectively to prevent this kind of damage. This speculation is consistent with the low consumption of fresh produce which has been noted among gastric cancer patients. Two stages are thus envisioned in the development of gastric cancer. This first, whether the result of a mutagenic transformation of the stomach mucosa or of "biochemical breakdown" of the mucous barrier, would lead to intestinal transformation of the mucosa and rise in pH. These conditions might favor exposure to and damage by various carcinogens. A second stage would be characterized by clear malignant transformation. The emphasis on the role of polysaccharides is consistent with reports that gastric cancer patients consume larger than expected amounts of starchy foods. While it is suggested that persons with blood group A might be more vulnerable to the biochemical sequence outlined, the findings of Correa *et al.* (1973) suggest that, at least in Japan, blood group A may be associated with diffuse stomach cancer rather than the intestinal form required by the polysaccharide damage model. While tentative, these theories integrate several disparate lines of investigation into a coherent sequence and should be pursued and refined.

12. References

Aird, I., Bentall, H. H., and Roberts, J. A. F., 1953, A relationship between cancer of the stomach and the ABO blood groups, *Br. Med. J.* **1**:799–801.

Ashley, D. J. B., 1969, Gastric cancer in Wales, *J. Med. Genet.* **6**: 76–79.

Ashley, D. J. B., and Davies, H. D., 1966, Gastric cancer in Wales, *Gut* **7**:542–548.

Balfour, D. C., and McCann, J. C., 1930, Sarcoma of the stomach, *Surg. Gynecol. Obstet.* **50**:948.

Bazaz-Malik, G., and Gupta, D. N., 1967, Sarcoma of the stomach, *Am. J. Gastroenterol.* **48**:512–522.

Berg, J. W., 1958, Histological aspects of the relation between gastric adenomatous polyps and gastric cancer, *Cancer* **11**:1149–1155.

Buckwalter and Knowler, 1958, Blood donor controls for blood group disease researches, *Am. J. Hum. Genet.* **10**:164–174.

Buell, P., and Dunn, J. E., Jr., 1965, Cancer mortality among Japanese Issei and Nisei of California, *Cancer* **18**:656–664.

Buell, P., Dunn, J. E., and Breslow, L., 1960, The occupational-social class risks of cancer mortality in men, *J. Chron. Dis.* **12**:600–621.

Burbank, F., 1971, Patterns in cancer mortality in the United States: 1950–1967, *Natl. Cancer Inst. Monogr.*, No. 33.

Choi, N. W., Entwistle, D. W., Michaluk, W., and Nelson, N., 1971, Gastric cancer in Icelanders in Maitoba, *Israel J. Med. Sci.* **7**:1500–1507.

Colcher, H., 1974, Cancer of the gastrointestinal tract: Gastric cancer diagnostic fiber optic Gastroscopy, *J. Am. Med. Assoc.* **228**:891–892.

Correa, P., Cuello, C., and Duque, E., 1970, Carcinoma and intestinal metaplasia of the stomach in Colombian migrants, *J. Natl. Cancer Inst.* **44**:297–306.

Correa, P., Sasano, N., Stemmerman, G. N., and Haenszel, W., 1973, Pathology of gastric carcinoma in Japanese populations: Comparisons between Miyagi Prefecture, Japan and Hawaii, *J. Natl. Cancer Inst.* **51**: 1449–1459.

Correa, P., Haenszel, W., Cuello, C., Tannenbaum, S., and Archer, M., 1975, A model for gastric cancer epidemiology, *Lancet* **2**:58–60.

Creagan, E. T., and Fraumeni, J. F., Jr., 1973, Familial gastric cancer and immunologic abnormalities, *Cancer* **32**:1325–1331.

Creagan, E. T., Hoover, R. M., and Fraumeni, J. F., 1974, Mortality from stomach cancer in coal mining regions, *Arch. Environ. Health* **28**:28–30.

Cutler, S. J., and Young, J. L., 1975, Third national cancer survey: Incidence data, *Natl. Cancer Inst. Monogr.*, No. 41.

Doll, R., 1969, The geographical distribution of cancer, *Br. J. Cancer* **23**:1–8.

Dungal, N., 1961, The special problem of stomach cancer in Iceland—With particular reference to dietary factors, *J. Am. Med. Assoc.* **178**:789–798.

Dunham, L. J., and Bailar, J. C., III, 1968, World maps of cancer mortality rates and frequency ratios, *J. Natl. Cancer Inst.* **41**:155–203.

Enterline, P., DeCoufle, P., and Henderson, V., 1972, Mortality in relation to occupational exposure in the asbestos industry, *J. Occup. Med.* **14**:897–903.

Fleiss, J. F., 1973, *Statistical Methods for Rates and Proportions*, Wiley, New York.

Glober, G. A., Cantrell, E. G., Doll, R., and Peto, R., 1971, Interaction between ABO and Rhesus blood groups, the site of origin of gastric cancers, and the age and sex of the patient, *Gut* **12**:570–573.

Goldsmith, J. R., and Miller, G. L., 1975, *Abstracts and Indexes to Selected Literature on Occupational and Environmental Carcinogenic Hazards,* The Franklin Institute Research Laboratories, Philadelphia.

Graham, S., and Lilienfeld, A. M., 1958, Genetic studies of gastric cancer in humans: An appraisal, *Cancer* **11**:945–958.

Graham, S., Lilienfeld, A. M., and Tidings, J. E., 1967, Dietary and purgation factors in the epidemiology of gastric cancer, *Cancer* **20**:2224–2234.

Graham, S., Schotz, W., and Martino, P., 1972, Alimentary factors in the epidemiology of gastric cancer, *Cancer* **30**:927–938.

Gregor, O., Toman, R., Prusova, F., Drnkova, V., and Pastorova, J., 1969, Geographical distribution of stomach cancer in Czechoslovakia, *Gut* **10**:150–154.

Griffith, G. W., 1968, The sex ratio in gastric cancer and hypothetical considerations relative to aetiology, *Br. J. Cancer* **22**:163–172.

Haenszel, W., Kurihara, M., Segi, M., and Lee, R. K. C., 1972, Stomach cancer among Japanese in Hawaii, *J. Natl. Cancer Inst.* **49**:969–988.

Haenszel, W., Kurihara, M. Locke, F. B., Shimuzu, K., and Segi, M., 1976, Stomach cancer in Japan, *J. Natl. Cancer Inst.* **56**:265–274.

Hagy, G. W., 1954, Familial study of gastric carcinoma, *Am. J. Hum. Genet.* **6**:434–447.

Hakama, M., 1972, Trends in stomach cancer incidence for male cohorts in Finland, *Ann. Clin. Res.* **4**:300–403.

Hammond, E. C., and Seidman, H., 1974, Epidemiology of gastric cancer, in: *Cancer Detection and Prevention,* Proceedings of the Second International Symposium on Cancer Detection and Prevention, pp. 70–80.

Hems, G., 1968, Susceptibility to stomach cancer, *Br. J. Cancer* **22**:461–465.

Hill, M. J., Hawksworth, G., and Tattersall, G., 1973, Bacteria, nitrosamines and cancer of the stomach, *Br. J. Cancer* **28**:562–567.

Hirayama, T., 1976, Metal material workers and lung cancer in Japan, *Ann. N.Y. Acad. Sci.* **271**:269–272.

Hirohata, T., and Kuratsune, M., 1969, The geographical comparison of mortality from cancer of the stomach and ulcer of the stomach in Japan, *Br. J. Cancer* **23**:465–479.

Hoffman, N. R., 1970, The relationship between pernicious anemia and cancer of the stomach, *Geriatrics,* pp. 90–95, April.

Hoskins, L. C., Loux, H. A., Britten, A., and Zamcheck, N., 1965, Distribution of ABO blood groups in patients with pernicious anemia, gastric carcinoma and gastric carcinoma associated with pernicious anemia, *N. Engl. J. Med.* **273**:633–637.

Hughes, E. S. R., 1966, Carcinoma of the stomach, *Med. J. Aust.,* pp. 663–665, April.

Imai, T., Kubo, T., and Watanabe, H., 1971, Chronic gastritis in Japanese with reference to high incidence of gastric carcinoma, *J. Natl. Cancer Inst.* *47:*179–195.

Jenner, A. W. F., 1939, Perniziöse Anämia und Magenkatzinom, *Acta Med. Scand.* **102**:529–590.

Kaplan, H. S., and Rigler, L. G., 1945, Pernicious anemia and carcinoma of the stomach—Autopsy studies concerning their relationship, *Am. J. Med. Sci.* **209**:339–348.

Kawashima, S., 1966, Early gastric cancer in Japan, *Scand. J. Gastroenterol.* **1**:248–252.

King, H., and Haenszel, W., 1973, Cancer mortality among foreign and native-born Chinese in the United States, *J. Chron. Dis.* **26**:623–646.

Kovi, J., Viola, M. V., Connelly, C. A., and Vohra, R., 1974, Gastric cancer in American Negroes, *Cancer* **34**:765–770.

Kraus, A. S., Levin, M. L., and Gerhardt, P. R., 1957, A study of occupational associations with gastric cancer, *Am. J. Public Health* **47**:961–970.

Kubo, T., 1971, Histologic appearance of gastric carcinoma in high and low mortality countires: Comparison between Kyushu, Japan and Minnesota, U.S.A., *Cancer* **28**:726–734.

Kubo, T., 1973, Gastric carcinoma in New Zealand: Some epidemiologic-pathologic aspects, *Cancer* **31**:1498–1507.

Lauren, P., 1965, The two histological main types of gastric cancer: Diffuse and so-called intestinal-type carcinoma: An attempt at a histo-clinical classification, *Acta Pathol. Microbiol. Scand.* **64:**31–49.

Levin, D. L., Devesa, S. S., Godwin, J. D., II, and Silverman, D. T., 1974, "Cancer Rates and Risks," DHEW Pub. No. (NIH) 76-691, U.S. Gov't Printing Office, Washington, D.C.

Lilienfeld, D. E., Garagliano, C. F., and Lilienfeld, A. M., 1976, A model for gastric cancer epidemiology (letter), *Lancet* **1:**45.

Logan, W. P. D., 1976, Cancers of the alimentary tract: International mortality trends, *WHO Chron.* **30:**413–419.

Lynch, H. T., 1972, *Skin, Heredity, and Malignant Neoplasms,* Medical Examination Publishing Co., New York.

Lynch, H. T. (ed.), 1976, *Cancer Genetics,* Thomas, Springfield, Ill.

Lyon, J. L., Klauber, M. R., Gardner, J. W., and Smart, C. R., 1976, Cancer incidence in Mormons and Non-Mormons in Utah, 1966–1970, *N. Eng. J. Med.* **294:**129–133.

Macklin, M. T., 1960, Inheritance of cancer of the stomach and large intestine in man, *J. Natl. Cancer Inst.* **24:**551–571.

Maddock, C. R., 1966, Environment and heredity factors in carcinoma of the stomach, *Br. J. Cancer* **20:**660–669.

Manuila, A., 1958, Blood groups and disease—Hard facts and delusions, *J. Am. Med. Assoc.* **167:**2047–2053.

Mason, T. J., McKay, F. W., Hoover, R., Blot, W. J., and Fraumeni, J. R., Jr., 1975, *Atlas of Cancer Mortality for U.S. Counties: 1950–1969,* DHEW Pub. No. (NIH) 75-780, Bethesda, Md.

Matolo, N. M., Klauber, M. R., Gorishek, W. M., and Dixon, J. A., 1972, High incidence of gastric carcinoma in a coal mining region, *Cancer* **29:**733–737.

Matsudo, H., Hodgkin, N., and Tanaka, A., 1974, Japanese gastric cancer, *Arch. Pathol.* **97:**366–368.

McConnell, R. B., 1966, The genetics of carcinoma of the stomach, in: *The Genetics of Gastrointestinal Disorders,* Oxford University Press, London.

McMichael, A. J., Andjelkovic, D. A., and Tyroler, H. A., 1976, Cancer mortality among rubber workers: An epidemiologic study, *Ann. N.Y. Acad. Sci.* **271:**125–142.

Merliss, R. R., 1971, Talc-treated rice and Japanese stomach cancer, *Science* **173:**1141–1142.

Milham, S., Jr., 1976, Neoplasia in the wood and pulp industry, *Ann. N.Y. Acad. Sci.* **271:**294–300.

Ming, S. C., 1974, Gastric cancer: Histogenesis and premalignant lesions, *J. Am. Med. Assoc.* **228:**886–888.

Ming, S. C., and Goldman, H., 1965, Gastric polyps: A histogenic classification and its relation to carcinoma, *Cancer* **18:**721–726.

Modan, B., Lubin, F., Barell, V., Greenberg, R. A., Modan, M., and Graham, S., 1974, The role of starches in the etiology of gastric cancer, *Cancer* **34:**2087–2092.

Mosbech, J., 1960, ABO blood groups in patients with stomach cancer, *Acta Unis. Int. Cancer.* **16:**1750–1755.

Mosbech, J., and Videbaek, A., 1950, Mortality from and risk of gastric carcinoma among patients with pernicious anemia, *Br. Med. J.* **2:**390–394.

Muñoz, N., and Asvall, J., 1971, Time trends in intestinal and diffuse types of gastric cancer in Norway, *Int. J. Cancer* **8:**144–157.

Muñoz, N., and Connelly, R., 1971, Time trends of intestinal and diffuse types of gastric cancer in the United States, *Int. J. Cancer* **8:**158–164.

Muñoz, N., Correa, P., Cuello, C., and Duque, E., 1968, Histologic types of gastric carcinoma in high- and low-risk areas, *Int. J. Cancer* **3:**809–818.

Newill, V. A., 1961, Distribution of cancer mortality among ethnic subgroups of the white population of New York City, 1953–58, *J. Natl. Cancer Inst.* **26:**405–417.

O'Gara, R. W., Stewart, L., Brown, J., and Hueper, W. C., 1969, Carcinogenicity of heated fats and fat fractions, *J. Natl. Cancer Inst.* **42:**275–284.

Raineri, R., and Weisburger, J. H., 1975 Reduction of gastric carcinogens with ascorbic acid, *Ann. N.Y. Acad. Sci.* **258:**181–189.

Roberts, J. A. F., 1959, Some associations between blood groups and disease, *Br. Med. Bull.* **15:**129–133.

Rønnov-Jessen, V., Ahlgren, P., and Qvist, C. F., 1965, Incidence of gastric cancer in medically treated patients with gastric ulcer, *Acta Med. Scand.* **178:**141–153.

Rubin, P., 1974, Cancer of the gastrointestinal tract: Gastric cancer diagnosis, *J. Am. Med. Assoc.* **228:**883–884.

Ruddell, W. S. J., Bone, E. S., Hill, M. J., Blendis, L. M., and Walters, C. L., 1976, Gastric-juice nitrite: A risk factor for cancer in hypochlorhydric stomach? *Lancet* **2:**1037–1039.

Saknyn', A. V., and Shabynina, N. K., 1973, Epidemiology of malignant neoplasms in nickel refineries, *Gig Tr. Prof. Zabol.* **9:**25–29 (abstr.) (in Goldsmith and Miller, 1975).

Salmela, H., 1968, Smooth muscle tumors of the stomach: A clinical study of 112 cases, *Acta Chir. Scand.* **134:**384–391.

Sander, J., Burkle, G., and Schweinsberg, F., 1972, Induction of tumors by nitrite and secondary amines or amides, in: *Topics in Chemical Carcinogenesis* (W. Nakahara, S. Takayama, T. Sujimura, and S. Odashima, eds.), pp. 292–312, University Park Press, Baltimore.

Schade, R. O. K., 1974, Cancer of the gastrointestinal tract. C. Gastric cancer diagnosis, cytology in early diagnosis, *J. Am. Med. Assoc.* **228:**890–891.

Schottenfeld, D., 1975, *Cancer Epidemiology and Prevention: Current Concepts,* Thomas, Springfield, Ill.

Selikoff, I. J., and Hammond, E. C., 1973, Multiple factor etiology of occupational lung cancer, in: *Cancer Detection and Prevention,* Int. Congr. Ser. No. 322, ISBN 9021902281.

Selikoff, I. J., Hammond, E. C., and Churg, J., 1968, Asbestos exposure, smoking and neoplasia, *J. Am. Med. Assoc.* **204:**104–110.

Sievers, M. L., 1973, Unusual comparative frequency of gastric carcinoma, pernicious anemia, and peptic ulcer in Southwestern American Indians, *Gastroenterology* **65:**867–876.

Sigurjonsson, J., 1966, Geographical variations in mortality from cancer in iceland, with particular reference to stomach cancer, *J. Natl. Cancer Inst.* **37:**337–346.

Silverberg, E., and Holleb, A. I., 1975, Major trends in cancer: 25 year survey, *Ca* **25:**2–20.

Sokoloff, B., 1938, Predisposition to cancer in the Bonaparte family, *Am. J. Surg.* **40:**673–678.

Staszewski, J., 1971, Migrant studies in alimentary tract cancer, *Recent Results Cancer Res.* **39:**85–97.

Staszewski, J., McCall, M. G., and Stenhouse, N. S., 1971, Cancer mortality in 1962–66 among Polish migrants to Australia, *Br. J. Cancer* **25:**599–610.

Stemmermann, G. N., 1967, Comparative study of histochemical patterns in non- neoplastic and neoplastic gastric epithelium: A study of Japanese in Hawaii, *J. Natl. Cancer Inst.* **39:**375–383.

Stemmermann, G. N., and Hayashi, T., 1968, Intestinal metaplasia of the gastric mucosa: A gross and microscopic study of its distribution in various disease states, *J. Natl. Cancer Inst.* **41:**627–634.

Sterup, K., and Mosbech, J., 1971, Sex ratio of gastric cancer related to site of the tumor, *Scand. J. Gastroenterol. Suppl* **9:**87–89.

Terris, M., and Hall, C. E., 1963, Decline in mortality from gastric cancer in native-born and foreign-born residents of New York City, *J. Natl. Cancer Inst.* **31:**155–162.

Thorsteinsson, T., 1969, Polycyclic hydrocarbons in commercially and home-smoked foods in Iceland, *Cancer* **23:**455–460.

Thorsteinsson, T., and Thordarson, G., 1968, Polycyclic hydrocarbons in singed food in Iceland, *Cancer* **21:**390–392.

Tomatis, L., 1976, The IARC program on the evaluation of the carcinogenic risk of chemicals to man, *Ann. N.Y. Acad. Sci.* **271:**396–409.

Tsuchiga, K., 1967, Role of environmental factors in cancer production, *Keio Igaku* **44:**709–717 (in Goldsmith and Miller, 1975).

Tulchinsky, D., and Modan, B., 1967, Epidemiological aspects of cancer of the stomach in Israel, *Cancer* **20:**1311–1317.

Van Wayjen, R. G. A., and Linschoten, H., 1973, Distribution of ABO and Rhesus blood groups in patients with gastric Carcinoma with reference to its site of origin, *Gastroenterology* **65:**877–883.

Videbaek, A., and Mosbech, J., 1954, Aetiology of gastric carcinoma elucidated by study of 302 pedigrees, *Acta Med. Scand.* **149:**137–159.

Weisburger, J. H., and Raineri, R., 1975, Assessment of human exposure and response to

N-nitroso compounds: A new view on the etiology of digestive tract cancers, *Toxicol. Appl. Pharmacol.* **31**:369–374.
Wenger, J., Brandborg, L. L., and Spellman, F. A., 1971, Cancer. Part I: Clinical aspects, *Gastroenterology* **61**:598–605.
Whitehead, R., Skinner, J. M., and Heenan, P. J., 1974, Incidence of carcinoma of stomach and tumour type, *Br. J. Cancer* **30**:370–573.
Woolf, C. M., 1956, Further study on familial aspects of carcinoma of stomach, *Am. J. Hum. Genet.* **8**:102–109.
Woolf, C. M., 1961, The incidence of cancer in the spouses of stomach cancer patients, *Cancer* **14**:199–200.
Woolf, C. M., and Isaacson, E. A., 1961, An analysis of 5 "stomach cancer families" in the State of Utah, *Cancer* **14**:1005–1016.
Wynder, E. L., Kmet, J., Dungal, N., and Segi, M., 1963, An epidemiological investigation of gastric cancer, *Cancer* **16**:1461–1496.
Young, M., and Russell, W. T., 1926, An investigation into the statistics of cancer in different trades and professions, M. Res. Council Spec. Rep. No. 99, His Majesty's Stationery Office, London (in Kraus *et al.*, 1957).
Zaldivar, R., 1970, Geographic pathology of oral, esophageal, gastric and intestinal cancer in Chile, *Ztschr. Krebsforsch.* **75**:1–13.
Zamcheck, N., Grable, E., Ley, A., and Norman, L., 1955, Occurrence of gastric cancer among patients with pernicious anemia at the Boston City Hospital, *N. Eng. J. Med.* **252**:1103–1110.

9

Epidemiology of Colorectal Cancer

David Schottenfeld and Joanna F. Haas

1. Introduction

In the following discussion the terms "colorectal cancer," "cancer of the large intestine," and "cancer of the large bowel" will be used to indicate that tumors classified according to the Eighth Revision of the International Classification of Disease (Public Health Service, 1968) as ICD 153 (cancer of the colon, excluding rectum) and ICD 154 (cancer of the rectum and rectosigmoid junction) are being considered in the aggregate. Where there are references to "cancer of the colon," it will be understood that this is colon (ICD 153), excluding the rectum and rectosigmoid, and "cancer of the rectum" (ICD 154) will be understood to include the rectosigmoid junction. Some authors (Logan, 1976) use the term "cancer of the intestine" to include cancers of the small intestine (ICD 152) as well as cancer of the colon (ICD 153). While generally cancers of the small intestine contribute such a small proportion of the total that this makes little difference, in some countries this is not the case. In Belgium, with high rates at both sites, small intestinal neoplasms make up 10% of cancer of the intestine defined in this way. In Japan, where mortality from colon cancer is low and mortality from small intestine cancer is rather high, the latter constitutes 30% of all cancers of the two sites combined. Unless otherwise specified, small intestine cancers will not be included in this review.

2. Magnitude of the Problem

Cancer of the large intestine continues to be a major cause of illness and death in the United States. In 1973, the probability of a white female develop-

David Schottenfeld • Chief, Epidemiology and Preventive Medicine, Memorial Sloan-Kettering Cancer Center, New York, New York 10021, and Professor of Public Health, Cornell University Medical College, New York, New York 10021. *Joanna F. Haas* • Assistant Professor of Public Health, Cornell University Medical College, New York, New York 10021.

Table 1. Frequency of Colorectal Cancer in the United States[a]

	White males	Black males	White females	Black females
Lifetime probability of eventually developing colorectal cancer (1973)	4.4%	2.9%	5.2%	3.6%
Lifetime probability of eventually dying from colorectal cancer (1973)	2.2%	1.5%	2.8%	2.0%
Estimated new cases in 1976	44,000	4,000	47,000	4,000
Incidence of colorectal cancer per 100,000[b]	44.0	37.7	34.7	32.6
Death rate for colorectal cancer per 100,000 (1973)	23.2	18.5	18.0	17.3
Colorectal cancer cases as percent of all new cancer (1976)	14.7%	10.3%	15.4%	12.9%

[a]Source: Seidman *et al.* (1976) and Cutler and Young (1975).
[b]Average annual incidence adjusted to 1950 U.S. standard (Third National Cancer Survey, 1969–71).

ing the disease at some time in her life was 5.2% and of her dying from it was 2.8% (Table 1). For white men, the corresponding figures were 4.4% and 2.2% (Seidman *et al.*, 1976). Some 99,000 cases identified annually make it the most common newly diagnosed malignancy, and despite fairly high relative survival rates there were 49,000 deaths from colorectal cancer in the United States in 1976. Colorectal cancer constituted 15.4% of all newly diagnosed cancer cases in white women and 14.7% in white men (excluding nonmelanotic skin cancer and carcinoma *in situ* of uterine cervix). Fifteen percent of all cancer deaths in females and 12% in males were due to colorectal cancer (American Cancer Society, 1977).

3. Anatomical and Histological Distribution of Colorectal Malignancies

During 1969–1971, the Third National Cancer Survey (3rd NCS) reported new cancer cases in ten areas of the United States with a total population of 21,003,451. The age-adjusted incidence rate for colorectal cancer was 38.6 per 100,000 per year (Cutler and Young, 1975) (Table 2). Of 26,598 cancers of the large intestine, 69.3% were in the colon and 30.7% were in the rectum or rectosigmoid junction. Within the colon itself, the largest number were located in the sigmoid. The majority of tumors of the rectum or rectosigmoid junction were in the rectum.

Of the 26,598 cancers of the large intestine reported, 24,127 had been microscopically confirmed. In the colon, 89.3% of 18,427 cases had been microscopically confirmed. For cancer of the rectum the proportion was higher, 93.5% of 8171 cases. Of all microscopically confirmed cases of cancer of the large intestine, 94% were adenocarcinomas (including mucin-secreting adenocarcinomas) and 4.3% were designated only as "malignant" or "carcinoma." There were 106 sarcomas (0.4%) and 136 carcinoids (0.6%). For the most part, histological type did not vary strikingly with the anatomical location

Table 2. Distribution of Cancers of the Large Intestine by Segment According to the Third National Cancer Survey[a]

Site	Number of cases	Percent of all cancers of the large intestine cases	Incidence[b]
Colon excluding rectum	18,427	69.3	26.6
Transverse colon	2,935	11.0	4.3
Descending colon	1,611	6.1	2.4
Sigmoid colon	6,266	23.6	9.2
Caecum	3,335	12.5	4.7
Appendix	160	0.6	0.3
Ascending colon	2,420	9.1	3.5
Large intestine, segment unspecified	1,700	6.4	2.3
Rectum and rectosigmoid junction	8,171	30.7	12.0
Rectosigmoid junction	2,299	8.6	3.4
Rectum	5,872	22.1	8.6
All large intestinal cancers	26,598	100.0	38.6

[a]Source: Cutler and Young (1975).
[b]Average annual incidence per 100,000 (adjusted to 1950 U.S. standard), males and females, all races.

within the large intestine (Table 3). Adenocarcinomas were overwhelmingly the most common histological type throughout. Carcinoid tumors were most frequently encountered in the appendix (58), rectum (33), and caecum (20).

Comparable findings have been reported from the End Results Group Registry. Of 60,193 cases of microscopically confirmed cancers of the large intestine collected since 1940, 93.3% were carcinomas, 0.4% were sarcomas (including lymphomas), and 0.5% were carcinoids (Berg and Godwin, 1974).

There is some evidence that mucin-producing tumors of the large intestine may differ epidemiologically and clinically from other adenocarcinomas. Tumors specifically described as mucin-producing or signet-ring cell adenocarcinomas constituted 7.8% of microscopically verified colorectal cancers reported in the Third National Cancer Survey. Such tumors composed 4.7% of the End Results Group Registry Series, while in other studies their reported frequency ranged from 9% to 27% (Berg *et al.*, 1969; Symonds and Vickery, 1976; Berezkin and Neishtadt, 1969). These tumors are reported to constitute a higher proportion of colorectal cancers among patients under 30 than in older age groups (Berg and Godwin, 1974). Mucin-producing tumors were relatively more common among blacks in both the 3rd NCS and the End Results Group Registry. In the 3rd NCS, mucin-producing adenocarcinomas and signet-ring cell carcinomas constituted 7.7% of tumors among whites and 11.2% among blacks. The corresponding proportions among cases from the End Results Group Registry were 4.4% among whites and 9% among blacks. Mucin-producing carcinomas of the large intestine appear to be characterized by poor survival regardless of their site (Symonds and Vickery, 1976). This may contribute to the shorter survival times reported among blacks with large bowel malignancies.

Table 3. Distribution of Colorectal Cancer by Histological Type[a]

Histological type	Site: Appendix		Colon		Rectosigmoid		Rectum		All sites combined	
I. All carcinomas	99	62%	16,153	99%	2,135	99%	5,410	98%	23,797	99%
Adenocarcinomas[b]	57		13,949		1,937		4,832		20,775	
Mucin-producing adenocarcinoma[c]	36		1,461		127		262		1,886	
Carcinoma, miscellaneous[d]	6		743		71		316		1,136	
II. Sarcoma	2	1%	78	0.5%	2	0.0%	24	0.4%	106	0.4%
Malignant lymphoma[e]	1		59		0		12		71	
Leiomyosarcoma	0		19		0		12		20	
Other sarcoma[f]	1		0		2		1		36	
III. Carcinoid	58	36%	43	0.3%	2	0.0%	33	0.6%	136	0.6%
IV. Miscellaneous										
NOS[g]	1		47	0.3%	9	0.0%	21	0.4%	78	0.3%
Melanoma	0	0.0%	0		0		10		10	
All types combined	160	100%	16,321	100%	2,148	100%	5,498	100%	24,127	100%

[a]Only microscopically confirmed cases have been included. Source: Cutler and Young (1975).
[b]Adenocarcinoma NOS (19,844); adenocarcinoma in adenomatous (420) or multiple polyps (14), papillary adenocarcinoma (493), duct adenocarcinoma (1).
[c]Mucin-producing adenocarcinoma and signet-ring cell carcinoma (20).
[d]Carcinoma NOS (954), papillary carcinoma (26), squamous cell carcinoma NOS (85), transitional cell carcinoma (38), carcinoma simplex (5), granular cell carcinoma (1), medullary carcinoma (2), adenosquamous carcinoma (3), adenocarcinoma with squamous metaplasia (12), carcinosarcoma (1), acinar cell carcinoma (1), small cell carcinoma (7).
[e]Lymphoma NOS (3), lymphosarcoma NOS (18), lymphocytic lymphosarcoma (8), lymphoblastic lymphosarcoma (11), reticulum cell sarcoma NOS (32), Burkitt's tumor (2).
[f]Mesothelioma (1), sarcoma NOS (1).
[g]NOS, Not otherwise specified.

In summary, among colorectal malignancies, adenocarcinomas are overwhelmingly most common. Histological subgroups of mucin-producing tumors may be of both etiological and prognostic importance. Tumors of nonepithelial origin are less frequently encountered. To the extent that adenocarcinoma is the dominant histological type, international comparisons of large bowel cancer frequencies are essentially comparisons of rates of adenocarcinomas. Detailed histological information is not often available for population-based statistics, and one must be aware of the possibility that rates of large bowel cancer in some areas may be influenced by different distributions of tumor histology.

4. *Geographical Pathology*

The practice of including cancer of the rectosigmoid with that of the rectum is troublesome, since cancers which develop in the rectosigmoid have much in common with those occurring in the more proximal colon. Moreover, the demarcation of the rectum and sigmoid is not universally agreed upon and varies with time, and from hospital to hospital. The definition of the junctional location between the rectum and sigmoid colon may vary when reported by the pathologist rather than by the surgeon or sigmoidoscopist. The surgeon generally locates the junction at the level of the lower margin of the sacral promontory. The rectosigmoid lies at or above the peritoneal reflection and may occur between 10 and 15 cm from the anal orifice on sigmoidoscopy. A further discrepancy often occurs between the reported diagnosis of an incident rectal cancer case by a registry or morbidity survey and the death certificate diagnosis for the same individual. The diagnosis of rectal cancer may be reassigned to colon or large intestine cancer on the death certificate. These factors introduce another element of uncertainty in international and time trend comparisons of the distribution of neoplasms along the lower gastrointestinal tract.

Incidence and mortality rates of colorectal cancer vary widely throughout the world. A number of consistencies are evident, however. High rates are characteristic of highly developed countries in the West. Lower rates are observed in Eastern Europe and still lower rates in developing countries. The geographical correlation of colon cancer and rectal cancer rates is quite high for the whole population and for males and females considered independently (Berg and Howell, 1974). Within most countries the correlation of male and female rates is very high (Logan, 1976).

Recent incidence rates for colon cancer from cancer registries around the world range from 1.3 cases per 100,000 in Ibadan, Nigeria, to 30 per 100,000 in the state of Connecticut in the United States. For cancer of the rectum, rates ranged from 1.2 per 100,000, again in Ibadan, to 18.2 per 100,000 in Connecticut. Table 4 lists rates of cancer of the colon and of cancer of the rectum. Rates for both sites have been adjusted to the 1950 world standard population for major cancer incidence registries throughout the world. Ad-

Table 4. Incidence of Colon and Rectum Cancer in Males in Selected Countries[a]

Country	Colon (ICD 8th revision 153)		Rectum (ICD 8th revision 154)	
	Adjusted[b]	Truncated[c]	Adjusted[b]	Truncated[c]
Nigeria: Ibadan	1.3	3.4	1.2	3.4
Bulawayo: African	7.0	4.5?[d]	1.3	3.6?
Brazil: Recife	2.8	3.5	2.7	4.3
Sao Paulo	8.7	12.1	6.9	12.8
Canada: Alberta	17.1	22.0	10.6	15.2
British Columbia	23.5	29.6	15.9	21.5
Manitoba	20.7	27.8	13.7	22.2
Maritime Provinces	19.3	26.0	13.5	19.8
Newfoundland	24.7	32.4	13.1	19.1
Quebec	16.2	21.6	12.7	17.5
Saskatchewan	17.8	22.5	13.8	21.4
Colombia: Cali	3.2	5.8	3.1	5.1
Cuba	6.9	7.7	4.2	5.1
Jamaica: Kingston[c]	9.1	15.5	4.9	7.5
United States				
Alameda: White	25.3	29.4	15.0	21.7
Black	23.0	34.9	10.7	15.9
Bay Area: White	28.3	32.3	15.2	20.0
Black	24.0	33.2	10.8	15.6
Chinese	23.5	26.8	19.5	24.4
Connecticut	30.1	35.8	18.2	26.0
Iowa	24.8	34.5	13.4	19.6
Detroit: White	26.2	33.5	16.0	23.2
Black	24.5	35.3	13.8	24.8
New Mexico: Spanish	8.7	11.2	6.7	8.6
Other white	23.3	27.0	12.1	15.9
American Indian	1.7	3.7?	4.9	12.1?
New York State	24.6	30.2	13.7	18.9
El Paso: Spanish	9.3	11.2	5.5	4.1?
Other white	15.4	23.6	6.8	12.8
Puerto Rico	6.0	9.9	4.2	7.5
Utah	16.3	23.9	9.2	13.0
India: Bombay	4.6	5.7	4.4	6.1
Israel: All Jews	11.6	15.9	10.6	15.1
Born in Israel	8.7	15.6	5.1	12.3
Born in Europe or America	12.9	17.2	11.9	15.1
Born in Africa, Asia	5.1	7.2	4.2	8.1
Non-Jews	2.3	3.8	3.8	6.0
Japan: Miyagi	5.6	7.8	6.8	9.5
Okayama	5.0	6.4	7.0	10.9
Osaka	6.3	8.7	6.9	9.0
Singapore: Chinese	11.9	16.6	10.0	16.3
Malay	3.4	6.8	4.7	9.9
Indian	5.0	12.4	6.4	11.7
Denmark[d]	16.2	18.9	16.7	20.6
Finland	7.9	9.7	7.7	9.3
German Democratic Republic	9.6	14.1	11.3	15.9

Continued

Table 4. Continued

Country	Colon (ICD 8th revision 153)		Rectum (ICD 8th revision 154)	
	Adjusted[b]	Truncated[c]	Adjusted[b]	Truncated[c]
Federal Republic of Germany: Hamburg	13.6	16.6	12.0	13.6
Saarland	15.5	16.6	16.9	21.8
Hungary: Szabolcs	3.1	6.1	5.2	7.5
Vas	9.1	14.6	11.0	16.1
Iceland[e]	12.3	17.0	7.9	10.4
Malta	7.0	9.0	10.1	13.3
Norway: Urban	15.0	18.2	11.2	14.4
Rural	11.2	15.5	9.4	12.5
Poland: Cieszyn	4.9	8.4	8.7	10.0
Cracow	6.0	9.9	6.0	8.5
Katowice	6.8	10.6	6.6	11.4
Warsaw, city	10.9	14.4	7.7	10.1
Warsaw, rural	4.2	7.1	3.8	5.3
Rumania: Timis	3.0	5.1	8.1	16.0
Spain: Zaragoza	6.5	7.9	6.9	9.4
Sweden	15.8	19.2	10.5	13.2
Switzerland: Geneva	18.9	24.1	13.8	15.0
U.K.: Birmingham	16.5	21.3	16.1	20.5
Oxford	15.7	20.4	13.1	17.1
Sheffield	13.8	17.7	13.3	18.0
Southwest	14.7	20.1	12.7	17.1
South Metropolitan Region	13.9	19.0	11.2	14.3
Liverpool	17.1	22.3	15.1	19.8
Ayrshire	16.6	20.6	14.0	19.8
Yugoslavia: Slovenia	6.0	8.8	11.4	16.7
New Zealand: Maori	7.4	14.8	4.6	5.8?
Non-Maori	23.0	36.1	15.4	23.8

[a]Source: Waterhouse *et al.* (1976).
[b]Adjusted to 1950 world standard population.
[c]Truncated rates are cases per 100,000 population in the 35–64 year age range.
[d]?, Rates are based on fewer than ten cases.
[e]ICD 7th revision.

justment to this young population standard lowers the apparent magnitude of the rates and may thereby not fully emphasize the importance of these neoplasms, in industrialized countries where a high proportion of the population is in the older age group. Use of incidence data permits comparison of the frequency of disease occurrence independent of different survival rates. Mortality rates reflect both the frequency of the disease and the likelihood of dying from it. Table 4 also lists truncated incidence rates. Truncated incidence rates are based on the experience of persons 35–64 years old and better reflect true differences in cancer incidence since they exclude the older age groups among which diagnostic reliability falls (Doll and Cook, 1967).

Scrutiny of factors which may introduce diagnostic bias is essential in interpreting differences between countries. The fact that incidence and mortality of colon cancer and of rectum cancer are 2–2.5 times higher in Denmark than in Finland prompted just such an examination on a case-by-case basis. Review of the frequency of other reportable gastrointestinal diseases revealed very similar patterns in both countries, suggesting that registration differences were not the explanation. The clinical evidence used in documenting colonic and rectal cancers was similar in both countries, and the surprisingly large difference in rates was apparently not explicable by reporting or diagnostic bias (Jensen *et al.,* 1974).

In Europe incidence rates* for colon cancer are highest for Northern and Western European countries [Sweden, 15.8 per 100,000; Switzerland (Geneva), 18.9], and somewhat lower in Eastern European countries including Poland (4.9), Rumania (3.0), and Yugoslavia (6.0). This may represent differences in economic development and its social correlates as much as geography. The rates for the city of Warsaw in Poland (10.9) and for East Germany (9.6) are intermediate between those of the rest of Central and Eastern Europe and the West. For cancer of the rectum, incidence rates range from 16.9 per 100,000 in Saarland, West Germany, to a low of 5.2 in Szabolcs, Hungary.

High rates of both colon and rectal cancer prevail in North America. In Canada and the United States, colonic cancer incidence rates are substantially higher than corresponding rates of rectal cancer. In South America, incidence data are available only for a few limited areas. Colombia reports quite low annual incidence rates for both neoplasms, with colon cancer incidence only 3.2 per 100,000 and that of rectal cancers 3.1 per 100,000. In Brazil, reported incidence rates are higher in the industrialized region of Sao Paulo (8.7 per 100,000 for colon and 6.9 per 100,000 for rectum) than in the poor coastal region of Recife (2.8 colon and 2.7 rectal cancer cases per 100,000). Data from the Inter-American Investigation of Mortality (Puffer and Griffith, 1967), an intensive study of mortality in ten Latin American cities plus San Francisco and Bristol, England, demonstrated considerable variation in mortality rates from large intestinal cancer in the Americas. Low death rates from both colon and rectal cancers were reported in the Colombian cities of Bogota and Cali and in Guatemala City and Mexico City. By contrast, in Argentina, La Plata had mortality rates for both colon and rectal cancer so high that they were comparable to those of San Francisco. Colon cancer deaths were almost 3 times as common as rectal cancers in La Plata, in contrast to a more equal distribution in cities with lower mortality from large bowel neoplasms. The similarities between rates in La Plata and in North America are especially interesting in light of suggestions that high colon cancer rates are related to high levels of beef consumption. As a major cattle-producing country, the per capita consumption of beef in Argentina is high.

In Asia, incidence rates for colon and rectal cancer vary markedly be-

*Note that these rates are adjusted to the 1950 world standard population (Waterhouse *et al.,* 1976).

tween countries and between population groups, although for the most part they are low. The Bombay Cancer Registry in India reports 4.6 cases per 100,000 for colon and 4.4 per 100,000 for rectum. In Singapore, incidence of colon and rectal cancer in the Malay and Indian populations is low, whereas among Singapore Chinese rates are substantially higher. Three areas of Japan report low incidence rates of both tumors, approximately 6 cases per 100,000 for colon cancer and 7 per 100,000 for rectal cancer. In the Yamanashi district of Japan, in which schistosomiasis japonica is prevalent, cancer of the colon is relatively common (Wynder *et al.,* 1969). In Japan, in contrast to most industrialized countries, rectal cancer occurs more commonly than colon cancer.

In summary, the ratio of colon cancer to rectal cancer incidence rates is correlated with overall incidence of large intestine cancer. The proportion of colon cancers is highest in high-incidence areas. Where the rates for both tumors are low, the proportion of rectal cancers is relatively high.

5. *Regional Variation within Countries*

Even within countries marked variation may occur in the frequency of cancers of the large intestine. Study of these differences may help distinguish etiological influences of the social from the physical environment. In the United States, mortality from cancer of the colon and cancer of the rectum shows marked concentration in the Northeast for males and females, for nonwhites and whites. Among whites and nonwhites the greatest concentration is in the North Atlantic coastal counties, with high-death-rate areas found in New Jersey, Massachusetts, southern New York State, and urban areas near the Great Lakes. In the South and Southwest, large areas experience rates of cancer of the large intestine significantly below the U.S. average (Mason *et al.,* 1975, 1976).

In an effort to explain some of these regional differences, detailed analysis of large bowel cancer mortality by county in the United States from 1950 to 1969 was undertaken (Blot *et al.,* 1976). High-rate counties tended to have a large population, higher income, higher educational levels, and a greater proportion of the population reported to be of Irish, German, or Czech descent. Separate measures of "urbanness" or "ruralness" did not further explain differences in county rates. Regional differences between the Northeast and Southeast persisted after adjustment for socioeconomic differences. For rectal cancer, high rates were also noted in heavily populated counties and those with high median incomes. Rectal cancer was highest in countries with a large percentage of residents of Greek, Irish, or German descent. No meaningful pattern was found when data on alcohol or beer consumption by county were correlated with colon or rectal cancer mortality rates. Substantial regional variation in colon and rectal cancer mortality rates exists in the United States and is not readily accounted for by demographic differences. This variation is especially noteworthy since per capita consumption of specific food products is fairly uniform throughout the United States and mortality differences may reflect nondietary factors.

In Canada, colon cancer incidence rates are higher than rectal cancer rates in each province. High colon cancer rates in British Columbia and Newfoundland are reminiscent of the coastal concentrations of high colon cancer mortality observed in the United States.

Rates of colon and rectal cancer from the United Kingdom are high but fairly uniform, with the exception of Scotland, where for decades cancers of the large bowel have been known to be especially common. The Scots eat large amounts of beef compared to the English, and it has been suggested that this may be related to the high frequency of cancer of the colon. Colorectal cancer rates for both Scotland and England have declined since the 1950s (Berg and Howell, 1974).

6. *Trends in Colon Cancer Occurrence*

The overall mortality from colon cancer among U.S. whites has been nearly stable for the past three decades. This stability is deceptive, since rates for women have declined while those for men have increased during this period. Such trends for white males and white females are observed in both the Northeast and the Southeast and in communities with populations greater than and less than 75,000. Thus the decline in female rates and the increase among males appear to be independent of geographical region and the size of the population group considered (Blot *et al.,* 1976). Among nonwhites of both sexes there has been a consistent increase in colon cancer mortality since 1950. In 1950 colon cancer mortality rates among nonwhites were less than 65% as high as those of whites, whereas by 1967 they had risen steeply and were approaching rates prevailing among whites (Burbank, 1971) (Fig. 1).

Rectal cancer mortality in the United States has been marked by consistent decline for both males and females, whites and nonwhites (Fig. 2). These trends have been discernible since the early 1950s in each age group over 40. The decline in U.S. rectal cancer mortality in the Northeast occurred in both sexes and was independent of the size of the reporting unit. In the Southeast, however, for males the decline in rectal cancer mortality was confined to communities with population over 75,000 (Blot *et al.,* 1976).

Connecticut Tumor Registry incidence data provide a longitudinal view of occurrence of new cases of colon cancer in that state since the late 1930s. This provides a somewhat different picture from national mortality data. It should be recalled that Connecticut is part of the high colon cancer mortality region of the North Atlantic coast. Colon cancer incidence has risen in Connecticut among females as well as males, although the increase among women since 1950 has been modest. For males and females, cancer incidence increased in descending, transverse, ascending, and sigmoid segments of the colon. During the same time period, Connecticut, like other regions in the

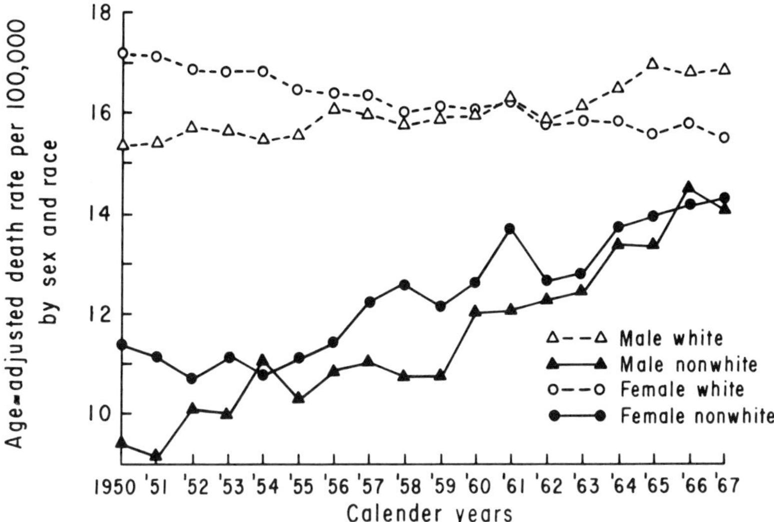

Fig. 1. Trends in colon cancer mortality, United States, average annual mortality rates, 1950–1967. Source: Burbank (1971).

United States, experienced a steep decline in stomach cancer incidence in both sexes (Eisenberg and Shambaugh, 1968).

As for rectal cancer, the Connecticut experience suggests that overall incidence rates have been nearly stable from 1940 to 1973. However, some increase occurred among males over 65 years of age. The proportion of all

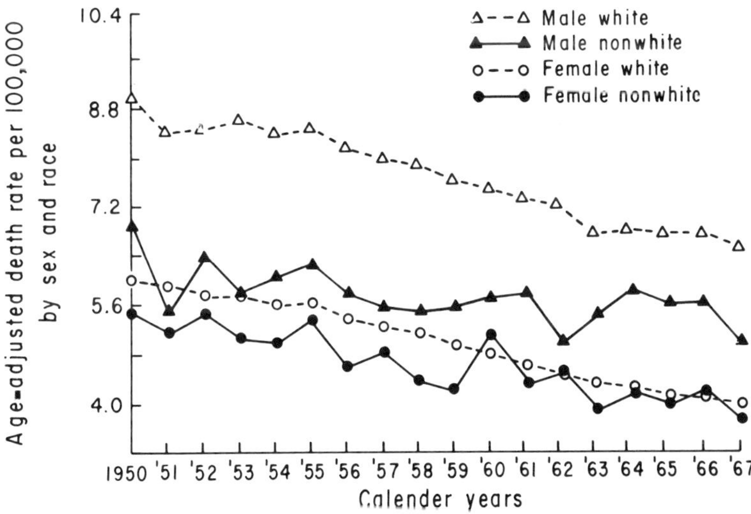

Fig. 2. Trends in rectal cancer mortality, United States, average annual mortality rates, 1950–1967. Source: Burbank (1971).

digestive tract cancers due to tumors of the rectum remained stable at about 19% during this period (Snyder *et al.,* 1977).

Incidence data from cancer registries outside the United States generally have shown slight increases in colon cancer rates during the last two decades (Fig. 3). The three reporting periods are not precisely coincident for all counties, but trends for the last decades can be distinguished. Some of the increase may reflect improved diagnosis and registration. Only Cali, Colombia, reported a decline in colon cancer incidence rates between the first and last reporting periods. In Kingston, Jamaica, and in Birmingham, England, rates in the middle period are somewhat higher than in the most recent interval.

International incidence trends for rectal cancer are shown in Fig. 4. Again, the tendency has generally been toward moderate increases in rates from first to last reporting period, with the exception of Newfoundland, Canada, where a sharp increase was reported. Only in Ibadan, Nigeria, a very low-incidence area, did a slight overall decline appear to have occurred.

Trends in mortality from colorectal malignancies are rather different and may reflect in part the effects of medical care. Between 1952 and 1967 Scotland and England experienced considerable declines in the male mortality from cancer of the colon, U.S. rates were more or less stable, and those of Western Germany, Italy, and Japan rose (Berg and Howell, 1974). Declines in mortality in the presence of increased incidence suggest that survival may have improved during this time.

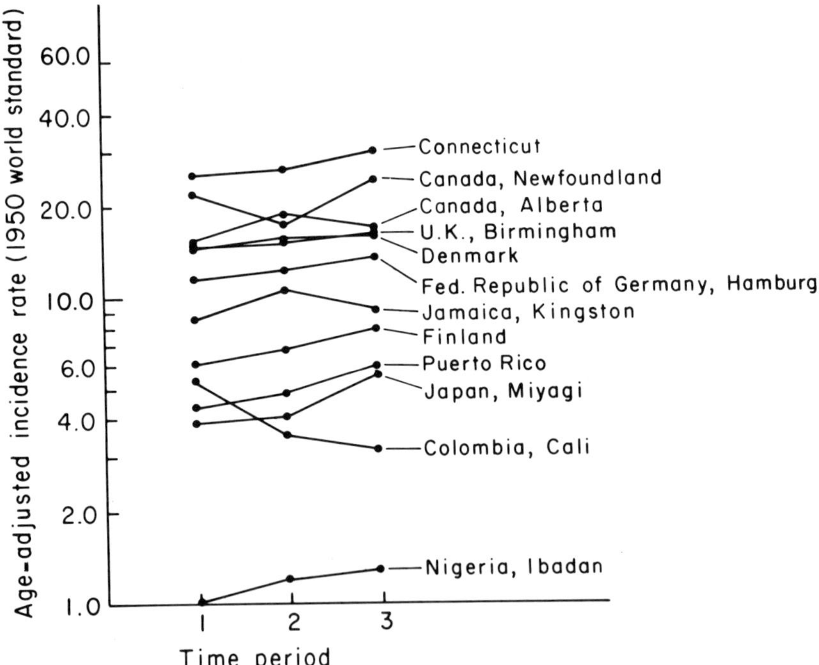

Fig. 3. International trends in colon cancer incidence. Sources: Waterhouse *et al.* (1976), and Doll *et al.* (1966, 1970).

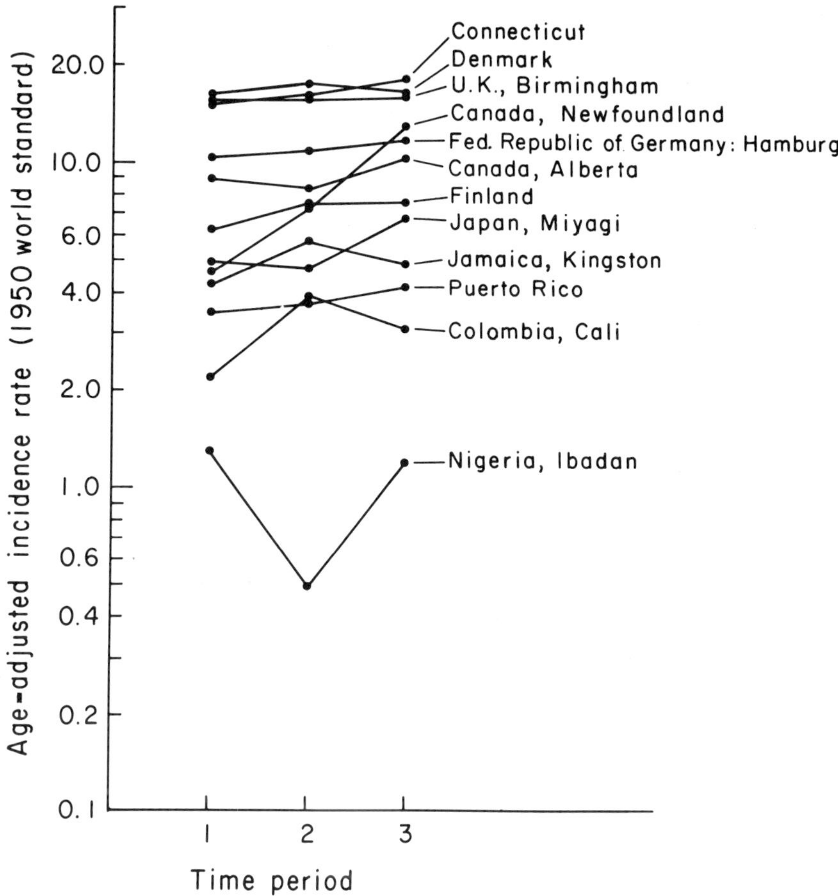

Fig. 4. International trends in rectal cancer incidence. Sources: Waterhouse *et al.* (1976) and Doll *et al.* (1966, 1970).

7. *Trends in Anatomical Localization*

Countries subject to high incidence of colon cancer demonstrate a relatively higher frequency of sigmoid cancers, whereas in low-risk countries cancers of the caecum and ascending colon predominate. An analysis of colorectal carcinoma reported by the Connecticut Tumor Registry from 1940 through 1973 demonstrated that the proportion of right colon lesions increased gradually from 13% to 22%. The proportion of colorectal cancers potentially within the view of the 25-cm proctosigmoidoscope diminished from 69% to 61%. During the 30-year period of the survey, age-adjusted cancer incidence increased 2.4 times in the ascending colon and 1.7 times in the sigmoid colon. The most significant increases above the rectosigmoid occurred in the men and women who were older than 65 years at the time of diagnosis. During the most recent calendar period (1970–1973), the incidence per 100,000 of carcinoma of the ascending colon and caecum in men over 65 years (93.4) exceeded, for the first time, that reported in women (85.3) (Snyder *et al.*, 1977).

Correa and Haenszel (1975) proposed the following hypothetical model for trends in the anatomical localization of colon cancers:

1. In low-risk countries (Eastern Europe, Asia, Africa, and South America), the cancers are concentrated in the caecum and ascending colon, women are at higher risk, and the maximum incidence has occurred by ages 50–55.
2. With the introduction of a new etiological factor, a new pattern emerges which is expressed initially as an increase in sigmoid cancers among older men in the context of rising rates of colon cancer.
3. A rise in sigmoid cancers among older women then follows.
4. After more intensive and prolonged exposure to the etiological factor(s), a later phase is characterized by an increase in cancers of the caecum and ascending colon. This upward displacement of colon cancers is ultimately more marked in men.

This pattern of shift to the right within the colon with rising incidence of colon cancer can occur independently of changes in the incidence of rectal cancer. In Connecticut from 1940 through 1973 overall rates of rectal cancer in both sexes remained nearly constant during the period despite the changing patterns of anatomical location of colon cancer. When all large intestine cancers are considered, the percentage in the rectum accessible to digital examination in the office has declined. The increasing number and proportion of right-sided colonic carcinomas underscore the need for screening and diagnostic procedures capable of discerning these lesions (Winawer *et al.*, 1976).

8. Personal Characteristics Affecting Colorectal Cancer Frequency

8.1. Age

The age-specific incidence rates of both colon and rectal cancer rise steadily from ages 10–14 to 80–84 (Figs. 5 and 6). There is a decline in rates in the age 85+ group, probably representing incomplete ascertainment of cases. The rate of increase in incidence is rather steady until age 70–75. In data from the 1969–1971 Third National Cancer Survey, age-specific incidence rates for males and females of both black and white populations are similar for colon cancer, particularly from ages 30 to 65, reflecting converging trends in colon cancer among blacks and whites in the United States. Rectal cancer incidence rates increase slowly after age 70 and decline over 85 (Cutler and Young, 1975). Average age-specific mortality rates in the United States from 1950 to 1969 appear to plateau for blacks of both sexes, beginning at age 65, but this may largely represent reporting and classification error (Burbank, 1971).

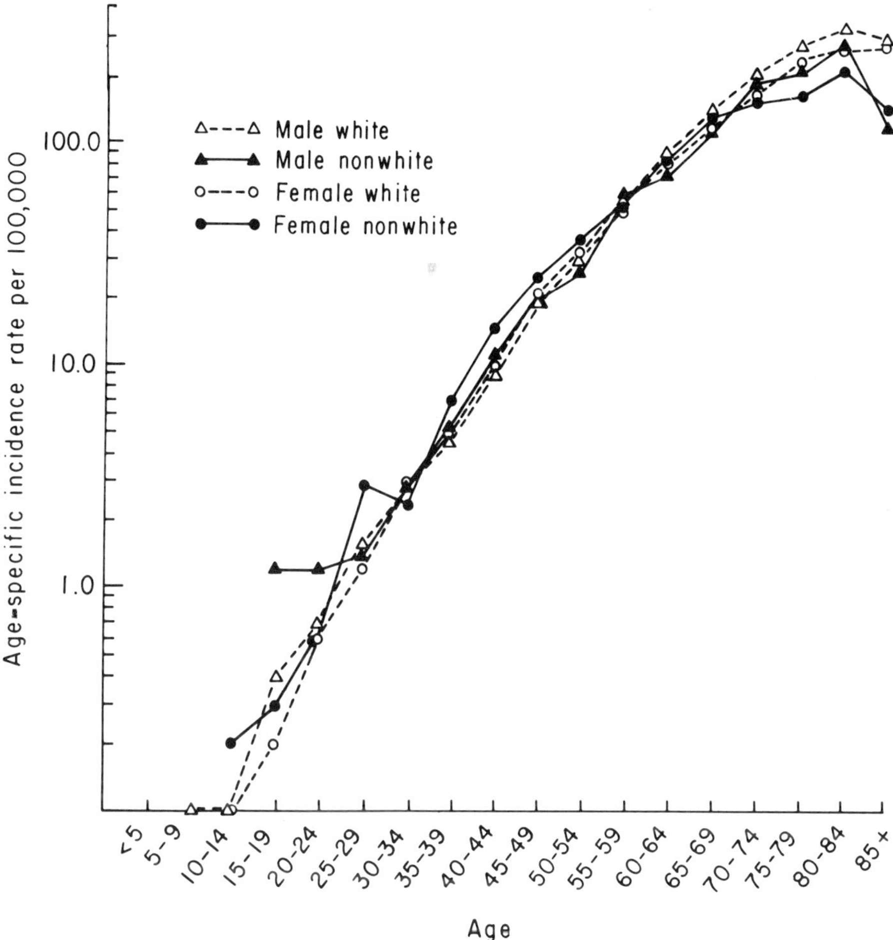

Fig. 5. Age-specific incidence rates for colon cancer. Source: Cutler and Young (1975).

During the 3 years of the Third National Cancer Survey, in which a population of 21,003,451 was surveyed, there were nine cases of cancer of the colon and one of cancer of the rectum in children under 15 years of age. Twenty cases of cancer of the colon, one of cancer of the rectum, and one of cancer of the rectosigmoid occurred in the 15–19 year age group. The corresponding average annual age-specific incidence rates for large intestinal cancer are 0.6 per million under age 15 and 4.5 cases per million for ages 15–19. These figures are higher than estimates based on mortality rates from large bowel cancer in persons under 20 derived from national death certificate data. The average annual mortality rate for colorectal cancer under age 15 was 0.2 per million (50 deaths during 1960–1968) and 2.3 per million for ages 15–19 (76 deaths during 1965–1968) (Chabalko and Fraumeni, 1975).

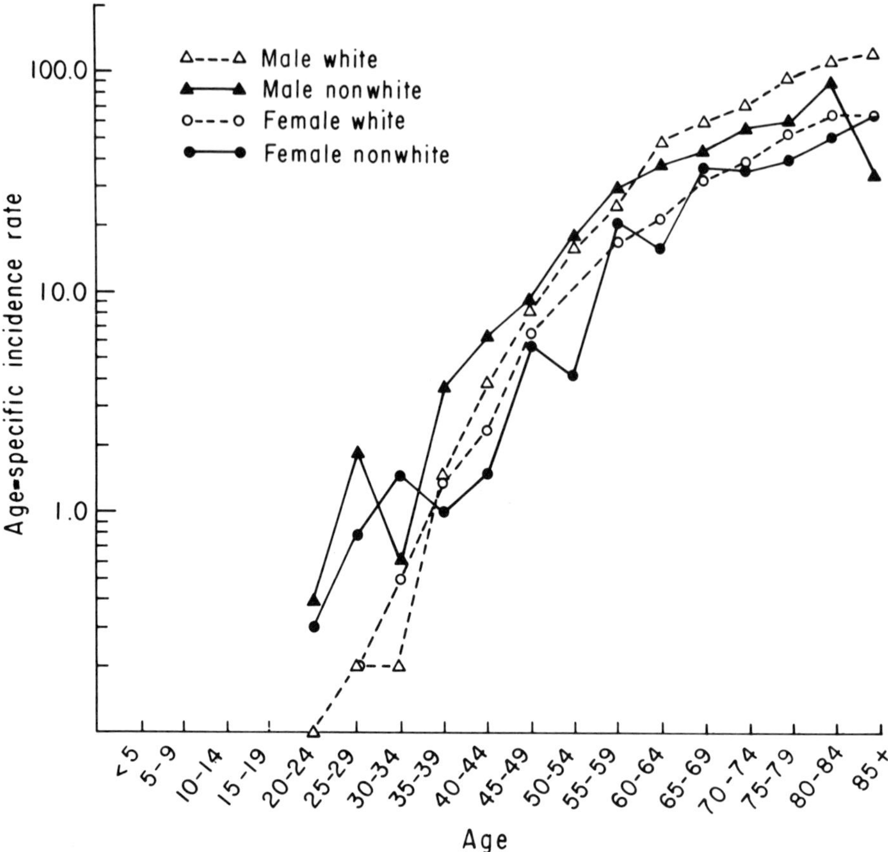

Fig. 6. Age-specific incidence rates for rectal cancer. Source: Cutler and Young (1975).

The incidence of colorectal tumors among blacks under 20 is 1.58 times that among whites of the same age group. Mortality rates have been 3–4 times as high among black youngsters under 20 compared to white children in the same age group.

Colorectal neoplasms in children differ from those in adults in several ways. They may be more often located in the colon, a higher percentage are associated with identifiable predisposing factors, and the histological pattern differs from that in adults. Among 76 children with colorectal cancer identified by hospital survey, familial polyposis occurred in 5.3%, ulcerative colitis in 3.9%, and granulomatous colitis in 1.3% (one case). Thus 10.5% of pediatric patients with colorectal cancers had known predisposing disease, while other children came from families which may represent so-called cancer families (Chabalko and Fraumeni, 1975).

Between one-third and one-half of children with colorectal cancer have mucinous adenocarcinomas, compared to adults in whom this histological type occurs in only about 5%. An unusually high proportion of younger cancer patients have been reported to have colloid-type histology, although questions of terminology haunt such comparisons (Cain and Longino, 1970). Among patients reported to the End Results Group Registry with carcinomas of the large bowel who were under 30 at the time of diagnosis, 13% had colloid-type carcinomas, compared to 4.6% of all patients reported. In this group, cases in males were significantly overrepresented (33 males, 13 females). The aggressive character of colloid tumors contributes to the overall poor survival of young patients with cancer of the large intestine. Only 11% of patients under 30 with colloid carcinomas of the large intestine survived 5 years, whereas in the older age groups with colloid cancers the 5-year survival was 37% (Berg and Godwin, 1974).

8.2. Sex

The rank order of large bowel cancer incidence and mortality in men as compared with women is closely correlated in most countries (Logan, 1976). This is true for colon cancer and rectal cancer when considered separately (Berg and Howell, 1974). Correlations between selected environmental variables and cancer of the colon rates are similar for males and females, although less so for rectal cancer (Armstrong and Doll, 1975). The sex ratios of colon cancer and rectal cancer differ, with rectal cancer being distinctly more common among males in most countries, whereas colonic cancer affects both sexes at rather similar rates (Wynder and Shigematsu, 1967). In the United States, colon cancer rates are slightly higher for males among whites, whereas among blacks the rates are nearly equal for males and females. Among young patients with colon and rectal cancer, males predominate.

8.3. Race

Racial differences between whites and nonwhites in the United States in the frequency of mortality from cancer of the colon were quite marked before 1950, but subsequent years have seen a steady convergence as a result of increasing rates among nonwhites. Mortality from cancer of the rectum is more common in whites than in nonwhites, although males of both races have higher rates than females. Moderate declines in rectal cancer mortality occurred among whites and nonwhites between 1950 and 1969, although the rate of decline was somewhat steeper for whites (Burbank, 1971). Incidence rates of colon cancer and rectal cancer of whites and blacks, determined by the Third National Cancer Survey, shown in Table 5, are higher for whites. In the younger age group, however, this pattern is reversed. Mortality and incidence rates for cancer of the large bowel in blacks under 20 are higher than rates for whites. Among blacks the incidence of large intestinal cancer cases among persons under age 20 was 2.0 per million, for whites 1.3 per million.

The extent to which racial differences are influenced by ascertainment differences is not fully resolved. Review of 16,105 autopsies performed in Los Angeles County Hospital from 1953 to 1959 suggests that only modest differences exist by race in the prevalence of undiagnosed cancer of the large

Table 5. Incidence of Colon Cancer and Rectal Cancer by Race and Sex[a]

	Colon	Rectum
All races		
Total	26.6	12.0
Male	28.2	15.4
Female	25.4	9.3
Whites		
Total	26.7	12.0
Male	28.5	15.5
Female	25.3	9.4
Blacks		
Total	24.7	10.4
Male	24.6	13.1
Female	24.9	7.7

[a]Average annual incidence per 100,000 population 1969–1971, Third National Cancer Survey, adjusted to 1950 U.S. standard population. Source: Cutler and Young (1975).

bowel found at autopsy. Overall, latent cancers found at autopsy differed little among blacks, Mexicans, Orientals, and whites (Berg *et al.,* 1970).

The marked racial differences in incidence of colon and rectum cancer in Hawaii are shown in Table 6. Rates of colon cancer among Hawaiians and Filipinos are low compared to those for Caucasians. Japanese males have colon cancer rates closer to Hawaiian Caucasians, while colon cancer rates for Chinese males are highest. Colon cancer rates among females are highest for Caucasians followed by Chinese and Japanese. The ratio of male to female

Table 6. Incidence of Colon Cancer and Rectal Cancer in Hawaii and San Francisco Bay Area by Race[a]

	Colon			Rectum		
	Male	Female	M/F ratio	Male	Female	M/F ratio
Hawaii[b]						
Hawaiian	14.1	16.9	0.83	9.4	2.9	3.24
Caucasian	23.9	22.9	1.04	13.5	12.0	1.13
Chinese	28.7	20.9	1.37	20.4	5.9	3.46
Filipino	16.8	15.3	1.09	14.5	0.0	—
Japanese	22.2	18.8	1.18	16.3	10.1	1.61
San Francisco Bay Area[c]						
Caucasian	28.3	24.0	1.18	15.2	10.4	1.46
Black	24.0	21.2	1.13	10.8	7.8	1.38
Chinese	23.5	13.8	1.70	19.5	9.4	2.07

[a]Incidence rates per 100,000 are adjusted to the 1950 world population standard. Classification is according is according to the ICD 7th edition. Source: Waterhouse *et al.* (1976).
[b]ICD 7th revision.
[c]ICD 8th revision.

colon cancer incidence rates in Hawaii ranges from 0.83 for ethnic Hawaiians to 1.37 for the Chinese population. In the San Francisco Bay area the rates for colon cancer show less variation except for Chinese females, who have lower levels of colon cancer.

Variations in cancer of the rectum by racial group are also marked. Chinese males have rates of colon cancer considerably higher than Caucasians. Rectal cancer rates among females vary in Hawaii, with very low rates among Filipinos and Hawaiians. The sex ratio for rectal cancer is much more variable than for colon cancer (Waterhouse *et al.,* 1976).

9. Migration

Ethnic and racial differences in colon cancer rates reinforce the concern that environmental factors play a major role in colon cancer etiology. In such situations migrant studies are of particular interest in estimating latency periods and defining environmental factors. Comparison of the experience with stomach and colon neoplasms of Japanese migrant and indigenous populations illustrates this. In migrant Japanese men and women (Issei), stomach cancer mortality under age 75 years was considerably higher than in U.S. Caucasians but only slightly less than in Japan. Among the male first-generation Japanese offspring (Nisei), age-specific mortality was lower than that observed in the Issei. Therefore, for the older Japanese migrants, stomach cancer mortality related more to the country of origin than to the country of destination. In the Japanese migrants to the United States, the mortality from colon cancer (excluding rectum) was more nearly that of the host country than that of the country of birth. Japanese in the United States have 2½ times greater risk of colorectal cancer than their counterparts in Japan (see Tables 4 and 6). These differences suggest that whereas environmental factors in stomach cancer determine susceptibility early in life, environmental influences later in life can affect the risk of colon cancer.

Colon cancer frequency has also been recorded in Puerto Rican migrants to New York City. Colon cancer mortality in 1960 among migrants to New York City was about the same as that for Puerto Ricans living on the island. About 1965, however, rates for Puerto Ricans on the United States mainland increased substantially in males but stabilized thereafter. Interpretation of these changes is especially difficult because of continuous to-and-fro migration of Puerto Ricans between New York City and Puerto Rico as well as a paucity of information on dietary habits of this population (Monk and Warshauer, 1975).

Jews of European origin seem to have high rates of colon cancer. In New York City, cancer of the colon mortality was about 30% higher among Jews aged 45 and older of both sexes compared with white Protestants and Catholics. For cancer of the rectum, there was no difference among the three religious groups (Newill, 1961). In Israel, population-based incidence studies demonstrated an intermediate incidence of large intestinal cancer, 22.2 per

100,000. Among Jewish males the incidence of cancer of the colon was 11.6 per 100,000, and that for cancer of the rectum 10.6 per 100,000. Among Jews born in Europe and America, large intestine cancer occurred almost 3 times more often than among Asian- and African-born Jews. The experience of the Israeli-born was intermediate between that of the European and non-European groups. Rates of colon cancer and rectal cancer were extremely low for non-Jews in Israel (Mass and Modan, 1969; Waterhouse *et al.*, 1976).

Information is available on cancer rates in Poland and among Polish migrants to the United States and to Australia. In Poland, rates of cancer of the colon and of the rectum are low compared to those of the native-born population of the United States. There is also an urban–rural gradient with higher rates in the urban population. Intestinal cancer mortality in Poland increased between 1959 and 1969. This increase was especially marked in the rural areas and among the elderly, and may represent improved reporting. Nonetheless, at the end of that interval, the risk for intestinal neoplasms was still low compared to the United States and Western Europe. By contrast, mortality rates for colon and rectal cancer among Polish-born migrants living in the United States were comparable to those of native whites. The risk of colon and rectum cancer among Poles who had migrated to the United States was thus considerably higher than among those in Poland, particularly considering that the rural background of most of these migrants put them at lower risk than average. In addition to the overall increase in risk of cancer of the large intestine, a higher proportion of colon cancers compared to rectal cancers occurred among Polish-born individuals dying in the United States during 1959–1961. This too is more consistent with the pattern of large bowel cancer in the United States than in their native Poland (Staszewski, 1972). The experience of Polish migrants to Australia is somewhat different from that of migrants to the United States, although because of small numbers this must be cautiously interpreted. The indigenous Australian population experiences high rates of cancer of the large intestine. The rates of these neoplasms in Polish men who have migrated to Australia are somewhat higher than those in Poland, but much lower than the Australian rates. For female migrants to Australia, rates are very close to the Australian experience and considerably higher than those in Poland. This is in contrast to Puerto Rican and Japanese populations migrating from low- to high-incidence areas, where male rates of colorectal cancer have increased before those of females. Complicating any comparison is the fact that social characteristics of Poles migrating to Australia were quite different from those going to the United States. Poles migrating to Australia were, for the most part, drawn from higher socioeconomic groups and urban areas. Moreover, the peak in migration to Australia occurred several decades later than the migration to America (Staszewski *et al.*, 1971).

Differing colon and rectal cancer rates among different ethnic groups living in the same region suggest the impact of undefined factors in the social environment. While a role for constitutional differences among the populations could be postulated, they are unlikely to be a major factor since large intestine cancer rates for different racial groups living in the same area tend to converge over time and migrating groups tend to reflect the rates of large intestine cancer in the new host country. It is interesting to contrast this behavior with that of stomach cancer. Countries with high rates of stomach cancer tend to have low rates of colorectal cancer. First-generation migrants from areas with high stomach cancer and low colorectal cancer tend to retain much of the excess risk from stomach cancer while assuming the higher colorectal cancer risk of the new environment. Studies of migrant populations suggest greater male susceptibility or exposure to factors causally related to colorectal cancer, and also suggest that such factors can operate after comparatively short latency.

10. Social Class and Occupational Level

As described previously, higher risks for esophageal and stomach cancer are evident in the lower socioeconomic groups. Although colorectal cancer is relatively uncommon in those countries at high risk of gastric cancer, the social class gradient for large bowel cancer is less constant and of lesser magnitude. Studies in Japan, Colombia (Cali), and the United States (Omaha-Douglas County) demonstrated higher colon cancer incidence among individuals of the upper social classes (Wynder and Shigematsu, 1967; Haenszel *et al.*, 1975; Lynch *et al.*, 1975).

Colorectal cancer is generally not viewed as an occupational disease, although it has been observed to occur more often than expected in asbestos workers. Berg and Howell (1975) reasoned that occupational factors should be studied to explain why the incidence of large bowel cancer in men over 55 is more than 30% higher than the incidence in women. A statistically and biologically significant relationship with a particular occupational group may be linked causally with a complex of social class factors (nutrition, other environmental factors, quality of medical care services, diagnostic reporting, etc.) or a specific exposure within the work setting. Of United States and United Kingdom industries with elevated colorectal cancer death rates, those composed of white-collar workers predominated. Among these occupational groupings, there was a positive correlation with mortality due to coronary heart disease and the malignant lymphomas. The standardized mortality ratios and proportionate mortality ratios were excessive among those occupations concerned with metalwork, yarn or textiles, and leather goods. The chemical exposures among the metalworkers (machinists, jobsetters, toolmakers, die makers and setters) may have included chlorinated cutting oils, lubricating oils, and cleansing solvents. The aggregate of workers in textiles and leathergoods have been exposed to dyes, solvents, and metallic compounds. One such agent, acrylonitrile, has been shown to be a carcinogen in rats. Recent preliminary investigations have suggested an excess of large intestine and lung tumors among textile workers exposed to this substance (American

Occupational Medical Association, 1977). Careful epidemiological surveillance of these various groups of workers will serve to identify the nature and extent of risks more precisely.

11. Diseases Associated with Cancer of the Large Intestine

11.1. Ulcerative Colitis

Among persons with severe, extensive, and long-enduring ulcerative colitis, the risk of carcinoma of the colon is increased. Analysis of survival of 396 persons whose symptoms had commenced prior to age 14 and in whom ulcerative colitis had been proctoscopically and radiologically confirmed at the Mayo Clinic between 1919 and 1965 showed that only 39% were alive 30 years after the onset of disease compared to some 95% expected. Fifty-two patients had developed carcinoma of the large intestine. Actuarial analysis demonstrated that the likelihood of developing cancer increased with duration of the disease, and it was estimated to reach 43% at 35 years after onset of ulcerative colitis. Cancer occurred in 30% during the first 10 years after onset, and after that an additional 20% developed the disease with each passing decade. More extensive colon involvement was associated with substantially greater risk of cancer, particularly in the first three decades after diagnosis of ulcerative colitis. For ulcerative colitis which, at the initial Mayo Clinic evaluation, was confined to the rectum, increased risk of rectal cancer did not become apparent until 30 years after onset. No consistent differences in risk by sex were noted. When onset of ulcerative colitis occurred at ages 5–9, the cumulative probability of colon cancer was significantly higher after 15 years than when onset had occurred at an earlier or later age in childhood (Devroede *et al.*, 1971).

The risk of colon cancer after adult onset of ulcerative colitis was assessed in a British study of 465 patients treated during 1952–1963. Eight patients, 1.7%, developed frank invasive carcinoma of the colon or rectum while under medical surveillance. The age- and sex-adjusted death rate from colorectal cancer in this group was 11 times that expected in the generation population. Actuarial analysis of the onset of colon cancer by person-years of observation among patients with different extent of colonic involvement suggested that the overall figure underestimated the risk in long-standing severe cases. The cumulative incidence after 25 years of symptomatic colitis was 25.6%, and, if only those patients with extensive colitis were considered, the estimated cumulative incidence of carcinoma afer 25 years was 41.8%. The risk of large bowel cancer in enduring extensive adult cases of ulcerative colitis was thus comparable to that of similar cases with childhood onset (deDombal *et al.*, 1966). Multifocal carcinoma of the bowel has been described in patients with long-quiescent ulcerative colitis (Farmer and Brown, 1964). Other series in the

Anglo-American literature (Farmer *et al.*, 1971; Welch and Hedberg, 1965) suggest similar overall risk of large bowel malignancies in patients with ulcerative colitis. It is of interest that some European observers have denied the existence of such an association based on review of ulcerative colitis series reported from Central Europe. These areas are at lower risk both for ulcerative colitis and for cancer of the large intestine than the United States and the United Kingdom. Whether the association between ulcerative colitis and colorectal cancer is not so strong in this region or whether these reports reflect differences in patient population and follow-up is not clear (Henning, 1967).

Several explanations might account for the additional risk of colorectal cancer in ulcerative colitis. Pathogenetic events in ulcerative colitis may directly or as a result of the repair process dispose to neoplastic changes in the bowel mucosa. Alternatively, a common factor may predispose individuals to both ulcerative colitis and colorectal cancer. These processes need not be mutually exclusive, and both might occur independently or synergistically. Ulcerative colitis accounts for only a small fraction of all colorectal cancers, and, conversely, only a minority of all patients who have ever had ulcerative colitis go on to develop colorectal cancer. Nonetheless, there are parallel features in the epidemiological pattern of each disease. Ulcerative colitis, like colon cancer, is generally regarded as a disease of industrialized countries, in which it may be occurring with increasing frequency. It is more common in females than males (in a ratio of 3:2) and is more common in whites than nonwhites, and possibly more common in Jews in the United States than in other whites (deDombal, 1971; Mendeloff *et al.*, 1970). There is evidence that, like colon cancer, ulcerative colitis mortality may be more frequent in the Northeast and North Central regions of the United States (Acheson, 1959). The peak period of onset of ulcerative colitis is in young adult life, decades earlier than the usual age at onset of large bowel cancer. The clinicopathological features of carcinoma of the large bowel occurring in patients with ulcerative colitis may be distinguished from those identified in patients with colorectal cancer not associated with ulcerative colitis. Cancer of the large intestine associated with ulcerative colitis is more likely to be mucinous and associated with a poorer survival than colorectal cancer in general. Multiple primary colorectal carcinomas are seen more often and right-sided lesions occur more commonly than observed in the general population. The peak age at onset of cancers in persons with ulcerative colitis is about 20 years younger than expected. There is a bimodal character to the curve which describes age at onset of colorectal cancer in ulcerative colitis patients. The second peak is at about 70 years of age (Welch and Hedberg, 1965). It is possible that cancers associated with ulcerative colitis may be of two types: one group, with unusual features, occurring in younger patients and the result of the pathogenetic events of ulcerative colitis and the second, in older persons, not very different from that occurring in the general population, and perhaps reflecting shared risk or etiological factors between ulcerative colitis and cancer of the large intestine.

11.2. Crohn's Disease

The relationship between Crohn's disease and large bowel intestinal cancer has been demonstrated fairly recently. Several case series suggested that adenocarcinomas of the small bowel could complicate Crohn's disease in up to 0.3% of cases (Goldman *et al.*, 1970; Valdes-Dapena *et al.*, 1976; Lightdale *et al.*, 1975). Colon and rectum cancer occurred in about 1.8% of Crohn's disease patients (Editorial, 1973). A follow-up study of 449 patients with long-standing Crohn's disease provides the best evidence for an association between Crohn's disease and cancer of the large intestine. All 449 patients had registered at the Mayo Clinc under age 21 between 1919 and 1965 and had Crohn's disease in the large and/or small intestine. A nearly complete follow-up was achieved and life table methods showed that the overall survival was considerably less than expected (70% surviving at 30 years). Eight patients developed colon (7) or rectal (1) cancer. All these patients had Crohn's involvement of the colon. Such cancers developed at quite young ages. The mean age was 33 years, and four patients were under 30. This was 20 times the expected number of colon cancers in a group of comparable age and sex based on Connecticut Tumor Registry incidence for the same period. Since this group included patients with Crohn's enteritis alone, the actual risk experienced by patients with Crohn's disease of the colon is probably greater (Weedon *et al.*, 1973). It is clear that in addition to excess risks of small intestinal cancer there is an increase in large intestinal cancer in patients with Crohn's disease.

12. Familial and Hereditary Factors in Large Intestine Cancer

Familial adenomatous polyposis of the colon, Gardner's syndrome, and Turcot's syndrome are associated with the development of adenomatous polyps in the colon and rectum. With the exception of Turcot's syndrome, all have autosomal dominant modes of inheritance. It is in familial adenomatous colonic polyposis that the risk of cancer of the large intestine is greatest, reaching 80% in untreated patients. As is commonly the case in genetically determined cancer, the neoplasms occur early in life. Two-thirds of patients with this disorder have had one or multiple primary intestinal cancers before age 40. Because of the high penetrance of the gene, evaluation and surveillance of family members of diagnosed patients are imperative. Surgical management of proven cases is effective in controlling mortality from this disease. New mutations are estimated to account for some 20% of the cases diagnosed in the general population, and occur with an estimated frequency of one in 6850 to one in 23,790 live births (DeCosse *et al.*, 1977; Erbe, 1976; Belleau and Braasch, 1966).

Gardner's syndrome is estimated to occur about half as frequently as familial polyposis and also carries a high risk of intestinal cancer (McKusick, 1974). The components of the syndrome, intestinal polyposis, soft tissue abnormalities, and bone abnormalities, are often not expressed in a single patient, and study of the family may be necessary to separate Gardner's syndrome from familial polyposis. Carcinoma occurs in the small intestine, as well as in the large bowel (Schnur *et al.,* 1973). Recently, efforts have been made to identify family members with the gene before they are symptomatic. There is evidence that tetraploidy in skin cultures containing epithelioid and fibroblastic cells occurs in most affected family members and in about half of asymptomatic family members who are at risk. Follow-up studies will confirm the predictive value of this technique in identifying individuals who will develop Gardner's syndrome (Danes and Krush, 1977).

Carcinoma is not common in the hereditary syndromes with hamartomatous polyps of the large bowel: the Peutz-Jegher syndrome and generalized juvenile polyposis. Tumors associated with the Peutz-Jegher syndrome most often involve the duodenal region and the risk of gastrointestinal cancer is estimated at 2–3% (Reid, 1974). In generalized juvenile polyposis, an increased risk of gastrointestinal cancer is suspected but the magnitude is uncertain.

So-called cancer families—in which adenocarcinomas occur with high frequency, at an early age, and at times at multiple primary sites within the individual—develop colorectal carcinomas, most commonly in association with adenocarcinomas of the endometrium and breast. In seven such families an autosomal dominant pattern of predisposition to cancer was suggested by pedigree analysis (Lynch and Krush, 1967; Law *et al.,* 1977).

For the "sporadic" cancers of the large intestine there is also evidence for increased risk in family members. Study of families of 145 patients suggested that there was an increase in large bowel cancer above rates expected in the general population. There were 78 cases observed compared to 27.2 expected. No excess of gastric cancer was observed in the families of large intestinal cancer patients. On the other hand, excesses of gastric cancer, but not intestinal cancer, were observed in the families of patients with gastric cancer (Macklin, 1960). Another report, in which death certificates of parents and sibs of 242 probands with large intestine cancer were reviewed, revealed 26 cases of cancer of the large intestine compared to eight for controls. The comparison group consisted of family members of a decedent without colorectal cancer who had been matched by age, sex, and year of death with the intestine cancer proband (Woolf, 1958). In both these studies it was felt that few, if any, familial polyposis families had been included and that accidental inclusion of such cases could not have been responsible for the results. These reports suggest that familial aggregation of intestinal cancer occurs even among sporadic cases that are not part of defined genetic syndromes. Such aggregation can of course reflect both environmental and gentic factors (Sherlock, 1967).

13. Dietary Factors in the Etiology of Carcinoma of the Large Intestine

The role of diet in the etiology of cancer has received a great deal of experimental and epidemiological attention throughout this century (Modan,

1977). Dietary intake directly shapes the environment of the gastrointestinal lumen and is a logical target for investigation of environmental determinants of neoplasms of the gastrointestinal mucosa. Diet composition has been compared among populations with divergent indices of gastrointestinal cancer. For cancer of the colon in males and in females, incidence rates in 23 countries were strongly correlated with per capita meat and animal fat consumption as well as with GNP. Mortality statistics for 32 countries showed similar results. Cereal consumption was negatively correlated with colon cancer incidence and mortality (although positively correlated with stomach cancer incidence and mortality). Patterns similar to those observed for colon cancer were reported for rectal cancer, although the magnitude of the correlations was lower. High meat and rather low cereal consumption is the norm in high GNP per capita countries where large intestine cancer is common (Armstrong and Doll, 1975).

Beyond narrow limits, one component of the diet can be augmented only if another is reduced. The increased intake of food of animal origin, especially meat, in developed countries has been at the expense of food of vegetable origin, and, along with carbohydrates, dietary fiber has decreased. It has been postulated that intestinal bacteria produce carcinogens from bile acids, dietary fats, or other ingested substrates, and that the geographical variations in colon cancer incidence reflect the interacting differences in diet and indigenous intestinal microflora. In the ensuing discussion the carcinogenic implications for human populations of low-fiber high-fat diets and alteration in gut metabolism ensuant to alteration of the microbial flora will be considered separately.

The concept of fiber deficiency as an etiological factor in cancer of the large intestine evolved on the basis of broadly drawn comparisons of patterns of lower intestinal disease in Western and traditional African societies. Observers of clinical disease in diverse parts of Africa affirmed the rarity of appendicitis, diverticular disease of the colon, polyps, and lower gastrointestinal malignancy in rural African populations with high fiber intake. With the introduction of Western dietary influences, the incidence of appendicitis is said to have increased. Similar evidence has been marshalled from the historical record of industrialized countries to show that diverticular disease of the colon emerged only late in this century as a clinically important disease (Painter and Burkitt, 1971).

In addition to historical trends and geographical correlations, the low-fiber-diet hypothesis must be tested in observational studies. One such study of the relationship between diverticular disease and fiber intake noted that British patients with diverticular disease reported lower daily crude fiber intake and more frequently had experienced hemorrhoids, varicose veins, hiatus hernia, gallstones, and abdominal hernia than controls (Brodribb and Humphreys, 1976). While the mean fiber intake reported by patients (2.6 g per day) was significantly lower than that reported by controls (5.2 g per day), these results cannot be accepted without further comment. The dietitians who took the diet history from which fiber content of diet was estimated also selected two controls for each patient who were age- and sex-matched. Many controls were co-employees, family, or friends of the dietitians. The absence of blinding procedures and the fact that at least some of the subjects were aware of the hypothesis may have led to distortion of patient recall. Patients with diverticular disease may have previously been advised to adhere to a low-residue diet and the temporal relationship between eating habits and bowel symptoms therefore rendered uncertain. The fact that the diverticular disease patients were attending university clinics exposed them to more sophisticated diagnostic inquiry and might have led to interviewer bias and greater awareness of hiatus hernias, gallstones, and abdominal hernias. The failure of the healthy control group to report such conditions with the same frequency cannot be interpreted as evidence for real differences in the prevalence of such conditions between the two groups.

A systematic effort has been made in studies coordinated by the International Agency for Research on Cancer (IARC) to investigate the dietary concomitants of the marked differences in rates of cancer of the colon and cancer of the rectum noted for Denmark and Finland (Jensen *et al.*, 1974). Two areas were selected for detailed study of diet, transit time, and stool bacterial content: Kuopio, a rural farming area of Finland, and Copenhagen, Denmark, which has colorectal cancer rates fourfold those of Kuopio. Diet histories were taken on a random sample of males aged 55–64 drawn from population registers in both areas, and participants were asked to keep 5-day diaries of food intake. Duplicate portions of 1 day's intake were also collected and analyzed for content. Results of this detailed investigation documented higher meat intake and beer consumption in Copenhagen and higher fiber intake and milk consumption in Kuopio. The authors warn that seasonal variation in fiber content in the diet of rural Finns may not have been fully reflected in this analysis. Interaction between high meat intake and low dietary fiber content may result in conditions particularly likely to result in intestinal malignancy. This study is noteworthy in having objectively documented differences in fiber intake consistent with the low-fiber hypothesis in geographically and culturally related areas which have large differences in intestinal cancer frequency.

Other support for the low-fiber hypothesis comes from a carefully designed case-control study in Israel. A study group of 198 cases of cancer of the colon and 77 cases of rectal cancer was assembled from six Tel Aviv hospitals. Cancers of the rectosigmoid were excluded. Two groups of controls were used. Controls were selected from surgical patients (with neither malignancy nor known gastrointestinal disorders), and a second set of neighborhood controls was selected from voting lists. Both sets of controls were matched with the colon cancer patient by age, sex, country of origin, and length of stay in Israel. Interviewers were not aware of the diagnosis of hospitalized patients and questions about food consumption frequency emphasized dietary habits up to a year before interview to avoid distortion from illness-induced changes in dietary practices. Reliability of diet history reporting was confirmed by reinterviewing a sample of the patients. Composition of food groups had been determined prior to analysis of data. Colon cancer patients reported significantly lower consumption of the group of foods with fiber content of more than 0.5%. For the great majority of foodstuffs in this group and for the food group as a whole, colon cancer patients reported significantly lower consumption frequency than either surgical or neighborhood controls. No such differences were observed during concurrent study of gastric cancer and rectal cancer patients (Modan *et al.,* 1975). The design and findings of this study strongly suggest that in this population consumption of fiber has been lower among persons who develop colon cancer than among those who do not.

One model for the mechanism whereby low-fiber diets might lead to increased risk of cancer of the colon depends on an increase in bowel transit time. In this model, prolonged exposure leads to prolonged contact between gut mucosa and carcinogenic metabolites of bacterial action on bile acids. To support this view, Burkitt has emphasized that, in contrast to Europeanized populations, rural Africans with high-fiber diets have frequent soft, bulky stools and rapid bowel transit.

Studies of bowel transit time in different populations have not supported a straightforward relation between cancer risk and transit time. Bowel transit times in two populations with similar colon cancer risk have been shown to vary (Glober *et al.,* 1974). Japanese living in Hawaii were found to have an incidence of colon cancer close to that of the Hawaiian Caucasians. Despite similarities in colon cancer risk, transit times in these two groups appear to be quite different. Among healthy males of Japanese ancestry living in Hawaii, bowel transit times were significantly shorter (mean of 30.8 hr) than among age-matched Caucasian controls (mean of 53.8 hr). There was no difference between the bowel transit times of first-generation Japanese compared to second-generation. Reported mean stool frequency among Japanese was somewhat higher than among Caucasians. The dietary fiber content was not estimated for either Caucasian or Japanese populations in this investigation.

In the inquiry previously alluded to concerning antecedents of differing colon cancer risk in Copenhagen and rural Finland (IARC, 1977), no differences were noted in mean transit time in males despite the higher fiber intake of the Finns. A bimodal distribution of transit times with the main peak at 30 hr and a second peak at 60 hr was noted for both Kuopio and Copenhagen. This bimodal distribution suggests the presence of metabolically different subpopulations and has not previously been noted.

The failure to find differences in transit time despite documented differences in fiber intake and other diet components, in two populations with markedly different cancer rates, suggests that the simple model of altered bowel transport characteristics does not adequately explain any association between diet fiber intake and bowel cancer risk. Moreover, the manner in which added fiber affects the bowel transit time of individuals on low-fiber diets is variable. In normal individuals and persons with diverticular disease on low-fiber diets who originally have delayed transit, addition of fiber has been shown to speed transit and increase stool weight (Burkitt *et al.,* 1974; Brodribb and Humphreys, 1976). However, in normals and patients with diverticular disease whose transit time was from the onset short, addition of fiber prolonged the transit time. The response of the bowel to the addition of fiber does not suggest that changes in transit time adequately explain any effect of low-fiber diet on colon cancer risk.

It has been suggested that examination of the chemical and bacterial content of feces might distinguish high-risk from low-risk populations. Individuals on a high-fat diet may have a different intestinal microflora and different levels of specific bacterial enzymes. The intestinal microflora has been shown experimentally to influence metabolically the potency of various types of chemical carcinogens. For example, the glucoside of cycasin when given orally to germ-free rats was excreted in the feces and urine almost entirely within 48 hr in its conjugated form and in a manner as if it had been administered intravenously. When fed to conventional rats with indigenous intestinal microflora, only 18–35% of the conjugated compound was recovered, and, in a number of instances, within a 2-year period adenocarcinomas appeared in the large intestine, kidney, liver (in association with diffuse centrilobular necrosis), and biliary passages. It was later shown that the cycasin glucoside had been hydrolyzed or deconjugated and converted to its aglycone, methylazoxymethanol. This product of cycasin hydrolysis was then demonstrated to be a potent carcinogen in germ-free animals (Laqueur, 1964, 1965).

Hill *et al.* (1971, 1975) observed that the Western diet was correlated with a higher fecal concentration of neutral and acid steroids derived, respectively, from endogenous cholesterol and bile salts. Subsequently, Reddy and Wynder (1973) confirmed that the excretion of cholesterol metabolites, coprostanol and coprostanone, and bile acid metabolites was higher in Americans consuming a high-meat diet than in American Seventh Day Adventists consuming a nonmeat diet, American vegetarians, and Chinese and Japanese immigrants. β-Glucuronidase activity was used as an index of fecal bacterial activity and was found to be higher in the group on the Western-type diet (Wynder and Reddy, 1973; Reddy *et al.*, 1977).

Nigro *et al.* (1973) and Chomchai *et al.* (1974) observed that an increase of bile acid metabolites in the large intestine of rats, induced either by feeding cholestyramine or by surgically diverting bile to the middle of the same intestine, enhanced axozymethane-induced tumors in the colon. Taurodeoxycholic, deoxycholic, and lithocholic acids appear to function as tumor promoters in conventional and germ-free rodent models. Historically, certain bile acids and neutral sterols are of interest because of their steric similarity to the carcinogenic polycyclic aromatic hydrocarbons.

Various mechanisms have been proposed by which intestinal bacteria, particularly those characterized as anaerobes, produce carcinogens or cocarcinogens from bile or fatty acid substrates. By means of dehydrogenase and dehydroxylase enzymes, certain anaerobic bacteria may alter the double bond configuration of the bile acid nucleus to yield structural analogues of methylcholanthrene, a known carcinogen. β-Glucuronidase may also be produced by specific intestinal bacteria and serve to convert procarcinogens into more active metabolites. In addition to the steroid metabolites, phenolic products of tyrosine and tryptophan metabolism may serve to augment experimentally induced colonic tumors (Alcantara and Speckmann, 1976).

The international epidemiological studies of dietary intake and fecal characteristics by Hill and associates were conducted on populations with apparent differences in life-style and economic development. In the IARC (1977) investigation previously described, the objective was to conduct metabolic epidemiological studies in two geographical areas (Copenhagen and Kuopio) with similar cultures but marked differences in the incidence of colon cancer. The dietary history of the population sample in Denmark was characterized by a higher (50%) meat intake, significantly lower mean intake of dietary fiber, and a significantly higher anaerobe/aerobe ($\log_{10}$) bacterial fecal excretion ratio. Fecal bile acid and neutral steroid excretion concentrations were not significantly different, which was at variance with the studies conducted in the United States, United Kingdom, Japan, Uganda, and India. The $\log_{10}$ mean excretion count of lactobacilli was signficiantly higher in the rural population from Finland (IARC, 1977). Studies are currently in progress to determine the effects of products containing lactobacilli on the intestinal microflora and bacterial enzyme systems. It has been suggested, for example, that yogurt may contain antitumor properties.

The role of diet in the pathogenesis of large bowel cancer has been described in relation to the distribution of individual nutrients in the diet and their secondary effects on endogenous metabolic processes. No specific carcinogen associated with the production, preservation, and manufacture of food has been identified. Geographical diversity in the incidence of colorectal cancer may be due to differences in the levels of exposure to various dietary factors and/or differences in the prevalence of factors protecting the host against the effects or protracted exposure to chemical carcinogens. Ingested chemicals, such as the antioxidants, and genetic factors may serve to protect the bowel mucosa.

Wattenberg (1974) listed various antioxidants that inhibited experimentally in the mouse and rat the carcinogenic action of polycyclic hydrocarbons on the forestomach, liver, lung, and breast. The antioxidants include butylated hydroxyanisole (BHA), butylated hydroxytoluene (BHT), α-tocopherol, and ethoxyquin. The phenolic antioxidants, BHA and BHT, are added to many foods and are widely used as food preservatives; α-tocopherol is present in natural produces such as wheat germ oil, and ethoxyquin is used as an antioxidant in many commercial animal diets. Although the exact mechanism or mechanisms by which the various antioxidants inhibit chemical carcinogenesis have not been determined, Shamberger has suggested that one important biological effect is inhibition of peroxidation. Peroxidation enhances the attachement of a carcinogen to deoxyribonucleic acid.

Selenium, a human trace element, is a potent antioxidant. Shamberger *et al.* (1973) reported that blood levels of selenium were significantly lower in patients with early-stage carcinoma of the stomach, pancreas, liver, and colon, but were normal in patients with carcinoma of the rectum and breast. The geographical distribution of age-adjusted cancer mortality, particularly in relation to the gastrointestinal tract (including rectum) and the kidney and urinary bladder, varied inversely with the concentration of selenium in the water and soil of U.S. cities. Although these studies are quite preliminary, they illustrate the complex and dynamic nature of inducing, augmenting, and inhibiting chemical factors that may mingle within the microecology of the intestinal tract.

14. References

Acheson, E. D., 1959, On the mortality ascribed to ulcerative colitis, *J. Chron. Dis.* **10:**469–487.

Alcantara, E. N., and Speckmann, E. W., 1976, Diet, nutrition, and cancer, *Am. J. Clin. Nutr.* **29:**1035–1047.

American Cancer Society, 1977, Cancer Statistics. *Ca* **27:**26–41.

American Occupational Medical Association, 1977, *NIOSH Advises Handling Acrylonitrile as Though a Human Carcinogen,* AOMA Report, July/August.

Armstrong, B., and Doll, R., 1975, Environmental factors and cancer incidence and mortality in different countries with special reference to dietary practices, *Int. J. Cancer* **15:**617–631.

Axtell, L. M., and Chiazze, L., Jr., 1966, Changing relative frequency of cancers of the colon and rectum in the United States, *Cancer* **19:**750–754.

Belleau, R., and Braasch, J. W., 1966, Genetics and polyposis, *Med. Clin. N. Am.* **50:**379–392.

Berezkin, D. P., and Neishtadt, E. L., 1969, Clinicomorphologic differences in two forms of colloid cancers in the rectum and sigmoid, *Vop. Onkol.* **15:**25–29. Cited by Berg and Godwin (1974).

Berg, J. W., and Godwin, J. D., II, 1974, The epidemiologic pathology of carcinomas of the large bowel, *J. Surg. Oncol.* **6:**381–400.

Berg, J. W., and Howell, M. A., 1974, The geographic pathology of bowel cancer, *Cancer* **34:**807–814.

Berg, J. W., and Howell, M. A., 1975, Occupation and bowel cancer, *J. Toxicol. Environ. Health* **1:**75–89.

Berg, J. W., Schottenfeld, D., Hutter, R. V. P., and Foot, F. W., 1969, *Histology, Epidemiology, and End Results: The Memorial Hospital Cancer Registry,* Memorial Hospital for Cancer and Allied Diseases, New York.

Berg, J. W., Downing, A., and Lukes, R. J., 1970, Prevalence of undiagnosed cancer of the large bowel found at autopsy in different races, *Cancer* **25:**1076–1080.

Blot, W. J., Fraumeni, J. F., Jr., Stone, B. J., and McKay, F. W., 1976, Geographic patterns of large bowel cancer in the United States, *J. Natl. Cancer Inst.* **57:**1225–1231.

Brodribb, A. J. M., and Humphreys, D. M., 1976, Diverticular disease: Three studies (Parts I, II, and III), *Br. Med. J.* **1:**424–430.

Burbank, F., 1971, Patterns in cancer mortality in the United States: 1950–1967, *Natl. Cancer Inst. Monogr.,* No. 33.

Burkitt, D. P., Walker, A. R. P., and Painter, N. W., 1974, Dietary fiber and disease, *J. Am. Med. Assoc.* **229:**1068–1074.

Cain, A. S., and Longino, L. A., 1970, Carcinoma of the colon in children, *J. Pediatr. Surg.* **5:**527–532.

Chabalko, J. J., and Fraumeni, J. F., Jr., 1975, Colorectal cancer in children: Epidemiologic aspects, *Dis. Colon Rectum* **18:**1–3.

Chomchai, C. C., Bhadrachari, N., and Nigro, N. D., 1974, The effects of bile on the induction of experimental intestinal tumors in rats, *Dis. Colon Rectum* **17:**310–312.

Correa, P., and Haenszel, W., 1975, Colon and rectum cancer—Comparative international incidence and mortality, in: *Cancer Epidemiology and Prevention: Current Concepts* (D. Schottenfeld, ed.), pp. 386–403, Charles C. Thomas, Springfield.

Cutler, S. J., and Young, J. L., Jr., 1975, Third National Cancer Survey: Incidence data, *Natl. Cancer Inst. Monogr.,* No. 41.

Danes, B. S., and Krush, A. J., 1977, The Gardner syndrome: A family study in cell culture, *J. Natl. Cancer Inst.* **58:**771–775.

DeCosse, J. J., Adams, M. B., and Condon, R. E., 1977, Familial polyposis, *Cancer* **39:**267–273.

deDombal, F. T., 1971, Ulcerative colitis: Epidemiology and aetiology, course and prognosis, *Br. Med. J.* **1:**649–650.

deDombal, F. T., Watts, J. McK., Watkinson, G., and Goligher, J. C., 1966, Local complications of ulcerative colitis: Stricture, pseudopolyposis, and carcinoma of colon and rectum, *Br. Med. J.* **1:**1442–1447.

Devroede, G. J., Taylor, W. F., Sauer, W. G., Jackman, R. J., and Stickler, G. B., 1971, Cancer risk and life expectancy of children with ulcerative colitis, *N. Engl. J. Med.* **285:**17–21.

Doll, R., and Cook, P., 1967, Summarizing indices for comparison of cancer incidence data, *Int. J. Cancer* **2:** 269–279.

Doll, R., Payne, P., and Waterhouse, J. A. H. (eds.), 1966, *Cancer Incidence in Five Continents, I,* Springer-Verlag, Berlin.

Doll, R., Muir, C. S., and Waterhouse, J. A. H., 1970, *Cancer Incidence in Five Continents, II,* U.I.C.C., Geneva.

Editorial, 1973, Does Crohn's disease predispose to intestinal cancer? *Br. Med. J.* **2:**3.

Eisenberg, H., and Shambaugh, E., 1968, Cancers of the gastrointestinal tract: Trends in incidence and mortality rates, in: *Sixth Annual Cancer Conference Proceedings,* Lippincott, New York.

Erbe, R. W., 1976, Inherited Gastrointestinal polyposis syndromes, *N. Engl. J. Med.* **294:**1101–1104.

Glober, G. A., Klein, K. L., Moore, J. O., and Abba, B. C., 1974, Bowel transit-times in two populations experiencing similar colon-cancer risks, *Lancet* **2:**80–81.

Farmer, R. G., and Brown, C. H., 1964, Colonic carcinoma and ulcerative colitis, *Arch. Intern. Med.* **113:**153–157.

Farmer, R. G., Hawk, W. A., and Turnbull, R. B., 1971, Carcinomas associated with mucosal ulcerative colitis, and with transmural colitis and enteritis (Crohn's disease), *Cancer* **28:** 289–292.

Goldman, L. I., Bralow, S. P., Cox, W., and Peale, A., 1970, Adenocarcinoma of the small bowel complicating Crohn's disease, *Cancer* **26:**1119–1125.

Haenszel, W., and Dawson, E., 1965, A note on mortality from cancer of the colon and rectum in the United States, *Cancer* **18:**265–272.

Haenszel, W., Correa, P., and Cuello, C., 1975, Social class differences among patients with large-bowel cancer in Cali, Colombia, *J. Natl. Cancer Inst.* **54:**1031–1035.

Henning, N., 1967, Carcinoma of the colon in ulcerative colitis: What is the risk? *Ger. Med. Mon.* **12:**402–403.

Hill, M. J., Crowther, J. S., Drasar, B. S., *et al.,* 1971, Bacteria and etiology of cancer of the large bowel, *Lancet* **1:**95–100.

Hill, M. J., Drasar, B. S., Williams, R. E. O., *et al.,* 1975, Fecal bile acids and clostridia in patients with cancer of the large bowel, *Lancet* **1:**535–538.

IARC, 1977, Dietary fibre, transit-time, faecal bacteria, steroids, and colon cancer in two Scandinavian populations: Report from the International Agency for Research on Cancer Intestinal Microecology Group, *Lancet* **2:**207–212.

Jensen, O. M., Mosbech, J., Salaspuro, M., and Jhamaki, T., 1974, A comparative study of the diagnostic basis for cancer of the colon and cancer of the rectum in Denmark and Finland, *Int. J. Epidemiol.* **3:**183–186.

Laqueur, G. L., 1964, Carcinogenic effects of cycad meal and cycasin, methylazoxymethanolglycoside in rats and effects of cycasin in germfree rats, *Fed. Proc.* **23:**1386–1387.

Laqueur, G. L., 1965, The induction of intestinal neoplasms in rats with the glycoside cycasin and its aglycone, *Virchows Arch. Pathol. Anat.* **340:**151–163.

Law, I. P., Herberman, R. B., Oldham, R. K., Bouzoukis, J., *et al.,* 1977, Familial occurrence of colon and uterine carcinoma and of lymphoproliferative malignancies, clinical description, *Cancer* **39:**1224–1228.

Lightdale, C. J., Sternberg, S. S., Posner, G. and Sherlock, P., 1975, Carcinoma complicating Crohn's disease: Report of seven cases and review of the literature, *Am. J. Med.* **592**:262–268.

Logan, W. P. D., 1976, Cancers of the alimentary tract: International mortality trends, *WHO Chronicle* **30**:413–419.

Lynch, H. T., and Krush, A. J., 1967, Heredity and adenocarcinoma of the colon, *Gastroenterology* **53**:517–527.

Lynch, H. T., Guirgis, H., Lynch, J., Brodkey, F. D., and Magee, H., 1975, Cancer of the colon: Socioeconomic variables in a community, *Am. J. Epidemiol.* **102**:119–127.

Macklin, M. T., 1960, Inheritance of cancer of the stomach and large intestine in Man, *J. Natl. Cancer Inst.* **24**:551–571.

Mason, T. J., McKay, F. W., Hoover, R., Blot, W. J., and Fraumeni, F. J., Jr., 1975, *Atlas of Cancer Mortality for U. S. Counties: 1950–1969,* DHEW Publ. No. (NIH) 75–780.

Mason, T. J., McKay, F. W., Hoover, R., Blot, W. J., and Fraumeni, J. F., Jr., 1976, *Atlas of Cancer Mortality Among U.S. Nonwhites: 1950–1969,* DHEW Publ. No. (NIH) 76-1204.

Mass, N., and Modan, B., 1969, Epidemiological aspects of neoplastic disorders in Israeli migrant population. IV. Cancer of the colon and rectum, *J. Natl. Cancer Inst.* **42**:529–536.

McKusick, V. A., 1974, Genetics and large-bowel cancer, *Digest. Dis.* **19**:954–958.

Mendeloff, A. I., Monk, M., Siegel, C. I., and Lilienfeld, A., 1970, Illness experience and life stresses in patients with irritable colon with ulcerative colitis: An epidemiologic study of ulcerative colitis and regional enteritis in Baltimore, 1960–1964, *N. Eng. J. Med.* **282**:14–17.

Modan, B., 1977, Dietary role in cancer etiology, *Cancer* **40**:1887–1891.

Modan, B., Barell, V., Lubin, F., Modan, M., Greenberg, R. A., and Graham, S., 1975, Low-fiber intake as an etiologic factor in cancer of the colon, *J. Natl. Cancer Inst.* **55**:15–18.

Monk, M., and Warshauer, M. W., 1975, Stomach and colon cancer mortality among Puerto Ricans in New York City and Puerto Rico, *J. Chronic Dis.* **28**:349–358.

Newill, V. A., 1961, Distribution of cancer mortality among ethnic subgroups of the white population of New York City, 1953–58, *J. Natl. Cancer Inst.* **26**:405–417.

Nigro, N. D., Bhadrachari, N., and Chomchai, C., 1973, A rat model for studying colonic cancer: Effect of cholestyramine on induced tumors, *Dis. Colon Rectum* **16**:438–443.

Painter, N. S., and Burkitt, D. P., 1971, Diverticular disease of the colon: A deficiency disease of Western civilization, *Br. Med. J.* **2**:450–454.

Public Health Service, 1968, *Eighth Revision International Classification of Diseases, Adapted for Use in the United States,* DHEW Public Health Service Publ. No. 1693.

Puffer, R. R., and Griffith, G. W., 1967, *Patterns of Urban Mortality: Report of the Inter-American Investigation of Mortality,* PAHO Scientific Publ. No. 151.

Reddy, B. S., and Wynder, E. L., 1973, Large bowel carcinogenesis: Fecal constituents of populations with diverse incidence rates of colon cancer, *J. Natl. Cancer Inst.* **50**:1437–1442.

Reddy, B. S., Mastromarino, A., and Wynder, E., 1977, Diet and metabolism: Large-bowel cancer, *Cancer* **29**:1815–1819, April Suppl.

Reid, J. D., 1974, Intestinal Carcinoma in the Peutz-Jeghers syndrome, *J. Am. Med. Assoc.* **229**:833–834.

Schnur, P. L., David E., Brown, P. W., Beahrs, O. H., ReMine, W. H., and Harrison, E. G., Jr., 1973, Adenocarcinoma of the duodenum and the Gardner syndrome, *J. Am. Med. Assoc.* **223**:1229–1232.

Seidman, H., Silverberg, E., and Holleb, A. I., 1976, Cancer statistics 1976: A comparison of white and black populations, *Ca* **26**:2–29.

Shamberger, R. J., Rukovena, E., Longfield, A. K., Tytko, S. A., *et al.,* 1973, Antioxidants and cancer. I. Selenium in the blood of normals and cancer patients, *J. Natl. Cancer Inst.* **50**:863–870.

Sherlock, P., 1967, Genetics and gastrointestinal disease. *Gastroenterology* **53**:575–677.

Silverberg, E., 1970, *Statistical Data on Cancer of the Colon and Rectum,* American Cancer Society, New York.

Snyder, D. N., Heston, J. F., Meigs, J. W., Flannery, J. T., 1977, Changes in site distribution of colorectal carcinoma in Connecticut, 1940–73, *Am. J. Digest Dis.* **22**:791–797.

Staszewski, J., 1972, Migrant studies in alimentary tract cancer, in: *Current Problems in the*

Epidemiology of Cancer and Lymphomas (E. Grandmann and H. Tulinius, eds.), Spring-Verlag, New York.

Staszewski, J., McCall, M. G., and Stenhouse, N. S., 1971, Cancer mortality in 1962–1966 among Polish migrants to Australia, *Br. J. Cancer* **25:**599–610.

Stemmermann, G. N., 1966, Cancer of the colon and rectum discovered at autopsy in Hawaiian Japanese, *Cancer* **19:**1567–1572.

Symonds, D. A., and Vickery, A. L., Jr., 1976, Mucinous carcinoma of the colon and rectum, *Cancer* **37:**1891–1900.

Valdes-Dapena, A., Rudolph, I., Hidayat, A., Roth, J. L. A., and Laucks, R. B., 1976, Adenocarcinoma of the small bowel in association with regional enteritis—Four new cases, *Cancer* **37:**2938–2947.

Waterhouse, J., Muir, C., Correa, P., and Powell, J. (eds.), 1976, *Cancer Incidence in Five Continents, III,* IARC Scientific Publications, Lyon.

Wattenberg, L. W., 1974, Potential inhibitors of colon carcinogenesis, *Digest Dis.* **19:**947–953.

Weedon, D. D., Shorter, R. G., Ilstrup, D. M., Huizenga, K. A., and Taylor, W. F., 1973, Crohn's disease and cancer, *N. Eng. J. Med.* **289:**1099–1103.

Welch, C. E., and Hedberg, S. E., 1965, Colonic cancer in ulcerative colitis and idiopathic colonic cancer, *J. Am. Med. Assoc.* **191:**815–818.

Winawer, S. J., Sherlock P., Schottenfeld, D., and Miller, D. G., 1976, Screening for colon cancer, *Gastroenterology* **70:**783–789.

Woolf, C. M., 1958, A genetic study of carcinoma of the large intestine, *Am. J. Hum. Genet.* **10:**42–47.

Wynder, E. L., and Reddy, B., 1973, Studies of large-bowel cancer: Human leads to experimental application, *J. Natl. Cancer Inst.* **50:**1099–1106.

Wynder, E. L., and Shigematsu, T., 1967, Environmental factors of cancer of the rectum and colon, *Cancer,* **20:**1520–1561.

Wynder, E. L., Hyams, L., and Shigmatsu, T., 1967, Correlations of international cancer death rates, *Cancer* 20:113–126.

Wynder, E. L., Kajitani, T., Ishikawa, S., Dodo, H., and Takano, A., 1969, Environmental factors of cancer of the colon and rectum. II. Japanese epidemiological data, *Cancer* **23:**1210–1220.

10

Heredity and Gastrointestinal Tract Cancer

Henry T. Lynch and Patrick M. Lynch

1. Historical Review

The study of cancer genetics in man has been steeped in controversy. Undoubtedly most of these problems center around the complexity of man himself as a subject for cancer genetic investigations; man's matings cannot be controlled, he has relatively few progeny, and his generation span is longer than that of most other animal species. In addition, it is difficult to obtain reliable information about his medical history, particularly histological verification of cancer one or more decades after treatment. In the study of gastrointestinal tract cancer, such verification is exceedingly important since the assessment of cancer of interal organs may be hampered significantly in the absence of such information. The pervasive fear of cancer among the populace compounds these difficulties; in some circumstances the investigations of a cancer-prone family may have to be curtailed or even abandoned when overpowering fear and denial cause certain patients to refuse further cooperation. Perhaps the most difficult obstacle in elucidating genetic patterns of cancer susceptibility is the omnipresence of environmental and dietary factors, the differential clustering of which may doggedly mimic a genetic model.

Notwithstanding these problems, phenomenal advances have been made during the past half century in the recognition of the role of host factors in cancer etiology (Lynch, 1976). The observations of Boveri (1914) relevant to chromosomal imbalance (aneuploidy) in cancer, followed in the early 1950s and 1960s by advances in cytogenetics, have been of inestimable influence in

Henry T. Lynch and Patrick M. Lynch • Department of Preventive Medicine/Public Health, Creighton University School of Medicine, Omaha, Nebraska 68178.

cancer genetics (Ohno, 1974). Thus we now find an increasing number of cytogenetic disorders with variable clinical manifestations, including an excess frequency of cancer of specific anatomical sites, including those of the gastrointestinal tract (Lynch, 1976).

Meticulous attention to clinical findings and histological verification of all varieties of cancer in extended kindreds have recently demonstrated that many Mendelian inherited diseases have hitherto unknown cancer associations. An estimate by Mulvihill (1975) suggests that 9% of the more than 2000 diseases listed in McKusick's (1975) catalogue *Mendelian Inheritance in Man* have a neoplastic association.

Modern research in cancer genetics has emphasized host–environmental interactions in cancer etiology. This interaction has been described clearly in the field of pharmacogenetics, and an extension of this reasoning in cancer is evidenced by the term "ecogenetics" (Mulvihill, 1976). This concept emphasizes such potentially important host–environmental interactions as arylhydrocarbon hydroxylase (AHH) inducer status in association with cigarette smoking and numerous other noxious environmental exposures in the production of pulmonary cancer; α_1-antitrypsin deficiency, with its predisposition to chronic obstructive pulmonary disease in the presence of environmental factors such as cigarette smoking, would be another example. Indeed, α_1-antitrypsin deficiency has been implicated with hepatomas and is of pertinence to this chapter (Berg and Eriksson, 1972).

Our major purpose will be to survey the role of genetic factors in the etiology of cancers of the gastrointestinal tract. Known environmental carcinogens will be discussed from the standpoint of their interaction with primary host factors, as will the cancer control implications of these ecogenetic factors. Table 1 catalogues those disorders of the gastrointestinal tract in which host factors have been etiologically demonstrated or suggested. Such conditions as Torre's disease may be exceedingly rare and the genetic etiology questionable. On the other hand, there are relatively frequently occurring disorders such as familial adenomatous polyposis coli, for which voluminous evidence has been accumulated in support of primary genetic factors. Caution must be used when interpreting this table, in that heredity may directly contribute to only a very small fraction of the total frequency of cancer which affects a particular organ. This is true particularly in the esophagus and liver, where host factors appear to be of very minuscule etiological importance when compared to the enormous impact of the environment.

2. *Oral Cavity Cancer*

Approximately 8% of all cancer diagnosed annually in the United States involves the oral cavity (Gardner and Rothman, 1969). The overwhelming majority of cancers of the oral cavity involve a strong environmental etiological component; with respect to carcinoma of the lips, sunlight and tobacco appear to be the principal causal factors. Nonetheless, skin pigmentation, a quantitative genetic trait, is of significant consequence. Thus ultraviolet radiation exposure appears to be more injurious to lightly pigmented individuals, with maximum protection from lip cancer being afforded blacks (Gardner and Rothman, 1969).

Cancer of the tongue, gingiva, buccal mucosa, hard and soft palate, and pharynx appears to be strongly influenced by all varieties of tobacco products. Heavy alcohol consumption accentuates this effect, but its role seems limited to that of a carcinogenic promoter, acting only in the presence of cigarette smoking and other tobacco use (Wynder *et al.*, 1957, 1976). In India, the Philippines, and parts of southern Russia, the chewing of betel nut quid, with a variety of products including slaked lime, is a major factor in oral cancer (Moore, 1965; Reddy, 1967; Orr, 1963). Systematic studies of such carcinogenic exposures in the context of host factors will help determine whether certain individuals are more susceptible to specific carcinogenetic insults, due to inherent biochemical, physiological, or anatomical aberrations. In a related manner, study of individuals who manifest apparently "spontaneous" neoplasms of the oral cavity, in the *absence* of the mentioned exposures, may indicate the presence of primary genetic factors (or hitherto unsuspected environmental agents). Pedigree studies may shed light on this problem.

Notwithstanding the predominance of environmental factors in oropharyngeal carcinoma, at least one exceedingly rare primary genetic cancer predisposing disorder may be cited. Dyskeratosis congenita, Scoggins type (Scoggins *et al.*, 1971), was described in a black family through three generations with male-to-male transmission. The disorder was inherited as an autosomal dominant. Clinical features included hyperpigmentation of the skin, palmar hyperkeratosis, dystrophic nails, osteoporosis, anemia, and premalignant leukokeratosis of the oral mucosa. In addition, these patients also have hematological, immunological, and chromosomal changes (endoreduplication) which are very similar to those found in the sex-linked recessive dyskeratosis congenita (Addison and Rice, 1965). This latter disorder is also characterized by cutaneous pigmentation, dystrophy of the nails, premalignant leukoplakia of the oral mucosa, and chromosomal changes, but includes frequent thrombocytopenia and testicular atrophy as well. Cancer may arise in areas of leukoplakia of the mouth and anus, or it may occur in the skin (Addison and Rice, 1965; Milgrom *et al.*, 1964; Sirinavin and Trowbridge, 1975).

3. Esophagus

The incidence rates of esophageal carcinoma vary markedly in different areas of the world (Burrell, 1969; Fortuine, 1969; Higginson and Oettle, 1960). This disease is associated with certain cultural patterns such as diet, smoking, and alcohol consumption, and it is clustered in lower socioeconomic groups (Cliffton, 1969; Mosbech and Videbaek, 1955; Wynder and Bross, 1961). Congenital anomalies (achalasia, congenital stenosis, and webs) and

Table 1. Familial/Genetic Clustering of Cancer of Gastrointestinal Tract

Syndrome and/or predominant cancer(s) association	Genetic/familial etiology	Associated lesions	Biological markers/specific specific diagnostic signs
Dyskeratosis congenita Scoggin's type (premalignant leukokeratosis of oral mucosa)	Autosomal dominant	Hyperpigmentation of the skin, palmar hyperkeratosis, dystrophic nails, osteoporosis	Chromosomal changes (breaks, rearrangements, endoreduplication)
Dyskeratosis congenita (premalignant leukokeratosis of oral mucosa, cancer of oral mucosa, pharynx, skin, and anus)	Sex linked	Hyperpigmentation of the skin, dystrophic nails, anemia (similar to Fanconi's aplastic anemia), testicular atrophy	Chromosomal changes (breaks, rearrangements, endoreduplication)
Scleroatrophic and keratotic dermatosis of limbs (sclerotylosis) (visceral tumors of tongue, tonsils, breast, uterus, and colon)	Possible autosomal dominant	Atrophic fibrosis of the skin of limbs, keratoderma of the palms and soles, hypoplasia of the nails	None, except characteristic phenotype
Tylosis palmaris et plantaris (esophageal carcinoma)	Autosomal dominant	Hyperkeratosis of the palms and soles	None, except characteristic phenotype
Gastric cancer	Increased empirical risk to first-degree relatives of proband, possible autosomal dominant in rare occurrences	None	None
Ataxia-telangiectasia (stomach cancer, lymphosarcoma, reticuloendotheliosis, Hodgkin's disease, medulloblastoma)	Autosomal recessive (stomach cancer also occurred in an obligate heterozygote)	Oculocutaneous telangiectasia, cerebellar ataxia, multiple additional neurological, cutaneous, and immunological aberrations	Deficient IgA, immunoglobulins, abnormal cellular immunity
Pernicious anemia (gastric carcinoma)	Familial, possible autosomal dominant in certain families	Multisystem manifestations, vitiligo in some that show gastric carcinoma	Positive Schilling test
Pancreatic cancer (exclusive of pancreatitis)	Single report of occurrences in four siblings	None	None

Hereditary pancreatitis (pancreatic carcinoma)	Autosomal dominant	Pancreatitis, pseudocysts	Cystinelike amino acid in the urine
Pancreatic cancer (in relatives heterozygous for ataxia-telangiectasia)	Autosomal recessive	None in heterozygous carriers	None
Diabetes mellitus (associated with pancreatic cancer exclusive of hereditary pancreatitis)	Familial, Mendelian inheritance not established, increased empirical risk	Retinopathy, uropathy, neuropathy, capillary vascular changes	Abnormal glucose tolerance curve
Multiple endocrine adenomatosis (islet cell tumors of pancreas)	Autosomal dominant, although sporadic occurrences are common	Medullary thyroid carcinoma and pheochromocytoma	Elevated calcitonin
Hepatoblastoma	Unknown, rare occurrences in siblings	Congenital defects in children	None consistent, α-fetoprotein elevation may be helpful
Hepatocellular carcinoma	Increased empirical risk	None	α_1-Antitrypsin deficiency, Australia antigen in several cases
Hemochromatosis (hepatocellular carcinoma)	Autosomal dominant	Systemic due to iron deposition in multiple organs	Serum iron elevation
Tyrosinemia (hepatocellular carcinoma)	Autosomal recessive	Cirrhosis of liver, features of Fanconi's syndrome	Elevation of blood tyrosine levels
α_1-Antitrypsin deficiency (hepatoma)	Autosomal recessive	Pulmonary emphysema	α_1-Antitrypsin deficiency
Gallbladder carcinoma	Increased empirical risk, prevalence among Indians in southwestern United States	Association with gallstones	None
Duodenal carcinoma	Rare familial occurrences, possible excess in autosomal dominantly inherited Peutz-Jeghers syndrome	As in Peutz-Jeghers syndrome	Cutaneous signs of Peutz-Jeghers syndrome when P-J is associated
Celiac disease (lymphoma, including small bowel involvement, esophageal carcinoma)	Possible autosomal dominant, sex influence	Steatorrhea	None

Continued

Table 1. Continued

Syndrome and/or predominant cancer(s) association	Genetic/familial etiology	Associated lesions	Biological markers/specific specific diagnostic signs
Torre's syndrome (multiple sebaceous tumors and visceral cancer, and miscellaneous cancers of the gastrointestinal tract, including colon and ampulla of Vater)	Rare familial occurrence, insufficient data to document inherited mechanism	Cutaneous lesions (multiple sebaceous cysts)	Cutaneous signs
Familial adenomatous polyposis coli (colon cancer)	Autosomal dominant	None	Consider colonic mucosa proliferation index in all of the following disorders involving colon cancer
Gardner's syndrome (colon cancer, sarcomas) (rare occurrences of thyroid carcinoma and retroperitoneal sarcoma)	Autosomal dominant	Soft tissue (sebaceous cysts, fibromas) and bone lesions (osteomas of mandible, sphenoid, and maxilla)	
Turcot's syndrome (colon cancer, central nervous system cancer)	Autosomal recessive	None	
Peutz-Jeghers syndrome (duodenal, colon, and ovarian cancer)	Autosomal dominant	Melanin spots of oral and vaginal mucosa and distal portions of fingers, generalized gastrointestinal polyps, primarily hamartomas	
Solitary polyps (colon cancer)	Autosomal dominant	Polyps	
Ulcerative colitis (colon cancer)	Possible autosomal dominant in certain families	Occasionally arthritis, systemic manifestations, and psychological aberrations	

Site-specific colon cancer exclusive of multiple polyposis coli (predominant proximal colon involvement)	Autosomal dominant	None
Cancer family syndrome (colon, endometrial, and other adenocarcinomas)	Autosomal dominant	None
Generalized gastrointestinal juvenile polyposis (cancer of small and large bowel)[a]	Not established	None
Generalized gastrointestinal adenomatous polyposis (cancer of colon, possibly of stomach and small bowel)[b]	Possible autosomal dominant	Desmoid reported
Cronkhite-Canada syndrome	No known familial reports	Skin pigmentation, atrophy of nails, hypoproteinemia
Familial combined breast and colon cancer	Possible autosomal dominant	None

[a]Reports of families typically included features of *mixed* juvenile and adenomatous polyps (Haggitt and Pitcock, 1970; Stemper *et al.*, 1975; Veale, 1965).
[b]No cancer reported.

acquired lesions (inflammatory stenosis, peptic stenosis, and lye stricture) have all been associated with esophageal cancer. Earlier age at onset frequently occurs in such affected individuals (Just-Viera and Haight, 1969; Lortat-Jacob *et al.,* 1969; Mosbech and Videbaek, 1955).

A total of 16 patients with histologically verified primary carcinoma of the esophagus were identified in Omaha, Nebraska, in 1964 and studied intensively (Lynch *et al.,* 1971). Particular interest was focused on environmental and occupational exposures to carcinogens, socioeconomic status, race, ethnic factors, cultural practices, alcohol consumption, and details of family history.

The socioeconomic level of all of the patients was distinctly below the median of the community where they resided. Interestingly, distribution of this lesion was restricted to the lowest socioeconomic census tracts, an area characterized by the greatest unemployment and lowest income per family in the city. Of additional interest was the fact that eight of the 16 affected individuals were black. This represented a significant difference at the 10% level between blacks and whites. Finally, no familial occurrences of esophageal cancer were found in this relatively small series. The sex ratio of 13 men to three women was in accordance with U.S. statistics, which indicate a greater incidence in men (Wynder and Bross, 1961). The association with alcoholism has been noted previously, although the etiological role may be linked to the specific type of alcoholic beverage consumed and its level of contaminants such as nitrosamines, zinc, lead, and other possible carcinogenic agents (McGlashan, 1969; Reilly and McGlashan, 1969).

The only firm association between carcinoma of the esophagus and hereditary factors has been found in autosomal dominantly inherited tylosis palmaris et plantaris (Harper *et al.,* 1970; Howel-Evans *et al.,* 1958; Shine and Allison, 1966). Howel-Evans *et al.,* (1958) were the first investigators to observe tylosis (hyperkeratosis) of the palms and soles (as shown in Fig. 1) in association with esophageal cancer in a large number of patients from two families. A life table of these families showed that 95% of the relatives with tylosis developed carcinoma of the esophagus by age 65. These findings were updated by Harper *et al.,* (1970). During the 12-year interval from 1958 to 1970, the predicted 95% occurrence of carcinoma of the esophagus in those patients showing tylosis was unfortunately occurring completely in accordance with the previous predictions. Six new cases of esophageal carcinoma occurred and each individual had the tylosis marker. There were no occurrences of esophageal cancer in patients who did not show tylosis, although in some individuals the tylosis was confined to the feet (as was found in two of the women who died of esophageal cancer since the original 1958 report). The tylosis in these families occurred at a later age than that found in the usual hereditary form (which lacks this cancer association); several members developed tylosis as late as middle age. Conversely, the associated esophageal cancer occurred about 10 years earlier than expected in the general population.

Measures undertaken to achieve the earliest possible diagnosis of esophageal cancer in these families have included barium swallow, esophagos-

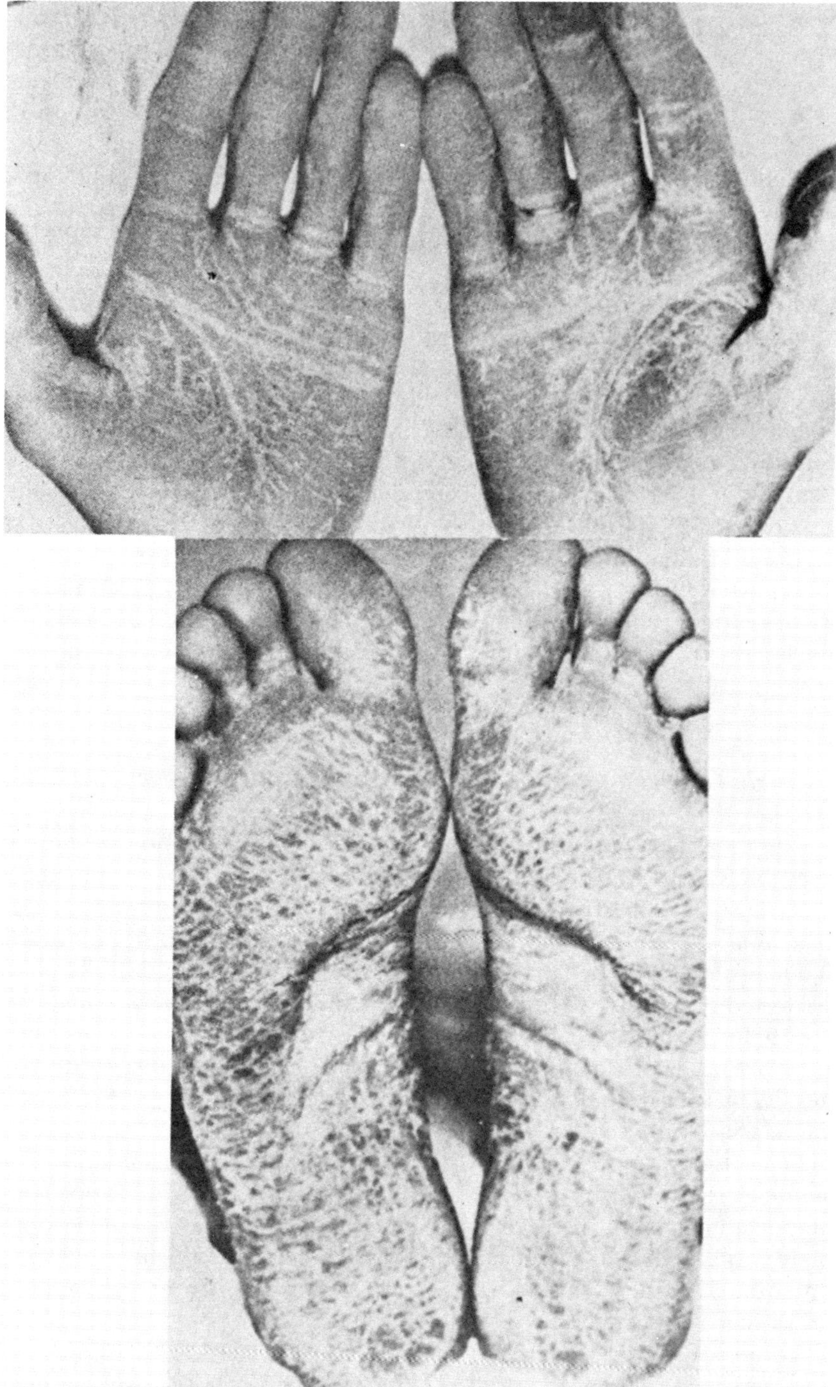

Fig. 1. Cutaneous manifestations of tylosis (hyperkeratosis) palmaris et plantaris. Reprinted from *Quarterly Journal of Medicine,* Vol. 27, 1958, with permission of the publishers.

copy, and, recently, esophageal exfoliative cytology studies. However, concern has been expressed about the possible deleterious effect of X-ray exposure on an esophagus that is already predisposed to cancer. In addition, family members have been advised not to smoke and to minimize their alcohol consumption. Not unexpectedly, it was found that these latter admonitions were not being followed by many members of the families. Since one of the youngest individuals to develop esophageal cancer (age 30) neither smoked nor drank, serious questions were raised as to the efficacy of stressing restrictions on smoking and consuming alcohol.

Shine and Allison (1966) described a family with tylosis whose index patient had a congenital abnormality of the esophagus and subsequently developed esophageal cancer. Congenital abnormality of the esophagus and tylosis were present in two and possibly three generations of this family. An autosomal dominant inheritance pattern was hypothesized.

In the United States, esophageal cancer in the absence of tylosis has failed to show any significant familial tendency (Lynch, 1976; Mosbech and Videbaek, 1955). However, in the already high-incidence region of Iran (Kmet and Mahboubi, 1972), one such esophageal cancer-prone kindred has been reported by Pour and Ghadirian (1974), who documented as many as 13 cases of esophageal carcinoma in an inbred family. Although a genetic factor is likely, the role of environment and diet as promoters certainly merits thorough study.

4. *Gastric Cancer*

There has been a significant decline in gastric cancer among whites in the United States during the past 40–50 years. For example, age-adjusted incidence rates for males in the State of New York, exclusive of New York City (Ferber *et al.*, 1962), reveal a decline from 23.5 per 100,000 in 1941 to 15.5 per 100,000 in 1960. This decline has been noted in both sexes, although males are still affected twice as frequently as females. Current incidence rates per 100,000 are 12.5 for males and 7.4 for females, according to the Third National Cancer Survey (1975). In contrast to the decline of this lesion in the United States, its incidence remains exceedingly high in Japan, Finland, Costa Rica, Iceland, and Chile.

This disease appears to be influenced by many environmental factors (Lilienfeld, 1972). For example, a patient's socioeconomic status appears to be an important variable, the poor having an incidence of gastric cancer approximately 3 times that of the more affluent. Immigrants to the United States from countries where this disease is prevalent have higher incidence rates from stomach cancer than the native-born.

Studies of dietary habits (which may also correlate with socioeconomic status) reveal increased gastric carcinoma in areas where people eat fewer green vegetables and citrus fruits but consume more starchy foods (Bjelke, 1974). An excess consumption of smoked fish and other dietary idiosyncrasies have been suspected in gastric cancer etiology (recall the above-mentioned high-risk countries). Soil has been analyzed in areas where gastric cancer occurs excessively, with special attention devoted to trace metals. Air quality, particularly occupational exposures in the textile and mining industries, and nitrate content of well waters and nitrate excretion by the population have also come under increasing scrutiny. A higher average intake of nitrogen has been observed in populations at high risk for stomach cancer, with nitrosamines receiving critical attention (Cuello *et al.*, 1976).

5. Genetics and Gastric Carcinoma

Genetic factors in gastric cancer have received considerable attention, although specific mechanisms of inheritance have not been identified (Graham and Lilienfeld, 1958). Historically, the most renowned family showing an increased aggregation of gastric carcinoma was that of Napoleon Bonaparte. Napoleon died in 1821 from gastric carcinoma, and it has been stated that his grandfather, his father, his brothers, and his three sisters all had been affected with carcinoma of the stomach (Sokoloff, 1938).

Pernicious anemia and blood group A appear to be associated with gastric carcinoma (Buckwalter *et al.*, 1957; Hoskins *et al.*, 1965; Mosbech, 1953; Mosbech and Videbaek, 1950; Shearman and Finlayson, 1967).

Identical twin studies have contributed little to our understanding of this disease, having revealed only a weak tendency for concordance of gastric cancer in monozygous as opposed to dizygous twins (Gorer, 1938; Lee, 1971). Stomach cancer appears to be associated with autosomal recessively inherited ataxia-telangiectasia, as shown by Haerer *et al.* (1969), who reported two siblings with ataxia-telangiectasia, each of whom developed mucinous adenocarcinoma of the stomach before age 20. Their mother also developed gastric cancer. The mother would have to be heterozygous (a carrier) for the gene for ataxia-telangiectasia, since the mode of inheritance is that of an autosomal recessive and her two affected children would necessarily be homozygous for this disease. The occurrence of gastric carcinoma in the mother suggests the possibility of a heterozygote effect of the deleterious recessive gene.

Carcinoma of the stomach in children is an exceedingly rare occurrence. Siegel *et al.* (1976) recently reported a 20-month-old white girl who manifested mucinous adenocarcinoma of the lesser curvature of the stomach and who died 3½ months following diagnosis. Autopsy disclosed a severely dysplastic thymus demonstrating complete absence of Hassall's corpuscles. There was also microscopic evidence of atrophy of the cerebellum with small folia and a thin granular layer. The combination of pathological lesions of the thymus and cerebellum suggested a diagnosis of ataxia-telangiectasia. However, neither gross cerebellar atrophy, ataxia, nor telangiectasia was present.

There appears to be a threefold increased empirical risk for gastric cancer among relatives of gastric cancer probands over that in the general population (Videbaek and Mosbech, 1954; Woolf, 1956). These figures do not indicate whether elevated risk is due to shared environmental exposures or to primary genetic factors.

Mosbech (1953) reported increased occurrences of achlorhydria, pernicious anemia, and gastric carcinoma among the relatives of patients with stomach cancer. Videbaek and Mosbech (1954) reasoned that possibly the tendency to achlorhydria was inherited and that this in turn predisposed the patients to both gastric cancer and pernicious anemia.

Atrophic gastritis has been suggested to be under genetic influence and to have a strong precancerous phenotype. In Finland, Varis (1971) found 23% of first-degree relatives of atrophic gastritis patients to manifest the condition themselves, compared to 3% of controls. Siurala *et al.* (1966) had previously demonstrated the association between atrophic gastritis and gastric carcinoma, nine of 100 previously diagnosed gastritis patients having subsequently manifested gastric carcinoma. The generally high rates for gastric carcinoma in the Finnish population suggest caution in interpreting these figures.

Creagan and Fraumeni (1973) described an inbred kindred in which 12 members developed stomach cancer, through four generations. The family resided in a rural area where the gastric cancer incidence was signifcantly higher than in surrounding areas. A search for environmental influences failed to reveal any specific factors which could be etiologically implicated. A battery of laboratory studies was performed in an attempt to elucidate mechanisms of familial susceptibility to stomach cancer. Many family members showed evidence of cell-mediated immunodeficiency, as evidenced by impaired lymphocyte transformation *in vitro,* skin test anergy, and lymphocytopenia. A number of relatives showed antibodies to gastric parietal cells. The authors suggested that mechanisms of autoimmunity and immunodeficiency, consistent with a genetic defect of T lymphocytes, might be involved in this family's proclivity to gastric cancer. One of the family members had pernicious anemia. Because several family members showed parietal cell antibodies and macrocytosis, the authors also suggested a subclinical process related to pernicious anemia. They also speculated that possibly a genetically mediated autoimmune gastritis, such as that reported by Taylor *et al.* (1962), had predisposed the patients to stomach cancer.

6. Cancer of the Small Intestine

Cancer of the small intestine is rare. This point is particularly relevant considering the large amount of surface area of the small intestine compared to the large bowel.

Maurer *et al.* (1976) described four patients with malignant lymphoma in a single family (three of five brothers and the son of one of their sisters). In three of these affected individuals, the primary tumor arose in the small intestine; in the fourth, the origin was the retroperitoneum. Low levels of immunoglobulins were found in one patient, and a second showed partial impairment of cellular immunity during a recurrence of his tumor, as measured by his failure to react to delayed hypersensitivity skin tests. Unaffected family members failed to show defects in their immunological system. Interestingly, the histological appearance of the tumors was similar, according to tissue sections available for review from three of the four patients. The tumor was classified as malignant lymphoma, diffuse, mixed-cell type (lymphocytic and histiocytic). These investigators suggested the possibility of a hereditary immune deficiency disease such as X-linked agammaglobulinemia. The authors reviewed previously reported familial lymphoma cases of the alimentary tract, especially of the small intestine or cecum, and found a 4:1 predominance of males over females. This contrasts with the sex incidence of nonfamilial intestinal lymphoma in adults where the sex ratio is equal and in children where the male-to-female ratio is 10:1. It is of interest that patients with primary immunodeficiency diseases show an approximately 10,000-fold cancer excess *vis-à-vis* the general age-matched population (Gatti and Good, 1971).

Pridgen *et al.* (1950) report multiple occurrences of cancer of the small intestine (jejunum and ileum) in relatives from the same family.

6.1. Carcinoma of the Duodenum

Carcinoma of the duodenum is exceedingly rare and constitutes only about 0.25% of all malignant neoplasms (Bockus, 1944). Ungar (1949) described duodenal carcinoma, histologically confirmed at autopsy, in three siblings (brothers ages 16 and 18 and their 19-year-old sister). It was of further interest that each of these siblings manifested polyposis of the small intestine and isolated polyps of the colon. Unfortunately, since no other details were given of physical findings, it is not known whether cutaneous manifestations might have been present, such as osteomas or sebaceous cysts as seen in Gardner's syndrome, or buccal or digital melanin pigmentation as in Peutz-Jeghers syndrome (Lynch, 1976), where duodenal carcinoma has also been described (Reid, 1965).

6.2. Peutz-Jeghers Syndrome

Peutz-Jeghers syndrome (P-J) was described originally by Peutz (1921) and was established as a clinical entity by Jeghers *et al.* (1949). This disorder is characterized by polyposis of the entire gastrointestinal tract, exclusive of the esophagus. Rarely, urinary tract, bronchial, and nasal polyps may occur. The polyps have usually been considered hamartomas and the question of malignant transformation in them has been controversial. The characteristic melanin pigmentation of the oral mucosa and the distal portions of the fingers distinguishes this disorder from generalized gastrointestinal polyposis (Fig. 2). Occassionally melanin pigmentation will also be found in the vaginal mucosa (Peutz, 1921).

A review of the literature on P-J syndrome yielded several documented

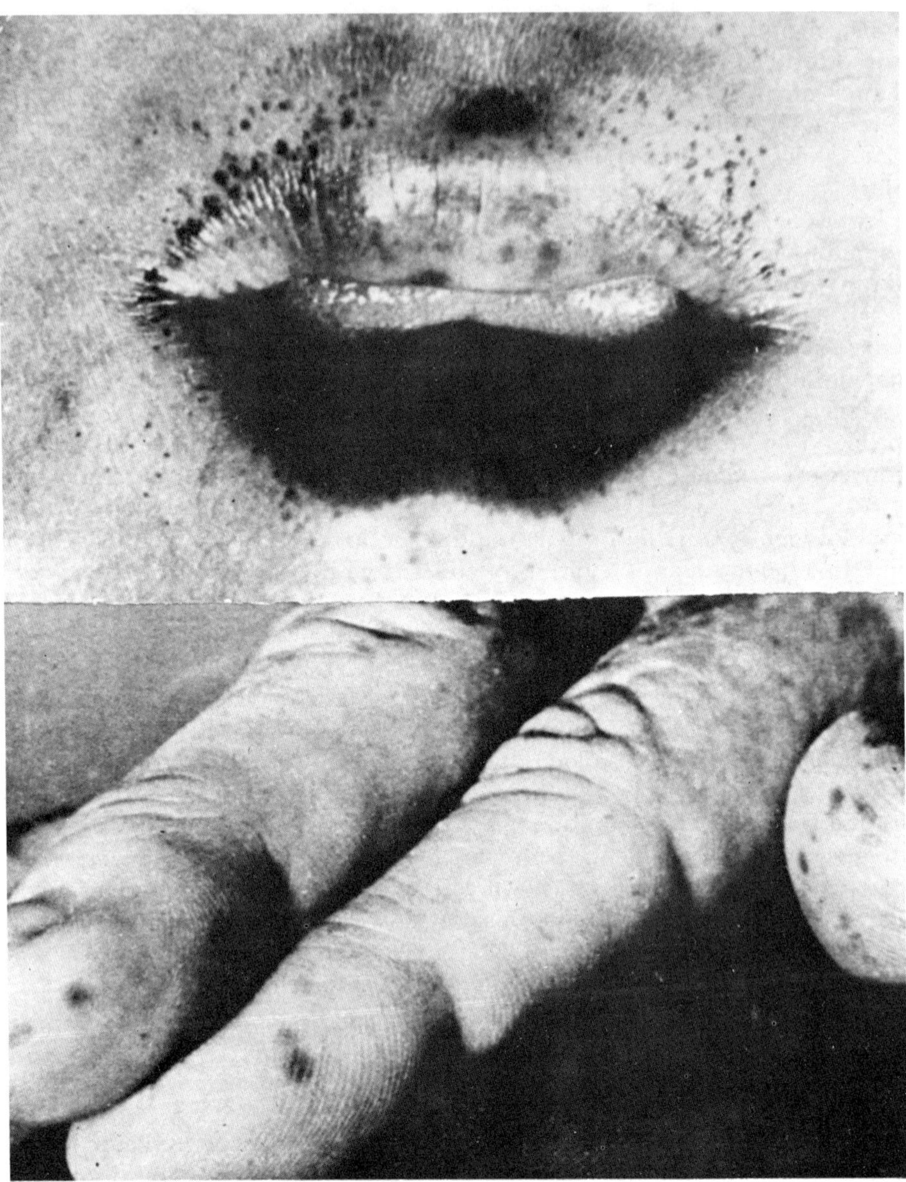

Fig. 2. Melanin pigmentation of buccal mucosa and distal fingers in Peutz-Jeghers syndrome. Reprinted from Butterworth and Strean, *Clinical Geno Dermatology,* 1962, with permission of The Williams and Wilkins Company.

cases of metastatic adenocarcinoma arising from malignant polyps of the gastrointestinal tract (particularly the duodenum) in affected patients (Lynch, 1967, 1976). Humphries *et al.* (1966) reported a woman with adenocarcinoma in a resected polyp from the transverse colon. This patient also had a previous histological diagnosis of papillary cystadenoma of an ovary. Ovarian carcinoma is believed to occur in excess in this syndrome, as reported by Christian (1971). In literature reviews, Reid (1965) found carcinoma of the duodenum in four of six cases of P-J syndrome and Bailey (1957) found small intestinal cancer in 13 of 67 cases from the literature. However, Morson and Dawson (1972) found little such risk.

The largest and most systematic investigation of P-J syndrome (and its possible cancer association) which we have encountered was that of Utsunomiya *et al* (1974*b*). This was part of a nationwide survey (Japan) of P-J syndrome in conjunction with an epidemiological study of polyposis of the digestive tract. Two hundred and twenty-two patients with the P-J syndrome were investigated. Twenty-eight of these 222 patients showed histological verification of cancer, including 15 early cancers (three gastric, eight small intestine, four colon) and 11 advanced cancers (three gastric, one small intestine, six colon, and one both colon and small intestine). Mortality among these patients was less than in patients with familial polyposis coli but higher than that for the general population. These investigators concluded that P-J syndrome patients showed an increased risk for the development of cancer, particularly of the colon. Because of involvement of the entire gastrointestinal tract, exclusive of the esophagus, it was suggested that the P-J syndrome be treated conservatively.

Because of intussusception, the patient may undergo repeated intestinal operations in his lifetime. Polypectomy must therefore be performed at these operations since ischemic damage occurring after repeated attacks of intussusception may require further intestinal resection. This problem has been the major cause of death from P-J syndrome in younger patients in Japan. During such operations, injury to intestinal mucosa should be avoided as much as possible since such injury may be associated with growth of new polyps (Utsunomiya *et al.,* 1974*b*).

6.3. Celiac Disease (Nontropical Sprue, Gluten-Induced Enteropathy)

There has been mounting evidence suggesting that celiac sprue is inherited in certain families. An autosomal dominant gene with incomplete penetrance has been suggested (MacDonald *et al.,* 1965), but a review by Stokes *et al.* (1976) notes a disparity among the several reported families and therefore proposes a multifactorial model. A sex-influenced factor must be considered since women are affected twice as frequently as men. The specific pathogenetic mechanism accounting for this sex ratio is unknown.

Gough *et al.* (1962) identified an association between celiac sprue and cancer. This was initially found to be intestinal reticulosis. This cancer association was confirmed by Harris *et al* (1967) in a study of 202 patients with adult celiac disease and idiopathic steatorrhea. They observed that 6.9% of these patients developed either lymphoma or carcinoma of the gastrointestinal tract (predominantly carcinoma of the esophagus). The mean duration of symptoms of celiac disease prior to the diagnosis of lymphoma in these patients was 21.2 years and for carcinoma of the gastrointestinal tract 38.5 years. Several other investigators (Gupte *et al.*, 1971; Tonkin, 1963; Whitehead, 1968) have documented a cancer association with celiac disease. When steatorrhea occurs with malignant lymphoma, the tumor is most often found in the proximal small intestine. As a general rule (Harris *et al.*, 1967), it has been stated that lymphoma is most likely to develop in a male, over age 40, with a history of celiac disease for more than 10 years, who is *not* on a gluten-free diet. While it has been suggested that a gluten-free diet might diminish the risk of malignant transformation in patients with celiac disease, evidence found by Holmes *et al.* (1976) casts doubt on this assumption.

The possible role of autoimmune factors (Asquith *et al.*, 1969; Hobbs and Hepner, 1968) in celiac disease (and consequently in malignant transformation) has been supported by the finding of immunoglobulin disturbances in affected patients.

7. *Pancreas Carcinoma*

Fraumeni (1975) reviewed the epidemiology of carcinoma of the pancreas and found marked geographical differences, the highest frequency being in Western or industrial countries (international studies suggest that the Western diet may be implicated). All racial groups appear to show a male predominance. In both sexes, blacks have higher rates than whites (Levin and Connelly, 1973). An approximately twofold increased risk for pancreatic cancer was found in cigarette smokers, and an association with moderate or heavy alcohol intake has been suggested. Occupational factors, including exposure to β-naphthylamine and benzidine, have been correlated with an excess of pancreatic cancer among chemists belonging to the American Chemical Society. Similarly, individuals working in metal industries are observed to be at increased risk.

Diabetics (particularly females) have a twofold increased risk for pancreatic cancer (Kessler, 1970). It is therefore not surprising that population groups which show high rates of pancreatic cancer are also prone to diabetes. These include the Maoris, Hawaiians, Jews, American Indians, and blacks (Fraumeni, 1975).

One of the interesting statistical aspects of this problem is the unexplained yet consistent inverse relationship between gastric cancer and pancreatic carcinoma. In the United States, the incidence of pancreatic carcinoma has increased as gastric cancer has decreased (Krain, 1970; Silverberg and Holleb, 1971; Stephenson, 1972). Forty years ago, stomach cancer occurred approximately 12 times more frequently than pancreatic cancer in the United States, while today the relationship between these two malignancies is reversed (Silverberg and Holleb, 1971; Stephenson, 1972). On an international scale, countries with a high incidence of gastric cancer have a low incidence of pancreatic cancer, and *vice versa.* This is found in strikingly high relief in Japan, where some of the highest rates of gastric cancer in the world have been observed with some of the lowest rates of pancreatic cancer (Segi *et al.*, 1969).

An interesting observation which may partially explain the inversely related incidence rates over time is the significant urban preponderance of pancreatic cancer and the gastric cancer excess in rural populations (Stephenson, 1972). Finally, the average age at onset of gastric cancer appears to be increasing, while that for pancreatic cancer appears to be decreasing.

Although the role of host factors in pancreatic carcinoma is probably rather limited, the autosomal dominantly inherited hereditary pancreatitis (Davidson *et al.*, 1968) first described by Comfort and Steinberg (1952) does appear to show an association with pancreatic carcinoma (Castleman, 1972). Eight cases of carcinoma of the pancreas have been described in patients with hereditary pancreatitis, the youngest of whom was a 39-year-old male. Seven of the tumors were adenocarcinoma of the pancreas and one was a cystadenocarcinoma.

The onset of hereditary pancreatitis usually occurs between ages 10 and 15. The clinical picture of this disease is variable and consists of episodes of mild abdominal pain with elevation of serum amylase in some of the patients. Others may manifest a severe hemorrhagic pancreatitis. Pseudocysts of the pancreas have been found in some patients. Of the 18 kindreds reported in the literature, members in about one-half of the families were found to excrete a cystinelike amino acid in their urine, but this does not appear to affect the clinical course of the disease (Appel, 1974).

Familial occurrences of pancreatic cancer unassociated with hereditary pancreatitis are exceedingly rare. MacDermott and Kramer (1973) described pancreatic carcinoma in four siblings. Autopsy or surgical proof of adenocarcinoma of the pancreas was obtained in two brothers and one sister, while carcinoma of the pancreas was found at surgical exploration in another brother. Significantly, there was no clinical evidence of hereditary pancreatitis in this family.

Pancreatic islet cell tumors have been found as a component of autosomal dominantly inherited multiple endocrine adenomatosis (Johnson *et al.*, 1967). Pancreatic cancer has also been reported in a survey of individuals heterozygous for the gene for ataxia-telangiectasia (Sholman and Swift, 1972), while patients who are homozygous for ataxia-telangiectasia seem to be more frequently predisposed to lymphoma. Pancreatic carcinoma has not been identified in individuals who are homozygous for this trait. Note that we have also referred to the association between ataxia-telangiectasia and gastric carcinoma both in individuals homozygous and in those heterozygous for this deleterious gene.

8. Gallbladder Carcinoma

With the exception of a firm association with gallstones, the etiology of carcinoma of the gallbladder is unclear (Lieber, 1952). One interesting feature of this disease is its prevalence among American Indians in the southwestern United States (Brown and Christensen, 1967; Kravetz, 1964; Nelson *et al.*, 1971; Sampliner and O'Connell, 1968; Sievers and Marquis, 1962).

Autopsies from several Indian tribes in the area have shown a 40% incidence of gallbladder disease. This is more than twice that found in American non-Indian populations. Nelson *et al* (1971) reviewed the medical records of the Fort Defiance Hospital on the Navajo Reservation in northern Arizona and found an inordinately high incidence of gallbladder disease of all varieties, a high rate of common duct stones, and a high incidence of gallbladder cancer (6% of patients undergoing laparotomy for gallbladder disease). Rates for gallbladder cancer from other reports of various southwestern Indian tribes range from 3% to 3.8% (Kravetz, 1964). These figures are higher than the generally accepted 1–2% incidence in the non-Indian population (Briele *et al.*, 1969; Derman *et al.*, 1961; Newman and Northup, 1964).

It would be prudent to conduct a genetic analysis on susceptibility to gallbladder disease and gallbladder cancer among individual families of the southwestern American Indian population, with particular attention given to potentially important familial associations such as diabetes mellitus (which could in part predispose to gallbladder disease and subsequently to cancer); consanguinity and exogenous factors such as diet should also be meticulously evaluated.

9. *Liver Cancer*

Hepatoblastoma has been found to be associated with certain congenital defects, particularly hemihypertrophy, which is also associated with neoplasms of the adrenal cortex and kidney in children (Fraumeni *et al.*, 1967, 1968; Fraumeni and Miller, 1967). Fraumeni *et al.* (1969) described two infant sisters (from a sibship of four) with hepatoblastoma. It was of interest that α-fetoprotein persisted in the serum of one of the affected infants.

Familial occurrences of hepatocellular carcinoma are rare. Hedinger (1915) reported familial occurrences of primary hepatic carcinoma in two sisters who died within a week of each other. Primary hepatocellular carcinoma was subsequently described by Kaplan and Cole (1965) in three siblings of Jewish extraction, ages 64, 64, 49. Consanguinity was absent in that family. Denison *et al.* (1971) described a family with concurrent Australia antigen and familial hepatoma. Sutnick *et al.* (1971) quoted data from two Japanese kindreds showing an excess of hepatoma, postnecrotic cirrhosis, chronic hepatitis, and persistent Australia antigen (Ohbayashi *et al.*, 1971, 1972). Upon close examination, transmission was found to be maternal only.

α_1-Antitrypsin deficiency is inherited as an autosomal recessive and has been associated with chronic obstructive pulmonary disease (Fagerhol and Laurell, 1970). Sharp *et al.* (1969) were the first to document an association between cirrhosis and α_1-antitrypsin deficiency. These observations have now been confirmed by Berg and Eriksson (1972). Moreover, these authors have shown an association between α_1-antitrypsin deficiency and primary hepatoma.

Hemochromatosis may predispose to primary carcinoma of the liver. The liver may be indurated and nodular, and should a sudden and unexpected improvement of the diabetes occur in association with weight loss, fever, anemia, and leukocytosis in a patient with hemochromatosis, then coexistent hepatoma should be suspected (Robbins, 1974).

Hemochromatosis appears to show an autosomal dominant mode of inheritance (Balcerak *et al.,* 1966; Johnson and Frey, 1962). In addition, juvenile hemochromatosis has been suggested by Debre *et al.* (1958) to be inherited as an autosomal recessive.

While primary etiological considerations in hepatoma appear to be environmental, its association with Australia antigen (Ohbayashi *et al.,* 1972), α_1-antitrypsin deficiency (Berg and Eriksson, 1972), and hemochromatosis (Robbins, 1974) suggests that host factors account for at least a fraction of the observed cases.

10. Colon Cancer

Cancer of the colon and rectum is the most frequently occurring visceral malignancy in the United States. Genetic factors have been implicated in site-specific colon cancer (with or without polyposis) as well as in syndromes where it is associated with disorders and tumors of other organs and systems (Lynch, 1976). Table 1 lists these multifarious conditions; when known, the mode of inheritance is given.

11. Cancer Family Syndrome

The criteria for the cancer family syndrome are as follows: (1) increased frequency of adenocarcinomas of all varieties in high-risk patients, with particular predominance of carcinoma of the colon and endometrium; (2) early age at cancer onset when compared to the same histological varieties occurring in the general population; (3) increased frequency of multiple primary malignant neoplasms; (4) segregation ratios consistent with an autosomal dominant mode of inheritance; and (5) predominance of *proximal* colonic lesions.

The first family reported in the literature with features consistent with these criteria was family "G." This family was originally studied by Dr. Aldred Warthin in 1895 (Warthin, 1913, 1925). Dr. Warthin was Chairman of Pathology at the University of Michigan School of Medicine, and it was therefore only logical that he would pay meticulous attention to pathological verification of cancer in this kindred. This same diligence was followed by his colleagues (Hauser and Weller, 1936) who updated family "G." A further evaluation of the kindred was begun by Weller in 1955, but was not completed due to his death. We were given all of the data accumulated by these past investigators and proceeded to update the family (Lynch and Krush, 1971). Vertical transmission of susceptibility to cancer was found to be perpetuated in accordance with early predictions.

Table 2. Risk for Colon Cancer in Offspring of Affected Parents

Family	Total number of relatives ascertained	Risk % of syndrome to progeny of affected parent in age interval ($\bar{x}$ ± 2 SD)
033	931	48 ± 5
120	177	54 ± 13
051	184	47 ± 9
001	1139	59 ± 6
200	79	59 ± 13
196	127	53 ± 9
(5 small kindreds)	124	60 ± 8
198[a]	232	54 ± 9
Totals	2993	54 ± 5

[a]Site-specific colon cancer. All others are consistent with cancer family syndrome.

The cancer family syndrome has been identified in several additional families in the United States (Lynch, 1974; Lynch and Krush, 1972, 1973; Lynch *et al.*, 1972, 1975; Smith, 1970), and it has also been observed by investigators in Europe (Bieler and Heim, 1965; Heinzelmann, 1964; Savage, 1956).

Table 2 presents the risk of colon or endometrial cancer to offspring of affected parents, among the families which compose our resource. The most relevant points with respect to these kindreds are the consistently early mean age at cancer onset (47 years ± 4 years), high risk for colorectal or endometrial cancer among offspring of affected parents, and extraordinary risk for multiple primary cancer in cancer-affected individuals. The excess risk for offspring of affected parents, relative to offspring of unaffected parents (nearly 50%), is strongly suggestive of an autosomal dominant mode of inheritance. The early age at onset and high frequency of multiple primary cancer are consistent with findings in classical hereditary precancerous disorders, such as familial adenomatous polyposis coli.

It is now possible, in light of the growing number of reported "cancer family syndrome" kindreds and improved statistical techniques, to classify this syndrome as an established genetic entity despite the persistent lack of genetic markers. Further studies are under way in an attempt to identify biological markers (Lynch, 1976). Indeed, concordance for HLA-A 2-12 and cancer in family "N" (Lynch *et al.*, 1975) has been shown, although the strength of the correlation lacks meaningful predictive capability.

12. Hereditary Site-Specific Colon Cancer

Hereditary site-specific colon cancer in the absence of multiple polyposis coli was first described in a kindred by Woolf and Gardner (1955). In this

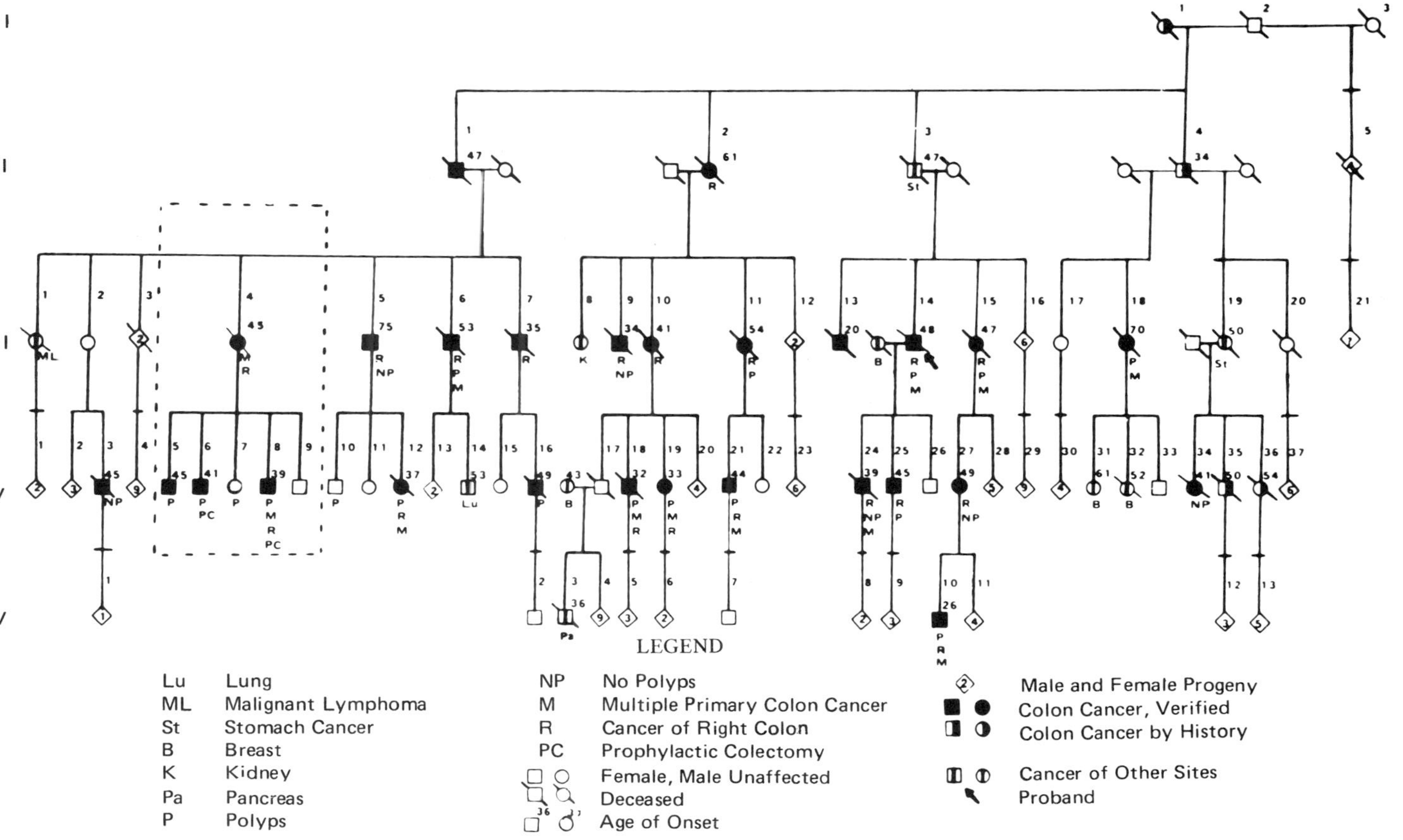

Fig. 3. Pedigree of kindred "R."

family there were discrete colon polyps with an excess of colorectal cancer. Thorough review of the pertinent literature yields a number of somewhat similar kindreds in the United States (Smith, 1970; Stemper *et al.*, 1975; Miller *et al.*, 1976), Great Britain (Savage, 1956; Fielding, 1969; Dunstone and Knaggs, 1972; Lovett, 1976), Norway (Kluge, 1964), Finland (Peltokallio and Peltokallio, 1966), Yugoslavia (Glidzic and Petrovic, 1968), and Switzerland (Mathis, 1962). We have recently studied a large kindred, family "R" (H. T. Lynch *et al.*, 1977), which shows features rather similar to those reported over the years (Fig. 3).

Genetic analysis of family "R" revealed that colon cancer risk was segregating with ratios strongly consistent with that of a single autosomal dominant gene with complete penetrance (only one of the 33 family members with gastrointestinal tract cancer did *not* have a similarly affected parent).

Two individuals in the family who had had verified colon cancer in 1969 and 1971, respectively (treated by hemicolectomy), recently underwent prophylactic removal of their remaining colon segments upon our recommendation. One of these individuals was found to have an occult adenocarcinoma of the cecum. This patient had been completely asymptomatic. We advised prophylactic surgery because patients from this family who developed carcinoma of the colon (treated conservatively via local resection or hemicolectomy) showed an inordinate risk for subsequent primary malignant neoplasms of the colon (approximately 50%).

There exists a striking proclivity to cancer of the proximal colon in this kindred (P. M. Lynch *et al.*, 1978), in most pedigrees manifesting the cancer family syndrome, and in those kindreds cited from the literature above (Table 3) (P. M. Lynch *et al.*, 1977). A more comprehensive analysis of this phenomenon is in progress. Based on preliminary review, the mean frequency of proximal colon cancer in these pooled families (approximately 65%) is significantly higher than figures expected in the general population (15–35% depending on which of the many sources one considers). Perhaps more compelling, this frequency reflects a fourfold increase over the figures reported by Bussey (1975), describing the site distribution of colon cancer among familial polyposis coli patients. The mean age at onset in the families with hereditary site-specific colon cancer is approximately 41 years, including family "R." The internal consistency of the findings in the kindreds reported constitutes an important consideration for etiology, carcinogenesis, and cancer control. It is obvious that surveillance of such patients at high risk for cancer of the proximal colon would be incomplete if it involved only proctosigmoidoscopic examination. Since the right colon is so commonly involved, it would be essential that barium enema be performed with particular attention given to visualization of the right colon and caecum. In addition, colonoscopy would be of immense value. Since early onset of cancer is characteristic, such examinations should begin at a relatively early age—possibly between ages 25 and 30. The lack of clinical signs or biochemical markers adds to the problem of surveillance of high-risk patients from families of this type. Possible segregation of patients into high- and low-risk

Table 3. Frequency of Proximal Colon Cancer in Colon Cancer—Prone Kindreds with Mean Age at Onset

Family	Number of members	First occurrence in proximal colon		Mean age at colon cancer onset
		Number	Percent	
001	6	6	100	48
033	27	11	40.7	52
051	6	3	50	48
120	7	5	71.4	52
196	11	4	36.4	44
200	7	6	85.7	47
30, 35, 115	8	7	87.5	44
198	26	21	80.8	45
Lovett (1976)	6	4	66.7	41
Miller *et al.* (1976)	4	3	75.0	35
Mathis (1962)	7	5	71.4	38
Dunstone and Knaggs (1972)	23	13	56.5	—
Fielding (1969)	5	4	80.0	41
Kluge (1964)	5	2	40.0	44
Stemper *et al.* (1975)	5	5	100	—
Peltokallio and Peltokallio (1966)	9	5	55.5	31
Glidzic and Petrovic (1968)	7	6	85.7	44
Savage (1956)	3	2	66.7	59
Bieler and Hein (1965)	2	2	100	51
Totals	174	114	66	46

classes according to variation in cell proliferation of the colonic mucosa, as developed by Lipkin and Deschner (1976), could aid in the recognition of patients destined to develop carcinoma of the colon. Similarly, karyotyping of cultured cells from mucosal brushing (acquired at sigmoidoscopy) may hold promise (Xavier *et al.*, 1971).

13. Familial Adenomatous Polyposis Coli

According to Shiffman (1962), the first recognition of diffuse polyposis coli was recorded in 1847. The familial nature of this disease was first described by Cripps (1881). The high frequency of malignant transformation in the colon and a more detailed description of the syndrome's natural history were noted by Lockhart-Mummery (1925) and by Dukes (1930). Those of us interested in this disease owe a great debt to Drs. Lockhart-Mummery and Dukes for the painstaking effort which they have given to this subject through many years of investigation and follow-up of families at the St. Mark's Hospital in London, England.

Of all the hereditary precancerous diseases, familial adenomatous polyposis coli (FPC) harbors one of the greatest risks of ultimate cancer occurrence (Morson and Bussey, 1970).

Notwithstanding the impressive body of knowledge now possessed regarding the disorder, many challenges remain, not least of which is the need to comprehend the increasing number of phenotypic presentations (Christian, 1971; Humphries *et al.*, 1966; Jeghers *et al.*, 1949; Peutz, 1921; Reid, 1965; Utsunomiya *et al.*, 1974*a*). Polyps may occur in organs other than the large bowel, including the small bowel and stomach, but questions remain as to how many of those polyps are true adenomas and should therefore be considered premalignant (Hoffman and Goligher, 9171; Utsunomiya *et al.*, 1974*a*).

Gardner's syndrome (Gardner, 1951), with its cutaneous and osseous manifestations (Fig. 4), and Turcot's syndrome (Baughman *et al.*, 1969; Turcot *et al.*, 1959), where intestinal polyposis is associated with central nervous system malignant neoplasms, probably constitute distinct genetic entities, given their extragastrointestinal features. Similarly, Peutz-Jeghers syndrome and juvenile polyposis coli (Stemper *et al.*, 1975) merit special treatment because of the nonadenomatous nature of the associated polyps. Table 1 provides a more full listing.

Carcinoma has been observed in as many as 50% of the initially diagnosed cases of FPC; in some patients carcinoma may precipitate the first recognizable symptoms of the disorder (Veale, 1965). The youngest recorded onset of symptoms in FPC was 4 months. The average age at onset of symptoms is 31.7 years (LeFevre and Jacques, 1951), although Dukes (1952) has indicated a mean age at onset of 21.1 years.

Adenocarcinoma of the colon has been found as early as age 11 by Yonemoto *et al.* (1969), who described generalized gastrointestinal polyposis in three children: a girl 9 years of age, her 10-year-old brother, and an unrelated 11-year-old girl. In each case, polyposis was demonstrated in the stomach, small bowel, and colorectum. It was of interest that the father of the 9- and 10-year-old siblings died at age 39 with adenocarcinoma of the colon and at autopsy extensive polyposis of the colon was found. There was no additional family history recorded. In the third case (an 11-year-old girl), the child's mother was known to have had polyposis of the colon and died of metastic adenocarcinoma of the colon. The maternal grandfather and two maternal uncles also died of carcinoma of the bowel, although no other history was available. Biopsies taken at the 7-cm level during sigmoidoscopy revealed adenocarcinoma in this young girl. Abdominal perineal resection with a total colectomy (including the terminal ileum) and an abdominal ileostomy were performed.

We are currently studying a family with FPC in which an 11-year-old girl and her 13-year-old cousin underwent total colectomies for adenocarcinoma of the colon. The disease has been manifested in two and perhaps three generations. The pedigree at present is incomplete, as the study has recently been initiated.

Recent findings show that polyposis of the entire gastrointestinal tract

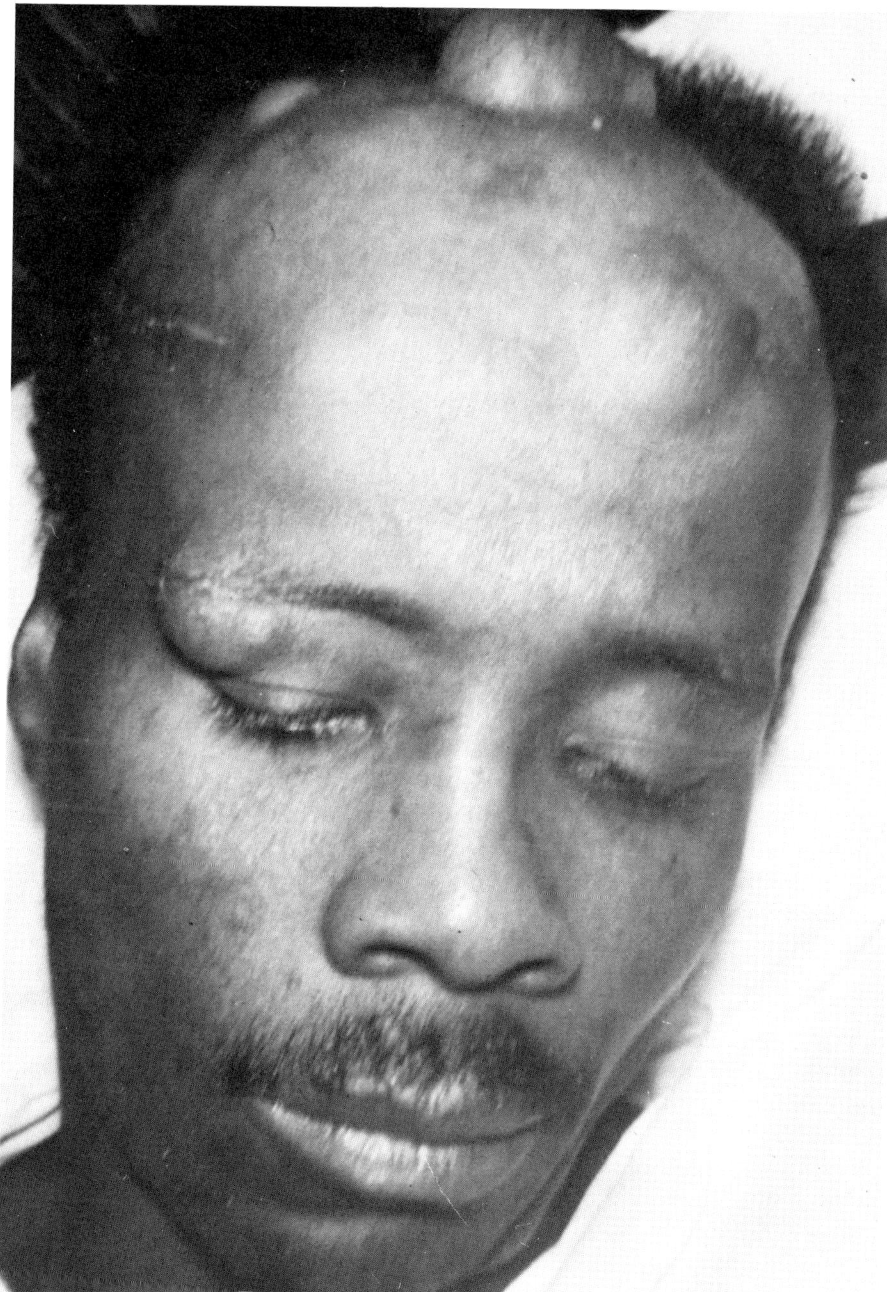

Fig. 4. A 36-year-old black male with a diagnosis of Gardner's syndrome. Note the presence of multiple soft and hard tumors of the face and head. Reprinted from an article by Dunning and Ibrahim in *Annals of Surgery 161*:563, April 1965, by permission of J. B. Lippincott Company.

may occur in some family members while polyposis is restricted to the colon in others. It is therefore important that the evaluation of patients with FPC include examination of the stomach and small bowel. Yonemoto *et al.* (1969) estimate that 5% of all cases of FPC involve extracolonic segments of the gastrointestinal tract.

Management of FPC and related disorders has long been a subject of considerable controversy. This has centered primarily around the propriety of performing abdominal colectomy with ileorectal anastomosis as opposed to total coloproctostomy. A study by Schaupp and Volpe (1972), wherein follow-up of a relatively large series of patients with FPC was available, suggested that the optimal treatment was abdominal colectomy with ileorectal anastomosis. These authors suggest frequent sigmoidoscopic evaluation of such patients with removal of all recurrent polyps. They advise excision of the rectum with ileostomy if carcinoma subsequently develops.

14. Presacral Teratomas

Certain hereditary neoplastic disorders may *indirectly* affect the gastrointestinal tract. One such example concerns the familial variety of presacral teratomas. These are relatively rarely occurring congenital tumors which harbor all three germinal layers. Ashcraft and Holder (1965) described a tumor complex composed of presacral teratoma and sacrococcygeal defect. In an updating of this work, Hunt *et al.* (19744) described radiographic findings in those patients originally described by Ashcraft and Holder (1974) and added additional members from six families. The syndrome included variable occurrences of vesicoureteral reflux, skin dimples, retrorectal abscess, and anorectal stenosis. The age at diagnosis ranged from 1 month to 89 years. The mode of inheritance was consistent with an autosomal dominant mode of transmission. Of 26 affected patients, six presented initially with abscesses; five of these abscesses extended immediately posterior to the anus. The most common symptom was constipation, which occurred in 22 of 26 patients. It is important to note that tumors in young individuals may not be evident initially because of slow differential growth. Thus periodic examination of members at high risk is strongly indicated. One of the patients, who had a large benign tumor removed, died 10 years later of malignant recurrent teratoma.

Features which distinguish the present disorder from the more commonly occurring nonfamilial sacrococcygeal teratomas include the almost equal sex incidence, lower potential for malignant transformation, lack of visible soft tissue calcification, presacral presentation, sacroccygeal defects, and of course excess occurrence of the disorder in members of a family. In the case of nonfamilial sacroccygeal teratomas, the lesions are seen more commonly in females, approximately 60% show visible calcification, and the incidence of malignancy increases with advancing age. While the low rate of malignancy has been observed in the familial variety, the fact that a malignant change did occur in a young individual calls attention to the need for resection of these tumors.

15. Summary and Conclusions

We have surveyed many of the known familial and hereditary factors in the etiology of cancer in each of the several organs composing the gastrointestinal tract. In doing so, the profound role of environmental factors has been conceded; with respect to such anatomical sites as the oral cavity, esophagus, liver, and pancreas, environmental factors appear to be responsible for the overwhelming majority of malignant neoplasms. Nevertheless, one must always remain cognizant of the fact that environmental factors, no matter how significant, act on hosts which vary significantly in cancer susceptibility or resistance, as determined by the genotype. Indeed, we find powerful evidence for the role of heredity in tylosis palmaris et plantaris, hereditary pancreatitis, and autosomal dominantly inherited conditions predisposing to carcinoma of the esophagus and pancreas.

The familial variety of gastric carcinoma usually does not show evidence of simple inheritance. While population studies show that first-degree relatives of an affected proband harbor an empirical stomach cancer risk which is 3 times that expected in the general population, any assessment of its genetic significance must control for the effect of shared environmental influences. This obviously would require rigorous case-by-case evaluation; yet such diligent investigation is extremely difficult to conduct on the large populations required to generate empirical risk figures.

Nevertheless, certain remarkable kindreds such as those exhibiting ataxia-telangiectasia do have an identifiable gastric cancer association. Others, as reported by Creagan and Fraumeni (1973), have shown gastric carcinoma to be manifested through multiple generations with evidence of immunodeficiency in high-risk relatives. Still other traits or diseases have shown association with gastric cancer in the general population, including blood group A, pernicious anemia, atrophic gastritis, and achlorhydria, each of which appears to have a familial or genetic component.

Autosomal dominantly inherited Peutz-Jeghers syndrome and celiac disease appear to predispose to cancer of the small intestine and possibly other anatomical sites. The reason for their proclivity to several cancer sites is unknown; a multidisciplinary inquiry is needed in these and other precancerous hereditary disorders. In the case of colorectal carcinoma, a number of distinct hereditary etiologies have been confirmed, even though approximately 80–90% of the occurrences of colon cancer are presumed to be the result of predominantly environmental factors. Classical syndromes associated with increased colon cancer susceptibility include familial polyposis coli, as well as those disorders with extracolonic manifestations as in Gardner's syndrome, Turcot's syndrome, and generalized gastrointestinal polyposis. Moreover, we see other hereditary colon cancer syndromes which lack identifiable stigmata such as adenomatous polyps or osseous or cutaneous signs. These include the cancer family syndrome and hereditary site-specific colon cancer. With respect to these latter disorders, a remarkable proclivity for carcinoma of the proximal colon has been observed; this fact mandates that more aggressive cancer control measures be utilized in the evaluation of high-risk patients, such as barium enema and colonoscopy, in addition to proctosigmoidoscopy. There remains a compelling need to identify biological preclinical markers in these syndromes.

The role of genetic factors in cancer of the gastrointestinal tract is still subject to controversy. While a few primary genetic associations have been described, the variable interaction of environmental and genetic factors undoubtedly influences the cancer frequency, i.e., penetrance of the particular deleterious gene(s), age at onset, as well as other biological aspects of the particular malignant neoplasms including perhaps even their degree of virulence. When more biochemical and physiological parameters are identified (such as greater refinement of the proliferation index of colon mucosa), a more clear recognition of genetic susceptibility to cancer should be at hand. The clinician might then more effectively incorporate this knowledge into his cancer control program. Problems on the horizon include the need to identify patients who may show particular susceptibility to certain environmental carcinogens. Of greater cogency, however, is the need to institute routine management programs in kindreds whose members' risk status has been or could be reasonably well established. With respect to the latter, a national registry of cancer-prone families, with full documentation of cancer risk status for specific varieties of cancer (when known) and mechanism for communication of findings to family physicians, could significantly expedite this goal.

Acknowledgments

This study was supported in part by a grant from The Fraternal Order of Eagles and by National Cancer Institute Grant No. 5 RO1 CA18480-02. We acknowledge with gratitude the technical support provided by our devoted secretary, Mary Bourque, and we thank Milton J. Swartz, M.D., Associate Professor of the Department of Preventive Medicine/Public Health, Creighton University School of Medicine, Omaha, Nebraska, for critically reviewing the manuscript.

16. References

Addison, M., and Rice, M. S., 1965, The association of dyskeratosis congenita and Fanconi's anemia, *Med. J. Aust.* **1**:797–799.

Appel, M. F., 1974, Hereditary pancreatitis: Review and presentation of an additional kindred, *Arch. Surg.* **108**:63–65.

Ashcraft, K. W., and Holder, T. M., 1965, Congenital anal stenosis with presacral teratoma, *Ann. Surg.* **162**:1091–1095.

Ashcraft, K. W., and Holder, T. M., 1974, Hereditary presacral teratoma, *Pediatr. Surg.* **9:**691–697.

Asquith, P., Thompson, R. A., and Cooke, W. T., 1969, Serum-immunoglobulins in adult coeliac disease, *Lancet* **2:**129–131.

Bailey, D., 1957, Polyposis of the gastrointestinal tract: The Peutz syndrome, Br. Med. J. **2:**433–439.

Balcerak, S. P., Westerman, M. P., Lee, R. E., and Doyle, A. P., 1966, Idiopathic hemochromatosis: A study of 3 families, *Am. J. Med.* **40:**857–873.

Baughman, Jr., F. A., *et al.*, 1969, The glioma-polyposis syndrome, *N. Eng. J. med.* **281:**1345–1346.

Berg, N. O., and Eriksson, S., 1972, Liver disease in adults with alpha_1 antitrypsin deficiency, *N. Eng. J. Med.* **287:**1264–1267.

Bieler, V., and Heim, U., 1965, Doppelkarzinom bei geschwistern familiäre Haufung von genital und Intestinalkarzinomen, *Schweiz Med. Wochenschr.* **95:**496–497.

Bjelke, E., 1974, Epidemiologic studies of cancer of the stomach, colon, and rectum with special emphasis on the role of diet, *Scand. J. Gastroenterol.* **9:**1–253 (Suppl. 31).

Bockus, H. T., 1944, *Gastroenterology,* Vol. 2, 2nd ed. Saunders, Philadelphia.

Boveri, T., 1914, *Zur Frage der Enstehung maligner Tumoren,* Fischer, Jena.

Briele, H. A., Long, W. B., and Parks, L. C., 1969, Gallbladder disease and cholecystectomy: Experience with 1500 patients managed in a community hospital, *Am. Surg.* **35:**218–222.

Brown, J. E., and Christensen, C., 1967, Biliary tract disease among the Navajos, *Am. Med. Assoc.* **202:**1050–1052.

Buckwalter, J. A., Wohlwend, C. B., Colter, D. C., *et al.*, 1957, The association of the ABO blood groups to gastric carcinoma, *Surg. Gynecol. Obstet.* **104:**176–179.

Burrell, R. J. W., 1969, Distribution maps of esophageal cancer among Bantu in the Transkei, *J. Natl. Cancer Inst.* **43:**877–889.

Bussey, H. J. R., 1975, *Familial Polyposis Coli,* 104 pp., John Hopkins University Press, Baltimore.

Cancer in New York State (Exclusive of New York City), 1941–1960: A Review of Incidence, and Mortality, Probability, Survivorship, 1962 (B. Ferber, V. H. Handy, P. R. Gerhardt, M. Solomon), 379 pp., Bureau of Cancer Control, New York State Department of Health, New York.

Castleman, B., 1972, Case records of the Massachusetts General Hospital: Weekly clinicopathological exercises, *N. Eng. J. Med.* **286:**1353–1359.

Christian, D. D., 1971, Ovarian tumors: An extension of the Peutz-Jeghers syndrome, *Am. J. Obstet. Gynecol.* **111:**529–534.

Cliffton, E. E., 1969, Surgery and irradiation in the treatment of esophageal cancer, *Hosp. Pract.* **4:**88–98.

Comfort, M. W., and Steinberg, A. G. 1952, Pedigree of a family with hereditary chronic relapsing pancreatitis, *Gastroenterology* **21:**54–63.

Creagan, E. T., and Fraumeni, J. F., Jr., 1973, Familial gastric cancer and immunologic abnormalities, *Cancer* **32(6):**1325–1331.

Cripps, W. H., 1881, Two cases of disseminated polypus of the rectum, *Trans. Pathol. Soc. London* **33:**165–168.

Cuello, C., Correa, P., Haenszel, W., *et al.*, 1976, Gastric cancer in Columbia. I. Cancer risk and suspect environmental agents, *J. Natl. Cancer Inst.* **57:**1015–1020.

Davidson, P., *et al.*, 1968, Hereditary pancreatitis: A kindred without gross aminoaciduria, *Ann. Intern. Med.* **68:**88–96.

Debre, R., Dreyfusl, J. C., Frezal, J., *et al.*, 1958, Genetics of haemochromatosis, *Ann. Hum. Genet.* **23:**16–30.

Denison, E. K., Peters, R. L., and Reynolds, T. B., 1971, Familial hepatoma with hepatitis-associated antigen, *Ann. Intern. Med.* **74:**391–394.

Derman, H., Gerbarg, D., Kelly, J., *et al.*, 1961, Are gallstones and gallbladder carcinoma related? *J. Am. Med. Assoc.* **176:**450–451.

Dukes, C. E., 1930, Hereditary factor in polyposis intestini, or multiple adenomata, *Cancer Rev.* **5:**241–256.

Dukes, C. E., 1952, Familial intestinal polyposis, *Ann. Eugen. London* **17**:1–29.

Dunstone, G. H., and Knaggs, T. W. L., 1972, Familial cancer of the colon and rectum, *J. Med. Genet.* **9**:451–454.

Fagerhol, M. D., and Laurell, C. B., 1970, the Pi system-inherited variants of serum alpha$_1$ antitrypsin, *Progr. Med. Genet.* **7**:96–111.

Fielding, J. F., 1969, Familial non-polypotic carcinoma of the colon, *Br. Med. J.* **1**:512–513.

Fortuine, R., 1969, Characteristics of cancer in the Eskimos of southwestern Alaska, *Cancer* **23**:468–474.

Fraumeni, J. F., Jr., 1975, Cancers of the pancreas and biliary tract: Epidemiological considerations, *Cancer Res.* **35**:3437–3446.

Fraumeni, J. F., Jr., and Miller, R. W., 1967, Adrenocortical neoplasms with hemihypertrophy, brain tumors, and other disorders, *J. Pediatr.* **70**:129–138.

Fraumeni, Jr., J. F., Geiser, C. F., and Manning, M. D., 1967, Wilms' tumor and congenital hemihypertrophy: Report of 5 new cases and review of literature, *Pediatrics* **40**:886–889.

Fraumeni, J. F., Jr., Miller, R. W., and Hill, J. A., 1968, Primary carcinoma of the liver in childhood: An epidemiologic study, *J. Natl. Cancer Inst.* **40**:1087–1099.

Fraumeni, J. R., Jr., Rosen, P. J., Hull, E. W., *et al.*, 1969, Hepatoblastoma in infant sisters, *Cancer* **24**:1086–1090.

Gardner, A. F., and Rothman, M. A., 1969, Oral medicine seminar No. 16: Oral cancer, *J. Conn. State Dent. Assoc.* **42**:190–192.

Gardner, E. J., 1951, Genetic and clinical study of intestinal polyposis: Predisposing factor for carcinoma of colon and rectum, *Am. J. Hum. Genet.* **3**:167–176.

Gatti, R. A., and Good, R. A., 1971, Occurrence of malignancy in immunodeficiency disease, *Cancer* **28**:89–98.

Glidzic, V., and Petrovic, G., 1968, Observations sur le caractère héréditaire des cancers du colon, *Bull. Cancer* **55(4)**:511–516.

Gorer, P. A., 1938, Genetic interpretation of studies on cancer in twins, *Ann. Eugen.* **8**:219–232.

Gough, K. R., Read, A. E., and Naish, J. M., 1962, Intestinal reticulosis as a complication of idiopathic steatorrhea, *Gut* **3**:232–239.

Graham, S., and Lilienfeld, A. M., 1958, Genetic studies of gastric cancer in humans: An appraisal, *Cancer* **11**:945–958.

Gupte, S. P., Perkash, A., Mahajan, C. M., *et al.*, 1971, Acute myeloid leukemia in a girl with celiac disease, *Am. J. Digest Dis.* **16**:939–941.

Haerer, A. F., Jackson, J. F., and Evers, C. G., 1969, Ataxia-telangiectasia with gastric adenocarcinoma, *J. Am. Med. Assoc.* **210**:1884–1887.

Haggitt, R. C., and Pitcock, J. A., 1970, Familial juvenile polyposis of the colon, *Cancer* **26**:1232–1238.

Harper, P. S., 1975, Genetic problems in tumors of the gastrointestinal tract, *Schweiz Med. Wochenschr.* **105**:564–569.

Harper, P. S., Harper, R. M. J., and Howel-Evans, A. W., 1970, Carcinoma of the oesophagus with tylosis, *Q. J. Med.* **39**:317–333.

Harris, O. D., Cooke, W. T., Thompson, H., *et al.*, 1967, Malignancy in adult coeliac disease and idiopathic steatorrhea, *Am. J. Med.* **42**:899–912.

Hauser, I. J., and Weller, C. V., 1936, A further report on the cancer family of Warthin, *Am. J. Cancer* **27**:434–449.

Hedinger, E., 1915, Primary hepatic cancer in two sisters, *Centralbl. Allg. Pathol.* **26**:385–387.

Heinzelmann, F., 1964, A cancer-prone family: Discussion of the question of inheritability of colonic carcinoma, *Helv. Chir. Acta* **31**:316–324.

Higginson, J., and Oettle, A. G., 1960, Cancer incidence in the Bantu and "Cape Colored" races of South Africa: Report of a cancer survey in the Transvaal (1953–55), *J. Natl. Cancer Inst.* **24**:589–671.

Hobbs, J. R., and Hepner, G. W., 1968, Deficiency of γM-globulin in coeliac disease, *Lancet* **1**:217–220.

Hoffmann, D. C., and Goligher, J. C., 1971, Polyposis of the stomach and small intestine in association with familial polyposis coli, *Br. J. Surg.* **58**:126–128.

Holmes, G. K. T., Stokes, P. L., Sorahan, T. M., *et al.,* 1976, Coeliac disease, gluten-free diet, and malignancy. *Gut* **17:**612–619.

Hoskins, L. C., Loux, H. A., Britten, A., *et al.,* 1965, Distribution of ABO blood groups in patients with pernicious anemia, gastric carcinoma, and gastric carcinoma associated with pernicious anemia, *N. Eng. J. Med.* **273:**633–637.

Howel-Evans, A. W., McConnell, R. B., Clarke, C. A., and Sheppard, P. M., 1958, Carcinoma of the esophagus with keratosis palmaris et plantaris (tylosis): A study of two families, *Q. J.* **27:**413–429.

Humphries, A. L., Shepherd, M. H., and Peters, H. J., 1966, Peutz-Jeghers syndrome with colonic adenocarcinoma and ovarian tumor, *J. Am. Med. Assoc.* **197:**296–298.

Hunt, P. T., Davidson, K. C., Ashcraft, K. W., and Holder, T. M., 1977, Radiography of hereditary presacral teratoma, *Radiology* **122:**187–191.

Jeghers, H., McKusick, V. A., and Katz, K. H., 1949, Generalized intestinal polyposis and melanin spots of the oral mucosa, lips and digits: A syndrome of diagnostic significance, *N. Eng. J. Med.* **241:**1031–1036.

Johnson, G. B., Jr., and Frey, W. G., III, 1962, Familial aspects of idiopathic hemochromatosis, *J. Am. Med. Assoc.* **179:**747–751.

Johnson, G. J., Summerskill, W. H. J., Anderson, V. E., *et al.,* 1967, Clinical and genetic investigation of a large kindred with multiple endocrine adenomatosis, *N. Eng. J. Med.* **277:**1379–1385.

Just-Viera, J. O., and Haight, C., 1969, Achalasia and carcinoma of the esophagus, *Surg. Gynecol. Obstet.* **128:**1081–1095.

Kaplan, L., and Cole, S. L., 1965, Fraternal primary hepatocellular carcinoma in three male, adult siblings, *Am. J. Med.* **39:**305–311.

Kessler, I. I., 1970, Cancer mortality among diabetics, *J. Natl. Cancer Inst.* **44:**673–685.

Kluge, T., 1964, Familial cancer of the colon, *Acta Chir. Scand.* **127:**392–398.

Kmet, J., and Mahboubi, E., 1972, Oesophageal cancer in the Caspian littoral of Iran: Initial studies, *Science* **175:**846–852.

Krain, L. S., 1970, The rising incidence of carcinoma of the pancreas, *J. Surg. Oncol.* **2:**115.

Kravetz, R. E., 1964, Etiology of biliary tract disease in southwestern American Indians: Analysis of 105 consecutive cholecystectomies, *Gastroenterology* **46:**392–398.

Lee, F. I., 1971, Carcinoma of the gastric antrum in identical twins, *Postgrad. Med. J.* **47:**622–624.

LeFevre, H. W., Jr., and Jacques, T. F., 1951, Multiple polyposis in an infant of four months, *Am. J. Surg.* **81:**90–91.

Levin, D. L., and Connelly, R. R., 1973, Cancer of the pancreas: Available epidemiologic information and its implications, *Cancer* **31:**1231–1236.

Lieber, M. M., 1952, The incidence of gallstones and their correlation with other disease, *Ann. Surg.* **135:**493–405.

Lilienfeld, A., 1972, Epidemiology of gastric cancer, *N. Eng. J. Med.* **286:**316–317.

Lipkin, M., and Deschner, E., 1976, Early proliferative changes in intestinal cells, *Cancer Res.* **36:**2665–2668.

Lockhart-Mummery, J. P., 1925, Cancer heredity, *Lancet* **1:**427–429.

Lortat-Jacob, J. L., Richard, C. A., Feketer, F., *et al.,* 1969, Cardiospasm and esophageal carcinoma: Report of 24 cases, *Surgery* **66:**969–975.

Lovett, E., 1976, Familial cancer of the gastrointestinal tract, *Br. J. Surg.* **63:**19–2 63:19–22.

Lynch, H. T., 1967, Hereditary factors in carcinoma, in: *Recent Advances in Cancer Research* (P. Rentchnik, ed.), Vol. 12, Springer-Verlag, Berlin.

Lynch, H. T., 1974, Familial cancer prevalence spanning eight years: Family "N," *Arch. Intern. Med.* **134:**931–938.

Lynch, H. T., 1976, *Cancer Genetics,* 639 pp., Thomas, Springfield, Ill.

Lynch, H. T., and Krush, A. J., 1971, Cancer family "G" revisited: 1895–1970, *Cancer* **27(6):**1505–1511.

Lynch, H. T., and Krush, A. J., 1972, The cancer family syndrome and cancer control, *Surg. Gynecol. Obstet.* **132:**247–250.

Lynch, H. T., and Krush, A. J., 1973, Differential diagnosis of the cancer family syndrome, *Surg. Gynecol. Obstet.* **136**:221–224.

Lynch, H. T., Ewers, D. D., Krush, A. J., *et al.*, 1971, Esophageal cancer in a Midwestern community, *Am. J. Gastroenterol.* **55(5)**:437–442.

Lynch, H. T., Swartz, M., Lynch, J., *et al,* 1972, A family study of adenocarcinoma of the colon and multiple primary cancer, *Surg. Gynecol. Obstet.* **134**:781–786.

Lynch, H. T., Guirgis, H., Swartz, M., *et al.*, 1973, Genetics and colon cancer, *Arch. Surg.* **106**:669–675.

Lynch, H. T., Thomas, R. J., Terasaki, P. I., *et al.*, 1975, HL-A in cancer family "N," *Cancer* **36(4)**:1315–1320.

Lynch, H. T., Harris, R. E., Bardawil, W. A., *et al.*, 1977, Management of hereditary site-specific colon cancer, *Arch. Surg.* **112**:170–174.

Lynch, P. M., Lynch, H. T., and Harris, R. E., 1977, Hereditary proximal colonic cancer, *Dis. Colon Rectum* **20(8)**:661–668.

Lynch, P. M., Lynch, H. T., Harris, R. E., *et al.*, 1978. Heritable colon cancer and solitary adenomatous polyps, in: *Cancer Detection and Prevention* (in press).

MacDermott, R. P., and Kramer, P., 1973, Adenocarcinoma of the pancreas in four siblings, *Gastroenterology* **65**:137–139.

MacDonald, W. C., Dobbins, W. O., III, and Rubin, C. E., 1965, Studies of the familial nature of celiac sprue using biopsy of the small intestine, *N. Eng. J. Med.* **272**:448–456.

Mathis, M., 1962, Familiaeres colon Karzinom: Ein Stammbaum aus dem Kanton Aargau, *Schweiz. Med. Wochensch.* **51**:1673–1678.

Maurer, H. S., Gotoff, S. P., Allen, L., *et al.*, 1976, Malignant lymphoma of the small intestine in multiple family members: Association with an immunologic deficiency, *Cancer* **37**: 224–2231.

McGlashan, N. D., 1969, Oesophageal cancer and alcoholic spirits in central Africa, *Gut* **10**:643–650.

McKusick, V. A., 1975, *Mendelian Inheritance in Man: Catalogs of Autosomal Dominant, Autosomal Recessive, and X-Linked Pheotypes,* 4th ed., Johns Hopkins University Press, Baltimore.

Milgrom, H., Stoll, Jr., H. L., and Crissey, J. T., 1964, Dyskeratosis congenita: A case with new features, *Arch. Dermatol.* **89**:345–349.

Miller, M. S., Constanza, M. E., Li, F. P., *et al.*, 1976, Familial colon cancer, *Cancer* **37**:946–948.

Moore, C., 1965, Smoking and cancer of the mouth, pharynx and larynx, *J. Am. Med. Assoc.* **191**:283–286.

Morson, B. C., and Bussey, H. J. R., 1970, Predisposing causes of intestinal cancer, in: *Current Problems in Surgery,* Year Book Medical Publishers, Chicago.

Morson, B. C., and Dawson, I. M. P., 1972, *Gastrointestinal Pathology,* Blackwell, Oxford.

Mosbech, J., 1953, *Heredity in Pernicious Anemia: A Proband Study of the Heredity and the Relationship to Cancer of the Stomach,* Munksgaard, Copenhagen.

Mosbech, J., 1958, ABO blood groups in stomach cancer, *Acta Genet. Stat. Med.* **8**:219–227.

Mosbech, J., and Videbaek, A., 1950, Mortality from and risk of gastric carcinoma among patients with pernicious anaemia, *Br. Med. J.* **2**:390–394.

Mosbech, J., and Videbaek, A., 1955, On the etiology of esophageal carcinoma, *J. Natl. Cancer Inst.* **15**:1665–1673.

Mulvihill, J. J., 1975, Congenital and genetic disease, in: *Persons at High Risk of Cancer: An Approach to Cancer Etiology and Control,* Proceedings of a Conference, Key Biscayne, Fl., December 10–12, 1974 (J. F. Fraumeni, Jr., ed.), pp. 3–35, Academic Press, New York.

Mulvihill, J. J., 1976, Host factors in human lung tumors: An example of ecogenetics in oncology, *J. Natl. Cancer Inst.* **57**:3–7.

Nelson, B. D., Porvaznik, J., and Benfield, J. R., 1971, Gallbladder disease in southwestern American Indians, *Arch. Surg.* **103**:41–43.

Newman, H. T., and Northup, J. S., 1964, Gallbladder carcinoma in cholelithiasis: A study of probability, *Geriatrics* **19**:453–455.

Ohbayashi, A., Mayumi, M., and Okochi, K., 1971, Australia antigen in familial cirrhosis, *Lancet* **1**:244.

Ohbayashi, A., Okochi, M., and Mayumi, M., 1972, Familial clustering of asymptomatic carriers of Australia antigen and patients with chronic liver disease or primary liver cancer, *Gastroenterology* **62:**617–625.

Ohno, S., 1974, Aneuploidy as a possible means employed by malignant cells to express recessive phenotypes, in: *Chromosomes and Cancer* (J. German, ed.), pp. 77–93, Academic Press, New York.

Orr, I., 1963, Oral cancer in betel nut chrewers in Travancore; its aetiology, pathology and treatment, *Lancet* **2:**575–580.

Peltokallio, P., and Peltokallio, V., 1966, Relationship of familial factors to carcinoma of the colon, *Dis. Colon Rectum* **9:**367–370.

Peutz, J. L. A., 1921, A very peculiar familial polyposis of the mucous membrane of the digestive tract and the nasopharynx together with peculiar pigmentation of the skin and mucous membranes, *Ned. Maandschr. Geneesk.* **10:**134.

Pour, P., and Ghadirian, P., 1974, Familial Cancer of the esophagus in Iran, *Cancer* **33:**1649–1662.

Pridgen, J. E., Mayo, C. W., and Dockerty, M. B., 1950, Carcinoma of the jejunum and ileum exclusive of carcinoid tumors, *Surg. Gynecol. Obstet.* **90:**513–524.

Reddy, D. G., 1967, Experimental production of cancer with betel nut, tobacco, slaked lime mixture, *J. Indian M. A.* **49:**315–318.

Reid, J. D., 1965, Duodenal carcinoma in the Peutz-Jegher's syndrome: Report of a case, *Cancer* **18:**970–977.

Reilly, C., and McGlashan, N. D., 1969, Zinc and copper contamination in Zambian alcoholic drinks, *S. Afr. J. Med. Sci.* **34:**43–48.

Robbins, S. L., 1974, *Pathologic Basis of Disease*, 281 pp., Saunders, Philadelphia.

Sampliner, J. E., and O'Connell, D. J., 1968, Biliary surgery in the southwestern American Indian, *Arch. Surg.* **96:**1–3.

Savage, D., 1956, A family history of uterine and gastrointestinal cancer, *Br. Med. J.* **2:**341–343.

Schaupp, W. C., and Volpe, P. A., 1972, Management of diffuse colonic polyposis, *Am. J. Surg.* **124:**218–222.

Scoggins, R. B., Prescott, K. J., Asher, G. H., *et al.*, 1971, Dyskeratosis congenita with Fanconi-type anemia and other defects (abstr.), *Clin. Res.* **19:**409.

Segi, M., Kurihara, M., and Matsuyama, T., 1969, *Cancer Mortality for Selected Sites in 24 Countries*, No. 5 (1964–1965), pp. 66–67, Tohoku University School of Medicine, Sendai, Japan.

Sharp, H. L., Bridges, R. A., Krivit, W., *et al.*, 1969, Cirrhosis associated with alpha$_1$ antitrypsin deficiency: A previously unrecognized inherited disorder, *J. Lab. Clin. Med.* **73:**934–939.

Shearman, D. G., and Finlayson, N. D. C., 1967, Familial aspects of gastric carcinoma, *Am. J. Digest Dis.* **12(5):**529–534.

Shiffman, M. A., 1962, Familial multiple polyposis associated with soft- and hard-tissue tumors, *J. Am. Med. Assoc.* **179:**514–522.

Shine, I., and Allison, P. R., 1966, Carcinoma of the esophagus with tylosis (keratosis palmaris et plantaris), *Lancet* **1:**951–953.

Sholman, L., and Swift, M., 1972, Pancreatic carcinoma and diabetes mellitus in families of ataxia-telangiectasia probands (abstr.), *Am. J. Hum. Genet.* **24:**48(a).

Siegel, S. E., Hays, D. M., Romansky, S., *et al.*, 1976, Carcinoma of the stomach in childhood, *Cancer* **38:**1781–1784.

Sievers, M., and Marquis, J., 1962, The southwestern American Indian's burden: Biliary disease, *J. Am. Med. Assoc.* **182:**570–572.

Silverberg, E., and Holleb, A. I., 1971, Cancer statistics, 1971, *Cancer* **21:**13–31.

Sirinavin, C., and Trowbridge, A. A., 1975, Dyskeratosis congenita: Clinical features and genetic aspects (report of a family and review of the literature), *J. Med. Gene.* **12:**339–354.

Siurala, M., Varis, K., and Wiljasulo, M., 1966, Studies of patients with atrophic gastritis—A 10–15 year follow-up, *Scand. J. Gastroenterol.* **1:**40–48.

Smith, W. G., 1970, The cancer-family syndrome and heritable solitary colonic polyps, *Dis. Colon Rectum* **13(5):** 362–367.

Sokoloff, B., 1938, Predisposition to cancer in the Bonaparte family, *Am. J. Surg.* **40:**673–678.

Stemper, T. J., Kent, T. H., and Summers, R. W., 1975, Juvenile polyposis and gastrointestinal carcinoma: A study of a kindred, *Ann. Intern. Med.* **83:**639–646.

Stephenson, H. E., 1972, Cancer of the pancreas and stomach: A study in contrasts, *Surgery* **71:**307–308.

Stokes, P. L., Ferguson, R., Homes, G. K. T., and Cooke, W. T., 1976, Familial aspects of coeliac disease, *Q. J. Med. (n.s.)* **45(180):**567–582.

Sutnick, A. I., London, W. T., and Blumberg, B. S., 1971, Australia antigen: A genetic basis for chronic liver disease and hepatoma? *Ann. Intern. Med.* **74:**442–444.

Taylor, K. B., *et al.,* 1962, Autoimmune phenomena in pernicious anaemia-gastric antibodies, *Br. Med. J.* **2:**1347–1352.

Third National Cancer Survey: Incidence Data, 1975, National Cancer Institute Monograph 41, Biometry Branch, Division of Cancer Cause and Prevention, National Cancer Inst. (S. J. Cutler and J. L. Young, Jr., eds.), 454, pp., DHEW Pub. No. (NIH) 75–787, Bethesda, Md.

Tonkin, R. D. (Spracklen, F., for, 1963, Reticulosis of small bowel as a late complication of idiopathic steatorrhea, *Proc. R. Soc. Med.* **56:**167–168.

Turcot, J., Després, J. P., and St. Pierre, F., 1959, Malignant tumors of the central nervous system associated with familial polyposis of the colon: Report of two cases, *Dis. Colon Rectum* **2:**465–468.

Ungar, H., 1949, Familial carcinoma of the duodenum in adolescence, *Br. J. Cancer* **3:** 321–330.

Utsunomiya, J., *et al,* 1974*a,* Gastric lesion of familial polyposis coli, *Cancer* **34(3):**745–754.

Utsunomiya, J., Gocho, H., Miyanaga, T., *et al.,* 1974*b,* Peutz-Jeghers syndrome: Its natural course and management, *Johns Hopkins Med. J.* **136(2):**71–82.

Varis, K., 1971, A family study of chronic gastritis: Histological, immunological and functional aspects, *Scand. J. Gastroenterol.* **6:**1–50 (Suppl. 13).

Veale, A. M. O., 1965, *Intestinal Polyposis,* Cambridge University Press, London.

Videbaek, A., and Mosbech, J., 1954, The aetiology of gastric carcinoma elucidated by a study of 302 pedigrees, *Acta Med. Scand.* **149:**137–159.

Warthin, A. S., 1913, Heredity with reference to carcinoma as shown by the study of the cases examined in the pathological laboratory of the University of Michigan, 1895-1913, *Arch. Intern. Med.* **12:**546–555.

Warthin, A. S., 1925, The further study of a cancer family, *J. Cancer Res.* **9:**279–286.

Watne, A., 1972, Gardner's syndrome, in:*Skin, Heredity, and Malignant Neoplasms* (H. T. Lynch, ed.), Chap. 10, Medical Examinations Publ. Co., New York.

Whitehead, R., 1968, Primary lymphadenopathy complicating idiopathic steatorrhea, *Gut* **9:**569–575.

Woolf, C. M., 1956, A further study on the familial aspects of carcinoma of the stomach, *Am. J. Hum. Genet.* **8:**102–109.

Woolf, C. M., and Gardner, E. J., 1955, Carcinoma of the gastro-intestinal tract; in a Utah family, *J. Hered.* **41:**273–276.

Woolf, C. M., Richards, R. C., and Gardner, E. J., 1955, Occasional discrete polyps of the colon and rectum showing an inherited tendency in a kindred, *Cancer* **8:**403–408.

Wynder, E.L., and Bross, I. J., 1961, A study of etiologic factors in cancer of the esophagus, *Cancer* **14:**389–412.

Wynder, E. L., Bross, I. J., and Feldman, R. M., 1957, Study of etiological factors in cancer of the mouth, *Cancer* **10:**1300–1323.

Wynder, E. L., Covey, L. S., Mabuchi, K., and Muschinski, M., 1976, Environmental factors in cancer of the larynx: A second look, *Cancer* **38:**1591–1601.

Xavier, R. C., Prolia, J. C., and Kirsner, J. B., 1971, Tissue and cytogenetic studies in chronic ulverative colitis and carcinoma of the colon; clinical applications of a new technique, *J. Lab. Clin. Med.* **78:**835.

Yonemoto, R. H., Slayback, J. B., Byron, Jr., R. J., *et al.,* 1969, Familial polyposis of the entire gastrointestinal tract, *Arch. Surg.* **99:**427–434.

11

Familial Polyposis Coli

H. J. R. Bussey and Basil C. Morson

1. Introduction

Although it is now 250 years since intestinal polyposis was first reported, probably not until 1847 was the first account given, by Corvisart, of what is now known as "familial polyposis coli." Twelve years later, Chargelaigue described the disease in two patients, a 16-year-old girl and a man aged 21 years. Since then the main characteristics have been established by numerous other case reports. Harrison Cripps (1882) gave the first indication that polyposis coli might be familial when he diagnosed multiple rectal polyps in a brother and sister. Many similar observations since then have firmly established the inherited nature of the disease. A littler later, Handford (1890) appears to have been the first to notice the high incidence of associated carcinoma of the colon and rectum. This observation, also fully substantiated by many subsequent reports, has important consequences in the study of the etiology of intestinal cancer and gives polyposis coli an interest and value much greater than its rarity would seem to justify.

2. The St. Mark's Hospital Polyposis Register

The description of familial polyposis coli about to be given is based on the records of the St. Mark's Hospital Polyposis Register. This was started in 1925 when J. P. Lockhart-Mummery investigated three families suffering from polyposis coli and had been subsequently expanded to 80 families by Cuthbert Dukes at the time of his retirement in 1956. Since then many more families have been added, and, even with the stricter criteria now required, the total number of families is 221, containing 677 members considered to have had the disease.

H. J. R. Bussey and Basil C. Morson • St. Mark's Hospital, London, England.

A polyposis family is defined as one in which at least one member suffers from multiple polyps of the large intestine, the histological nature of which has been confirmed by microscopic examination to be adenomatous. "Multiple" in this connection is deemed to mean more than 100 polyps, a figure determined for reasons to be elaborated upon later.

The first member of the family usually presents with symptoms due to the intestinal polyps and is therefore the propositus. On confirmation of the diagnosis, he (or she) is questioned about his relatives and from the information provided a provisional family pedigree is constructed. If the disease has been inherited, it is usually obvious from which parent it has been derived. Every effort is then made to persuade all living blood relatives of the affected individuals to attend for examination, preferably at St. Mark's Hospital, but if this is not practicable then at a local hospital from which information can be subsequently obtained. The first relatives to be contacted are usually the children of the propositus and his brothers and sisters and then the search is continued for aunts and uncles on the affected parent's side and also their children. It is usual to postpone examination of young children until about the age of 14 years, as it is infrequent for the adenomas to develop before this age and even more rare for them to cause symptoms. Negative sigmoidoscopic examinations are repeated at 2-year intervals.

The disease is characterized by the presence of many hundreds, or even thousands, of adenomatous tumors in the colon and rectum. These often appear in the second and third decades of life but may be delayed to middle age or, rarely, later. It is also now firmly established that the lesions are genetic in origin, most victims having inherited the disease from a parent affected by it. Finally, and most important in the present context, there is a high incidence of intestinal cancer in patients with polyposis coli (Fig. 1). These points will be discussed in the following sections.

3. Sex and Age

The total of 677 family members recorded in the St. Mark's Hospital Polyposis Register who are considered to have suffered from polyposis coli includes 367 males (54.2%) and 310 females (45.8%). This proportion agrees roughly with the equal sex ratio expected in a non-sex-linked genetic characteristic.

It is generally believed that polyposis coli always affects the younger members of the community, and its occasional discovery in an older person causes clinicians to wonder if this can be the same disease. Analysis of the age distribution at diagnosis of 281 propositus cases is shown in Table 1. It will be seen that about one-third of all patients are diagnosed as having polyposis before the age of 30 years, a further third between 30 and 40 years of age, and the remainder after 40 years. The average age at diagnosis is approximately 35 years. These figures apply only to those patients presenting with symptoms and give little indication of the age at which adenomas commence to appear.

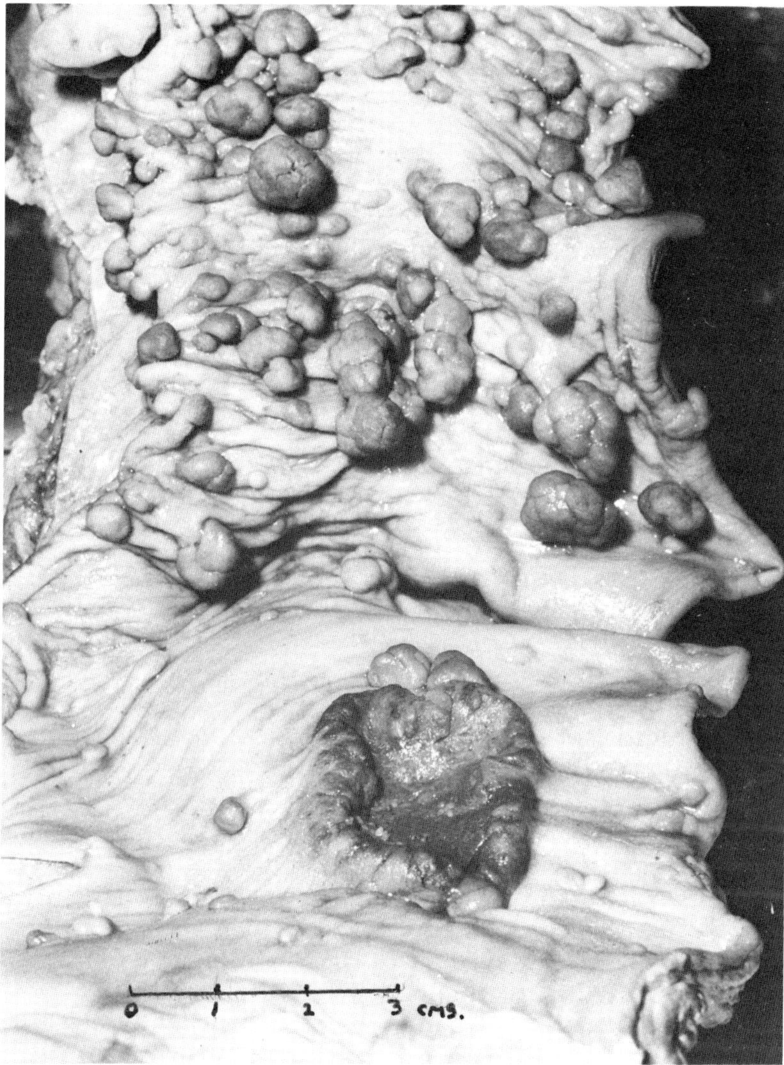

Fig. 1. Portion of a proctocolectomy specimen removed for polyposis coli. Numerous pedunculated adenomas of varying size are present as well as smaller mucosal nodules. An ulcerating adenocarcinoma is situated in the lower half of the photograph.

This is obtained more accurately by considering those family members who have been invited to attend for examination because near relatives have been found to have the disease. Among these "call-up" patients, some are found to have polyposis, although symptoms are frequently absent. The average age at diagnosis in 117 such call-up patients discovered to have polyposis was 24.5 years, with a range from 9 to 57 years, i.e., approximately 10 years earlier on the average than for propositus patients. However, more patients in the call-up group will have to be observed for a longer period before an accurate age

Table 1. Age Distribution at Diagnosis of Familial Polyposis Coli (281 Propositus Cases)

Age in years		Number of cases	Percentage
0–9		1	0.4
10–19		15	5.4
20–29		79	28.1
30–39		92	32.6
40–49		64	22.8
50–59		23	8.2
60–69		5	1.8
≥70		2	0.7
	Total	281	100.0

distribution curve can be constructed for the times at which adenomas start developing, particularly in the older age range.

4. Symptoms

The average age of the propositus patients at the time of diagnosis was 35.8 years and the average age at the onset of symptoms, as far as this can be asceratined, was 32.9 years. Patients in the call-up group with and without symptoms had mean ages of 25.5 years and 24.8 years, respectively. It is therefore probable that adenomas are present on the average for 10 years before giving rise to symptoms and that patients tolerate their symptoms for 3 years before seeking advice (Bussey, 1975).

Bleeding from the rectum is the commonest symptom and occurs in at least three-fourths of propositus patients. Diarrhea is nearly as frequent, but the incidence of both these symptoms is increased when intestinal cancer is also present. Mucus discharge and pain, mainly abdominal, are less frequent. Surprisingly, more than 5% of the propositus patients for whom clinical histories were available had emergency admissions for intestinal obstruction, perforation, severe hemorrhage, or terminal carcinomatosis.

4.1. Number of Adenomas

It is difficult to determine accurately the proportion of individuals in the general population who develop adenomas of the large intestine, but it seems probable that it is around 10%. There is certainly a wide variability in the number of adenomas present in different individuals. An analysis of the numerical distribution as seen at St. Mark's Hospital over a 12-year period suggests that the cases fall naturally into two groups (Bussey, 1975). In the first group, the number of adenomas in most patients was less than six, and less than 1% of a total of 1788 patients had more than this number. Of the 15 patients who did exceed this figure, none had more than 50 adenomas. Outside the series surveyed, rare examples of patients with up to 70 or 80 adenomas have been encountered.

On the other hand, colectomy specimens from polyposis coli patients average 1000 adenomas with a scatter of cases above and below this figure, giving a range from just over 100 to over 5000. It would therefore seem reasonable to suggest the figure of 100 adenomas as a convenient and useful marker for the boundary between patients with solitary or few tumors ("multiple adenomas") and those with familial polyposis coli. It had been thought possible that cases in which there were between 50 and 100 adenomas might represent polyposis with a low penetrance or expressivity, but so far no patient in this group has been found to have relatives with true familial polyposis coli.

4.2. *Size of Adenomas*

A survey of the size distribution of more than 14,000 adenomas in 13 colectomy specimens removed from propositus patients with polyposis showed that approximately 90% were less than 0.5 cm in dimeter and only 1% more than 1.0 cm in diameter. In 15 colectomy specimens removed from relatives of polyposis patients who were called up for examination because they were at risk and who were found to have polyps, there were 8600 tumors, 98% of which were less than 0.5 cm in diameter and fewer than 0.1% of which were over 1.0 cm in diameter. The two groups of patients differed in average age by approximately 10 years, indicating that intestinal adenomas are relatively slow-growing tumors. The size of adenomas has been shown to be related to malignancy (Muto *et al.,* 1975). It is infrequent for adenomatous tumors less than 1.0 cm in diameter to go malignant, and this probably explains the low number of cancers found relative to the large numbers of adenomas present. In about one-half of the cases in which there is associated cancer of the large bowel there is only one carcinoma, and although one patient had eight cancers, the majority do not have more than three malignant tumors.

4.3. *Distribution of Adenomas*

The adenomas in polyposis coli are for the most part confined to the colon and rectum. Reports of extension of the polyposis into the terminal ileum almost certainly refer to the presence of multiple enlarged lymphoid follicles in this region and not to adenomatous tumors. A solitary adenoma, 2 cm in diameter, has been seen in the terminal ileum in only one of the cases recorded in the St. Mark's Hospital Polyposis Register. Rare examples of adenomatous polyps in the small intestine have been recorded, but more recently the increased use of endoscopic examination of the duodenum has indicated that adenomas are much more commonly present in this area than was originally thought. Two cases of adenomatosis of the duodenum have been encountered, and these will be published. In general it may be said that extracolonic adenomas in polyposis patients are very uncommon.

The distribution of the adenomas around the large intestine is fairly even, although there is a slight tendency for the density to be somewhat less in the transverse colon. This is the site too at which the tumors are generally smaller. In most cases the tumors are larger in the descending and sigmoid colon. Occasionally, when exceptionally large numbers of polyps are present (i.e., 4000–5000) the whole mucosal surface is evenly carpeted throughout with similar-sized tumors. Although adenomatous polyps are not frequently found in the appendix, the intramucosal changes representing the earlier stages of adenoma formation may be seen, although probably less commonly than in the colon itself. In one particular family all six colectomy specimens removed so far have shown fewer and much smaller tumors in the ascending colon than in the remainder of the colon with a marked transition at the hepatic flexure.

The pattern for tumors in the rectum follows mainly that found in the sigmoid colon. Because of the policy adopted at St. Mark's Hospital of conservation of the rectum whenever possible, there is less opportunity for observation of the rectal polyps. If the rectum is removed, almost always a cancer is present and this may occupy much of the surface area. It must be stressed that, contrary to what has been stated to the opposite, the rectum of polyposis patients always contains adenomas. On one occasion only, these were few in number but still sufficed for a diagnosis of polyposis coli. It is this consistency in the presence of rectal polyps in polyposis coli patients which enables sigmoidoscopy to be a trustworthy method of diagnosing the disease, thus simplifying the follow-up and examination of family members. Colonoscopy or barium enema examination should then be used to provide further information about the extent of the lesions, but sigmoidoscopy is sufficient for preliminary diagnosis.

5. *Inheritance of Familial Polyposis Coli*

The genetic nature of polyposis coli has been gradually confirmed since Harrison Cripps's first observation of the disease in two siblings in 1882. It is now known that it is inherited as a dominant Mendelian character which is not sex linked and may be transmitted by either sex to either sex. Each child of a parent with polyposis coli is at a 50:50 risk of inheriting the disease. If, however, a child does not inherit the disease, he or she will not transmit it to future generations. In theory 50% of the children of polyposis patients will develop adenomas, but in practice the incidence rate is about 40–45% because of death occurring before the adenomas develop or cause symptoms. Because of the working of the laws of chance, there is an uneven incidence rate in families. For instance, there is a 1-in-32 risk that all the children in a five-sibship family will have polyposis and an equal chance that none will have it.

Clinicians are sometimes surprised to find that the relatives of an individual in whom polyposis has been diagnosed themselves show no evidence of the disease, even when the family may be a large one. Such cases are usually the result of the polyposis arising in that particular patient because of a new mutation. It is important to realize that the condition is genuine "familial" polyposis coli and may be transmitted to any children in exactly the same way as if a strong family history were present. Among the 221 families in the St. Mark's Hospital Polyposis Register, approximately half appeared to be of the "solitary" type when first encountered (Bussey, 1975). The proportion is probably inflated by the inclusion of families of relatively small size in which there is inadequate medical history.

6. *Incidence in the General Population*

The incidence of polyposis in the general population cannot be determined directly and its estimation by indirect methods introduces errors of unknown extent. Neel (1954) arrived at a figure of 1 in 29,000. Refinement of the method by Reed and Neel (1955) more than tripled this figure (1 in 8300). The estimate of 1 in 23,790 made by Veale (1965) was similar to Neel's first result, but Pierce (1968) and Alm and Licznerski (1973) gave higher values, 1 in 6850 and 1 in 7646, respectively. The St. Mark's Hospital Polyposis Register does not as yet include all cases occurring in the United Kingdom and the actual proportion is not known, so a direct incidence rate cannot be calculated from this source, except that it is at least 1 in 40,000.

7. *Diagnosis of Polyposis Coli*

So far there is no way of telling beforehand which members of the family will eventually develop adenomatosis. Blood groups (Veale, 1958), intracellular granules in the epithelial cells (Birbeck and Dukes, 1963), and fingerprints have been unsuccessfully considered as genetic markers. More recently, two further observations of possible genetic linkages have been made which may prove more useful in preselecting affected individuals. The first is a report of a high incidence of small subclinical osteomas within the mandibles of polyposis patients (Utsunomiya and Nakamura, 1975), and the second is the possibility that the polyposis gene may be carried on the same chromosome with HLA genes (Vargish *et al.*, 1975). Even if these findings are substantiated by further research, their clinical usefulness in predicting polyposis has yet to be established. Meanwhile, repeated sigmoidoscopic examination, backed by colonoscopy and barium enema examination, remains the only sure method of diagnosis.

8. *Differential Diagnosis*

The finding of multiple polyps in the colon and rectum does not automatically establish a diagnosis of familial polyposis coli. This can be made only when microscopic examination of one or more polyps confirms that they are adenomas. A number of conditions exist that produce multiple intestinal polyps, and these have to be considered when investigating a patient with colonic polyps. The main factors involved in making a diagnosis are clinical history, number of polyps and their distribution throughout the gastrointestinal tract, possible hereditary pattern, associated pathology, and, most important, histology of the polyps. It is vital, whenever possible, to excise several polyps in order to confirm the histology. The gastrointestinal polyposis conditions are classified below.

8.1. Inflammatory Polyposis

Polyps may arise as the result of any chronic inflammatory process and are most frequently found in the colon and rectum. In the Western world the commonest antecedent is chronic ulcerative colitis, and since this is sometimes accompanied by cancer of the large intestine the possibility of misdiagnosis is increased. The polyps, however, are composed of granulation tissue, aggregates of inflammatory cells, irregular tubules, glandular spaces, and fibrous tissue in varying proportions, and do not normally show any adenomatous epithelium, although villous adenomas may occasionally be seen in these patients who also develop intestinal cancers. Another form of multiple inflammatory polyps may be encountered in those areas of the world where schistosomiasis is endemic. These show histological changes similar to those described above but the mucosal tags formed frequently contain numerous bilharzial ova in the submucosa. Often there is a familial incidence of schistosomiasis and this may give a false impression of hereditary disease.

Enlargement of the lymphoid follicles in the gastrointestinal tract, due either to inflammation or to an allergic immunological response, is another form of polyposis which may affect the whole gastrointestinal tract or may be confined to segments such as the large intestine (Louw, 1968). This is more common in the younger age groups and can, in the absence of histological investigation, prove confusing, particularly if it should occur in a member of a family known to suffer from adenomatosis coli (Gruenberg and Mackman, 1972).

8.2. Polyposis Due to Hamartomatous Lesions

8.2.1. Peutz-Jeghers Syndrome

The Peutz-Jeghers syndrome is one in which polyps may be present throughout the gastrointestinal tract, or limited to various segments thereof, and in which the patient often exhibits a frecklelike pigmentation of the skin, mainly of the lips and buccal mucosa. The tumors frequently produce colicky abdominal pains and may give rise to intussusception of the small bowel, this being the part of the gastrointestinal tract where the polyps most commonly arise. The symptoms usually develop before puberty, the onset being in general earlier than with adenomatous polyposis coli. The polyps, which are not so numerous as in polyposis coli, are composed of normal mucus-secreting epithelium with a stroma which often contains much smooth muscle derived from the muscularis mucosae. There is no evidence of neoplastic hyperplasia and the tumors are considered to be hamartomas. The syndrome is genetic in nature, and although in a few reported cases this has been associated with gastrointestinal malignancy, usually of the stomach and duodenum, there is no strong premalignant potential such as is found in familial polyposis coli. However, it is said that ovarian tumors occur in 5% of females suffering from Peutz-Jeghers syndrome, these tumors being generally of the sex cord cell type described by Scully (1970).

8.2.2. Juvenile Polyposis

In 1966 Veale *et al.* reported a form of polyposis in which the tumors resembled the "juvenile" or "mucus-retention" polyps of children, but instead of being solitary or few in number could be present in hundreds. The polyps resemble those of Peutz-Jeghers syndrome in being hamartomas and in having either a generalized or a segmental distribution in the gastrointestinal tract. They differ, however, in not containing any smooth muscle element and in being more frequently confined to the large intestine. In about one-fourth of the families investigated, juvenile polyposis has been found in more than one family member, sugesting that genetic factors are involved to some degree. Further investigation of a larger series of cases accumulated since the original report in 1966 has indicated differences in the morphology and histology of the solitary type of juvenile polyp and that found in multiple juvenile polyposis. There is also some evidence of a possible association with cancer of the gastrointestinal tract, but its incidence rate and that of the possibly inheritable juvenile polyposis have yet to be determined.

8.2.3. Other Forms of Hamartomatous Polyposis

Less common conditions giving rise to multiple polyps of the gastrointestinal tract are neurofibromatosis and lipomatosis.

8.3. Polyposis Due to Neoplasms

The most commonly encountered neoplasm in the gastrointestinal tract is, of course, that being reviewed in this chapter, i.e., the adenoma, either as familial polyposis coli or as "multiple adenomas." The numerical distinction between these has already been discussed. In all respects, other than number, there seem to be no differences in the characteristics and behavior of the tumors in the two conditions. This gives support to the hypothesis set out by Veale (1965) that all adenomas have a genetic basis, familial polyposis coli being inherited as a dominant character and the less numerous "multiple adenomas" as a recessive character. This idea has recently received further support from the work of Lovett (1976), who found that deaths from intestinal cancer were 4–5 times greater among relatives of patients with cancer of the colon and rectum than in the general population.

Multiple lymphosarcomatous polyposis and leukemic polyposis are other neoplastic types rarely met with.

8.4. Miscellaneous Types of Polyposis

Hyperplastic (metaplastic) polyps are often found in small numbers in the large intestine, usually being concentrated in the lower sigmoid colon and rectum. Occasionally, however, they are of sufficient size and number as to be mistaken for adenomatosis, a possibility which may be compounded by associated intestinal carcinoma in the patient or a near relative.

Cystic pneumatosis of the large intestine and the Cronkhite-Canada syndrome produce lesions which may be described as polypoid rather than polyps and are usually discovered on radiological examination. In the first condition, a nodular appearance of the mucosa is produced by the submucosal gas cysts and in the second by mucus distension of the epithelial tubules and secondary inflammatory changes. In all three types of polyposis, biopsy and histological examination of the lesions will confirm the diagnosis.

9. Histology of Familial Polyposis Coli

The polyps present in the colon and rectum of patients suffering from polyposis coli are adenomas.

The general term "adenoma" is applied to any benign neoplastic tumor arising from the mucus-secreting cells of the intestinal mucosa. Within this group two distinct types are recognized, the tubular adenoma (adenomatous polyp) and the villous adenoma. The tubular adenoma is composed of branching convoluted tubules surrounded by lamina propria and forms a mainly solid tumor which is usually pedunculated. The villous adenoma is more commonly a sessile growth, often occupying a large surface are, with long, thin, fingerlike processes which show little or no branching. Between these two types there is a group of adenomas whose histological characters either are intermediate between tubular and villous or are a mixture of the two types, and for these the term "tubulovillous" is used. Among adenomas from nonpolyposis patients, the tubular type is most frequently encountered, forming 75% of the total, while 10% are villous and the remaining 15% tubulovillous (Muto *et al.,* 1975). In polyposis coli the adenomas have a similar distribution, the only difference being that there is probably a slightly increased proportion of tubular adenomas. This may be due to the fact that most of the tumors in polyposis are discovered at an early stage of development before their true characteristics have emerged.

No differences have been found in the structure and behavior of adenomas from polyposis patients and those from nonpolyposis patients. Because of this, familial polyposis coli can be regarded as a useful model from which to extract information about the life history of adenomas in general, and one aspect in which this is particularly helpful is in studying the early stages in their formation.

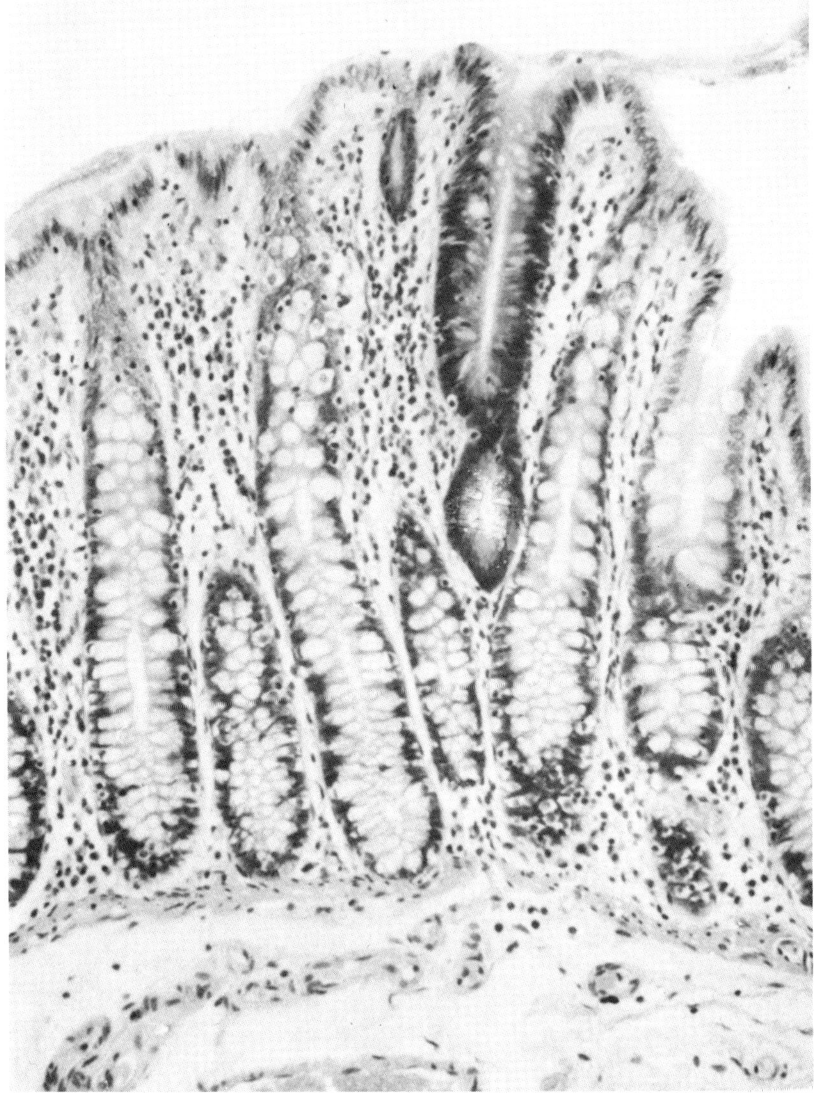

Fig. 2. Mucosa from a case of polyposis coli. A single tubule shows atypia of the epithelium similar to that seen in adenomas. ×175.

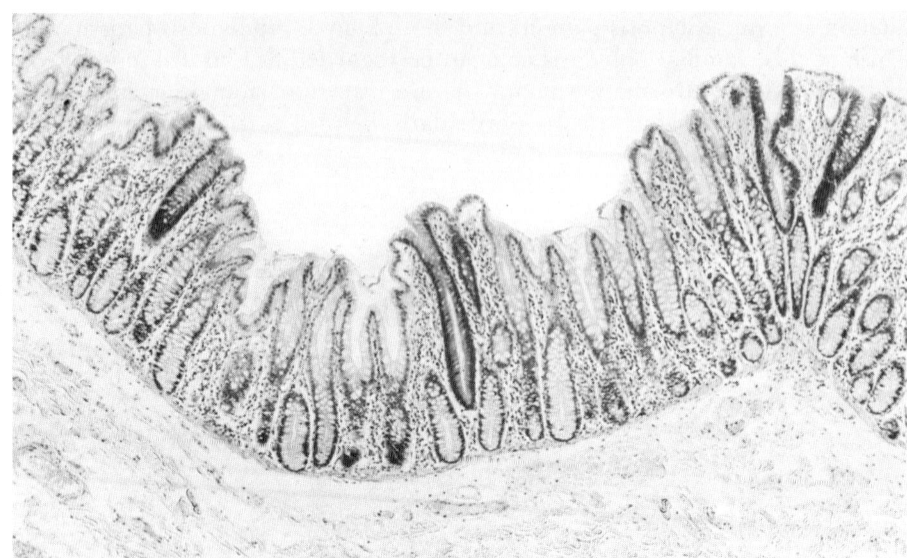

Fig. 3. Section of mucous membrane in which there are three foci of hyperplasia, hyperchromatism, and mild atypia of the epithelium. ×85, reproduced at 75%.

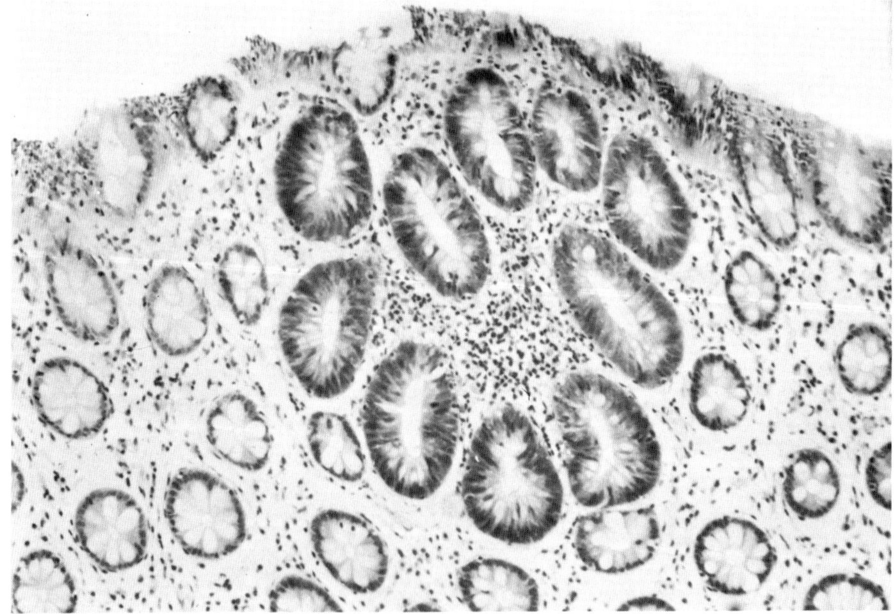

Fig. 4. Transverse section through a portion of mucosa taken from an area in which no obvious polyp was present. A group of ten adenomatous tubules represents an early stage in the formation of a polyp. ×180, reproduced at 75%.

10. Formation of Adenomas

Adenomas when found in nonpolyposis patients are not only relatively few in number but also at a relatively mature stage of development. In polyposis, the tumors are numerous and at all stages of development; because of this, the successive stages of formation are easily observed. Naked-eye inspection of a colectomy specimen removed for polyposis shows polyps and sessile mucosal nodules of decreasing size, but microscopic sections will in many cases reveal the stages which precede the formation of visible tumors. The earliest definite lesion discernible consists of a single tubule or crypt of Lieberkühn in which the normal epithelium is replaced by the type seen in adenomas, in which the main features are hyperchromatism, stratification of the epithelial cells, decreased mucus production, and increased mitotic activity (Fig. 2). These small lesions are usually few in number and relatively hard to find, but occasionally they may form a considerable proportion of the epithelial tubules (Fig. 3). At this stage the changes are completely intramucosal without thickening of the mucous membrane. The next step is for small groups of adjacent adenomatous tubules to form (Fig. 4), and at this stage the mucosa increases in depth due either to slight bulging or to early sprouting of the affected tubules above the mucosal surface (Fig. 5). When the lesion is about eight to ten tubules in width, as in Fig. 6, it becomes just visible to the naked eye as a small raised disk on the mucosal surface about 1 cm in diameter. From this point the growth enlarges by elongation and branching of the

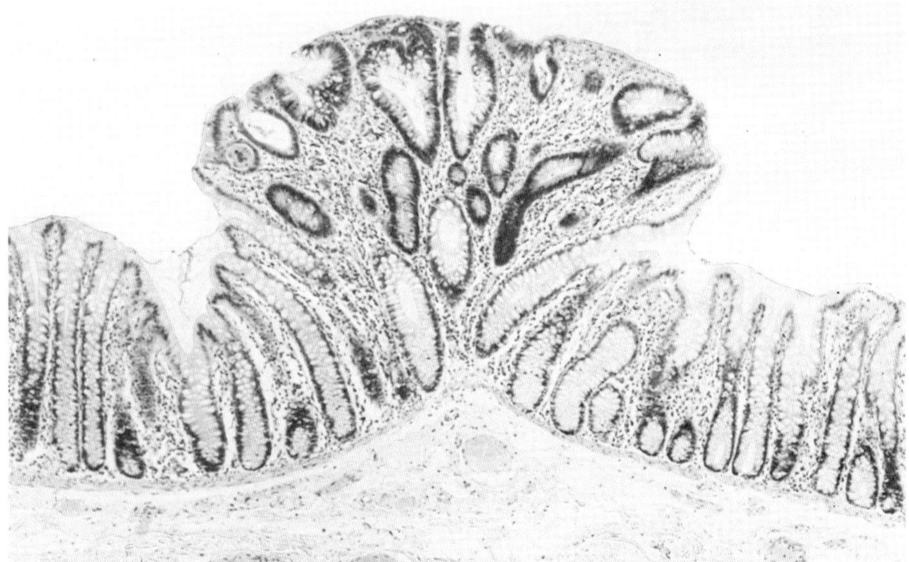

Fig. 5. Vertical section through a small lesion slightly larger than that seen in Fig. 4. It has acquired a polypoid shape but is still too small to be seen by the naked eye. ×85, reproduced at 80%.

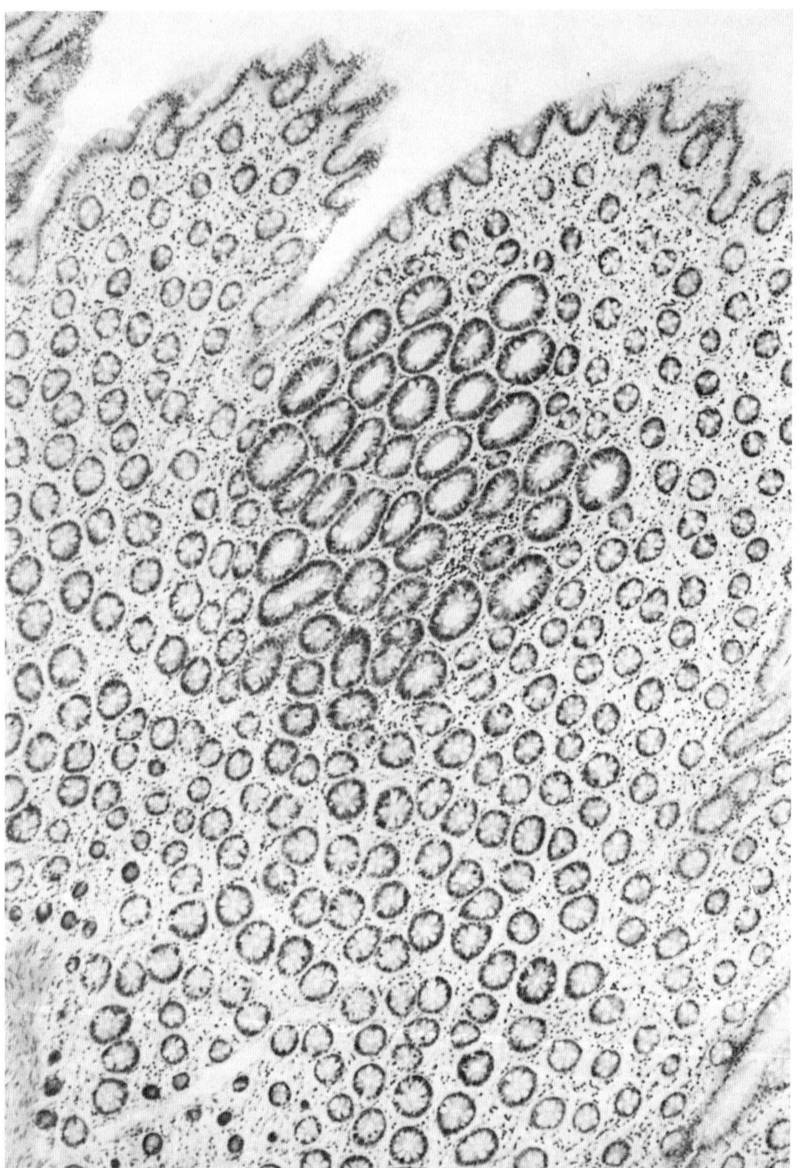

Fig. 6. Cluster of about 35 adenomatous tubules in a transverse section of the mucosa from a case of polyposis coli. It is about eight tubules in diameter and probably would have been just discernible on naked-eye inspection. ×70.

tubules and begins to exhibit the features of a small adenomatous polyp (Fig. 7). Less commonly, a much wider area of mucosa shows epithelial hyperplasia, particularly in the upper part of the tubules, and then the tumor is much more sessile, being perhaps 1–2 cm in diameter and only little raised above the surface of the mucous membrane. This growth pattern is almost certainly the

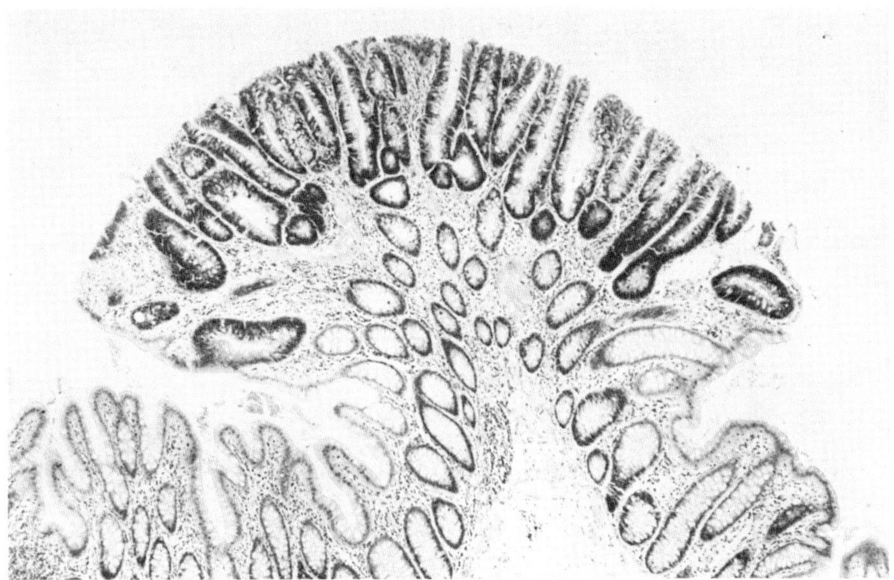

Fig. 7. Small adenomatous polyp about 20 tubules in diameter and measuring 1.8 mm across. At this size the tumor begins to acquire clinical significance. ×70, reproduced at 80%.

forerunner of the broad-based sessile villous adenoma. Both types of adenoma, the tubular and the villous, may proceed through increasing degrees of mild, moderate, and severe dysplasia to invasive carcinoma. Malignant change, however, is more likely to occur in adenomas in which the villous element is more prominent.

11. Malignancy and Familial Polyposis Coli

The high incidence of associated carcinoma with familial polyposis coli has long been noted. It is usually stated that the disease is one in which malignancy will eventually occur if the patient is not treated. In nearly 300 propositus cases recorded in the St. Mark's Hospital Polyposis Register, nearly two-thirds of the patients already had cancer when they first presented. Formerly, before colectomy or total protocolectomy was available and surgical treatment was more limited, some patients who initially had no ascertainable cancer developed malignancy later, raising the incidence rate almost to 90%. Analysis of a series of polyposis patients who either refused operation or received the limited treatment by surgery available at the time shows the increasing incidence of cancer with the increasing period of observation (Table 2). It will be seen that the cancer rate rises from 12% during the first 5 years of observation to over 50% at 20 years and that the only three patients observed for more than 20 years all developed carcinoma (Morson, 1974).

It is obvious that the untreated polyposis patients run a great risk of

Table 2. Familial Polyposis: Relationship between Incidence of Malignancy and Length of Observation

Period (yr)	Number of cases observed	Developed cancer	
		Number	Percent
0–5	59	7	11.9
5–10	39	10	25.6
10–15	19	6	31.6
15–20	9	5	55.6
Over 20	3	3	100.0

developing intestinal cancer. In itself, this fact does not support the thesis that cancer of the colon and rectum arises in preexisting adenomas, although the association is strongly suggestive. Much evidence has been accumulated supporting the adenomacarcinoma sequence (Morson and Bussey, 1970; Morson, 1974; Muto *et al.*, 1975), and this has been substantiated by observations on polyposis coli patients. Examination of nearly 2000 cancers of the colon and rectum seen at St. Mark's Hospital from 1957 to 1968 showed that over 14% had arisen from preexisting adenomas. With carcinomas associated with polyposis coli, the proportion is over one-third. The difference is largely due to the fact that more than half the polyposis patients with associated cancer have more than one malignant tumor. Since it is usually the most advanced cancer which produces the symptoms causing the patient to seek advice, any other cancers present are removed at earlier stages before the evidence of their origin in adenomas has been destroyed. In Section 13 further support for the adenoma–carcinoma sequence is found in the reduced incidence of cancer in the retained rectal stamp brought about by the periodic destruction of developing adenomas.

It is of interest that a comparison between carcinoma of the large intestine in polyposis patients and that arising in nonpolyposis patients shows no significant differences in histological grading, in staging by Dukes's method, in distribution around the intestine, or in survival rate. The only differences found in the polyposis patients were the higher proportion of carcinomas with proven origin in preexisting benign tumors, an incidence rate of about 50% of patients with synchronous multiple intestinal cancers, and the earlier onset of, and death from, cancer, all features which could reasonably be expected from the earlier appearance and multiplicity of adenomas in the polyposis population (Bussey, 1975).

12. Gardner's Syndrome

In the early 1950s Gardner and his co-workers recorded in a series of papers a family whose members suffered from multiple adenomas of the colon as well as a number of other extracolonic lesions. Many similar reports have followed, and the controversy as to the exact nature and relationship of these lesions to familial polyposis coli still continues.

In the early reports by Gardner, the syndrome, subsequently named after him, was stated to be a triad consisting of

1. Multiple adenomas of the colon and rectum.
2. Multiple epidermoid cysts and connective tissue tumors of the skin.
3. Multiple osteomas of the skull and mandible.

After a review of the family 20 years later, Gardner (1969) included additional lesions such as osteomas of the entire skeletal system, postoperative desmoids of the abdominal wall, and dental abnormalities. Many other conditions have been suggested by other authors for inclusion in the syndrome, but the most likely genuine candidates are carcinoma of the duodenum, particularly of the ampullary region, carcinoma of the thyroid, and malignant tumors of the central nervous system (Turcot's syndrome). There is no doubt that patients with Gardner's syndrome have a greatly increased potential for neoplastic growth which manifests in varying ways.

Controversy continues as to whether familial polyposis coli and Gardner's syndrome are entirely different diseases or whether Gardner's syndrome is just polyposis coli plus a further genetic abnormality responsible for the extracolonic lesions. It has also been suggested that the type of polyposis occurring in the two conditions differs in that fewer polyps are present in Gardner's syndrome. In the St. Mark's Hospital series considerable variation is found between individual colectomy specimens, but this variability is unrelated to the presence or absence of the extracolonic lesions. When sufficiently large series of colectomy specimens from both Gardner and non-Gardner polyposis patients are compared, no differences emerge. In any case, the distinction between the two types is often not easily made. Some patients have the skin and other stigmata of Gardner's syndrome in a very attenuated form, perhaps an osteoma in one patient and a cyst or two in another. Much depends on the energy and thoroughness of the investigator. Utsunomiya and Nakamura (1975) find that over 90% of polyposis patients have subclinical intramandibular bony opacities which are infrequently found in nonpolyposis patients. This, as well as other recent reports, makes it reasonable to think that perhaps all familial polyposis coli may be Gardner's syndrome with varying degrees of expressivity. Smith (1968) subscribes to this view when he states that "a single mutation is responsible for most of the various syndromes associated with multiple colonic polyposis." Investigation and follow-up of polyposis families for longer periods of time will be necessary before the many problems connected with Gardner's syndrome can be solved.

13. Treatment of Polyposis Coli

Basically the treatment of familial polyposis coli depends on the destruction of the adenomas. These are too numerous to permit use of the new techniques of colonoscopy and polypectomy, and it is therefore necessary to use surgical removal of the diseased bowel. This can be achieved by one of two alternatives. The whole large intestine from caecum to anus can be removed by total proctocolectomy, but this has the disadvantage of leaving the patient with a pertinent ileostomy. The alternative, which can be undertaken only if the rectum is free from cancer, is to resect the colon only and perform an ileorectal anastomosis. This gives the patient a natural bowel action but presents another problem in that the residual rectal mucosa still has the potentiality of producing further adenomas, requiring the patient to attend at about 6-monthly intervals for examination and destruction of any tumors found. There is little doubt that this latter method of treatment is the one preferred by most patients and is the one most commonly employed at St. Mark's Hospital.

Up to the end of 1975, colectomy and ileorectal anastomosis had been performed as a primary operation on 100 polyposis patients with one operation death. Six of the survivors have subsequently had the rectal stump excised. In four cases this was for carcinoma arising in the rectum and in one because of inability to control by diathermy the numerous adenomas which carpeted the rectal mucosa. These excisions were all carried out in St. Mark's Hospital. The sixth patient was operated on elsewhere for reasons unconnected with neoplastic disease of the rectum. Thus the apparent gross risk of subsequent rectal carcinoma is about 4%. This figure is, however, misleading in that it takes no account of the varying periods of exposure to risk. Some patients have only recently been operated on and others have succumbed either from recurrent colonic carcinoma or from unrelated diseases. In all, 68 have been observed over a period of 5 years, and of these 11 have gone on to survive more than 20 years. When these factors are taken into consideration, the accumulative risk, as calculated on an actuarial basis, is found to be about 7% over the 20-year period of observation. This is an acceptable figure which may be further reduced when analysis indicates the reasons why cancer appears in the rectum, such as failure of the patient to cooperate or of the surgeon to destroy all the adenomas. Of the four rectal cancers, two appeared in the first 5 years following colectomy and ileorectal anastomosis and one each in the second and third 5-year periods. In only one of the four cases had lymphatic spread occurred and in this to a single lymph node. Thus all the patients had a favorable prognosis and a good chance of permanent cure.

Schaupp and Volpe (1972) recorded only one case of rectal cancer in 48 patients who had undergone colectomy and ileorectal anastomosis. On the other hand, Moertel *et al.* (1970) condemned this operation as dangerous, citing an overall incidence of 22% of their patients with subsequent rectal cancer and an accumulative risk of 59% after 23 years of observation. This disparity is difficult to understand but may in part be due to the selection of the cases. The high incidence of deaths due to the rectal cancers (17 cases out of a total of 25 followed up for 5 years) is also surprising in a group of patients who were under surveillance because of the known risk of subsequent cancer.

From the acccount which has been given, it will appear that familial polyposis coli is a useful model from whose study many lessons could be effectively extrapolated to the problem of adenomas and carcinoma in the large intestine. It is a disease involving multiple adenomas indistinguishable from those found more generally in the nonpolyposis population. In particular, the adenomas from both sources can show progressively increasing epithelial atypia which finally equates with that seen in invasive carcinoma. The multiple adenomas of polyposis coli occur in a predictable fashion in a small compact group of the community within which the possible effect of environmental factors can be studied. Furthermore, the disease is closely associated with other growth patterns, mostly of a neoplastic nature, sometimes benign and sometimes malignant. The exact nature of these associations and of the possible effect of genetic and environmental factors still requires investigation, the outcome of which could prove of interest to oncologists, environmentalists, and geneticists alike.

14. References

Alm, T., and Licznerski, G., 1973, The intestinal polyposis, *Clin. Gastroenterol.* **2:**577–602.

Birbeck, M. S. C., and Dukes, C. E., 1963, Electron microscopy of rectal neoplasms, *Proc. R. Soc. Med.* **56:**793–798.

Bussey, H. J. R., 1975, *Familial Polyposis Coli,* Johns Hopkins University Press, Baltimore.

Chargelaigue, A., 1859, Des polyps du rectum, Thesis, Paris.

Corvisart, L., 1847, Hypertrophie partielle de la muqueuse intestinale, *Bull. Soc. Anat.* **22:**400.

Cripps, W. H., 1882, Two cases of disseminated polypus of the rectum, *Trans. Pathol. Soc. London* **33:**165–168.

Gardner, E. J., 1969, Gardner's syndrome re-evaluated after twenty years, *Proc. Utah Acad.* **46:**1–11.

Gruenberg, J., and Mackman, S., 1972, Multiple lymphoid polyps in familial polyposis, *Ann. Surg.* **175:**552–554.

Handford, H., 1890, Disseminated polypi of the large intestine becoming malignant, *Trans. Pathol. Soc. London* **41:**133.

Louw, J. H., 1968, Polypoid lesions of the large bowel in children with particular reference to benign lymphoid polyposis, *Pediatr. Surg.* **3:**195–209.

Lovett, E., 1976, Family studies in cancer of the colon and rectum, *Brit. J. Surg.* **63:**13–18.

Moertel, C. G., Hill, J. R., and Adson, M. A., 1970, The surgical management of multiple polyposis, *Arch. Surg.* **100:**521–526.

Morson, B. C., 1974, The polyp-cancer sequence in the large bowel, *Proc. R. Soc. Med.* **67:**451–457.

Morson, B. C., and Bussey, H. J. R., 1970, Predisposing causes of intestinal cancer, in: *Current Problems in Surgery,* Year Book Medical Publishers, Chicago.

Muto, T., Bussey, H. J. R., and Morson, B. C., 1975, The evolution of cancer of the colon and rectum, *Cancer* **36:**2251–2270.

Neel, J. V., 1954, Problems in the estimation of the frequency of uncommon inherited traits, *Am. J. Hum. Genet.* **6:**51.

Pierce, E. R., 1968, Some genetic aspects of familial multiple polyposis of the colon in a kindred of 1,422 members, *Dis. Colon Rectum* **11:**321–329.

Reed, T. E., and Neel, J. V., 1955, A genetic study of multiple polyposis of the colon (with an appendix deriving a method of estimating relative fitness), *Am. J. Hum. Genet.* **7:**236–263.

Schaupp, W. C., and Volpe, P. A., 1972, Management of diffuse colonic polyposis, *Am. J. Surg.* **124:**218–222.

Scully, R. E., 1970, Sex cord tumor with annular tubules: A distinctive ovarian tumor of the Peutz-Jeghers syndrome, *Cancer* **25:**1107–1121.

Smith, W. G., 1968, Familial multiple polyposis: Research tool for investigating the etiology of carcinoma of the colon? *Dis. Colon Rectum* **11**:17–31.

Turcot, J., Despres, J. P., and St. Pierre, F. 1959, Malignant tumors of the central nervous system associated with familial polyposis of the colon, *Dis. Colon Rectum* **2**:465–468.

Utsunomiya, J., and Nakamura, T., 1975, The occult osteomatous changes in the mandible in patients with familial polyposis coli, *Br. J. Surg.* **62**:45–51.

Vargish, T., Dawkins, H. G., Heise, E., and Myers, R. T., 1975, Serologic detection of persons at risk in familial polyposis coli, in: *Surgical Forum* Vol. 26, 61st Annual Congress, American College of Surgeons.

Veale, A. M. O., 1958, Possible autosomal linkage in man, *Nature (London)* **182**:409–410.

Veale, A. M. O., 1965, *Intestinal Polyposis,* Eugenics Laboratory Memoirs, Series 40, Cambridge University Press, London.

Veale, A. M. O., McColl, I., Bussey, H. J. R., and Morson, B. C., 1966, Juvenile polyposis coli, *J. Med. Genet.* **3**:5–16.

12

Defining the Precursor Tissue of Ordinary Large Bowel Carcinoma: Implications for Cancer Prevention

Nathan Lane, Cecilia M. Fenoglio, Gordon I. Kaye, and Robert R. Pascal

> The observations that atypism, carcinoma *in situ,* or intramucosal carcinoma is rarely seen except in adenomatous polyps and papillary adenomas and that invasive foci less than 5 millimeters in diameter are rarely seen except in these lesions, constitute evidence to support the belief that the vast majority of cancers arise in adenomatous polyps and papillary adenomas. (Grinnel and Lane, 1958)
>
> In the absence of any well-documented alternative, the presently available evidence suggests that intestinal cancers have a preceding benign or precancerous phase which presents morphologically as adenomatous or villous tumors which can be large or small, sessile or pedunculated. (Morson and Bussey, 1970)
>
> That there exists a relationship between adenomas and carcinomas of the large intestine becomes increasingly certain. In fact, it is probable that most, possibly even all, carcinomas arise in preexisting adenomatous tumors. One method of controlling intestinal cancer could be by attacking its precursor—the adenoma. (Bussey, 1975)

1. Introduction

To accomplish the purpose indicated in the title of this chapter, i.e., to define the precursor tissue of ordinary large bowel carcinoma, particular attention

---

Nathan Lane and Cecilia M. Fenoglio • Division of Surgical Pathology, Departments of Surgery and Pathology, College of Physicians and Surgeons, Columbia University, New York, New York 10032. ***Gordon I. Kaye*** • Albany Medical College, Albany, New York 12208. ***Robert R. Pascal*** • Veterans Administration Hospital, Tampa, Florida 33612.

has been given to terminology. We have attempted to use simple and accurate terms, with the help of diagrams and illustrations, so that internists, surgeons, radiologists, *and pathologists* will have the same mental image and hence the ease of communication so needed for proper diagnosis and treatment in this field.

Regarding the term "precursor tissue," this is synonymous with precancerous or preneoplastic lesion or tissue. These terms carry with them the implication not only that cancer may develop in such a lesion or abnormal tissue but also that cancer will develop in such an abnormal focus with far greater frequency than in the seemingly morphologically normal adjacent tissue. In the case of the large bowel the further implication of the term "precursor tissue" is that (until we learn how to avoid the development of this precursor tissue) its detection and removal will reduce the incidence of colorectal carcinoma.

This chapter will discuss only those benign lesions known as adenomas and hyperplastic polyps and only the ordinary moderately and well-differentiated adenocarcinomas. Excluded from consideration are the rare cases of undifferentiated carcinoma and carcinoma arising in ulcerative colitis. Also excluded are a variety of unrelated polypoid masses such as juvenile polyps, the polypoid hamartomas of Peutz-Jeghers syndrome, inflammatory pseudopolyps, polypoid leiomyomas, lymphoid masses, and lipomas. However, some insights gained from the study of familial polyposis cases will be mentioned.

2. *Basic Concepts*

The evolution of ordinary large bowel carcinoma from its precursor tissue is best understood if one recalls a few features of normal colonic histology and cell kinetics.

The flat nonvillous mucosa has simple test-tube-shaped glands—the crypts of Lieberkühn. The tissue between these crypts is the lamina propria. A thin layer of smooth muscle—the muscularis mucosae—is the boundary line between the mucosa and submucosa, and it is the structure which is used to distinguish between an intramucosal (or *in situ*) process and an invasive proliferation (Fig. 1).

Cell division is very active but is normally restricted to the deep one-half or one-third of the crypts (Fig. 2). Cells produced by this active division migrate "upward" and differentiate into two principal cell types, the goblet cells and the absorptive cells (Fig. 3).

In 3–4 days this dynamic process of division and migration is perfectly balanced by exfoliation from the free surface.

In brief, three points are important: (1) normally, cell division is restricted to the deep portion of the crypt; (2) normally, with migration there occurs differentiation into two main cell types, the goblet cell and the absorptive cell; (3) the muscularis mucosae is the dividing line between an intramucosal and an invasive process.

3. Benign Proliferations

If, in one or several crypts, an imbalance between cell division and exfoliation should bring about a net gain in the number of cells, a protrusion or "polyp" will result. In older adults, benign proliferations of this sort are very common. Therefore, in order to discern the precursor relationship of *some* of these proliferations to carcinoma, it is essential to classify them.

1. These proliferations (polyps) are divided into two basic biological types, the hyperplastic polyps and the adenomas.
2. Furthermore, the adenomas must be divided according to size, and it is desirable to specify their shape and histological pattern as well.
3. Finally, it is essential to appreciate not only the absolute frequency of these proliferations but especially the relative frequency of hyperplastic polyps to adenomas, and the relative frequency of small and large adenomas.

3.1. Two Basic Types

The two biological types of benign proliferations occurring in adults may be discussed in terms of hyperplasia and benign neoplasia, and it is because of

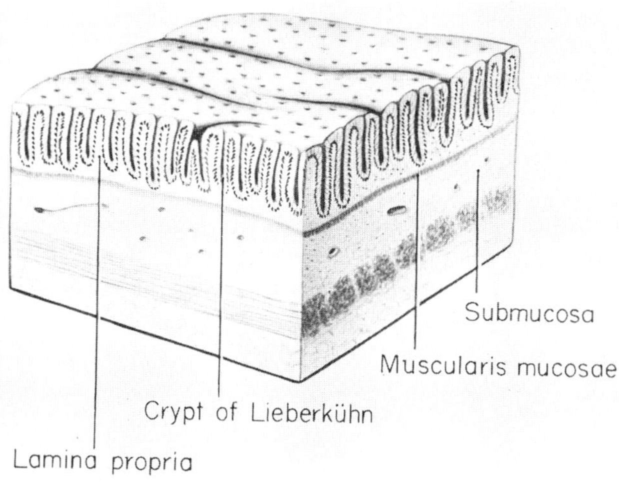

Fig. 1. Diagram of normal colon to emphasize the muscularis mucosae. It is of prime importance to remember that in neoplasia it is the muscularis mucosae that is used to distinguish between an intramucosal (*in situ*) and an invasive neoplasm.

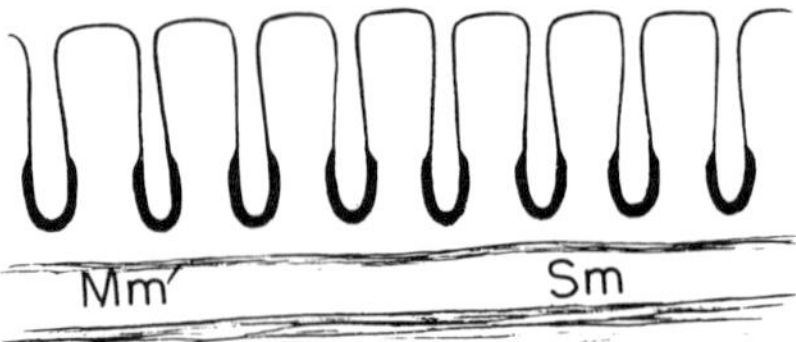

Fig. 2. Normal controlled replication is restricted to the deep portion of the crypts, as indicated by the heavy shading. Reprinted from *Cancer 34*:819–823 (1974).

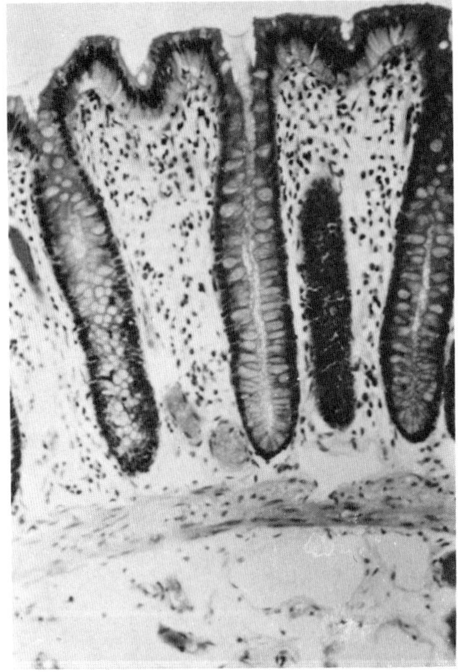

Fig. 3. Normally, cells migrate upward and differentiate into two main cell types; the goblet cells are prominent in the crypts and the absorptive cells are more evident on the free surface.

the different characteristics of hyperplasia vs. neoplasia that these two kinds of proliferations have such a different meaning in terms of the subsequent development of large bowel cancer. Fortunately, these two types are easily distinguished histologically (Lane and Lev, 1963; Lane *et al.*, 1971; Kaye *et al.*, 1973; Fenoglio and Lane, 1974).

3.1.1. *Hyperplasia*

Grossly, hyperplastic polyps appear as sessile discrete smoothly rounded "dewdrop" elevations and almost always are less than 5 mm (Fig. 4). Microscopically, the excessive number of cells results in papillary infoldings of the epithelium within the crypts, producing the typical serrated or corkscrew appearance of the glands (Fig. 5). In support of the idea that this is merely a hyperplastic process one sees that differentiation into goblet and absorptive

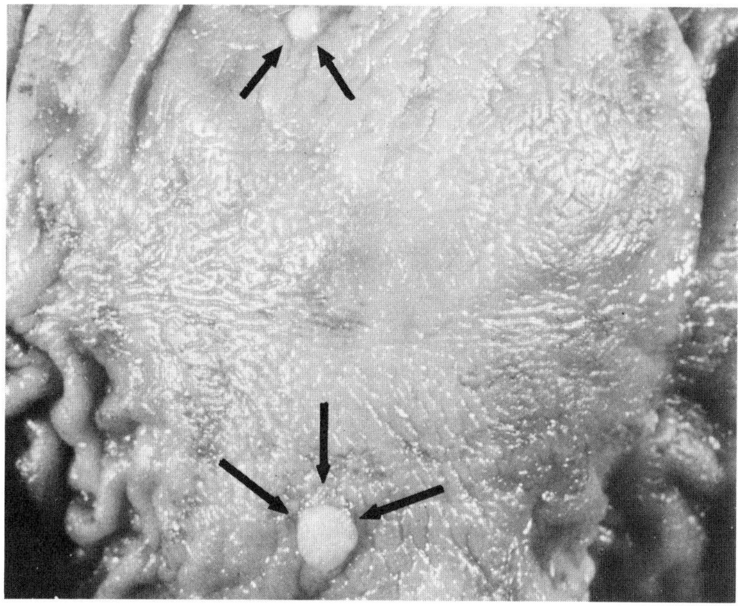

Fig. 4. Hyperplastic polyps usually measure a few millimeters in diameter and have a discrete "dewdrop" appearance.

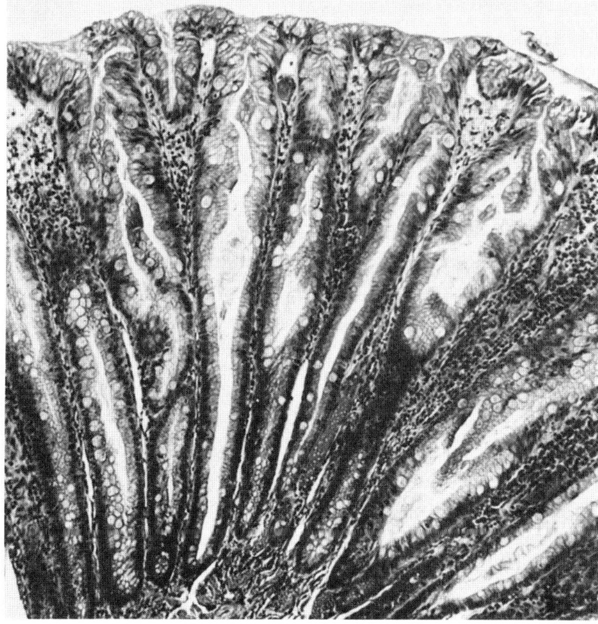

Fig. 5. In hyperplastic polyps, the papillary infolding of the epithelium is typical. The important point is that differentiation into goblet and absorptive cells is similar to normal.

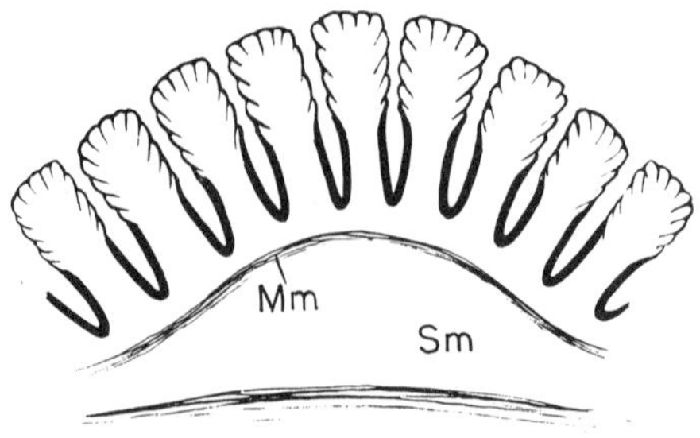

Fig. 6. The heavy lines show that in hyperplastic polyps, as in normal mucosa, the zone of replication remains restricted to the lower portion of the crypts. Reprinted from *Cancer 34*:819–823 (1974).

cells is indistinguishable from normal. This correlates with the fact that in this hyperplastic lesion, cell division remains restricted to the lower portions of the crypts—as in the normal (Fig. 6). Cell differentiation and restriction of cell division in a manner similar to the normal are important characteristics of nonneoplastic tissue.

An additional histological feature concerns an associated "hyperplastic" connective tissue change. Excess collagen production results in a thickening of the basement membrane beneath the surface epithelium. The dynamics of this phenomenon and how it contrasts with the situation in adenomas are discussed later and are illustrated in Fig. 17.

3.1.2. Benign Neoplasia

Grossly, adenomas are most commonly pedunculated. They may be bulky and sessile, or, rarely, flat and plaquelike (Fig. 7a,b,c). Unlike the hyperplastic polyps, their size may vary from minute to huge. Several histological patterns occur; either a tubular or a villous (papillary) appearance may be present, or these patterns may be combined (Fig. 8).

Regardless of the variety of gross and microscopic patterns, the basic characteristics of the cells composing the adenomas are the same. In general, the adenomatous epithelium is tall, very crowded, and produces a "picket fence" pattern with a marked increase in the nuclear cytoplasmic ratio (Fig. 9). Correlated with this nuclear change is a failure of orderly differentiation into goblet and absorptive cells. This in turn reflects the fact that in adenomas the control mechanisms governing DNA synthesis are largely lost, so that thymidine uptake and cell division occur at all levels in adenomatous tissue (Figs. 10 and 11). This last is perhaps the cardinal feature indicating the neoplastic nature of adenomas.

Both morphologically and dynamically these cells are indistinguishable from the partially differentiated cells which constitute the replicating population of the normal colonic crypt (Kaye *et al.*, 1973).

3.2. Associated Connective Tissue Features

Some years ago our group became interested in certain specific and contrasting connective tissue changes in hyperplastic polyps and adenomas (Pas-

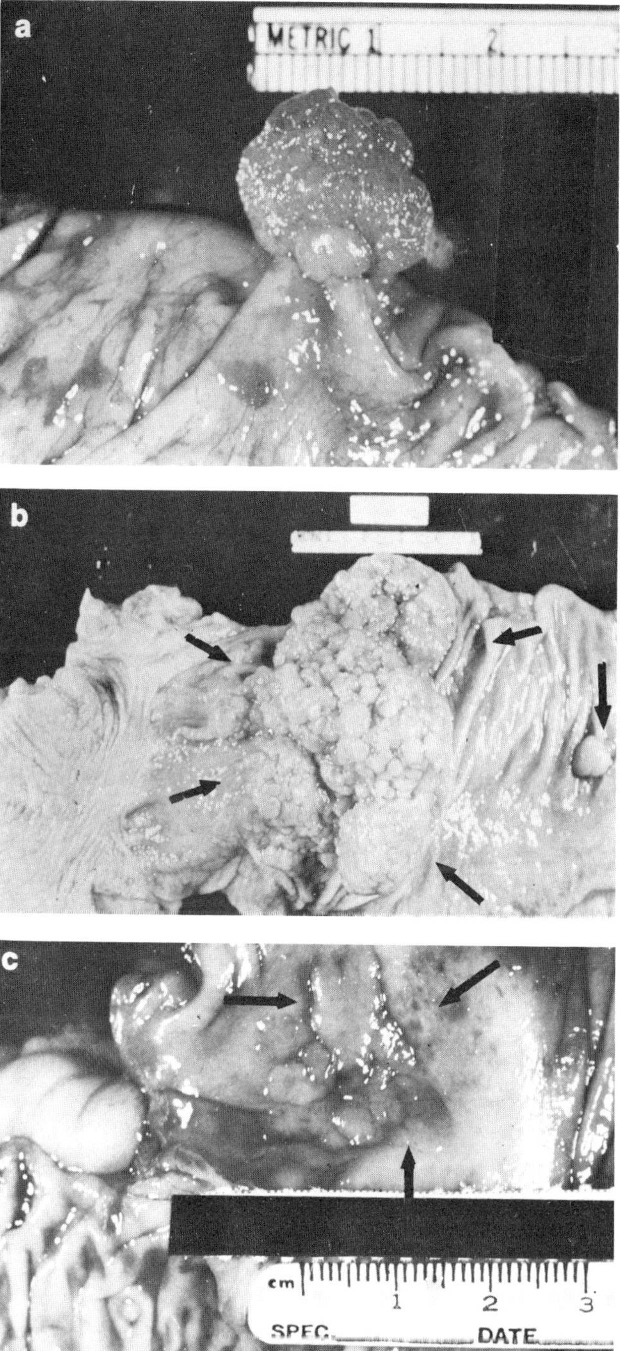

Fig. 7. The three typical gross appearances of adenomas. (a) Pedunculated adenoma. (b) Sessile adenomas. A bulky sessile adenoma, also known as papillary or villous adenoma, is in the center. A small rounded sessile adenoma is seen at the extreme right. (c) Flat, plaquelike adenoma.

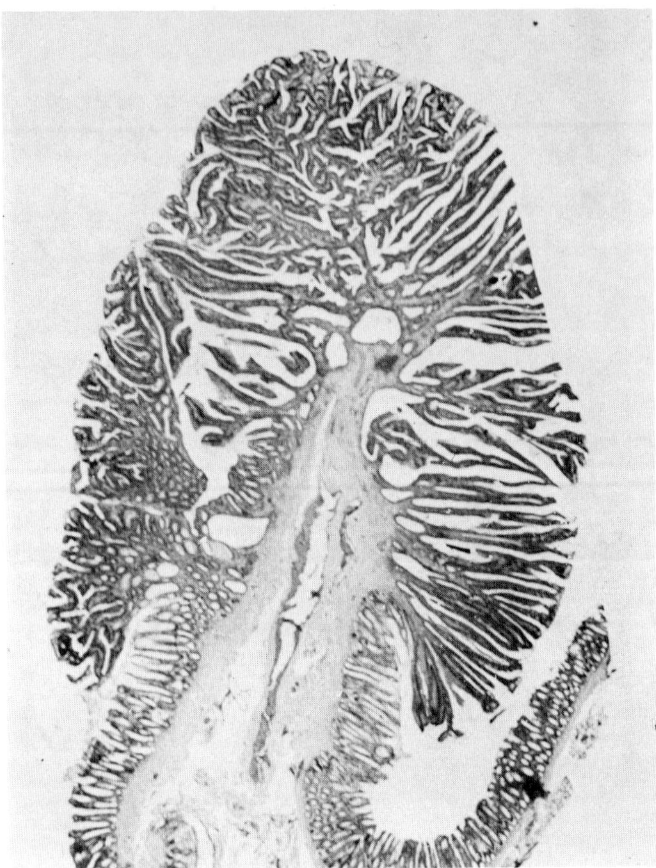

Fig. 8. Pedunculated adenoma with both papillary fronds and tubular areas. Reprinted from *Int Abstr. Surg. 106:*519–538 (1958).

cal *et al.,* 1968; Kaye *et al.,* 1968, 1971). The normal crypt is tightly invested by a sheath of fibroblasts, apparently directly apposed to the epithelium, with minimal collagen between the fibroblasts and epithelial cells (Fig. 12a,b). However, at the mouth of the crypt, and especially under the free surface epithelium, one observers a rather uniform band of collagen (Fig. 13). Because of its position, as though it were supporting the surface epithelium, we called this the collagen table. Based on autoradiographic and electron microscopic studies, it was noted that the fibroblasts around the bottom of the crypt picked up thymidine, indicating replication at the same crypt level at which the epithelial cells replicated. Furthermore, they migrated "upward" (and differentiated) synchronously with the epithelium. In the normal mucosa, as is the case with the epithelium, they lost the ability to pick up thymidine and replicate at the surface. These features are summarized in Fig. 14.

In adenomas the fibroblasts beneath the surface epithelium remain immature and show thymidine uptake—just like the adenomatous epithelium

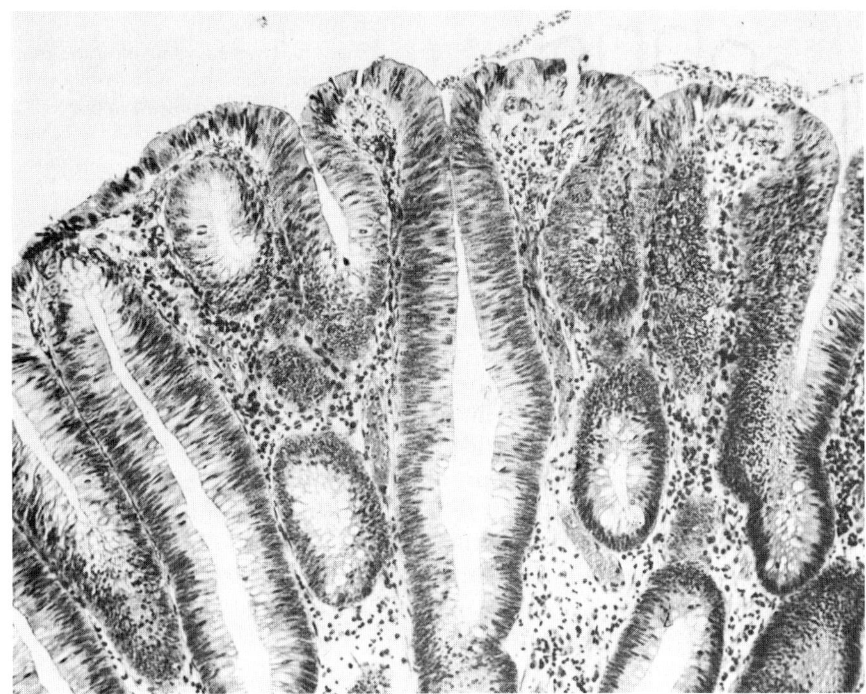

Fig. 9. In adenomas there tends to be uniformity of the epithelium. The crowding of elongated nuclei produces the typical "picket fence" appearance. Orderly differentiation into goblet and absorptive cells is largely lost. Reprinted from *Gastroenterology 60:*537–551 (1971).

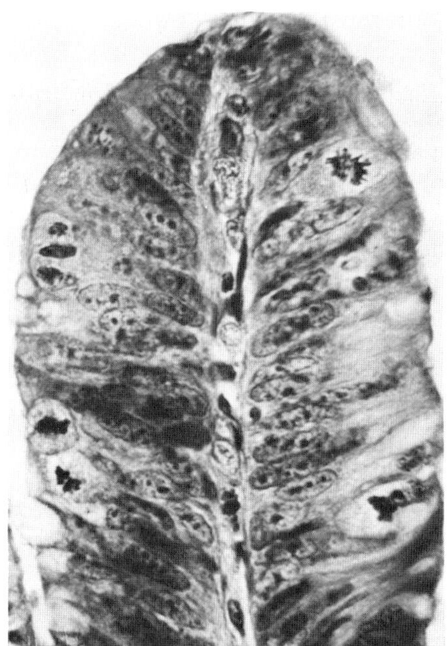

Fig. 10. In an adenoma, mitotic activity may be seen at all levels—even at the free surface. Reprinted from *Gastroenterology 60:*537–551 (1971).

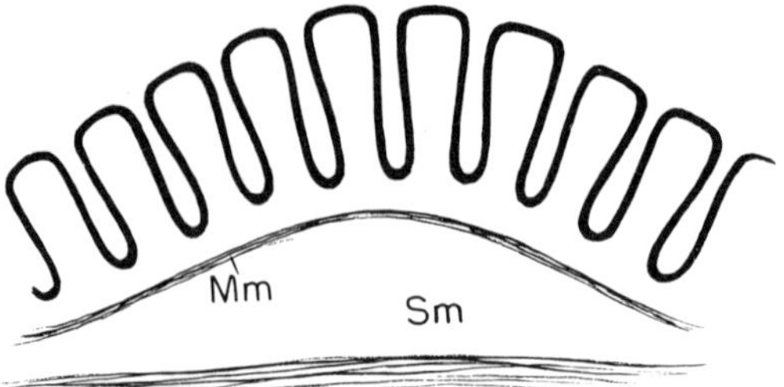

Fig. 11. The heavy line indicates that in adenomas the zone of cell replication is *not* restricted. In contrast to normal mucosa and hyperplastic polyps, cell replication occurs in all regions of adenomatous epithelium. The loss of control of replication confirms the neoplastic nature of adenomas. Reprinted from *Cancer 34:*819–323 (1974).

(Fig. 15). The collagen table is only minimally produced by these immature subepithelial fibroblasts, causing the collagen table to be *thinner* than that under the normal adjacent epithelium (Fig. 16). In contrast, in hyperplastic polyps, underneath the fully differentiated and hyperplastic surface epithelium, mature fibroblasts produce a collagen table that is also "hyperplastic" and, as in Fig. 17, is *thicker* than the adjacent normal collagen table. This epithelial–fibroblast partnership is further shown by the fact that the point of thickening or thinning of the collagen table corresponds precisely with the point of epithelial junction between normal and hyperplastic or normal and adenomatous epithelium.

These contrasting connective tissue changes further emphasize the fundamentally different nature of hyperplastic polyps and adenomas.

3.3. The Anatomical Origin of Adenomas

By using serial sections, Bussey (1975) has been able to detect adenomatous transformation of single crypts in grossly normal mucosal areas in familial polyposis specimens. In effect, he has demonstrated "unicryptal" adenomas. In similar grossly normal areas in familial polyposis cases, Deschner and Lipkin (1975) have found occasional crypts which, although histologically normal, show thymidine uptake continuing at or near the surface. This evidence suggests a failure of those control mechanisms in the deep portion of the crypt which normally restrict replication to this site. It may be the earliest known demonstration of an abnormality which reflects the transformation of normal to adenomatous epithelium.

Although adenomas ultimately may assume a wide variety of sizes, shapes, and histological patterns, it seems that at their inception all of them have the same morphology. In studying minute adenomas (Lane and Lev, 1963), one observes a small number of crypts which are completely adenomatous. Furthermore, the surface of these minute adenomas remains smooth (Fig. 18a). The latter indicates that at the outset no adenomatous tubules or papillary fronds preferentially grow from the free surface with preservation of normal colonic crypts below. When these minute adenomas (1–2 mm) are systematically studied with serial sections, one always observes that at the central point of origin of the lesion the *full depth* of a few crypts is adenomatous. It is only in random sections away from the center of the lesion that one may gain the misleading impression that the adenomatous epithelium has arisen in the upper portions of the crypts (Fig. 18b,c). This superficial position of the adenomatous epithelium toward the periphery of the adenoma is simply the result of spread of the adenomatous epithelium from the central nidus of origin (Fig. 19).

The above observations support the following hypothesis regarding the precise site of origin of adenomatous epithelium in a crypt. It is known that in normal growth, cell division, occurring deep in the crypt, is a controlled process which gives rise to daughter cells that have been programmed to migrate "upward" and *stop* synthesizing DNA. If, in this replicating zone, normal control mechanisms fail, an abnormal daughter cell population will result. Such cells will *continue* to synthesize DNA even after migrating "upwards." However, since it is in the deep one-third of the crypt that the original loss of control has taken place, this is the primary site of origin of the abnormally replicating adenomatous cell population. It is only subsequent to this that the ongoing cell division in the entire crypt results in a sufficient number of adenomatous cells so that we are able to recognize that an adenoma has developed.

3.4. Size, Shape, and Histological Pattern Relationships

In contrast to the hyperplastic polyps, almost all of which are minute and sessile, in various adenomas there are several statistical correlations to be noted among size, shape, and histological patterns (Morson, 1974).

The average small adenoma, i.e., in the size range of approximately 1–1.5 cm, tends to be pedunculated and to have a tubular pattern. Among larger adenomas, a greater proportion tend to be sessile and have a papillary (villous) pattern microscopically. As discussed below, it is the larger adenomas that are the most significant as a precancerous tissue.

3.5. Absolute and Relative Frequencies

Among older adults who are repeatedly examined sigmoidoscopically over many years, "polyps" may be found in as many as 25% (Gilbertsen *et al.*, 1965). Complete colon examination at autopsy has disclosed "polyps" in 50% of these specimens (Chapman, 1963).

However, of greater importance than absolute figures such as these is an understanding of *relative* frequency. Hyperplastic polyps are at least 10 times as frequent as all adenomas (Arthur, 1968) and in turn small adenomas (i.e., <1.5 cm) are about 10 times as common as large adenomas (Fenoglio and Lane, 1974). Thus the large adenomas represent only about 1% of all large bowel "polyps."

Since the frequency of all benign proliferations is so great, unless they are classified as described in the preceding pages according to their type, size, and relative frequency, no relationship to carcinoma is statistically discernible. Unfortunately, the term "polyp" is often used indiscriminately. However, with

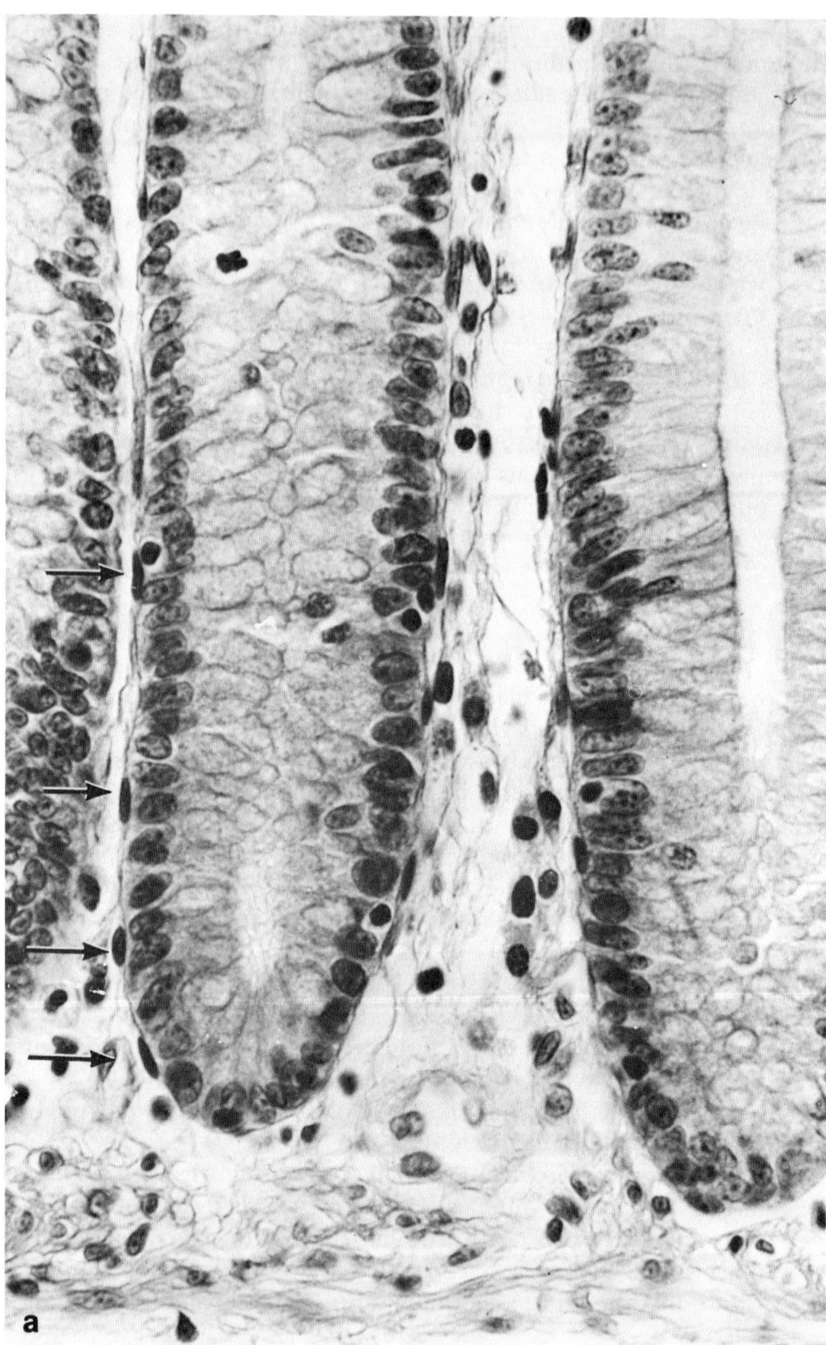

Fig. 12. Sagittal section (a) and cross-section (b) of normal colonic crypts. Note the sheath of flattened fibroblast nuclei closely investing the epithelium. These appear as a chain of elongated nuclei in (a) and as a complete ring in (b). Other cells of the lamina propria appear to be randomly distributed. Reprinted from *Gastroenterology 54:*835–851 (1968).

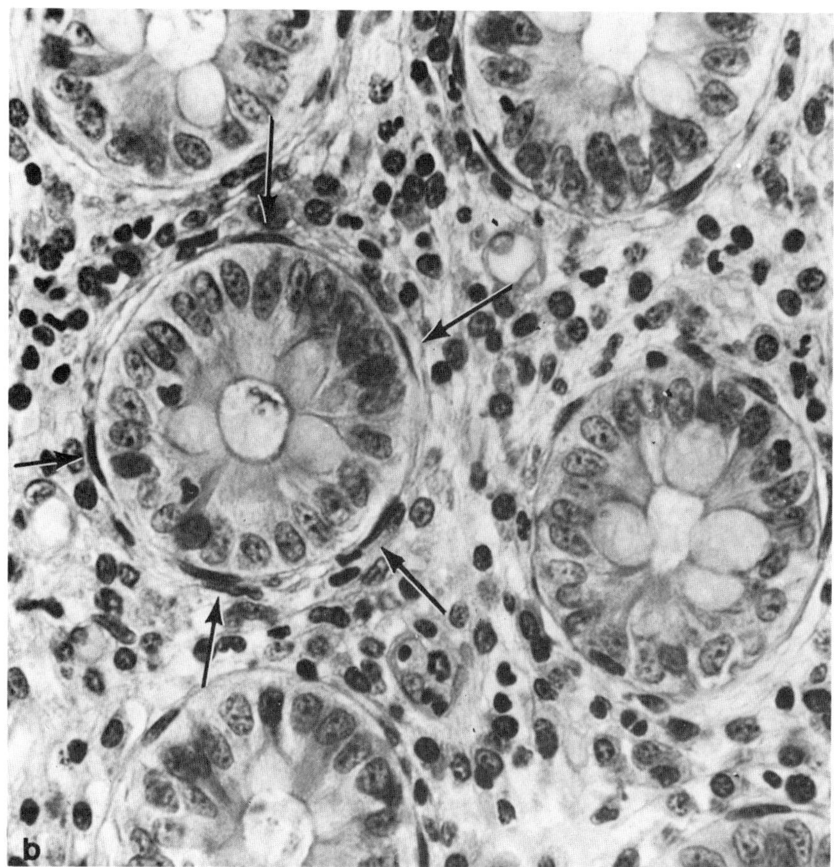

Fig. 12. *(continued)*

an understanding of their proper classification one can critically evaluate such questions as the overall frequency of "polyps," their distribution relative to carcinoma in the colon, and, most important, the incidence with which carcinoma may be found in "polyps."

4. *Focal Carcinoma in Benign Proliferations*

There are several practical anatomical features that clinicians and pathologists should understand concerning the frequency with which focal carcinoma may be found in benign proliferations.

The significance of hyperplastic polyps is readily disposed of since foci of carcinoma and/or adenoma are (almost) never found in these lesions. It is generally agreed that they have no statistically significant relationship as a precursor tissue to either carcinoma or adenoma; nonetheless, it seems to be correct that they are frequently found in colons bearing adenomas and/or carcinomas as anatomically separate lesions.

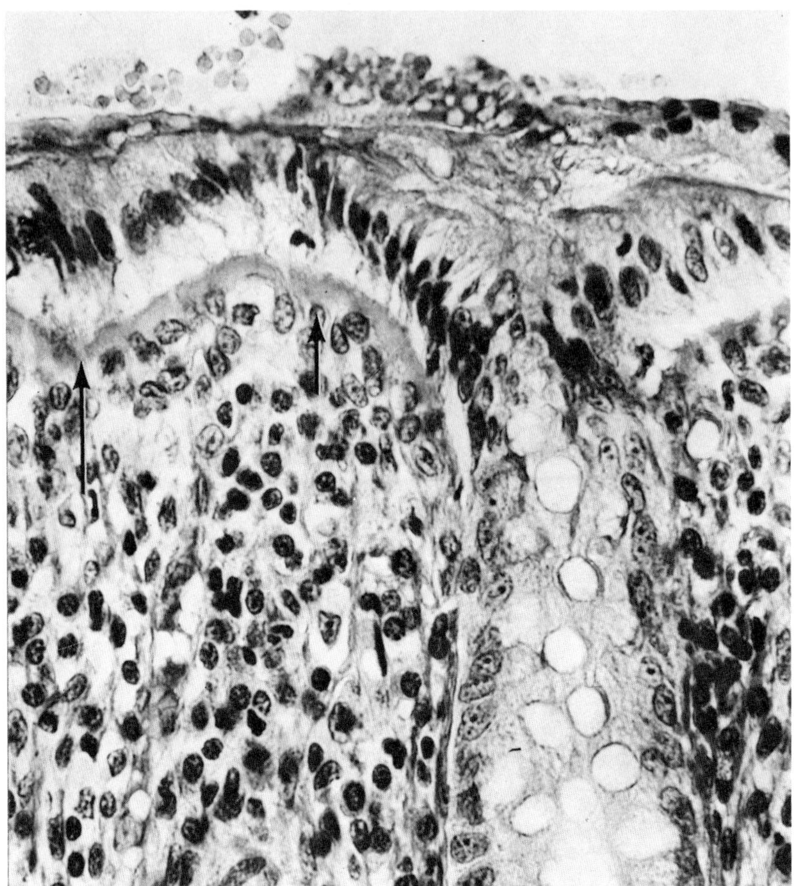

Fig. 13. At the surface of normal colonic mucosa, functional differentiation of the pericryptal fibroblast sheath is manifested by the production of a well-defined collagen table (arrows). Fewer fibroblast nuclei are seen under the absorptive epithelium of the surface. Reprinted from *Gastroenterology* *54*:835–851 (1968).

The question of focal carcinoma in adenomas is more complex. Clinically significant focal carcinoma is found with sufficient frequency in larger adenomas so that they may be considered to be precancerous lesions. However, to comprehend critically any claim as to the frequency with which carcinoma may be found in adenomas, it is mandatory to distinguish between intramucosal (*in situ*) and invasive carcinoma, since intramucosal carcinoma must be excluded for statistical purposes.

Clear-cut examples of intramucosal carcinoma *do* exist and are individually important because they are the most minimal form and stage in which carcinoma can be recognized. However, statistics that include intramucosal carcinoma in calculating the frequency of carcinoma in adenomas are without practical value, for two reasons. First, the distinction between atypia and in-

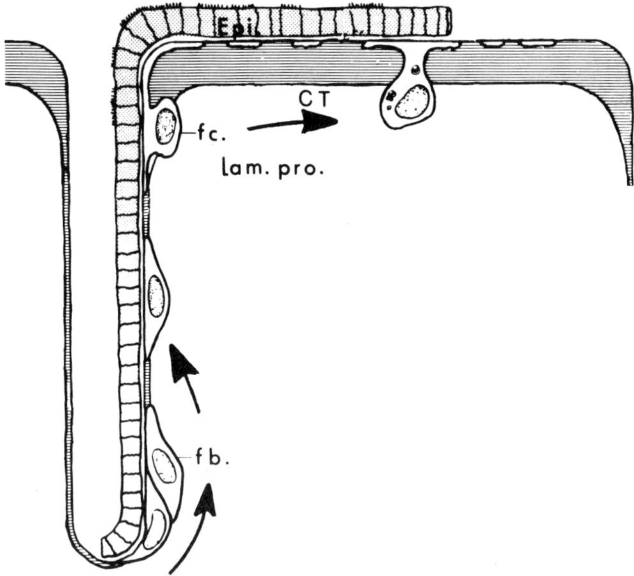

Fig. 14. Migration and maturation of the pericryptal fibroblast sheath in normal colonic mucosa. As in the epithelium, replication of fibroblasts (fb) is restricted to the deep zone of the crypt. As the fibroblasts migrate in synchrony with the epithelium, they too stop dividing and differentiate into functioning fibrocytes (fc), producing the normal collagen table (CT, hatched area).

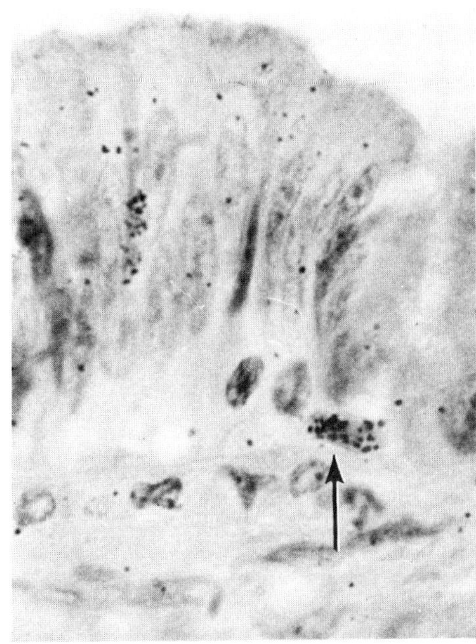

Fig. 15. Autoradiography of adenomatous mucosa shows uptake of tritiated thymidine by nuclei of both the surface adenomatous epithelial cells and subjacent immature fibroblasts (arrow). Reprinted from *Gastroenterology 54*:835–851 (1968).

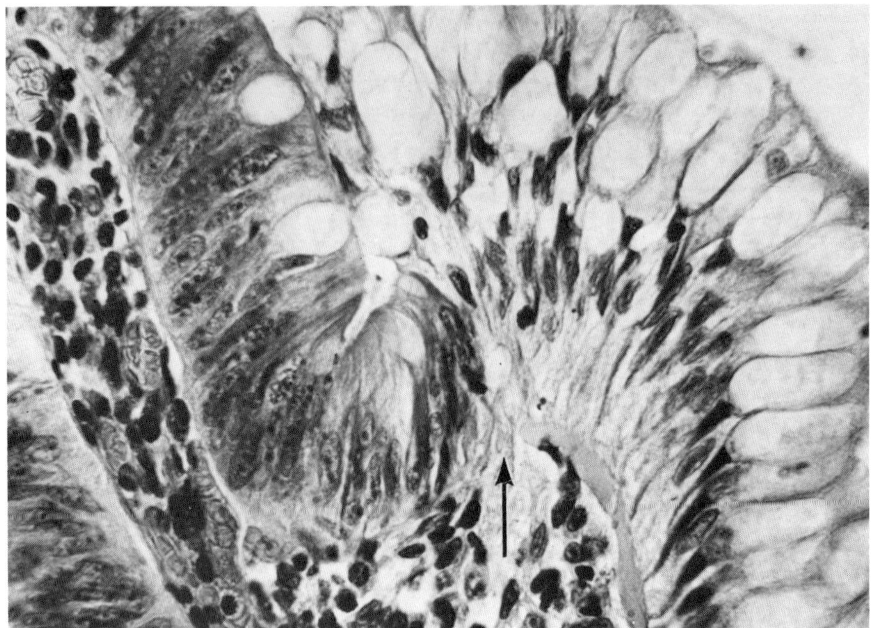

Fig. 16. Junction (arrow) of adenomatous (left) and normal (right) epithelium. There is so little collagen production under the adenomatous epithelium that the collagen table is thin and indistinct. A well-developed collagen table is seen under the normal epithelium. Reprinted from *Gastroenterology 60:*537–551 (1971).

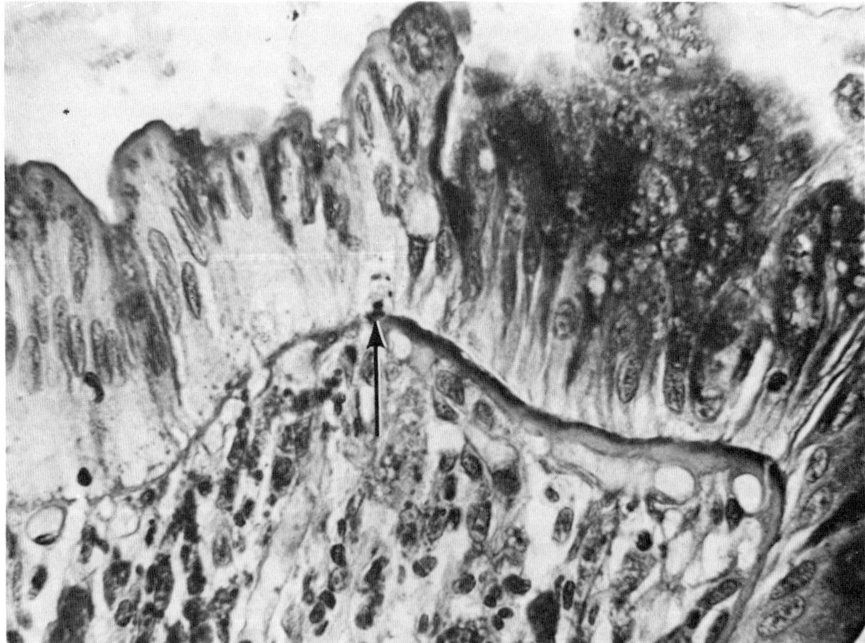

Fig. 17. Junction (arrow) of edge of hyperplastic polyp (right) and normal (left) epithelium. There is an overproduction of collagen, resulting in a greatly thickened collagen table under the surface epithelium of hyperplastic polyps. Reprinted from *Gastroenterology 60:*537–551 (1971).

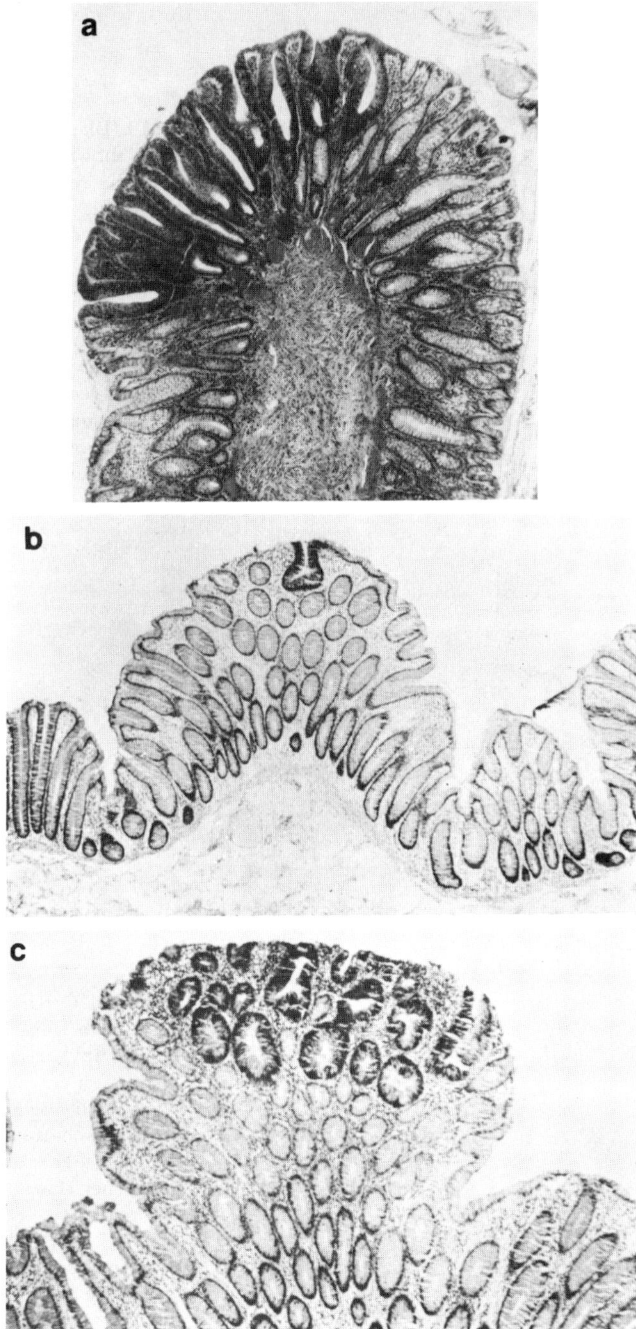

Fig. 18. Three sections through a small adenoma. (a) Sagittal section through the center of a minute adenoma. It is evident that the neoplastic cells extend from the bases of the crypts to the smooth surface. In (b), from the edge of the lesion, it would appear as if the adenomatous epithelium were arising in the superficial portion of a single crypt. In (c), closer to but not yet at the center of the lesion, the adenomatous crypts still appear to arise superficially. Reprinted from *Cancer 16:*751–764 (1963).

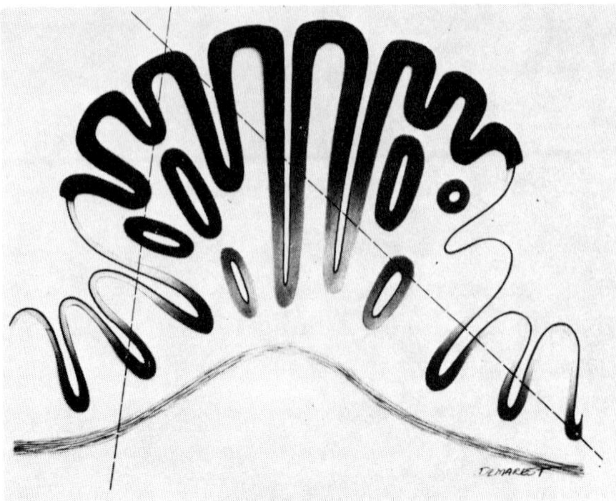

Fig. 19. Diagram of the adenoma shown in Fig. 18. The neoplastic cells, which probably arise in the base of one central crypt, spread centrifugally to replace other crypts. Histological sections not from the center of the lesion—such as indicated by the broken lines—can produce the appearances of Fig. 18b,c. Such off-center sections would give the misleading impression that adenomatous epithelium arises superficially. Reprinted from *Cancer 16:*751–764 (1963).

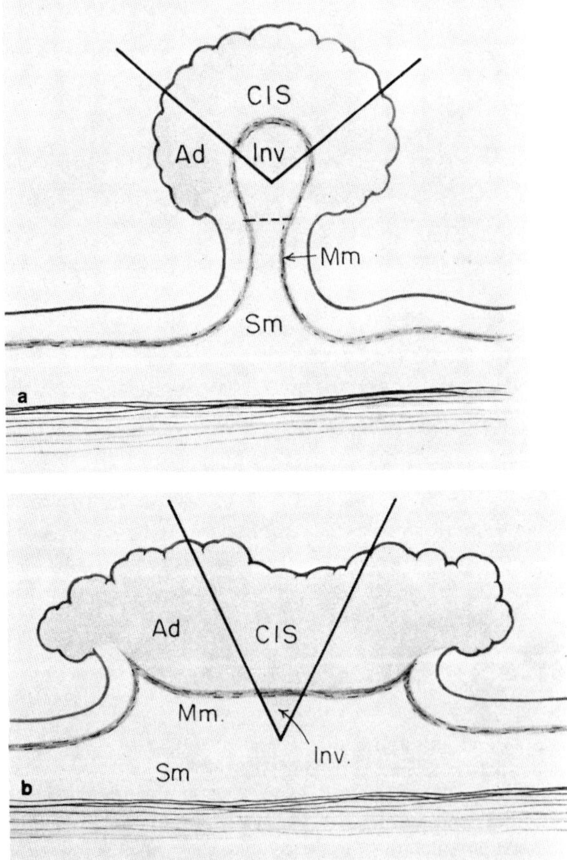

Fig. 20(a). Carcinoma *in situ* (CIS) with focal invasive carcinoma (Inv) arising in a pedunculated adenoma (Ad). The wedge of invasive cancer is confined to the submucosa of the head of the adenoma. At this stage, metastases can occur but are very rare. Reprinted from *Cancer 34:*819–823 (1974). (b) Focal invasive carcinoma arising in a sessile adenoma involves the submucosa of the bowel wall as soon as it crosses the muscularis mucosae. There is a greater frequency of metastasis from focal carcinoma in sessile (villous) adenomas than in pedunculated (polypoid) adenomas. Reprinted from *Cancer 34:*819–823 (1974).

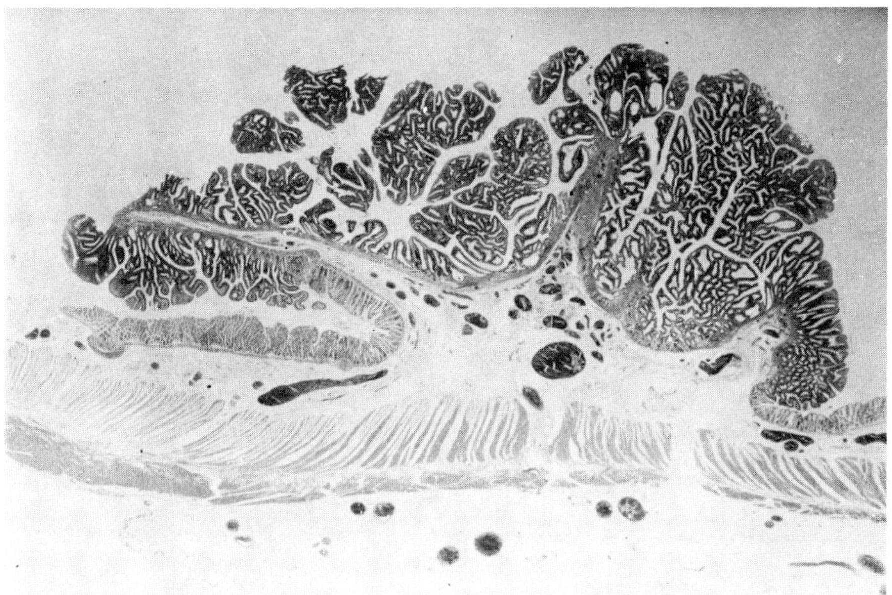

Fig. 21. A sessile adenoma of the papillary-villous type (note the proximity of the base of the lesion to the richly vascularized submucosa). This shows that with properly prepared sections one can precisely trace the muscularis mucosae, even when it follows a complex pathway, as in this specimen.

tramucosal carcinoma is imprecise. Second, intramucosal carcinoma by itself, i.e., without invasion across the muscularis mucosae, does not metastasize. Therefore, it is not *clinically* significant at the time it is observed in a specimen. Thus for the practical purpose of conservatively evaluating the frequency with which carcinoma may be found in adenomas, only lesions showing invasion should be counted as being clinically significant. Figures 20a, 20b, 21, 22a, and 22b show that, just as in the normal mucosa, in both pedunculated and sessile adenomas it is the muscularis mucosae that is the dividing line between an intramucosal and an invasive neoplasm.

Remembering that small adenomas are about 10 times as common as large adenomas, the frequency of focal invasive carcinoma is approximately as follows: Focal invasive carcinoma occurs but is very rare in small adenomas. However, it may be found in 10% or more of larger adenomas. The likelihood of finding carcinoma increases with the size of the adenomas together with the tendency of the larger adenomas to be sessile and have villous (papillary) features (Morson, 1974; Fenoglio and Lane, 1974). Thus the subgroup "larger adenomas" may be considered a statistically signfiicant precursor tissue for large bowel carcinoma.

The chance of encountering focal invasive cancer among *all* benign proliferations, including the hyperplastic polyps, is inconsequential—perhaps 0.1 of 1%. Hence the necessity to subclassify them as to type, frequency, and size. These relationships are summarized in Table 1.

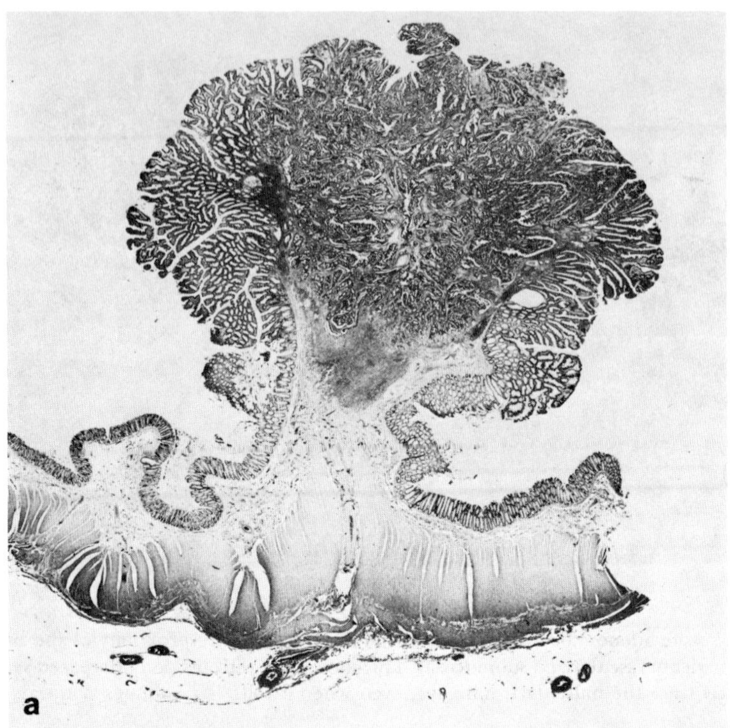

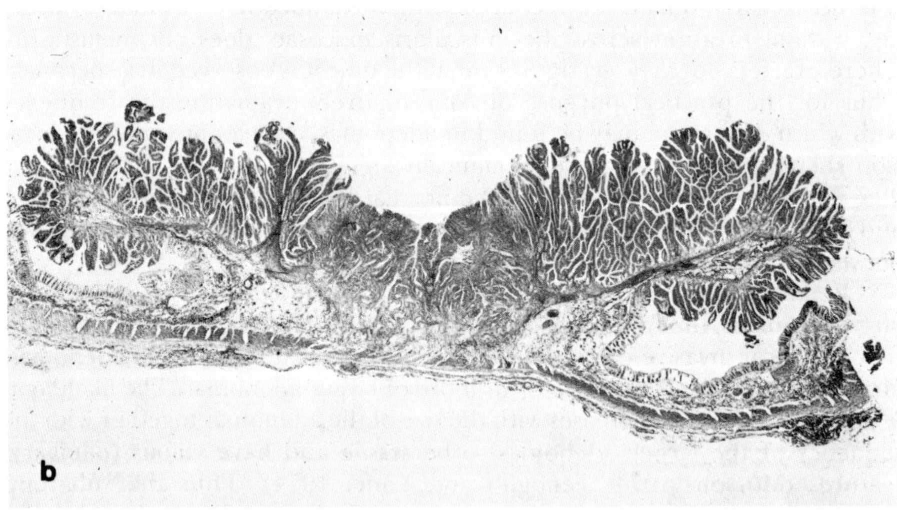

Fig. 22(a). Invasive carcinoma arising in a pedunculated adenoma. As diagrammatically illustrated in Fig. 20a, it is clear that the cancer has crossed the muscularis mucosae but has invaded only the submucosa of the head of the adenoma. Reprinted from *Gastroenterology 64:*51–66 (1974). (b). Again using the muscularis mucosae as a boundary, it is evident in this sessile adenoma that an invasive focus of cancer has invaded the colonic submucosa. This corresponds to the diagram in Fig. 20b.

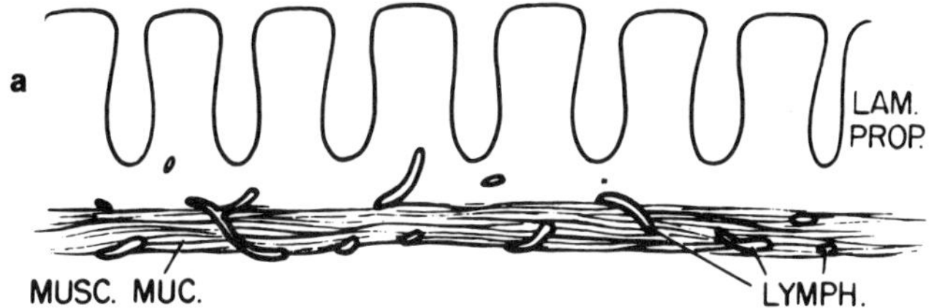

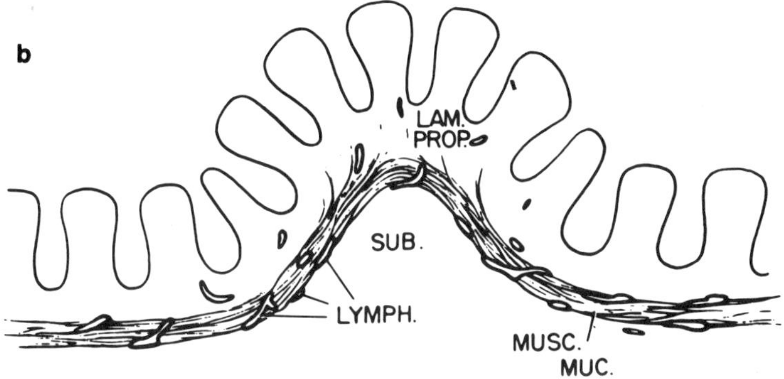

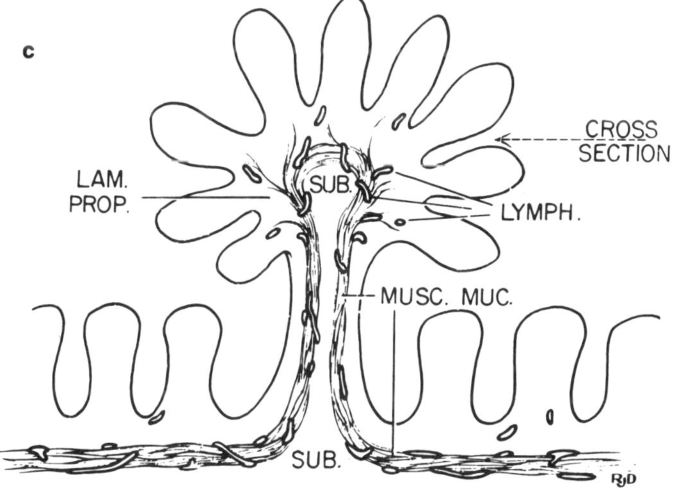

Fig. 23. Distribution of mucosal lymphatics in normal colon (a), hyperplastic polyps (b), and adenomas (c). (a) The normal colonic mucosa shows a lymphatic plexus around the muscularis mucosae. From this, some blind loops extend upward for a short distance into the lamina propria, but no lymphatics are seen above the level of the base of the crypts. (b) In hyperplastic polyps the basic anatomical relationships are preserved. The major change is an architectural one in which the fibers of the muscularis are elevated. (c) In the adenomas there is a disorganization of the fibers of the muscularis mucosae and the distribution of lymphatics is preserved. Reprinted from *Gastroenterology 64:*51–66 (1973).

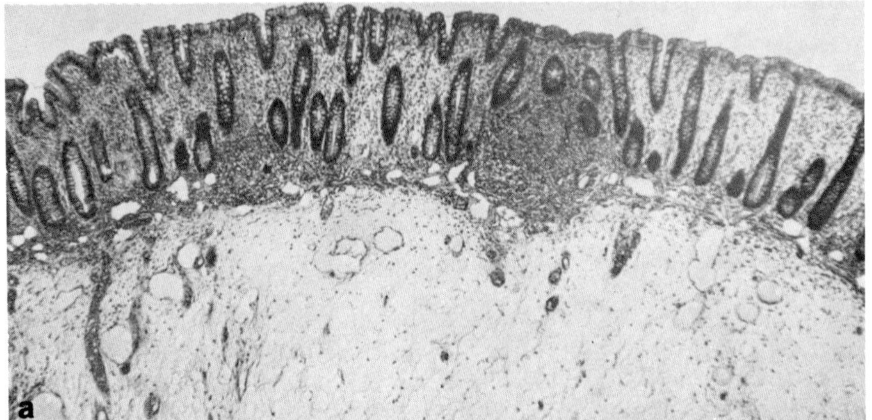
a
b

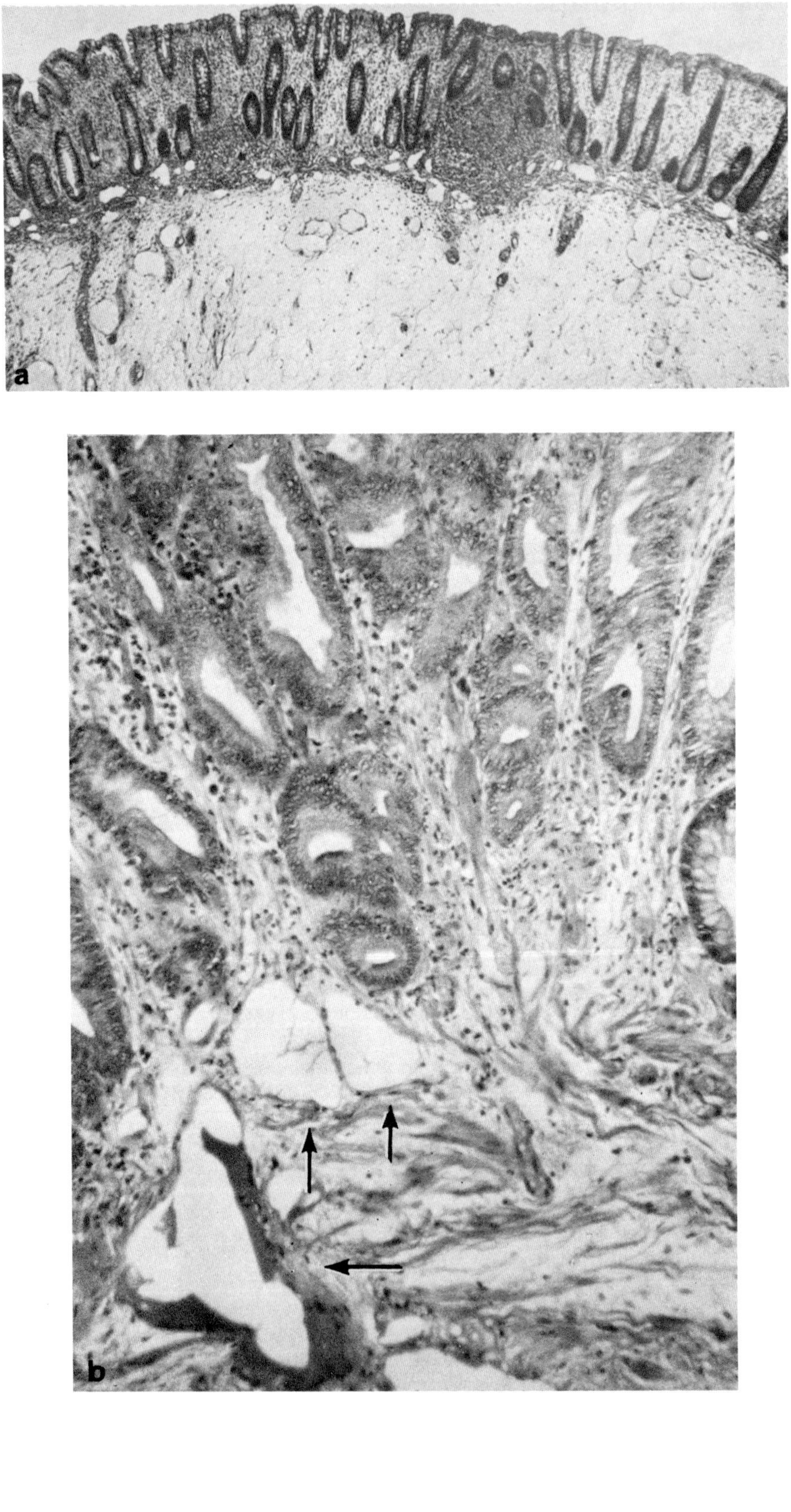

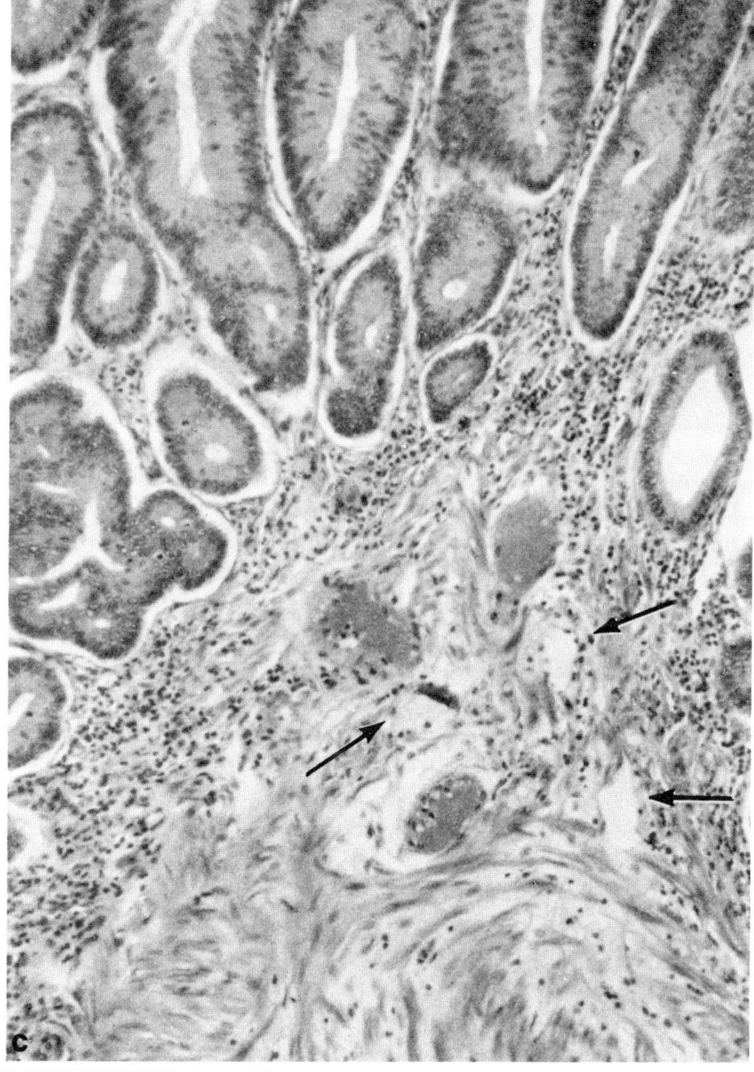

Fig. 24. (a) In normal mucosa the most superficial lymphatics form a plexus at the level of the muscularis mucosae. ×50. (b,c) At the base of the hyperplastic polyps (b) superficial fibers of the muscularis mucosae with their associated lymphatics may be "pulled up" a short distance toward the intercryptal lamina propria. In adenomas (c), elevation of the neoplastic crypts and "pulling up" of fibers of the muscularis mucosae (M) may be quite marked and lymphatics may accompany them (arrows). (b) ×88; (c) ×88. Reprinted from *Gastroenterology 61*:51–66 (1973).

Table 1. Classification and Approximate Frequency of Randomly Chosen "Polyps": Significance of Size

Of 1000 "polyps," there will be
900 hyperplastic polyps,
90 small adenomas (focal carcinoma is rare),
10 large adenomas, of which
1 will have invasive carcinoma.
Thus incidence of invasive carcinoma = 0.1% in all "polyps"
but = 10% in the large adenomas.

5. Relationship of Mucosal Lymphatics and Metastasis

Because the colonic mucosa is so richly vascularized, the absence of metastasis from intramucosal carcinoma in an adenoma is of some interest. A partial explanation emerged from a study of the distribution of colonic mucosal lymphatics, particularly in adenomatous tissue (Fenoglio *et al.,* 1973). Initially, specimens of colonic carcinoma showing extensive intramural lymphatic spread were studied. Even with extensive intramural lymphatic permeation by cancer cells, the lamina propria of the normal mucosa never showed lymphatic involvement. This enigma prompted a light and electron microscopic study of the lamina propria of more than 20 specimens each of normal mucosa, hyperplastic polyps, and adenomatous polyps. The ultrastructural criteria for distinguishing lymphatics from capillaries are well established (Fenoglio *et al.,* 1973). The findings in each tissue indicated that lymphatics are absent in the mucosal lamina propria superficial to the muscularis mucosa. Although electron microscopic observation proves this with the greatest precision, the results are best visualized in the dimensions of conventional histology (Figs. 23 and 24). In brief, the findings were that the lamina propria in each case is without lymphatics.

Thus intramucosal carcinoma in adenomas does not gain access to lymphatics until it reaches the level of muscularis mucosae. In most adenomas the distance from the adenomatous surface to its muscularis mucosae is many times the distance from the surface of normal mucosa to its muscularis mucosae (Figs. 20a, 20b, and 21). Therefore, should a focus of carcinoma arise near the surface of a large adenoma, it may grow to considerable size before reaching the muscularis mucosae and the lymphatics at this level. The lamina propria of adenomas is richly endowed with blood capillaries and why intramucosal carcinoma does not metastasize via these channels is completely unknown.

6. The Origin of Large Bowel Carcinoma

Has *de novo* carcinoma—as defined in modern terms of cellular dimensions—really been observed? Thus far in this chapter we have documented that certain adenomas, i.e., the larger ones, are a significant precursor tissue to ordinary large bowel carcinoma. The question remains

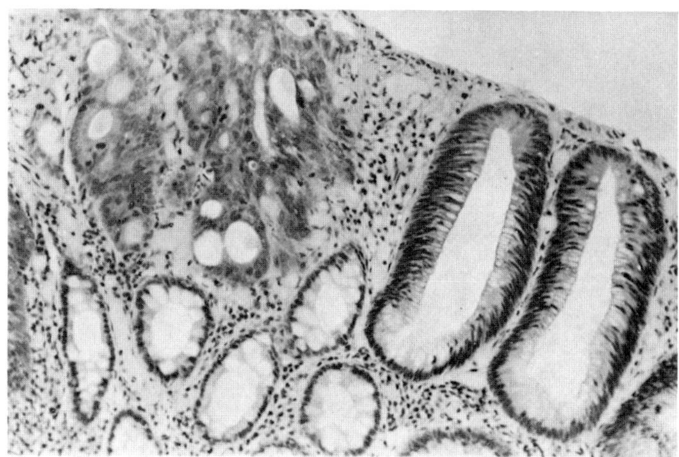

Fig. 25. A small focus of purely intramucosal carcinoma (upper left) arising in a flat adenoma under 0.5 cm in diameter. Further growth of the carcinoma would probably have obliterated the adenomatous epithelium on the right.

whether all or almost all ordinary carcinoma evolves via adenomatous tissue or whether it arises *de novo.* In terms of modern cell biology, the expression "*de novo* carcinoma" means that from the epithelium of a normal crypt(s) there occurs a direct one-step transformation into microscopically recognizable cancerous epithelium and glands.

Some years ago the *de novo* concept was given impetus by a study of 20 "small" cancers in which thorough study disclosed no associated adenomatous tissue (Spratt and Ackerman, 1962). "Small carcinomas," which were accepted as *de novo,* were defined as any lesion up to *2 cm.* At that time this was considered small enough to reflect the morphology of the neoplastic process at its origin. Actually, only two of the 20 carcinomas were 5 mm or less, while the majority were between 1 and 2 cm. All the lesions had already become invasive. When carcinomas have reached such a size and stage, they may no longer be an accurate reflection of the morphology of the neoplasm at the time of its cellular origin. Therefore, it is impossible to decide whether such carcinomas did or did not arise in antecedent adenomatous tissue, which was then destroyed by the growth of the carcinoma. Thinking in terms of the cellular origin of neoplasia, a 1–2 *cm* cancer is already a large lesion.

At present, attitudes on this subject are more in keeping with the minute, even microscopic dimensions that are involved in the cellular origins of cancer. Therefore, a "small" lesion, to be acceptable as representing the morphology of a neoplasm at its inception, should not be more than a few millimeters—or even a fraction of a millimeter—in size.

Our experience is the same as Morson's (1966); i.e., persisting adenomatous tissue is found in inverse proportion to the degree of advancement of the carcinoma. As had Morson, we too have observed residual adenomatous tissue quite commonly in small cancers, and we believe that as the invasive cancer progresses the adenomatous tissue is destroyed.

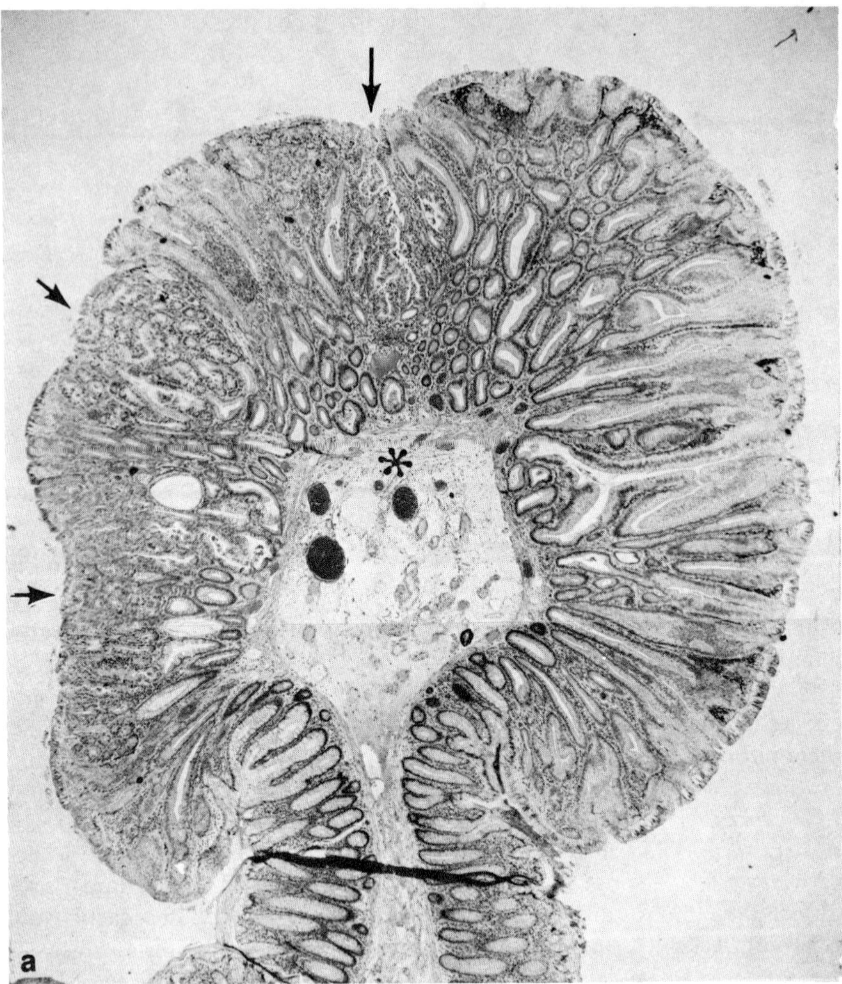

Fig. 26. Intraepithelial carcinoma plus focal invasive carcinoma, arising in a 5-mm adenoma (a). The intraepithelial carcinoma (arrows) has already replaced much of the adenomatous epithelium. At higher magnification (b), the disorganized, noninvasive carcinoma contrasts with the adenomatous glands. At one point in this adenoma [asterisk in (a)], but at a deeper level of sectioning, there was a focus of invasive carcinoma (c) which did not exceed 2 mm. Such foci of minute cancer (microcancer) have not been observed in normal, nonadenomatous mucosa.

Occasionally one encounters minute or microcancer in small adenomas. Such foci probably represent the most minimal stage or "degree" of cancer recognizable by present means. Figures 25 and 26 illustrate two examples of this phenomenon. The adenomas did not exceed 5 mm. One contained a zone of only intramucosal carcinoma (Fig. 25) while the other showed, in addition, an invasive focus, which did not exceed 2 mm (Fig. 26). Since neither adenoma exceeded 5 mm, it is evident that only minimal additional growth of

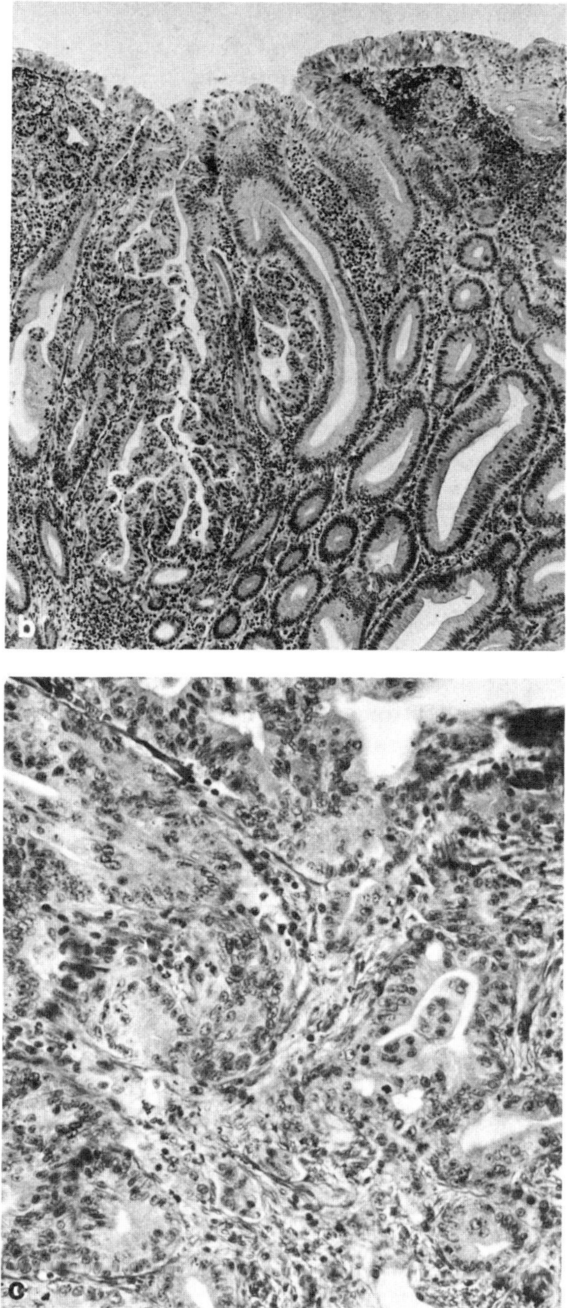

Fig. 26. *(continued)*

the carcinoma would have obliterated the evidence of the precursor adenomatous tissue.

Keeping in mind these very small dimensions, it seems that such foci of minute or microcancer are found only in adenomatous tissue. In this required minute size range, they simply have not been observed to date as a *de novo* process in normal nonadenomatous mucosa in spite of virtually unlimited opportunity to find them.

6.1. Relevance of Familial Polyposis

Familial polyposis is the natural human model for the study of ordinary bowel carcinomas since there is no known difference as far as morphogenesis is concerned between the adenomas and carcinomas in familial polyposis and in ordinary large bowel neoplasia.

The pathological evidence provided by familial polyposis specimens supports the idea that most carcinoma evolves via adenomatous tissue (Bussey, 1975). In such specimens minute and microscopic foci of carcinoma can be found—but they have been observed only in adenomas. On the other hand, foci of purely microscopic neoplasia, even as small as a single crypt, have been observed and proved to be only adenomas, not carcinomas. These observations are based on extensive microscopic study in polyposis cases of areas of grossly normal mucosa (Bussey, 1975). *De novo* carcinoma just does not seem to occur in familial polyposis—in spite of the tremendous predilection for carcinoma in this condition.

While much valuable information will be gained by the study of animal models, there is no evidence to suggest that large bowel neoplasms produced by carcinogen administration more accurately reflect the morphogenesis of ordinary large bowel cancer than what has been observed in familial polyposis. Indeed, unless new evidence causes us to downgrade familial polyposis as a model, it should be the yardstick against which experimental results should be measured.

6.2. Evidence from Periodic Sigmoidoscopy and Polypectomy in Relation to the Adenoma-Carcinoma Sequence

The 25-year study done at the University of Minnesota Cancer Detection Center appears to provide empirical proof for the contention that most ordinary adenocarcinoma arises from adenomatous tissue (Gilbertsen, 1974). That study involved periodic sigmoidoscopic examination of thousand of individuals with removal of mucosal protrusions. The statistically anticipated incidence of rectosigmoid carcinoma was reduced by 85%. It is not our purpose to discuss the pros and cons of the feasibility of such studies on a truly massive scale, but the experience from that clinic provides valuable empirical documentation for all the other evidence which suggests that the adenoma–carcinoma sequence is the usual pathway in the development of large bowel carcinoma.

7. Conclusion

From a *practical* point of view, the cardinal points of this chapter are concerned with ordinary moderately and well-differentiated adenocarcinoma and those benign proliferations of adults known as hyperplastic polyps and adenomas. These two benign lesions are separate and distinct, and their classification by type, size, and relative frequency is necessary. Hyperplastic polyps, which are unrelated to neoplasia, are 10 times as common as adenomas. In turn, small adenomas are 10 times as frequent as large adenomas so that these large adenomas constitute only about 1% of all the benign proliferations we are considering. Cancer, intramucosal and invasive, *can* occur in small adenomas, but only the large adenomas will harbor invasive cancer with significant frequency, i.e., 10% or more.

The cellular origin of cancer involves minute or microscopic dimensions. Hence a lesion to be acceptable as reflecting the morphology of a neoplasm at its inception must measure only a few millimeters or perhaps a fraction of a millimeter. *It is essential to accept the discipline of these minute dimensions,* and, in this case, we note that minute or microcancer is observed in adenomatous tissue but has not been reported as a *de novo* process in normal mucosa—in spite of unlimited opportunity to find it. The same applies to familial polyposis—even though there is a tremendous predilection for carcinoma in this condition. The University of Minnesota clinical study cited in the previous section of this chapter supports the above.

Until prevention of adenomas becomes an accomplished fact, the safe detection and removal of adenomatous tissue represent the most assured way of reducing the incidence of large bowel cancer.

8. References

Arthur, J. F., 1968, Structure and significance of metaplastic nodules in the rectal mucosa, *J. Clin. Pathol.* **21**:735–745.

Bussey, H. J. R., 1975, *Familial Polyposis Coli,* Johns Hopkins University Press, Baltimore.

Chapman, I., 1963, Adenomatous polypi of large intestine: Incidence and distribution, *Ann. Surg.* **157**:223–226.

Deschner, E. E., and Lipkin, M., 1975, Proliferative patterns in colonic mucosa in familial polyposis, *Cancer* **35**:413–418.

Fenoglio, C. M., and Lane, N., 1974, The anatomical precursor of colorectal carcinoma, *Cancer* **34**:819–823.

Fenoglio, C. M., Kaye, G. I., and Lane, N., 1973, Distribution of human colonic lymphatics in normal, hyperplastic, and adenomatous tissue, *Gastroenterology* **64**:51–66.

Gilbertsen, V. A., 1974, Proctosigmoidoscopy and polypectomy in reducing the incidence of rectal cancer, *Cancer* **34**:936–939.

Gilbertsen, V. A., Knatterud, G. L., Lober, P. H., and Wangensteen, O. H., 1965, Invasive carcinoma of the large intestine: A preventable disease? *Surgery* **57**:363–365.

Grinnell, R. S., and Lane, N., 1958, Benign and malignant adenomatous polyps and papillary adenomas of the colon and rectum. An analysis of 1,856 tumors in 1,335 patients, *Int. Abstr. Surg.* **106**:519–538.

Kaye, G. I., Lane, N., and Pascal, R. R., 1968, Colonic pericryptal fibroblast sheath: Replication, migration, and cytodifferentiation of a mesenchymal cell system in adult tissue, *Gastroenterology* **54:**852–865.

Kaye, G. I., Pascal, R. R., and Lane, N., 1971, The colonic pericryptal fibroblast sheath: Replication, migration, and cytodifferentiation of a mesenchymal cell system in adult tissue, *Gastroenterology* **60:**515–536.

Kaye, G. I., Fenoglio, C. M., Pascal, R. R., and Lane, N., 1973, Comparative electron microscopic features of normal, hyperplastic, and adenomatous human colonic epithelium, *Gastroenterology* **64:**926–945.

Lane, N., and Lev, R., 1963, Observations on the origin of adenomatous epithelium of the colon, *Cancer* **16:**751–764.

Lane, N., Kaplan, H., and Pascal, R. R., 1971, Minute adenomatous and hyperplastic polyps of the colon: Divergent patterns of epithelial growth with specific associated mesenchymal changes, *Gastroenterology* **60:**537–551.

Morson, B. C., 1966, Factors influencing the prognosis of early cancer of the rectum, *Proc. R. Soc. Med.* **59:**707.

Morson, B. C., 1974, The polyp-cancer sequence in the large bowel, *Proc. R. Soc. Med.* **67:**451–457.

Morson, B. C., and Bussey, H. J. R., 1970, *Predisposing Causes of Intestinal Cancer,* Year Book Medical Publishers, Chicago.

Pascal, R. R., Kaye, G. I., and Lane, N., 1968, Colonic pericryptal fibroblast sheath: Replication, migration, and cytodifferentiation of a mesenchymal cell system in adult tissue, *Gastroenterology* **54:**835–851.

Spratt, J. S., Jr., and Ackerman, L. V., 1962, Small primary adenocarcinomas of the colon and rectum, *J. Am. Med. Assoc.* **179:**337–346.

III

Use of Experimental Models

13

Experimental Stomach Carcinogenesis

Takashi Sugimura and Takashi Kawachi

1. Introduction

The stomach is the organ which specifically comes into contact with food. Although food differs greatly from country to country, it has been shown that food definitely contains carcinogens: naturally occurring ones (Evans and Mason, 1965), artifically added ones (Sano *et al.,* 1977), and contaminants (Shank *et al.,* 1972; Sugimura *et al.,* 1977). Epidemiological studies have revealed a close correlation between diet characteristics and the frequency of stomach carcinoma (Haenszel *et al.,* 1972; Oiso, 1975).

Stomach carcinoma is still very common in many countries of the world. In Western countries, the frequency of this cancer has declined during the past few decades (Muñoz and Asvall, 1971; Muñoz and Conneley, 1971). However, in some countries, such as Japan, Chile, Finland, Iceland, and several in Eastern Europe, stomach cancer is a dominant disease among many malignant diseases (Hirayama, 1975, 1977). Even in Western countries, a diffuse type of stomach carcinoma that is actually more malignant than the other type still occurs at a constant rate. This type of stomach cancer often afflicts the younger generation (Muñoz and Asvall, 1971).

As with most human cancers, the real causative agent of stomach cancer remains obscure. The histogenesis of carcinogenic processes also remains to be clarified, although there are many reports available on human cases (Morson, 1955; Järvi and Laurén, 1964). Exact follow-up of the stages of histogenesis, including those for many different types of stomach carcinomas, is necessary.

At present, in some countries like Japan, mass-screening radiographic

Takashi Sugimura and Takashi Kawachi • National Cancer Research Institute, Tokyo, Japan.

methods for detecting stomach cancer have been adopted as a first step (Oshima *et al.,* 1977). However, iatrogenic radiation hazard must be carefully considered (Yamada, 1977). From this viewpoint, serum tests, such as that for antiparietal cell antibody, should be explored in relation to stomach cancer and precancerous changes in the stomach epithelium (Stickland and MacKay, 1973). The establishment of a simple and reliable method of producing experimental stomach cancer has been awaited by scientists involved clinically and fundamentally in stomach cancer research.

Clinical techniques for early diagnosis of stomach cancer have developed tremendously in the past decade (Ichikawa *et al.,* 1971), mainly as a result of the development of double-contrast radiography and fiberscopic examination associated with biopsy. Carcinoma *in situ* has been defined, and atypical growth (frequently abbreviated "ATP") has been proposed by some pathologists (Murakami *et al.,* 1953, Monaco *et al.,* 1962; Nakamura *et al.,* 1966). However, evidence fully supporting the time course of these changes is not available because human beings cannot be subjected to precise scientific follow-up studies. In practical terms, there are many cases of far-advanced human stomach cancer available for surgical treatment. However, although these patients can certainly be given cancer chemotherapy, we must have animals with *stomach cancer in the stomach* for test purposes. The distribution and metabolism of drugs definitely differ from organ to organ. And there is no doubt about the inadequacy of tumors transplanted subcutaneously or intraperitoneally for such preparatory studies.

2. *Experimental Production of Stomach Carcinoma by N-Methyl-N′-nitro-N-nitrosoguanidine*

In the history of chemical carcinogenesis studies, the experimental production of stomach cancer was one of the most difficult problems to be overcome during the past five decades. Although some success was achieved (Klein and Palmer, 1941), the method was technically tedious and the manner of administration was not natural. The frequency of stomach carcinoma production was low. Under these circumstances, we were very fortunate to be able to find a method to produce stomach cancer in rats by administration of an aqueous solution of *N*-methyl-*N′*-nitro-*N*-nitrosoguanidine (MNNG) in drinking water (Sugimura and Fujimura, 1967). This method itself is easy and the incidence of stomach cancer is fairly high, ranging from 70% to 100% (Sugimura *et al.,* 1969, 1970; Sugimura and Kawachi, 1973). The results with this method are highly reproducible. The site specificity is fairly high, although stronger exposure results in the occurrence of malignant tumors in the duodenum and the upper part of the jejunum (Sugimura *et al.,* 1969; Fujimura *et al.,* 1970).

This method is applicable to dogs (Sugimura *et al.,* 1969, 1972; Sugimura and Kawachi, 1973, 1976). Because the dog stomach is fairly large and repeated radiological and endoscopic examinations are possible, dog stomach carcinoma can be regarded as a good clinical model for human stomach cancer (Sugimura and Kawachi, 1973). Furthermore, new experimental immunological and biochemical tests on stomach juice and serum can be made using this model animal system to examine stomach carcinomas or precancerous gastric changes.

3. Chemical Background of Stomach Carcinogenesis by MNNG

MNNG was reported to be strongly mutagenic in bacteria in by Mandell and Greenberg (1960) and was used by many geneticists and molecular biologists to yield mutants efficiently. Although the somatic mutation theory has a long history (Boveri, 1914; Bauer, 1928), it was not until 1966 that MNNG was also found to be carcinogenic independently by us (Sugimura *et al.,* 1966) and by Druckrey *et al.* (1966; Schoenthal, 1966). Subcutaneous injection into rats yielded many transplantable fibrosarcomas (Sugimura *et al.,* 1966).

MNNG is a stable compound in neutral aqueous solution (Sugimura *et al.,* 1969). The presence of a phosphate ion accelerates its breakdown to form *N*-methyl-*N'*-nitroguanidine (MNG) (McKay, 1948; McKay *et al.,* 1950; Lawley and Thatcher, 1970; Haga *et al.,* 1972). MNG is a fairly inert compound, not mutagenic and not carcinogenic (Sugimura *et al.,* 1976). In acidic conditions, MNNG is very quickly converted to MNG (McKay and Wright, 1947). In alkaline conditions, it is known that MNNG degrades to yield azoxymethane, which is a strong methylating agent (McKay, 1948; McKay *et al.,* 1969). Many tissues of animals, including the stomach epithelium, have the capacity, probably enzymatic, to convert MNNG to MNG (Sugimura *et al.,* 1969). The pH of the gastric juice of the rat is < 3–4; microlocally it is close to 1. All these conditions explain the fairly high specificity of MNNG for producing stomach cancer. MNNG acts directly on the epithelial cell. Excess MNNG in the stomach is mostly converted to MNG under acidic conditions. A large excess of MNNG may reach the duodenum, where alkaline conditions may result in the alkylation of nucleic acids in intestinal epithelial cells. Once MNNG is absorbed into tissues, it is quickly converted to MNG; therefore, it is unlikely that organs other than the stomach will be exposed to MNNG in its intact form. This fate of orally administered MNNG accounts for the specific production of stomach cancer. Of course, if MNNG is mixed in the diet, it can readily react with a dietary component, nucleic acids and proteins, and be degraded to MNG. It is rather difficult to give MNNG as an aqueous solution for the experimental production of stomach cancer. A device was made using *N*-ethyl-*N'*-nitro-*N*-nitrosoguanidine (ENNG, ethyl analogue of MNNG) (Kurihara *et al.,* 1974). ENNG was poured on a pellet diet for dogs, and the pellets were soaked in ENNG solution and immediately given to the animal. ENNG still remained active because its reactivity with nucleic acids and proteins is much lower than that of MNNG. It was found that feeding dogs twice a day with such a diet provided sufficient ENNG administration to produce specific stomach carcinoma (Kurihara *et al.,* 1974).

MNNG can produce methylation in nucleic acids and proteins. 7-Methylguanosine-O^6-methylguanosine, 3- and 1-methylguanosine, 1-methyladenosine, and 3-methylcytosine were isolated and identified (Craddock, 1968; Lawley, 1968; McCalla, 1968; Singer *et al.*, 1968; Loveless, 1969; Lawley and Thatcher, 1970). As previously mentioned, in this reaction, no enzyme was involved. MNNG can also catalyze the nitroamidination reaction of the α-amino group of the free amino acids and the ϵ-amino residue of a polypeptide chain (Skinner *et al.*, 1960; Sugimura *et al.*, 1968; Nagao *et al.*, 1969, 1971; McCalla and Reuvers, 1968).

However, the presence of the sulfhydryl compound enhances the rate of methylation of nucleic acids remarkably, as reported by Schulz and McCalla (1969). The sulfhydryl group was similarly nitroamidinated, and this nitroamidination reaction resulted in the concomitant activation of another part of the molecule, the *N*-methyl-*N*-nitroso moiety of MNNG.

Incidentally, the lysine residue in the polypeptide chain was converted to a nitrohomoarginine residue by nitroamidination (Skinner *et al.*, 1960). Since the p*K* value of nitrohomoarginine is lower than that of lysine, this change resulted in a definite change in the physiocochemical properties of the affected proteins (Sugimura *et al.*, 1969; Nagao *et al.*, 1969, 1971).

4. General Technical Aspects of MNNG and ENNG Stomach Carcinogenesis

MNNG and ENNG are commercially available (Aldrich Chemical Co., Inc., Milwaukee, Wisconsin). Chromatographically, both are fairly pure, although sometimes a small amount of MNG or ENG may be found. Both can be kept in the dark and in a dried condition.

A stock solution of 1 mg MNNG or ENNG per milliliter of deionized water can stand at least for a week in a light-tight refrigerator and can be diluted every 2 days with tap water. The bottle containing MNNG solution is carefully covered with aluminum foil.

Rats and dogs were given the MNNG solution as plain drinking water. No depression of body weight increase and peripheral blood cell count was observed, indicating the specific action of MNNG on gastric epithelium (Sugimura *et al.*, 1969).

5. Experiments on Rats

5.1. General Features of the Carcinogenic Processes

Wistar strain male rats, weighing about 100 g at the inauguration of experiment, were generally used. A pellet diet and drinking water solution containing 30 or 100 μg/ml of MNNG were administered *ad libitum.* A typical experiment involved the continuous administration of 83 μg/ml of MNNG (Sugimura *et al.*, 1969; Saito *et al.*, 1970; Sugimura and Kawachi, 1973). Three days later, a shallow erosion was found, mostly in the pyloric region. Three weeks later, regenerative hyperplastic changes were consistently found. Upward or downward adenomatous hyperplasia was observed 6 months after the inauguration of MNNG administration. Adenocarcinoma, showing cellular and structural atypism and indicating active infiltration through the musculus propria, was often observed after 12 months. The involvement of the serosa was observed in some cases, and in a few cases metastasis in the liver was found (Sugimura *et al.*, 1972; Sugimura and Kawachi, 1973).

The gastric cancer that developed was mainly differentiated-type adenocarcinoma, and diffuse-type and the signet-ring-cell-type adenocarcinomas were also produced. These gastric-type carcinomas metastasized in the adjacent lymph nodes (Sugimura *et al.*, 1969; Sugimura and Kawachi, 1973). This preference for different metastatic sites by different types of gastric carcinomas closely mimics the case of human gastric carcinoma.

Although the pylorus was a preferential site for the carcinomas, adenocarcinomas were also produced in the fundic portion. It is noteworthy that the forestomach was almost entirely unaffected by *ad libitum* administration of MNNG solution. Forced feeding of a more concentrated ethanolic solution of ENNG directly into the stomach by a stomach tube resulted in the formation of squamous cell carcinomas but not tumors in the glandular stomach (Schoenthal, 1966).

Tabuchi *et al.* (1975) observed very early changes after a one-pulse intragastric administration of MNNG at the rate of 100 mg/kg body weight. A remarkable finding was the fatty change in the surface mucous cells. Nongastric carcinogen failed to induce this mucosal change.

A well-differentiated adenocarcinoma in the glandular stomach of the Wistar rat produced by MNNG plus 4-nitroquinoline 1-oxide was successfully transplanted into newborn rats of the same strain (Hirose *et al.*, 1976).

5.2. Administration of MNNG during a Limited Period

Hirono and Shibuya (1972) reported that a single administration of MNNG aqueous solution yielded stomach carcinoma in the glandular stomach. In this case, the latent period was about 10 months.

In most carcinogenesis experiments using chemicals, a minimum time of exposure is observed. In the case of MNNG stomach carcinogenesis, about 7 months of administration of an 83 μg/ml solution is sufficient to yield a fairly high rate of stomach cancer (Fujimura *et al.*, 1970).

5.3. Observations Made during Stomach Carcinogenesis by MNNG

Under nembutal anesthesia, a barium sulfate suspension and air can be introduced into the rat stomach through a gastric tube. By application of a soft X-ray technique used for mammography, a beautiful demonstration of the presence of gastric carcinoma in rat stomach was made by Kurihara *et al.* (1971). The findings thus obtained radiographically coincided very well with the findings obtained at autopsy. This radiographic examination can be carried out repeatedly without sacrificing an animal, and it can serve as a technique for follow-up studies of the carcinogenic process.

5.4. Autoradiographic Examination of the Carcinogenic Process by MNNG

In the normal gastric mucosa, DNA synthesis occurs at the bottom part of the pyloric gland and at the neck part of the fundic gland. It is notworthy that DNA synthesis occurs in a certain area in this well-organized histological architecture. After the administration of MNNG, this strict localization of DNA synthesis is completely disturbed. Many DNA-synthesizing cells are observed by autoradiography to be scattered irregularly after the injection of tritiated thymidine. The actual rate of DNA synthesis per average preexisting DNA is considerably higher in regenerative hypertrophy than in normal epithelial conditions. It was observed that this high rate of DNA synthesis decreased when the tissue became really malignant (Sugimura *et al.*, 1969; Saito and Sugimura, 1973).

5.5. Strain Specificity

Bralow *et al.* (1971) reported that rats of the Buffalo strain were not susceptible to induction of stomach cancer by MNNG. A higher capacity to change MNNG to MNG, either by stronger acidic conditions or by more active enzyme, is a possibility, as is the presence of a greater amount of mucous material covering the glandular stomach epithelium and protecting it from MNNG exposure.

5.6. Effects of Other Factors and Conditions on Stomach Carcinogenesis by MNNG

Tatematsu *et al.* (1975) administered high concentrations of sodium chloride in the diet during and/or after the administration of MNNG. Sodium chloride was once thought to be a factor in the high incidence of stomach cancer in human beings (Sato *et al.*, 1959).

Oral administration of iodoacetamide in drinking water produced stomach ulcer in the fundic region of the stomach. MNNG administration after this treatment produced adenocarcinoma in the region where the ulcer formed. The incidence of adenocarcinoma in the pyloric region was not enhanced by iodoacetamide, which could not produce an ulcer in this area (Takahashi *et al.*, 1976). Fukushima *et al.* (1976) used glass beads, which most likely would not be able to pass through the pyloric ring. The presence of glass beads definitely enhanced the carcinogenic action of MNNG, possibly because the MNNG solution stayed in the stomach longer. Mechanical stimulation producing a damaging effect and a reactive regenerating process may also have played a role in this enhancement.

Dahm and Werner (1976) reported that the rat stomach subjected to gastrojejunostomy by Bilroth's method II developed more malignant cancer in the residual glandular stomach at the site of anastomosis than in ordinary conditions.

The effect of detergent on MNNG carcinogenesis in the glandular stomach of rat by MNNG was also studied by Fukushima *et al.* (1974). Benzene alkylsulfonate enhanced the incidence of a more malignant and anaplastic type of adenocarcinoma (Takahashi, 1970). The presence of the detergent may be effective to remove the mucous material from the glandular epithelium and also to help MNNG penetrate into cells.

Tatematsu *et al.* (1976) observed that 4% mucin added to the diet significantly suppressed the incidence of stomach cancer induced by MNNG plus a saturated sodium chloride solution given once a week through a gastric tube. More recently, attention has been focused on the findings on noncarcinogenic promoting agents. The administration of croton oil dissolved in drinking water plus Tween 80 enhanced the incidence of MNNG adenocarcinoma in the glandular stomach of the rat (Sano *et al.*, 1976). This definitely indicates that the two-step mechanism of carcinogenesis also occurs in stomach carcinogenesis. These experimental results indicate that chronic inflammation produced by noncarcinogenic promoting agents in food is responsible for the development of human stomach cancers.

Some carcinogens are reported to produce immunosuppression in animals. However, oral administration of MNNG for 30 weeks, which is sufficient to produce gastric carcinoma, scarcely suppressed antibody production in sheep red blood cells. This is because orally administered MNNG is quickly degraded to MNG by acidic gastric fluid and an MNNG-degrading enzyme in the gastric epithelium. Peripheral lymphocytes were not affected by MNNG. In accordance with this, the subcutaneous injection of MNNG produced immunosuppression (Saito *et al.*, 1976).

Tahara and Haizuka (1975) reported that 20 intraperitoneal injections of gastrin at a rate of 50 μg/kg at 3-day intervals resulted in a remarkable increase in the production of scirrhous carcinoma by MNNG. Neither serotonin, histamine, glucagon, nor insulin showed this kind of effect. Gastrin stimulated hydrochloric acid production, but the trophic action by gastrin on glandular stomach mucosa might be a more reasonable explanation for this effect.

5.7. *Chemotherapy Experiments Using Experimental Stomach Cancer Induced by MNNG*

Trial use of experimental stomach cancer for screening chemotherapeutic drugs was carried out by Umezawa and his associates. Rats were given MNNG solution in drinking water and were operated on following production of stomach cancer to allow photography of the inside of the stomach. Actual measurements of tumor sizes were made in each rat. Later, a control group was given a saline injection while the experimental group received injections of a bleomycin derivative and fluorouracil. Rats were killed in the

66th experimental week, and the growth of tumors was shown to be more effectively suppressed by bleomycin derivatives (Matsuda 1976).

5.8. Related Phenomena in Stomach Cancer Production: Experimental Production of Intestinalization

Human cancers frequently originate from intestinal metaplasia in the stomach. Intestinal metaplasia is commonly observed in countries where the incidence of stomach cancer is high. Many reports have indicated the close relation between intestinal metaplasia and adenocarcinoma of the stomach, especially the well-differentiated type (Morson, 1955; Järvi and Laurén, 1964; Nakamura *et al.*, 1968; Stemmermann and Hayashi, 1968; Imai *et al.*, 1971; Stemmermann and Brown, 1974).

During the course of stomach carcinogenesis in the glandular stomach of rats, intestinal metaplasia has been noted (Sugimura *et al.*, 1969, 1970). Sasajima *et al* (1976) found that *N*-propyl-*N'*-nitro-*N*-nitrosoguanidine (PNNG, propyl analogue of MNNG) is suitable for producing intestinal metaplasia in the rat glandular stomach. PNNG is mutagenic and also carcinogenic; however, it is less reactive with biological material and is a weaker carcinogen than MNNG. PNNG is probably a suitable substance for yielding stomach carcinoma from intestinal metaplasia in rats that closely mimics the situation of human stomach cancer.

6. Experiments on Dogs

6.1. Induction Method

As described in the introduction of this chapter, the large size of the dog stomach permits precise radiographic follow-up endoscopic examination. Also, dogs are very tame and can tolerate anesthetic procedures for diagnosis.

MNNG and ENNG are used as carcinogens. Method I is to administer a carcinogen in a drinking water solution (Sugimura *et al.*, 1971), and method II is to administer a carcinogen in dried dog food pellets that have been soaked with aqueous carcinogen solution. In method II, quantitative uptake of carcinogen can be achieved (Kurihara *et al.*, 1974).

At least 20 reports of experiments using beagles and mongrel dogs have been published, in all of them adenocarcinomas developed. The results have been collected and published in a review (Sugimura and Kawachi, 1976).

With method I, after the administration of MNNG at 83 μg/ml for 15 months to mongrel dogs, the development of stomach cancer was observed by autopsy at 17–34 months (Shimosato *et al.*, 1971). With a dose level of 60 μg/ml, administration for 27 months was sufficient to cause the presence of adenocarcinoma at autopsy between 30 and 43 months. Beagle dogs which received 83 μg/ml of MNNG for 6, 9, or 12 months showed adenocarcinomas on autopsy at around 20 months. Beagle dogs administered 150 μg/ml of ENNG for 9 months showed adenocarcinomas in the stomach on autopsy at between 15 and 22 months.

With method II, after the administration of 250 ml of ENNG at 150 μg/ml with 2% Tween 60 for 8 months, beagles which were killed at between 9 and 27 months had adenocarcinomas in the stomach.

As in the rat experiments, higher concentrations of carcinogen and longer exposure times produced tumors in other loci than the stomach. Squamous cell carcinoma in the lower part of the esophagus (Sasajima *et al.*, 1977; Sekizuka *et al.*, 1975) and leiomyosarcoma in the duodenum and the upper part of the jejunum were produced (Shimosato *et al.*, 1971) in dogs by overdosage.

A concentration of a little less than 150 μg/ml of ENNG with method I or 150 μg/ml of ENNG for 6–8 months would probably be sufficient to produce stomach cancer very specifically. More than 50 dogs are now under experimental observation. More information on the standard procedure for producing stomach cancer will be available soon.

6.2. *General Observations on Production of Dog Stomach Cancer*

Dog stomach cancer often developed in the antrum and pylorus, but the cardiac portion of the dorsal wall was also a preferential site. Histologically, they were the well-differentiated type and also the poorly differentiated type of adenocarcinoma.

A well-differentiated type of adenocarcinoma developed in the cardiac area, as well as in the antral and pyloric regions. Polypoids or elevated types of tumors developed mainly in the upper portion of the stomach and were histologically the well-differentiated type of adenocarcinoma. Poorly differentiated adenocarcinoma or signet ring carcinoma, which had a depressed form, developed mainly in the antral and pyloric regions.

A well-differentiated adenocarcinoma that was seen in a malignant ulcerated lesion in the antrum of a beagle dog given an ENNG solution metastasized to the liver. A poorly differentiated adenocarcinoma invading the muscle layer in the pylorus metastasized to a peripyloric lymph node in the same dog (Sasajima *et al.*, 1977). Lung metastasis of an anaplastic adenocarcinoma of the stomach of vagotomized beagle dog treated with MNNG was reported (Fujita *et al.*, 1974, 1975). Multiple metastatic carcinomatosis of canine stomach carcinoma (Borrmann type III) into liver, lung, bone, and skin was also reported (Kurihara *et al.*, 1975*a*).

A moderately differentiated type of gastric adenocarcinoma in a mongrel dog induced by MNNG was serially transplanted to nude mice (Taguchi *et al.*, 1975). Biopsied signet ring cells from ENNG-induced stomach carcinoma of a living beagle dog was serially transplanted to nude mice (Kurihara *et al.*, 1975*b*).

6.3. *Presentation of Typical Cases of Tumor Development and Clinical Applications*

Successive changes in the stomach of beagle dogs that been given MNNG in drinking water *ad libitum* were examined by endoscopy and biopsy. Hyperemia, erosion, and ulcers appeared progressively at the angulus in the antrum of the stomach during MNNG adminitration. Erosion and ulcers were rapidly cured, resulting in mucosal atrophy and an ulcer scar. Subsequently, adenocarcinomas developed at the ulcer scar. Subsequently, adenocarcinomas developed at the ulcer scar of the angulus. Autopsy revealed well-differentiated tubular adenocarcinoma with serosal invasion and lymph node metastasis (Saito *et al.,* 1977).

The progress of the lesions in the stomach of dogs that received MNNG or ENNG was followed by radiographic examination. The most common sites of these lesions were the antroangular portion near the lesser curvature and the cardiac portion near the greater curvature. Flat or ulcerative lesions seen by radiography were often found to be adenocarcinomas (Noguchi *et al.,* 1974).

The gross appearance and histological structure of the stomach in dogs are quite similar to those of the human stomach. The pyloric area is a little narrower in the dog stomach than in the human stomach, so that endoscopic examination is difficult. The gross appearance of dog stomach carcinoma is also quite similar to that of human stomach carcinoma, i.e., polypoid, protruded, flat, depressed, and ulcerative (Noguchi *et al.,* 1974). Various lesions similar to those in man develop mainly in the antroangular portion. The histological types of dog stomach carcinoma were found to resemble human stomach cancer (Sugimura nd Kawachi, 1973).

The availability of dogs having stomach cancer for use in follow-up experiments on the efficacy of chemotherapy is a great advantage. Beagle dogs given ENNG solution in the drinking water for some months develop prominent stomach carcinomas in the pyrolic and antral regions as detected by X-ray, endoscopy, and biopsy examinations. Treatment of dogs with stomach carcinoma by administration of chemotherapeutic drugs is now possible.

Detection of precancerous lesions or lesions related to stomach cancer is possible using dogs treated with carcinogens. In particular, biochemical examination of stomach juice and serum of dogs having stomach cancer or precancerous lesions should be conducted.

7. Future Problems

The incidence of human scirrhous carcinoma is about 5% of the incidence of stomach carcinoma in general, and the prognosis is worst. However, an induction method for experimental scirrhous-type stomach cancer has not yet been established. Methods to produce precancerous changes of the stomach such as atrophic gastritis and intestinal metaplasia can be established by administration of *N*-propyl-*N'*-nitro-*N*-nitrosoguanidine. Detailed studies on the relation between stomach cancer and these lesions are desirable.

The presence of early stomach cancer equivalent to human cancer should be surveyed carefully in animals and methods to produce it should be devised. By studies of the chronological changes in the behavior of early stomach cancer in animals, the exact relationship between it and advanced cancer can be clarified.

Stomach cancer in animals could be used in the screening of chemotherapeutic agents. That in big animals like the dog is a suitable model for repeated roentgenographic and endoscopic examination to evaluate the effect of chemotherapy.

Biochemically or immunologically detectable markers that might reflect precancerous changes or cancer of the stomach should be investigated in serum or gastric juice of animals.

Administration of croton oil in the drinking water increases the induction of stomach carcinoma in rats. This indicates the presence of carcinogenic agents of stomach cancer in food. It also suggests the possibility of inhibition of stomach cancer by the administration of agents inhibitory to the cocarcinogenic process. Establishment of an assay system to find cocarcinogens in our environment is necessary.

8. *References*

Bauer, K. H., 1928, *Mutationstheorie der Geschwulst-Entstehung, Übergang von K in Geschwulst-zellen durch Gen Änderung,* Springer-Verlag, Berlin.

Boveri, T., 1914, *Zur Frage der Entstehung maligner Tumoren,* Fischer, Jena.

Bralow, S. P., Gruenstein, M., and Meranze, D. R., 1971, Strain resistance to gastric adenocarcinoma in rats ingesting NG, *Proc. Am. Assoc. Cancer Res.* **12**:3.

Craddock, V. M., 1968, The reaction of *N*-methyl-*N'*-nitro-*N*-nitrosoguanidine with deoxyribonucleic acid, *Biochem. J.* **106**:921–922.

Dahm, K., and Werner, B., 1976, Susceptibility of the resected stomach to experimental carcinogenesis, *Ztschr. Krebsforsch.* **85**:219–229.

Druckrey, H., Preussmann, R., Ivankovic, S., So, B. T., Schmidt, C. H., and Bucheler, J., 1966, Zur Erzeugung subcutaner Sarkome an Ratten: Carcinogene Wirkung von Hydrazodicarbonzaure-bis-(Methylnitrosamid), *N*-Nitroso-*N*-n-butyl-harnstoff, *N*-Methyl-*N*-nitrosonitroguanidin und *N*-Nitroso-imidazolidon, *Ztschr. Krebsforsch.* **68**:87–102.

Evans, I. A., and Mason, J., 1965, Carcinogenic activity of bracken, *Nature (London)* **208**:913–914.

Evans, I. A., and Osman, M. A., 1974, Carcinogenicity of bracken and shikimic acid, *Nature (London)* **250**:348–349.

Fujimura, S., Kogure, K., Sugimura, T., and Takayama, S., 1970, The effect of limited administration of *N*-methyl-*N'*-nitro-*N*-nitrosoguanidine on the induction of stomach cancer in rats, *Cancer Res.* **30**:842–848.

Fujita, M., Taguchi, T., Takami, M., Usugane, M., Takahashi, A., and Shiba, S., 1974, Carcinoma and related lesion in dog stomach induced by oral administration of *N*-methyl-*N'*-nitro-*N*-nitrosoguanidine, *Gann* **65**:207–214.

Fujita, M., Taguchi, T., Takami, M., Usugane, M., and Takashi, A., 1975, Lung metastasis of canine gastric adenocarcinoma induced by *N*-methyl-*N'*-nitro-*N*-nitrosoguanidine, *Gann* **66**: 107–108.

Fukushima, S., Tatematsu, M., and Takahashi, M., 1974, Combined effect of various surfactants on gastric carcinogenesis in rats treated with *N*-methyl-*N'*-nitro-*N*-nitrosoguanidine, *Gann* **65**:371–376.

Fukushima, S., Hananouchi, M., Shirai, T., Tatematsu, M., Hirose, M., Yoshida, S., and Takahashi, M., 1976, Effect of plastic bead on gastric carcinogenesis in rats treated with *N*-methyl-*N'*-nitro-*N*-nitrosoguanidine, *Gann* **67**:197–205.

Haenszel, W., Kurihara, M., Segi, M., and Lee, R. K. C., 1972, Stomach cancer among Japanese in Hawaii, *J. Natl. Cancer Inst.* **49**:969–988.

Haga, J. J., Russell, B. R., and Chapel, J. F., 1972, The kinetics of decomposition of *N*-alkyl derivatives of nitrosoguanidine, *Cancer Res.* **32**:2085.

Hirayama, T., 1975, Epidemiology of cancer of the stomach with special reference to its recent decrease in Japan, *Cancer Res.* **35**:3460–3463.

Hirayama, T. (ed.), 1977, *Epidemiology of Stomach Cancer, Key Questions and Answers,* WHO Collaborating Center for Evaluation of Methods of Diagnosis and Treatment of Stomach Cancer, National Cancer Center, Tokyo.

Hirono, I., and Shibuya, C., 1972, Induction of stomach cancer by a single dose of *N*-methyl-*N'*-nitro-*N*-nitrosoguanidine through a stomach tube, in: *Topics in Chemical Carcinogenesis* (W. Nakahara, S. Takayama, T. Sugimura, and S. Odashima, eds.), pp. 121–132, University of Tokyo Press, Tokyo.

Hirose, M., Takahashi, M., Hananouchi, M., Tatematsu, M., Kinoshita, H., Fukushima, S., and Ito , N., 1976, Transplantation of chemically induced gastric cancer in Wistar rats, *Gann* **67:**365–369.

Ichikawa, H., Yamada, T., Horikawa, H., Doi, H., Matsue, H., Tobayashi, K., Sasagawa, M., and Haga, A., 1971, X-ray diagnosis of early gastric cancer, *Jpn. J. Clin. Oncol.* **1:**1–17.

Imai, T., Kubo, T., and Wantanabe, H., 1971, Chronic gastritis in Japanese with reference to high incidence of gastric carcinoma, *J. Natl. Cancer Inst.* **47:**179–195.

Järvi, O., and Laurén, P., 1964, On the role of heterotopias of the intestinal epithelium in the pathogenesis of gastric cancer, *Acta Pathol. Microbiol. Scand.* **29:**26–44.

Klein, A. J., and Palmer, W. L., 1941, Experimental gastric carcinoma: a critical review with comments on the criteria of induced malignancy, *J. Natl. Cancer Inst.* **1:**559–584.

Kurihara, M., Ichikawa, H., and Fujimura, S., 1971, X-ray diagnosis of cancer in the glandular stomach of rats, *Gann* **62:**225–229.

Kurihara, M., Shirakabe, H., Murakami, T., Yasui, A., Izumi, T., Sumida, M., and Igarashi, A., 1974, A new method for producing adenocarcinomas in the stomach of dogs with *N*-ethyl-*N'*-nitro-*N*-nitrosoguanidine, *Gann* **65:**163–177.

Kurihara, M., Izumi, T., Miyasaka, K., Shirakabe, H., Yasui, A., Kamano, T., and Kondo, S., 1975*a,* Diffuse metastatic carcinomatosis of dog stomach carcinoma induced with *N*-ethyl-*N'*-nitro-*N*-nitrosoguanidine, *Juntendo-Igaku (Tokyo)* **21:**408–414.

Kurihara, M., Izumi, T., Miyasaka, K., Suzuki, K., Sudo, K., Kasui, A., and Kamano, T., 1975*b,* Transplantation of experimental dog stomach adenocarcinoma to nude mice, *IRCS Med. Sci.* **3:**221.

Lawley, P. D., 1968, Methylation of DNA by *N*-methyl-*N*-nitrosourethane and *N*-methyl-*N'*-nitro-*N*-nitrosoguanidine, *Nature (London)* **218:**581.

Lawley, P. D., and Thatcher, C. J., 1970, Methylation of deoxyribonucleic acid in cultured mammalian cells by *N*-methyl-*N'*-nitro-*N*-nitrosoguanidine, *Biochem. J.* **116:**693–707.

Loveless, A., 1969, Possible relevance of *O*-6 alkylation of deoxyguanosine to the mutagenicity and carcinogenicity of nitrosamines and nitrosamides, *Nature (London)* **223:**206–207.

Mandell, J. D., and Greenberg, J., 1960, A new chemical mutagen for bacteria, 1-methyl-3-nitro-1-nitrosoguanidine, *Biochem. Biophys. Res. Commun.* **3:**575–577.

Matsuda, A., 1976, Experimental chemotherapy of chemically induced gastric cancer of rats with new bleomycin, *Proceedings of the U.S.-Japan Cooperative Cancer Research Program: Symposium on Bleomycin.*

McCalla, D. R., 1968, Reaction of *N*-methyl-*N'*-nitro-*N*-nitrosoguanidine and *N*-methyl-*N*-nitroso-*p*-toluenesulfonamide with DNA *in vitro, Biochim. Biophys. Acta* **155:**114–120.

McCalla, D. R., and Reuvers, A., 1968, Reaction of *N*-methyl-*N'*-nitro-*N*-nitrosoguanidine with protein: Formation of nitroguanido derivatives, *Can. J. Biochem.* **46:**1411–1415.

McKay, A. F., 1948, A new method of preparation of diazomethane, *J. Am. Chem. Soc.* **70:**1974–1975.

McKay, A. F., and Wright, G. F., 1947, Preparation and properties of *N*-methyl-*N'*-nitro-*N*-nitrosoguanidine, *J. Am. Chem. Soc.* **69:**3028–3030.

McKay, A. F., Ott, W. L., Taylor, G. W., Buchanan, M. U., and Crooker, J. F., 1950, Diazohydrocarbons, *Can. J. Res. Sect. B* **28:**683–688.

Monaco, A. P., Roth, S. I., Castleman, B., and Welch, C. E., 1962, Adenomatous polyps of the stomach: A clinical and pathological study of 153 cases, *Cancer* **15:**456–467.

Morson, B. C., 1955, Carcinoma arising from areas of intestinal metaplasia in the gastric mucosa, *Br. J. Cancer* **9:**377–385.

Muñoz, N., and Asvall, J., 1971, Time trends of intestinal and diffuse types of gastric cancer in Norway, *Int. J. Cancer* **8:**144–157.

Muñoz, N., and Connely, R., 1971, Time trends of intestinal and diffuse types of gastric cancer in the United States, *Int. J. Cancer* **8:**158–164.

Murakami, T., Nakamura, S., and Suzuki, T., 1953, On the histogenesis of gastric cancer based on observations on cancer of mucosa, *Gann* **44:**158–162.

Nagao, M., Yokoshima, T., Hosoi, H., and Sugimura, T., 1969, Interaction of *N*-methyl-*N'*-nitro-*N*-nitrosoguanidine with ascites hepatoma cells *in vitro, Biochim. Biophys. Acta* **192:**191–199.

Nagao, M., Hosoi, H., and Sugimura, T., 1971. Modification of cytochrome *c* with *N*-methyl-*N'*-nitrosoguanidine, *Biochim. Biophys. Acta* **237:**369–377.

Nakamura, K., Sugano, H., Takagi, K., and Fuchigami, A., 1966, Histopathological study on early carcinoma of the stomach: Criteria for diagnosis of atypical epithelium, *Gann* **57:**613–620.

Nakamura, K., Sugano, H., Takagi, K., and Kumakura, K., 1968, Carcinoma of the stomach in incipient phase: Its histogenesis and histological appearances, *Gann* **59:**251–258.

Noguchi, M., Yamada, T., Ichikawa, H., Tanaka, N., Kawachi, T., and Kogure, K., 1974, Radiological study of canine stomach cancer induced by *N*-methyl-*N'*-nitro-*N*-nitrosoguanadine, *Gann* **65:**93–102.

Oiso, T., 1975, Incidence of stomach cancer and its relation to dietary habits and nutrition in Japan between 1900 and 1975, *Cancer Res.* **35:**3254–3258.

Oshima, A., Sakagami, F., Hanai, A., and Fujimoto, I., 1977, Evaluation of a mass screening program for gastric cancer, in: *Epidemiology of Stomach Cancer: Key Questions and Answers* (T. Hirayama, ed.), WHO Collaborating Center for Evaluation of Methods of Diagnosis and Treatment of Stomach Cancer, National Cancer Center, Tokyo.

Saito, T., and Sugimura, T., 1973, Biochemical studies on carcinogenesis in the glandular stomach of rats with *N*-methyl-*N'*-nitro-*N*-nitrosoguanidine, *Gann* **64:**373–381.

Saito, T., Inokuchi, K., Takayama, S., and Sugimura, T., 1970, Sequential morphological changes in *N*-methyl-*N'*-nitro-*N*-nitrosoguanidine carcinogenesis in the glandular stomach of rats, *J. Natl. Cancer Inst.* **44:**769–783.

Saito, T., Nomoto, K., Tamada, R., and Inokuchi, K., 1976, Effect of *N*-methyl-*N'*-nitro-*N*-nitrosoguanidine on immune response in rats in stomach carcinogenesis, *Gann* **67:**339–345.

Saito, T., Sasaki, O., Tamada, R., Iwamatsu, M., and Inokuchi, K., 1977, Follow-up studies of carcinogenesis in the stomach of dogs, in: *Pathophysiology of Carcinogenesis in Digestive Organs* (E. Farber, T. Kawachi, T. Nagayo, H. Sugano, T. Sugimura, and J. H. Weisburger, eds.), University of Tokyo Press, Tokyo.

Sano, T., Kawachi, T., Sasajima, K., Sugimura, T., and Fukushima, S., 1976, Carcinogenic effect of croton oil on experimental stomach cancer in rats, *Proc. Jpn. Cancer Assoc.*, p. 30.

Sano, T., Kawachi, T., Matsukura, N., Sasajima, K., and Sugimura, T., 1977, Carcinogenicity of a food additive, AF-2, in hamsters and mice, *Ztschr. Krebsforsch.* **89:**61–68.

Sasajima, K., Kawachi, T., Matsukura, N., Sano, T., and Sugimura, T., 1976, Studies on experimental intestinal metaplasia by *N*-propyl-*N'*-nitro-*N*-nitrosoguanidine in rats, *Proc. Jpn. Cancer Assoc.*, p. 46.

Sasajima, K., Kawachi, T., Sano, T., Sugimura, T., Shimosato, Y., and Shirota, A., 1977, Esophageal and gastric cancers with metastases induced in dogs by *N*-methyl-*N'*-nitro-*N*-nitrosoguanadine, *J. Natl. Cancer Inst.* **58:**1789–1794.

Sato, T., Fukuyama, T., Urata, G., *et al.*, 1959, Studies of the causation of gastric cancer. 1. Bleeding in the glandular stomach of mice by feeding with highly salted foods, and a comment on salted foods in Japan, *Bull, Inst. Public Health* **8:**10–13.

Schoenthal, R., 1966, Carcinogenic activity of *N*-methyl-*N*-nitroso-*N'*-nitroguanidine, *Nature (London)* **209:**726–727.

Schulz, U., and McCalla, D. R., 1969, Reaction of cysteine with *N*-methyl-N-nitroso-*p*-toluenesulfonamide and *N*-methyl-*N'*-nitro-*N*-nitrosoguanidine, *Can. J. Biochem.* **47:**2021–2027.

Sekizuka, H., Doi, H., Sunagawa, M., Nagai, S., Kojima, S., Hiraide, H., Hoshi, K., and Murakami, T., 1975, Induction of esophageal cancer associated with gastric cancer in a dog by *N*-ethyl-*N'*-nitro-*N*-nitrosoguanidine, *Gann* **66:**683–688.

Shank, R. C., Wogan, G. N., and Gibson, J. B., 1972, Dietary aflatoxins and human liver cancer. I. Toxigenic moulds in foods and foodstuffs of tropical South-east Asia, *Food. Cosmet. Toxicol.* **10:**60–65.

Shimosato, Y., Tanaka, N., Kogure, K., Fujimura, S., Kawachi, T., and Sugimura, T., 1971, Histopathology of tumors of canine alimentary tract produced by *N*-methyl-*N'*-nitro-*N*-nitrosoguanidine, with particular reference to gastric carcinogenesis, *J. Natl. Cancer Inst.* **47:**1053–1070.

Singer, B., Fraenkel-Conrat, H., Greenberg, J., and Michelson, A. M., 1968, Reaction of nitrosoguanidineanidine (*N*-methyl-*N'*-nitro-*N*-nitrosoguanidine) with tobacco mosaic virus and its RNA, *Science* **160:**1235–1237.

Skinner, W. A., Gram, H. F., Greene, O. M., Greenberg, J., and Baker, B. R., 1960, Potential anticancer agents. XXXI. The relationship of chemical structure to antileukaemic activity with analogues of 1-methyl-3-nitro-1-nitrosoguanidine (NSC-9369), *J. Med. Pharm. Chem.* **2:**299–333 (1960).

Stemmermann, G. N., and Brown, C., 1974, A survival study of intestinal and diffuse types of gastric carcinoma, *Cancer* **33:**1190–1195.

Stemmermann, G. N., and Hayashi, T., 1968, Intestinal metaplasia of the gastric mucosa: A gross and microscopic study of its distribution in various disease states, *J. Natl. Cancer Inst.* **41:**627–634.

Stickland, R. G., and MacKay, I. R., 1973, A reappraisal of the nature and significance of chronic atrophic gastritis, *Am. J. Digest. Dis.* **18:**426–440.

Sugimura, T., and Fujimura, S., 1967, Tumour production in glandular stomach of rats by *N*-methyl-*N'*-nitro-*N*-nitrosoguanidine, *Nature (London)* **216:**943–944.

Sugimura, T., and Kawachi, T., 1973, Experimental stomach cancer, *Methods Cancer Res.* **7:**245–308.

Sugimura, T., and Kawachi, T., 1976, Das experimentelle Mager Karzinom, *Leber Magen Darm.* **6:**80–90.

Sugimura, T., Nagao, M., and Okada, Y., 1966, Carcinogenic action of *N*-methyl-*N'*-nitro-*N*-nitrosoguanidine, *Nature (London)* **210:**962–963.

Sugimura, T., Fujimura, S., Nagao, M., Yokoshima, T., and Hasegawa, S., 1968, Reaction of with protein, *Biochim. Biophys. Acta* **170:**427–429.

Sugimura, T., Fujimura, S., Kogure, K., Baba, T., Saito, T., Nagao, M., Hosoi, H., Shimosato, Y., and Yokoshima, T., 1969, Production of adenocarcinomas in the glandular stomach of experimental animals by *N*-methyl-*N'*-nitro-*N*-nitrosoguanidine, *Gann Monogr.* **8:**157–196.

Sugimura, T., Fujimura, S., and Baba, T., 1970, Tumor production in the glandular stomach and alimentary tract of rat by *N*-methyl-*N'*-nitro-*N*-nitrosoguanidine, *Cancer Res.* **30:**455–465.

Sugimura, T., Tanaka, N., Kawachi, T., Kogure, K., Fujimura, S., and Shimosato, Y., 1971, Production of stomach cancer in dogs by *N*-methyl-*N'*-nitro-*N*-nitrosoguanidine, *Gann* **62:**67.

Sugimura, T., Kawachi, T., Kogure, K., Nagao, M., Tanaka, N., Fujimura, S., Takayama, S., Shimosato, Y., Noguchi, M., Kuwabara, N., and Yamada, T., 1972, Induction of stomach cancer by *N*-methyl-*N'*-nitro-*N*-nitrosoguanidine: Experiments on dogs as clinical models and metabolism of this carcinogen, in: *Topics in Chemical Carcinogenesis* (W. Nakahara, S. Takyama, T. Sugimura, and S. Odashima, eds.), pp. 105–119, University of Tokyo Press, Tokyo.

Sugimura, T., Nagao, M., Kawachi, T., Honda, M., Yahagi, T., Seino, Y., Matsushima, T., Shirai, A., Sawamura, M., Sato, S., Matsumoto, H., and Matsukura, N., 1977, Mutagen-carcinogens in food with special reference to highly mutagenic pyrolytic products in broiled foods, in: *Origins of Human Cancer* (J. D. Watson and H. Hiatt, eds.), Cold Spring Harbor Laboratory, Cold Spring Harbor, N.Y.

Tabuchi, Y., Mitsumo, T., and Sugiyama, T., 1975, Mucosal damage induced by various gastric carcinogens in the glandular stomach of the rat, *J. Natl. Cancer Inst.* **55:**1395–1401.

Taguchi, T., Fujita, M., and Usugane, M., 1975, Heterotransplantation of a cinine gastric cancer induced by *N*-methyl-*N'*-nitro-*N*-nitrosoguanidine into nude mice, *Biken J.* **18:**175–177.

Tahara, E., and Haizuka, S., 1975, Effect of gastro-entero-pancreatic endocrine hormones on the histogenesis of gastric cancer in rats induced by *N*-methyl-*N'*-nitro-*N*-nitrosoguanidine; with special reference to development of scirrhous gastric cancer, *Gann* **66:**421–426.

Takahashi, M., 1970, Effect of alkylbenzenesulfonate as a vehicle for 4-nitroquinoline 1-oxide on gastric carcinogenesis in rats, *Gann* **61:**27–33.

Takahashi, M., Shirai, T., Fukushima, S., Hananouchi, M., Hirose, M., and Ito, N., 1976, Effect of fundic ulcers induced by iodoacetamide on development of gastric tumors in rats treated with *N*-methyl-*N'*-nitro-*N*-nitrosoguanidine, Gann **67:**47–54.

Tatematsu, M., Takahashi, M., Fukushima, S., Hanaouchi, M., and Shirai, T., 1975, Effects in rats of sodium chloride on experimental gastric cancers induced by *N*-methyl-*N'*-nitro-*N*-nitroso-guanidine or 4-nitroquinoline-1-oxide, *J. Natl. Cancer Inst.* **55:**101–106.

Tatematsu, M., Takahashi, M., Hananouchi, M., Shirai, T., Hirose, M., Fukushima, S., and Ito, N., 1976, Protective effect of mucin on experimental gastric cancer induced by *N*-methyl-*N'*-nitro-*N*-nitrosoguanidine plus sodium chloride in rats, *Gann* **67:**223–229.

Yamada, T., 1977, Studies on the evaluation of mass screening of gastric cancer, *Report to the Ministry of Health and Welfare, Japan.*

14

Experimental Colon Carcinogenesis

Morris S. Zedeck

1. Introduction

Probably the most significant contribution in recent years toward the understanding of colon carcinogenesis has been the introduction of several compounds having marked propensity for induction of colon tumors in laboratory animals. Single or relatively few doses of MAM,* DMH, AOM, MNNG, or MNU result in the induction of large numbers of colon tumors in most, if not all, of the treated animals within a relatively short time. The intestinal distribution and the histological characteristics of the tumors are remarkably similar to what is found in humans. Animal model systems have been developed with the use of these agents and are invaluable for studying the mechanism(s) of initiation of tumor development as well as, in the case of those agents effective after a single treatment, the sequential changes from the moment of initiation until the formation of a tumor. In addition, epidemiological studies of various populations of the world have led to the suggestion that dietary fat, intestinal flora, and bile acids may influence the induction of colon tumors. The modifying effects of these factors in the formation of colon tumors can now also be evaluated in reliable animal model systems. The basic aims of this chapter are to present data of studies directed at understanding why colonic epithelium is especially sensitive to induction of

*Abbreviations: MAM, methylazoxymethanol; DMH, dimethylhydrazine; AOM, azoxymethane; MNNG, *N*-methyl-*N*'-nitro-*N*-nitrosoguanidine; MNU, *N*-methyl-*N*-nitrosourea; DMNA, dimethylnitrosamine; i.v., intravenous(ly); s.c., subcutaneous(ly); i.r., intrarectal(ly).

Morris S. Zedeck • Laboratory of Pharmacology, Memorial Sloan-Kettering Cancer Center, New York, New York 10021.

tumors by these compounds and to present and consider the evidence obtained thus far of the role of dietary factors, intestinal flora, and bile acids in the induction of colon cancer. Other experimental systems that may prove useful in understanding colon carcinogenesis are also discussed.

2. *Historical Background*

Colon tumors can be induced in laboratory animals by classes of chemicals having diverse structures and properties. Much of the early work in colon carcinogenesis used agents such as 2′,3-dimethyl-4-aminobiphenyl, 3-methyl-2-naphthylamine, *N, N′*-2,7-fluorenylbisacetamide, benzidine, and bracken fern (*Pteridium aquilinum*), and several reviews on their use have been published (Weisburger, 1971, 1973; Pozharisski, 1973). Colon tumors are also found in animals treated with aflatoxin (Ward *et al.*, 1975) and with polycyclic hydrocarbons (Della Porta, 1961; Homburger *et al.*, 1972; Wynder and Reddy, 1973; H. Marquardt,* personal communication).

Studies of colon tumor induction by azoxy-containing compounds began when Laqueur (1965) reported the carcinogenicity of MAM and cycasin, methylazoxymethanol-β-D-glucoside. Cycasin is without effect following parenteral administration or when given orally to germ-free rats. It was soon realized that the intestinal flora cleaves the glucoside moiety of cycasin and liberates MAM; the aglycone MAM can induce tumors by any route of administration (Laqueur and Spatz, 1968). MAM degrades spontaneously, and the mechanism by which it forms a chemically reactive species has been reported (Nagasawa *et al.*, 1972). The synthesis of MAM acetate (Matsumoto *et al.*, 1965) provides a form of the carcinogen that is stable and effective parenterally. The findings of Laqueur (1965) that intestinal tumors are induced in rats by the aglycone MAM prompted Druckrey (1970) to study the carcinogenic activities of dialkylhydrazines and azo- and azoxyalkanes. Most notable in this series as inducers of colon tumors are DMH and AOM. These agents are administered either orally or parenterally and are metabolized in liver (Preussmann *et al.*, 1969; Wittkop *et al.*, 1969). Narisawa *et al.* (1971) reported that MNNG, which decomposes spontaneously, can induce colon tumors when given i.r. In addition, it has been found that colon tumors can be induced with MNU, given either orally or i.r., in rats (Leaver *et al.*, 1969; Reddy *et al.*, 1975*b*), mice (Narisawa and Weisburger, 1975), and guinea pigs (Narisawa *et al.*, 1975). The synthesis of these agents, their proposed metabolic pathways, the dosage schedules and species used, and the morphology and distribution of the induced tumors have been extensively reviewed (Laqueur and Spatz, 1968; Druckrey, 1970; Weisburger, 1971; Druckrey, 1972; Narisawa *et al.*, 1972; Weisburger, 1972). Many of the animal model systems useful in studies of colon carcinogenesis have been cited

*A single i.v. injection of 7,12-dimethylbenz[*a*]anthracene, 25 mg/kg, was given either to intact rats or to rats at 5 or 24 hr after partial hepatectomy; the incidence of colon tumors within 1–2 years is 3/23, 4/18, and 6/17, respectively.

(Zedeck and Sternberg, 1974). In addition, Narisawa and Nakano (1973) reported that treatment of rats with MAM acetate i.r. for only 7 days results in a high incidence of colon tumors without tumors in the small intestine. Also, Ward (1975) has shown that single doses of AOM can induce tumors of the gastrointestinal tract, ear canal, kidney, liver, and preputial gland, the incidence of tumors in each tissue depending on the dose employed. The colon was most sensitive to the carcinogenic effect of AOM.

3. Structure-Activity Relationships

The common feature among MAM, DMH, AOM, MNNG, and MNU is the eventual formation of a methylating moiety, either metabolically or spontaneously. Slight modifications of these structures result in compounds that are no longer capable of being activated to colon carcinogens. Diethylhydrazine, for example, cannot induce colon tumors, nor can the unsymmetrical 1,1-dimethylhydrazine (Druckrey, 1970, 1972). An analogue of AOM, methylazoxyoctane, induces pulmonary and bladder tumors without any tumors in intestine (Ward *et al.*, 1974). The presence of the aliphatic chain alters markedly the organotropy of the azoxy-containing carcinogen.

4. Selective Effects of Carcinogens in Colon and Duodenum

Gennaro *et al.* (1973) have shown that segments of colon transposed to mid-small intestine develop tumors following treatment of rats with AOM, while in the same animals segments of small intestine transposed to the colon are not affected. Such results suggest that the colon is inherently more sensitive to the tumor-inducing effects of these agents than the small intestine. In support of this suggestion is the fact that a single i.v. injection of MAM acetate can induce in rats more tumors of the colon than of the small intestine (Zedeck and Sternberg, 1974).

It was of interest to determine whether the colon and small intestine respond differently to the acute effects of carcinogens. We studied, therefore, carcinogen-induced pathological and biochemical alterations in both colon and small intestine during the first week of treatment. It is the aim of these studies to correlate acute changes with those requisite for eventual tumor development and to understand the mechanism responsible for the marked sensitivity of colonic epithelium to tumor induction.

4.1. Early Pathological and Biochemical Alterations

The response of intestinal epithelium to the necrotizing effects of the carcinogens occurs rapidly. At 6 hr after a carcinogenic dose of MAM acetate, 35 mg/kg, i.v., severe karyorrhexis is evident in duodenum and colon; the change is more marked in the duodenum. By 24 hr, much of the cellular debris has been removed, although uneven alignment and enlargement of crypt nuclei are still evident. No pathology is observed in jejunum or ileum as late as 24 hr after treatment. At 72 hr, edema, dilated crypts, and mucosal atrophy can be found in colon. At 7 days, there are occasionally increased numbers of inflammatory cells in the lamina propria in both duodenum and colon (Zedeck *et al.*, 1970; Zedeck andSternberg, 1975). At no time are there any histological abnormalities in either Peyer's patches of the small intestine or the lymphoid follicles of the colon.

Hawks *et al.* (1974) studied the acute pathological changes induced by DMH, and, in agreement with their findings, we find that the changes in duodenum and colon of rats treated with DMH are similar to those induced by MAM acetate. In studies of the acute effects of DMNA, a potent inducer of hepatic and renal tumors (Magee and Barnes, 1967), it is important to note that we could not find any pathological alterations up to 72 hr after treatment in either duodenum or colon.

Our initial biochemical studies dealt with measurement of DNA synthesis in both small intestine and colon. Inhibition of DNA synthesis, as determined by measuring [*methyl*-^{3}H]thymidine incorporation into DNA, is often a reflection of cell loss rather than of a specific alteration in the DNA biosynthetic pathways. Since in these studies karyorrhectic cells are found at times of max-

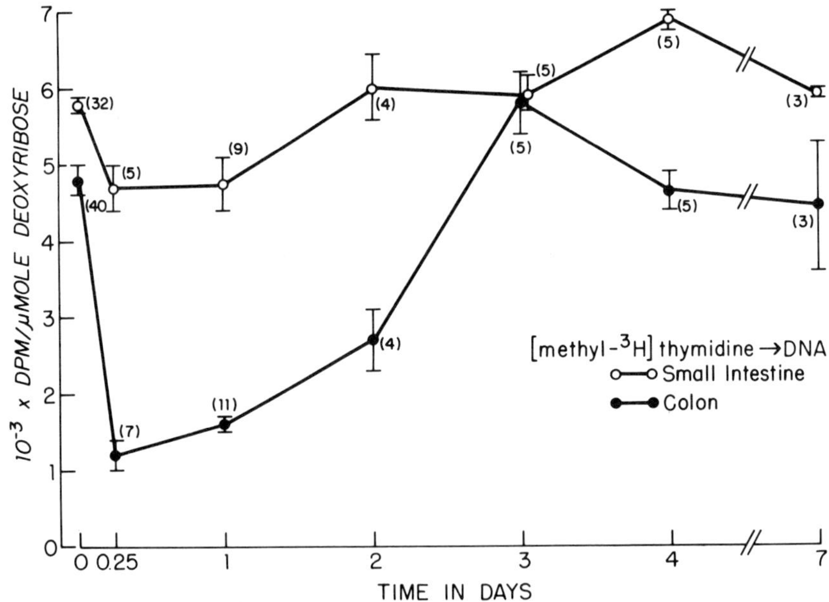

Fig. 1. Effect of MAM acetate, 35 mg/kg, i.v., on DNA synthesis in rat small intestine and colon. At various intervals after treatment, rats were injected i.v. with [*methyl*-^{3}H]thymidine (50μCi/2 μmol/kg) and killed 10 min later. The tissues were homogenized and the DNA was extracted as previously described (Zedeck *et al.*, 1970). The numbers in parentheses denote the number of rats studied at each interval. Data obtained from rats treated with saline were similar at each of the intervals studied and are collectively shown at 0 time. The data are expressed as the mean ±SEM.

imal inhibition of DNA synthesis, it cannot be stated with certainty which of these two phenomena is the direct effect of carcinogen treatment.

As shown in Fig. 1, MAM acetate inhibits DNA synthesis in small intestine approximately 20% by 6 hr. This effect is short-lived and by the second day after treatment DNA synthesis has returned to normal levels. In contrast, DNA synthesis in colon is inhibited approximately 75% by 6 hr and does not return to control values until the third day (Zedeck and Sternberg, 1975). The distribution of tumors in the small intestine is noteworthy in that those that do occur are predominantly in the duodenum (Zedeck and Sternberg, 1974). In view of the marked abnormality present in duodenum soon after treatment, it is likely that duodenal DNA synthesis is inhibited.

Since in the above study we assayed the entire small intestine, including jejunum and ileum, which are unaffected by MAM acetate, any effect on the duodenum could have been masked. DNA synthesis was determined, therefore, in each segment of the small intestine and, in addition, in the caecum and in the various segments of the colon. The data in Table 1 indicate that in small intestine DNA synthesis is inhibited in duodenum to a greater extent than in jejunum or ileum, and that caecum and each segment of the colon are similarly affected. The results suggest that a correlation exists between the segment of intestine in which DNA synthesis is acutely inhibited and the site of tumor formation. We have not regularly looked for cecal tumors in the past but in view of these data will examine the caecum carefully in future studies. Laqueur *et al.* (1967) and Ward *et al.* (1973*a*) have observed cecal tumors in rats treated with MAM and AOM, respectively.

Table 1. Effect of MAM Acetate on DNA Synthesis in the Various Segments of the Intestinal Tract[a]

	Percent of control[b]		
Intestinal segment	I	II	III
Duodenum[c]	41.7	37.0	39.6
Jejunum	69.3	55.3	66.5
Ileum	68.7	78.0	72.6
Caecum	37.4	26.4	37.5
Ascending colon	34.8	40.3	20.5
Transverse colon	28.0	41.3	14.8
Descending colon	34.1	34.9	28.7

[a]At 24 hr after treatment with either saline or MAM acetate, 35 mg/kg, i.v., weanling rats were given [*methyl*-^{3}H]thymidine (50 μCi/2 μmol/kg), i.v., and killed 10 min later. The tissues were homogenized and the DNA was extracted as described (Zedeck *et al.*, 1970).

[b]In each of three experiments (I, II, III), the segments of three control rats were pooled as were those of three treated rats. The results of each experiment are given.

[c]The first 5 cm of intestine from the pylorus is denoted duodenum; the remainder of the small intestine was cut in half to give jejunum and ileum. The colon between caecum and anus was divided into three equal segments.

Table 2. Effects of Various Treatments on DNA Synthesis in Rat Small Intestine and Colon

Treatment[a]	*n*	Small intestine	*n*	Colon
Saline	32	5.8 ± 0.1[b]	40	4.8 ± 0.2
MAM acetate	9	4.8 ± 0.3	11	1.6 ± 0.1
DMNA	3	4.8 ± 0.5	5	2.2 ± 0.3
DMH·diHCl	4	4.6 ± 0.2	6	2.5 ± 0.4
5FU	4	0.3 ± 0.0	6	0.3 ± 0.1
HN_2	3	1.1 ± 0.1	3	0.9 ± 0.0

[a] At 24 hr after receiving i.v. injections of either saline, 35 mg/kg MAM acetate, 35 mg/kg DMNA, 35 mg/kg DMH·diHCl, 100 mg/kg 5FU or 2 mg/kg HN_2, the rats received [*methyl*-^{3}H]thymidine (50 μCi/2 μmol/kg), i.v., and were killed 10 min later. The organs were removed and analyzed for incorporation of thymidine into DNA as previously described (Zedeck *et al.*, 1970).
[b] dpm/μmoles deoxyribose × 10^{-3} (x ± SEM).

We also studied the effects of DMH and DMNA on DNA synthesis, and as controls we tested 5-fluorouracil (5FU) and nitrogen mustard (HN_2), chemotherapeutic agents not considered intestinal carcinogens but having the ability to inhibit proliferating cells (Karnofsky and Clarkson, 1963). The data in Table 2 indicate that, like MAM acetate, DMH and DMNA inhibit DNA synthesis in colon to a greater extent than in small intestine. The fact that 5FU

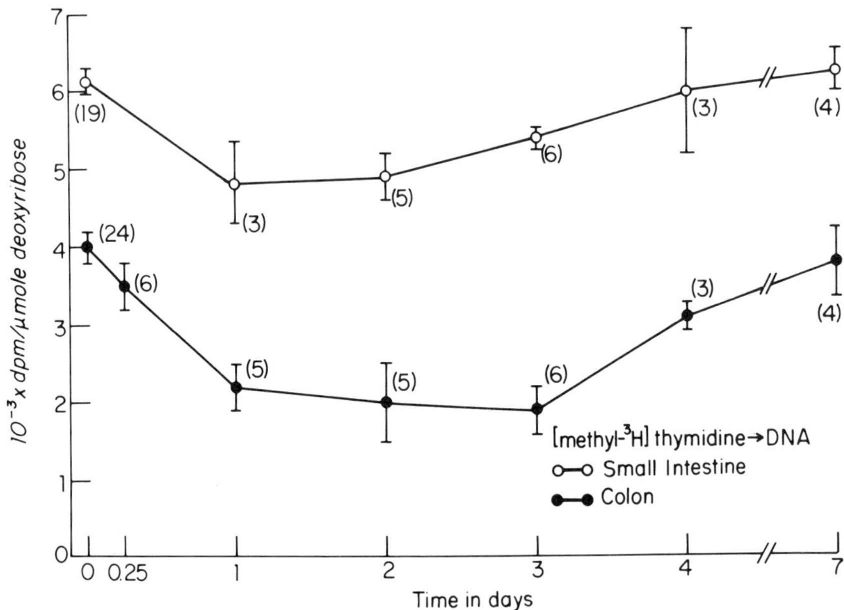

Fig. 2. Effect of DMNA, 35 mg/kg, i.v., on DNA synthesis in rat small intestine and colon. Details are given in the caption of Fig. 1.

and HN_2 inhibit DNA synthesis markedly in each tissue suggests that all segments of the intestine are similarly affected.

The data obtained with DMNA are of considerable interest, and the inhibition of DNA synthesis in small intestine and colon over a period of 7 days is shown in Fig. 2. The fact that DNA synthesis in colon is inhibited and no pathological changes are detectable suggests that DMNA may induce a specific alteration of DNA biosynthesis. In addition, these results suggest that the primary effect of MAM acetate is inhibition of DNA synthesis and that the presence of intestinal abnormality following treatment with MAM acetate may be attributable to, in contrast to the results with DMNA, the rapidity and extent of the induced inhibition. It appears, therefore, that rat colon can metabolize DMNA. Most studies of microsomal mixed-function oxidase activity in rat intestine were done with small intestine (Chhabra *et al.,* 1974; Wattenberg, 1971); enzyme activity, relative to liver, is very low. Wattenberg (1971) studied benzpyrene hydroxylase activity in rat small intestine and colon. Enzyme activity in colon was undetectable but could be induced. Intestinal enzyme activity should be determined using DMNA as substrate.

Rice *et al.* (1975) and Fahmy *et al.* (1975) studied the biological effects of methyl(acetoxymethyl)nitrosamine, which, when deesterified, yields methyl(hydroxymethyl)nitrosamine, the proximate carcinogenic form of DMNA. Genetic studies with this derivative (Fahmy and Fahmy, 1975) as well as with the acetoxy derivative of diethylnitrosamine (Fahmy *et al.,* 1975) indicate that the acetoxy derivatives are more potent mutagens than the parent compounds. Rats treated with the acetoxy derivative of DMNA develop tumors of the small intestine and colon (Rice *et al.,* 1975). These results suggest that resistance to tumor induction by DMNA in intestine may be due to the low levels of microsomal enzyme activity. Since it appears that the colon can metabolize a sufficient amount of DMNA to be able to inhibit DNA synthesis and other results suggest that colonic epithelium may directly activate DMH and AOM (see Section 10), extensive studies of microsomal mixed-function oxidase activity in rat colon should now be considered.

4.2. Deacetylation of MAM Acetate

Free MAM has also been evaluated as a carcinogen. In one study (Laqueur and Matsumoto, 1966) tumors arose predominantly in the liver, kidney, duodenum, and colon, while in another study (Laqueur *et al.,* 1967) tumors were also induced in jejunum and ileum. In our studies with MAM acetate, tumors are rarely noted in jejunum and ileum, and these segments of intestine are also resistant to the acute biochemical lesions induced by MAM acetate. Poynter *et al.* (1971/1972) have reported that deacetylation of MAM acetate is requisite for biological activity, and it is conceivable that the different responses observed may be due to varying activities of deacetylation among the different intestinal segments. Homogenates of the various segments of small intestine and colon, homogenates of liver and kidney, and dilutions of blood were assayed for esterase activity using MAM acetate as

Table 3. Measurement of Esterase Activity in Rat Organs with MAM Acetate as Substrate[a]

Organ	Units/mg protein[b]
Liver	329.0
Kidney	176.0
Duodenum	144.5
Jejunum	103.1
Ileum	78.4
Caecum	41.3
Colon	35.1
Blood	2.5

[a]Buffer (20 mM triethanolamine, 154 mM NaCl, pH 7.8) was used to homogenize organs or to dilute the blood. MAM acetate, 3 μmol, was added and the rate of deacetylation was determined by measuring the decrease in pH with time with a Radiometer pH meter having a single electrode and expanded scale. Standard curves of pH vs. acetate concentration were prepared using acetic acid.

[b]One unit of enzymatic activity can hydrolyze 1 nmol MAM acetate per minute at 35°C. Protein concentrations were determined by the method of Lowry *et al.* (1951).

substrate. The data in Table 3 indicate that all the tissues analyzed have more esterase activity than does blood, and that no correlation exists between tissue enzyme activity and sensitivity to the biochemical effects of MAM acetate. Both jejunum and ileum have considerably more enzyme activity than does colon, and kidney, which is relatively unaffected by MAM acetate (Zedeck *et al.,* 1970), has an even higher level of activity. In view of the deacetylase activity present in kidney, it is curious that rats treated with methyl(acetoxymethyl)nitrosamine, the proximate carcinogenic form of DMNA, do not develop renal tumors (Rice *et al.,* 1975).

In the event that MAM acetate does not distribute uniformly following parenteral treatment, we prepared and injected rats with free MAM. The extent of inhibition of DNA synthesis in each of the intestinal segments is similar to that observed with MAM acetate; the jejunum and ileum are least affected.

The above results suggest that the organotropic effects of MAM acetate are probably not the result of differences in deacetylation. It seems reasonable to propose that, in addition to its spontaneous decomposition, MAM can be metabolized to yield the reactive methylating moiety, and that some tissues may be more active in this process than other tissues. Such a mechanism could explain the organotropism exhibited by this carcinogen.

4.3. Late Pathological and Biochemical Alterations

Sequential studies of the changes induced in small intestine and colon of mice and rats treated repeatedly with DMH have been described (Springer *et al.,* 1970; Wiebecke *et al.,* 1973; Thurnherr *et al.,* 1973; Haase *et al.,* 1973). As early as 45 days after treatment is begun, cells active in DNA synthesis can be found at the uppermost portion of the crypt while in untreated animals only cells in the lowest two-thirds of the crypt synthesize DNA. By 3 months, cells incorporating tritiated thymidine into DNA are found at the luminal surface of the crypts, and labeled cells are also observed at the mucosal surface (Springer *et al.*, 1970; Thurnherr *et al.*, 1973). At this time, the colonic glands of mice and rats show abnormalities consisting of edema, inflammation, loss of mucus-producing cells, and elongation. The authors conclude that carcinogens affect proliferating crypt cells and result in their leaving the crypt without having differentiated and continue to progress along the villous as undifferentiated cells. A report by Pozharisski (1975) tends to support the concept that intestinal carcinogens exert their effects on proliferating cells. An increased labeling index in rat caecum was induced by applying a purse-string suture to form a diverticulum. This suture provided both a temporary and a permanent (as a ligature) source of injury to the caecum. Treatment with DMH results in an increased incidence of tumors, with the majority of them forming in the zone of the ligature. This author cannot but wonder whether other factors also play a role in the increased tumor incidence in this zone since proliferating cells in caecum are always present in abundant numbers. In addition, the increased rate of proliferation around the ligature is accompanied by an inflammatory reaction.

5. Role of Intestinal Flora in Colon Carcinogenesis

Induction of colon tumors in germ-free rats has been studied with MAM (Laqueur *et al.*, 1967), with DMH (Reddy *et al.*, 1974*b*, 1975*a*), with AOM (Reddy *et al.*, 1975*a*), and with MNNG (Reddy *et al.*, 1974*b*). In germ-free animals, MAM and DMH, although less effective, are still carcinogenic. When DMH is used, conventional rats develop approximately a twofold greater incidence of colon tumors than do germ-free rats; the duration of onset of the tumors is increased in the germ-free rats.

The decreased incidence of tumors noted in germ-free rats relative to conventional rats may be due to differences in the intestinal epithelium. Abrams *et al.* (1963) have shown that the height of crypt and villus is less in ileum of germ-free mice as compared to conventional mice; also, the rate of cell turnover is significantly decreased.

In experiments with AOM and MNNG, the number of rats in both the conventional and germ-free groups that develop tumors is similar, but the number of tumors is greater in the germ-free rats. Since in these studies MNNG and AOM were given i.r., it was suggested that in conventional rats some of the carcinogen does not reach the colonic mucosa. The fact that agents such as DMH and AOM are active in germ-free rats suggests that the metabolism of these agents by liver to MAM, the subsequent glucuronidation of MAM, and the eventual release of the carcinogen by the intestinal flora may not be as significant a metabolic pathway as discussed by Weisburger (1971). The reactive species of these agents may well be formed in the liver and then be transported to the colonic epithelium via the circulation. More likely, the carcinogens are activated by the colonic epithelium itself.

6. Role of Bile and Blood in Carcinogen Transport

Pozharisski *et al.* (1975) found DNA-associated radioactivity in rat colon as early as 1 hr after injection of ^3H-labeled DMH. These data suggest that the carcinogen can be absorbed by the colonic epithelium via the circulation. In fact, very little DMH or its metabolites are excreted via the bile (Hawks and Magee, 1974; Fiala and Weisburger, 1975). Within 24 hr after administration of ^{14}C-labeled DMH to rats, s.c., 60% of the radioactive dose is found in expired air; of this, approximately 10% is $^{14}CO_2$. Less than 1% is excreted via the bile, and after 24 hr 0.07–0.09% of the dose is detectable in colon. Data suggesting that these agents can induce tumors following a hematogenous distribution were provided by Wittig *et al.* (1971). They reported that tumors can arise in that portion of the colon remaining after colostomy in rats treated with DMH.

We have studied the inhibition of DNA synthesis in segments of small intestine and colon of rats treated with MAM acetate following cannulation of the bile duct. Within 3 hr, DNA synthesis in each segment of colon, in caecum, and in duodenum is inhibited approximately 80%, while in jejunum and ileum DNA synthesis is inhibited 50% and 30%, respectively. These results are qualitatively similar to those obtained in intact rats (Table 1). These data also indicate that the carcinogen can reach the colonic epithelium via the circulation, and that it can induce its effects rapidly.

7. Role of Bile Acids and Dietary Factors in Colon Carcinogenesis

Numerous studies of the etiology of human colon cancer have led investigators to strongly suggest dietary factors as causal agents. Much effort has been directed toward studies of beef fat consumption, vegetable fiber content, composition of the colonic flora, and fecal content of bile acids. The results of such studies suggest that populations consuming a high-fat diet are at greater risk for development of colon cancer and that metabolism of bile acids by colonic flora may also play a role. Much of the current thinking in all these areas has been published in *Cancer Research,* Vol. 35, No. 11, Part 2: Nutrition in the Causation of Cancer (1975), and the reader is referred to the cited volume for a review of the literature. While such epidemiological studies are not within the realm of this chapter, their findings have prompted many studies in laboratory animals and these experiments will now be discussed.

7.1. Bile Acids and Dietary Fat

Nigro *et al.* (1973) reported that feeding rats cholestyramine, a nonabsorbable ion-exchange resin with affinity for bile salts, while treating them with either DMH, AOM, or MAM results in a significant increase of colonic tumors. Such treatment results in greater secretion of bile salts and higher concentrations of bile acids in the feces. The bile acids may possibly act as carcinogens or cocarcinogens or be converted by the intestinal flora into such factors that enhance formation of colon tumors. To rule out any effect by cholestyramine itself, these investigators increased the content of fecal bile acids by shunting the bile flow from the duodenum to the mid-small intestine; this procedure also results in greater yields of colon tumors in AOM-treated rats (Chomchai *et al.,* 1974). The effect of dietary fat content on tumor incidence and fecal bile acid composition has been studied in rats (Reddy *et al.,* 1974*a*). Rats fed a diet containing 20% fat develop more tumors following treatment with DMH than do rats fed normal- or low-fat-content diets. In addition, rats fed high-fat diets excrete greater quantities of fecal neutral steroids and bile acids than do rats on low-fat diets. It is curious, however, that, while rats fed high-fat diets develop more colonic tumors than rats fed Purina Lab Chow, the latter group excrete even greater amounts of bile acids and neutral sterols. Nigro *et al.* (1975) treated rats repeatedly with AOM while maintaining them on a diet containing 35% beef fat. These rats, as compared to carcinogen-treated animals fed a normal diet, develop approximately twice as many tumors. Narisawa *et al.* (1974) treated rats once with MNNG, i.r., and then administered i.r. over prolonged periods either lithocholic or taurodeoxycholic acid. Rats receiving either bile acid following the carcinogen develop more tumors than those treated with carcinogen alone; rats receiving bile acids only do not develop colon tumors. It would appear from these studies that bile acids do play a modifying role in colon carcinogenesis.

7.2. Vitamin A and Lipotropic Agents

The effect of dietary constituents such as vitamin A and lipotropic agents on colon tumor induction in laboratory animals has been reviewed (Reddy *et al.,* 1975*b;* Rogers and Newberne, 1975). In brief, fat-enriched diets without the lipotropes choline and methionine or diets deficient in vitamin A can augment induction of colon tumors by chemical carcinogens. As reported in the two cited reviews, however, results differ with different carcinogens. It is as yet unclear whether the modifying effects of these dietary factors are due to alterations in metabolic activation of the carcinogen, altered sensitivity of the target tissue in need of the deficient constituent, or an effect on the lymphoid elements resulting in aberrant immunological responses (Rogers and Newberne, 1975).

7.3. Tryptophan and Indole

Chung *et al.* (1975) suggested that tryptophan metabolism by the intestinal flora may play a role in colon tumor induction. Indole, a metabolic product of tryptophan, has been found to be carcinogenic, and both tryptophan and indole can enhance tumor formation in animals receiving

2-acetylaminofluorene. Rats on an all-meat diet have elevated levels of tryptophan in the feces and an increase in tryptophanase activity. The authors suggest that the association between high-meat diet and increased incidence of colon tumors in humans may be related, in part, to the elevated levels of tryptophan and indole in the feces.

8. Studies on Inhibition of Colon Tumor Induction

The use of phenolic antioxidants for inhibition of chemical carcinogenesis has received considerable attention (Wattenberg, 1974). Thus far, however, few of these studies have dealt with inhibition of colon carcinogenesis. Wattenberg (1975) reported that feeding of disulfiram (Antabuse, tetraethylthiuram disulfide) results in complete protection against induction of colon tumors in mice treated with DMH. Under the same conditions, butylated hydroxyanisole (BHA) offers little protection. It is not certain, however, whether disulfiram directly affects the target tissue, reacts with the ultimate form of the carcinogen, or interferes with metabolic activation of DMH to its ultimate reactive species.

The effects of BCG (bacillus Calmette-Guérin) injection on the incidence of DMH-induced tumors in rats were investigated (Rogers and Gildin, 1975). Administration of BCG prior to treatment with DMH, or following the course of treatment with DMH, fails to elicit any effect on tumor incidence or rate of tumor development. In addition, injection of BCG directly into the colon tumors has no affect on tumor size. In another study (Kroes *et al.,* 1975), immunosuppression of rats by treatment with the γ fraction of antilymphocytic serum was found not to alter the incidence of colon tumors induced by AOM.

9. Other Experimental Systems

9.1. Transplantable Colon Tumors

Several transplantable colon tumors are available for such studies as determination of tumor growth kinetics, evaluation of potentially useful antitumor agents, and detection of tumor antigens. Transplantable colon tumors have been established in Buffalo rats (McCall and Cole, 1974), Fischer rats (Ward *et al.,* 1973*b*), BD-IX rats (Martin *et al.,* 1973), BALB/c and C57BL/6 mice (Corbett *et al.,* 1975), and NMRI mice (Double *et al.,* 1975). These tumors differ histologically, in their propensity for metastases, and in their growth rates. In all, this spectrum provides many different experimental conditions suitable for a variety of studies.

9.2. Organ Cultures

Another technique valuable for study of colon carcinogenesis is that of organ culture. Newborn rat and hamster colon (Schiff, 1975) and adult mouse colon (Defries and Franks, 1975) can be maintained in organ culture from 24 to 28 days. Such systems allow for sequential biochemical and pathological studies of colonic epithelium following treatment with chemical carcinogens *in vitro*.

10. Conclusions and Discussion

The data indicate that colon carcinogens are effectively transported to their target sites via the circulation. Experiments of Pozharisski *et al.* (1975) showing DNA-associated radioactivity in colon at 1 hr after giving [^{3}H]DMH, experiments of Wittig *et al.* (1971) showing tumorigenic effects of DMH in the remaining segments of colon after colostomy, and the fact that MAM acetate can inhibit colonic DNA synthesis in rats having cannulated bile ducts indicate that these agents do not require either transport by the bile or metabolism by intestinal flora to exert their biological effects. It is still uncertain whether that which reaches the target site via the circulation is the original compound or an activated form of the carcinogen released by the liver. Several facts can be cited, however, to support the concept that the target tissues directly convert the parent compounds into ultimate carcinogens.

It must be recognized that the class of carcinogens discussed herein exhibit marked organotropy. It is reasonable to suppose that, if the liver supplied the circulation with reactive species of the administered agent, then tumors would be seen in many tissues. In this regard, it is curious that animals treated with DMH or AOM develop colonic tumors more rapidly and in far greater numbers than they develop liver tumors (Druckrey, 1970; Ward *et al.*, 1973*a*).

Also, no tumors are found in the offspring of rats treated with either DMH or AOM during the period of gestation (Druckrey, 1972). The fact that tumors can be induced transplacentally by MAM (Spatz and Laqueur, 1967, 1968) suggests that activated carcinogens could have reached the fetus had they been excreted by the maternal liver into the circulation. These data also indicate that fetal tissues cannot metabolize DMH or AOM. It is of interest that diethylhydrazine induces tumors transplacentally, suggesting that this structural analogue of DMH can be activated by fetal tissues (Druckrey, 1972). Should it be proven that, in fact, DMH and AOM are activated in colon directly, the results would be in keeping with the concept that organotropism exhibited by chemical carcinogens is the result of selective activation by the target tissue (Druckrey, 1972).

The data obtained from studies of the acute effects of MAM acetate indicate that a correlation exists between that segment of intestine affected soon after treatment and the site of tumor development. While the observed acute biochemical and pathological lesions may not be related to the events requisite for tumor initiation, they indicate either that the segment so affected can selectively enhance the conversion of MAM to its ultimate carcinogenic form or that, for some still unknown reason, these segments are inherently more sensitive to any of the carcinogen-induced effects than is the remainder of the intestines. The fact that a single treatment with MAM acetate induces more tumors of the colon than of duodenum or caecum (Zedeck and Sternberg, 1974), even though DNA synthesis in each of these tissues is similarly inhibited, suggests that other factors play a modifying role in tumor development. In this regard, results of several lines of investigation indicate that the bile acids and/or bacteria may influence the formation of colon tumors.

The finding that small intestine and colon respond similarly to the toxic effects of both 5FU and HN_2 exaggerates even further the selective resistance of jejunum and ileum to the carcinogen-induced lesions. It is of interest to note that the offspring of rats fed cycasin during the first week of pregnancy develop tumors of the jejunum; no jejunal tumors are observed in the mothers or in the offspring of rats fed carcinogen during the later periods of gestation (Spatz and Laqueur, 1967). Such relationships between age and sensitivity to tumor induction may prove to be very significant in view of the suggestion presented herein that metabolic processes, the activity of which may be age related, may enhance the degradation of MAM to its ultimate carcinogenic form.

Much is yet to be learned if we are to understand the precise mechanism by which these simple chemical molecules can transform normal intestinal epithelium into cells no longer responsive to internal regulatory mechanisms of cell proliferation and differentiation. To this end, it has been shown that these agents can interact with nucleic acids (Matsumoto and Higa, 1966; Shank and Magee, 1967; Hawks and Magee, 1974; Pozharisski *et al.,* 1975; Lawley, 1972) and that DNA strand breakage can occur and, in some cases, persist for prolonged periods (Damjanov *et al.,* 1973). It has been reported that ligation of high molecular weight newly synthesized DNA is interfered with in the second phase of cell replication following treatment with MAM acetate (Van Den Berg, 1974). In a different direction, information regarding the mechanism of cell detachment at the mucosal surface of the intestine and the effects of carcinogens on this process may prove useful in understanding polyp formation.

It is hoped that further use of the animal model systems discussed herein will lead to an understanding of the mechanism of colon carcinogenesis, to the design of an assay system for identification of colon carcinogens within our environment, and to the successful treatment of colon cancer.

11. Addendum

Since the submission of the manuscript of this chapter, data given in Tables 1 and 3, Fig. 1, and Sections 4.1 and 6 have been published (M.S. Zedeck, D.J. Grab, and S.S. Sternberg, 1977, Differences in the acute response of the various segments of rat intestine to treatment with the intestinal carcinogen, methylazoxymethanol acetate, *Cancer Res. 37:*32–36).

ACKNOWLEDGMENTS

The studies described herein that were conducted in the Laboratory of Pharmacology at Memorial Sloan-Kettering Cancer Center were supported in part by Public Health Service Grants CA 08748 from the National Cancer Institute and CA 15637 from the National Cancer Institute through the National Large Bowel Cancer Project. Survey of the literature relevant to this review ended December 1975.

I would like to thank Dr. Stephen S. Sternberg for his interest and cooperation in evaluating countless numbers of histology slides relevent to all our studies of chemical carcinogenesis, and Miss Queng Hui Tan for her excellent technical assistance. The studies of tissue esterase activity and of the effects of free MAM were conducted by Mr. Dennis Grab as part of his thesis research project; full reports will be published elsewhere.

12. References

Abrams, G. D., Bauer, H., and Sprinz, H., 1963, Influence of the normal flora on mucosal morphology and cellular renewal in the ileum: A comparison of germ-free and conventional mice, *Lab. Invest.* **12:**355–364.

Chhabra, R. S., Pohl, R. J., and Fouts, J. R., 1974, A comparative study of xenobiotic-metabolizing enzymes in liver and intestine of various animal species, *Drug Metab. Dispos.* **2:**443–447.

Chomchai, C., Bhadrachari, N., and Nigro, N.D., 1974, The effect of bile on the induction of experimental intestinal tumors in rats, *Dis. Colon Rectum* **17:**310–312.

Chung, K.-T., Fulk, G. E., and Slein, M. W., 1975, Tryptophanase of fecal flora as a possible factor in the etiology of colon cancer, *J. Natl. Cancer Inst.* **54:**1073–1078.

Corbett, T. H., Griswold, D. P., Jr., Roberts, B. J., Peckham, J. C., and Schabel, F. M., Jr., 1975, Tumor induction relationships in development of transplantable cancers of the colon in mice for chemotherapy assays, with a note on carcinogen structure, *Cancer Res.* **35:**2434–2439.

Damjanov, I., Cox, R., Sarma, D. S. R., and Farber, E., 1973, Patterns of damage and repair of liver DNA induced by carcinogenic methylating agents *in vivo*, *Cancer Res.* **33:**2122–2128.

Defries, E. A., and Franks, L. M., 1975, Effects of age and carcinogen treatment on cell growth in organ cultures of adult mouse colon (abstr.), *Br. J. Cancer* **31:**265.

Della Porta, G., 1961, Induction of intestinal, mammary, and ovarian tumors in hamsters with oral administration of 20-methylcholanthrene, *Cancer Res.* **21:**575–579.

Double, J. A., Ball, C. R., and Cowen, P. N., 1975, Transplantation of adenocarcinomas of the colon in mice, *J. Natl. Cancer Inst.* **54:**271–275.

Druckrey, H, 1970, Production of colonic carcinomas by 1,2-dialkylhydrazines and azoxyalkanes, in: *Carcinoma of the Colon and Antecedent Epithelium* (W. J. Burdette, ed.), pp. 267–279, Thomas, Springfield, Ill.

Druckrey, H., 1972, Organospecific carcinogenesis in the digestive tract, in: *Topics in Chemical Carcinogenesis* (W. Nakahara, S. Takayama, T. Sugimura, and S. Odashima, eds.), pp. 73–103, University Park Press, Baltimore.

Fahmy, O. G., and Fahmy, M. J., 1975, Genetic properties of *N*-α-acetoxymethyl-*N*-methylnitrosamine in relation to the metabolic activation of *N,N*-dimethylnitrosamine, *Cancer Res.* **35:** 3780–3785.

Fahmy, O. G., Fahmy, M. J., and Wiessler, M., 1975, *N*,α-Acetoxyethyl-*N*-ethyl-nitrosamine: A precursor of the biologically effective metabolite of *N,N*-diethylnitrosamine, *Biochem. Pharmacol.* **24:**2009–2012.

Fiala, E. S., and Weisburger, J. H., 1975, On the metabolism of the carcinogen 1, 2-dimethylhydrazine in rats (abstr.), *Toxicol Appl. Pharmacol.* **33:**178.

Gennaro, A. R., Villanueva, R., Sukonthaman, Y., Vathanophas, V., and Rosemond, G. P., 1973, Chemical carcinogenesis in transposed intestinal segments, *Cancer Res.* **33:**536–541.

Haase, P., Cowen, D. M., Knowles, J. C., and Cooper, E. H., 1973, Evaluation of dimethylhydrazine induced tumours in mice as a model system for colorectal cancer, *Br. J. Cancer* **28:**530–543.

Hawks, A., and Magee, P. N., 1974, The alkylation of nucleic acids of rat and mouse *in vivo* by the carcinogen 1,2-dimethylhydrazine, *Br. J. Cancer* **30:**440–447.

Hawks, A., Hicks, R. M., Holsman, J. W., and Magee, P. N., 1974, Morphological and biochemical effects of 1,2-dimethylhydrazine and 1-methylhydrazine in rats and mice, *Br. J. Cancer* **30:**429–439.

Homburger, F., Hsueh, S.-S., Kerr, C. S., and Russfield, A. B., 1972, Inherited susceptibility of inbred strains of Syrian hamsters to induction of subcutaneous sarcomas and mammary and gastrointestinal carcinomas by subcutaneous and gastric administration of polynuclear hydrocarbons, *Cancer Res.* **32:**360–366.

Karnofsky, D. A., and Clarkson, B. D., 1963, Cellular effects of anticancer drugs, *Annu. Rev. Pharmacol.* **3:**357–428.

Kroes, R., Berkvens, J. M., and Weisburger, J. H., 1975, Immunosuppression in primary liver and colon tumor induction with *N*-hydroxy-*N*-2-fluorenylacetamide and azoxymethane, *Cancer Res.* **35:**2651–2656.

Laqueur, G. L., 1965, The induction of intestinal neoplasms in rats with the glycoside cycasin and its aglycone, *Virchows Arch. Pathol. Anat.* **340:**151–163.

Laqueur, G. L., and Matsumoto, H., 1966, Neoplasms in female Fischer rats following intraperitoneal injection of methylazoxymethanol, *J. Natl. Cancer Inst.* **37:**217–225.

Laqueur, G. L., and Spatz, M., 1968, Toxicology of cycasin, *Cancer Res.* **28:**2262–2267.

Laqueur, G. L., McDaniel, E. G., and Matsumoto, H., 1967, Tumor induction in germfree rats with methylazoxymethanol (MAM) and synthetic MAM acetate, *J. Natl. Cancer Inst.* **39:**355–371.

Lawley, P. D., 1972, The action of alkylating mutagens and carcinogens on nucleic acids: *N*-Methyl-*N*-nitroso compounds as methylating agents, in: *Topics in Chemical Carcinogenesis* (W. Nakahara, S. Takayama, T. Sugimura, and S. Odashima, eds), pp. 237–258, University Park Press, Baltimore.

Leaver, D. D., Swann, P. F., and Magee, P. N., 1969, The induction of tumours in the rat by a single oral dose of *N*-nitrosomethylurea, *Br. J. Cancer* **23:**177–187.

Lowry, O. H., Rosebrough, N. J., Farr, A. L., and Randall, R. J., 1951, Protein measurement with the Folin phenol reagent, *J. Biol. Chem.* **193:**265–275.

Magee, P. N., and Barnes, J. M., 1967, Carcinogenic nitroso compounds, *Adv. Cancer Res.* **10:**163–246.

Martin, M. S., Bastien, H., Martin, F., Michiels, R., Martin, M. R., and Justrabo, E., 1973, Transplantation of intestinal carcinoma in inbred rats, *Biomedicine* **19:**555–558.

Matsumoto, H., and Higa, H. H., 1966, Studies on methylazoxymethanol, the aglycone of cycasin: Methylation of nucleic acids *in vitro, Biochem. J.* **98:**20c–22c.

Matsumoto, H., Nagahama, T., and Larson, H. O., 1965, Studies on methylazoxymethanol, the aglycone of cycasin: A synthesis of methylazoxymethyl acetate, *Biochem. J.* **95:**13c–14c.

McCall, D. C., and Cole, J. W., 1974, Transplantation of chemically induced adenocarcinomas of the colon in an inbred strain of rats, *Cancer* **33:**1021–1026.

Nagasawa, H. T., Shirota, F. N., and Matsumoto, H., 1972, Decomposition of methylazoxymethanol, the aglycone of cycasin, in D_2O, *Nature (London)* **236:**234–235.

Narisawa, T., and Nakano, H., 1973, Carcinoma of the large intestine of rats induced by rectal infusion of methylazoxymethanol, *Gann* **64:**93–95.

Narisawa, T., and Weisburger, J. H., 1975, Colon cancer induction in mice by intrarectal instillation of *N*-methylnitrosourea, *Proc. Soc. Exp. Biol. Med.* **148:**166–169.

Narisawa, T., Sato, T., Hayakawa, M., Sakuma, A., and Nakano, H., 1971, Carcinoma of the colon and rectum of rats by rectal infusion of *N*-methyl-*N*′-nitro-*N*-nitrosoguanidine, *Gann* **62:**231–234.

Narisawa, T., Nakano, H., Hayakawa, M., Sato, T., and Sakuma, A., 1972, Tumors of the colon and rectum induced by *N*-methyl-*N*′-nitro-*N*-nitrosoguanidine, in: *Topics in Chemical Carcinogenesis* (W. Nakahara, S. Takayama, T. Sugimura, and S. Odashima, eds.), pp. 145–158, University Park Press, Baltimore.

Narisawa, T., Magadia, N. E., Weisburger, J. H., and Wynder, E. L., 1974, Promoting effect of bile acids on colon carcinogenesis after intrarectal instillation of *N*-methyl-*N*′-nitro-*N*-nitrosoguanidine in rats, *J. Natl. Cancer Inst.* **53:**1093–1097.

Narisawa, T., Wong, C.-Q., and Weisburger, J. H., 1975, Induction of carcinoma of the large intestine in guinea pigs by intrarectal instillation of *N*-methyl-*N*-nitrosourea, *J. Natl. Cancer Inst.* **54:**785–787.

Nigro, N. D., Bhadrachari, N., and Chomchai, C., 1973, A rat model for studying colonic cancer: Effect of cholestyramine on induced tumors, *Dis. Colon Rectum* **16:**438–443.

Nigro, N. D., Singh, D. V., Campbell, R. L., and Pak, M. S., 1975, Effect of dietary beef fat on intestinal tumor formation by azoxymethane in rats, *J. Natl. Cancer Inst.* **54:**439–442.

Poynter, R. W., Ball, C. R., Goodban, J., and Thackrah, T., 1971/1972, The influence of physostigmine on the activation of methylazoxymethanol acetate, a potent carcinogen, by a serum factor *in vitro*, *Chem. Biol. Interact.* **4:**139–143.

Pozharisski, K. M., 1973, Tumours of the intestines, in: *Pathology of Tumours in Laboratory Animals*, Vol. 1: *Tumours of the Rat*, Part 1 (V. S. Turusov, ed.), pp. 119–140, International Agency for Research on Cancer, Lyon.

Pozharisski, K. M., 1975, The significance of nonspecific injury for colon carcinogenesis in rats, *Cancer Res.* **35:**3824–3830.

Pozharisski, K. M., Kapustin, Y. M., Likhachev, A. J., and Shaposhnikov, J. D., 1975, The mechanism of carcinogenic action of 1,2-dimethylhydrazine (SDMH) in rats, *Int. J. Cancer* **15:**673–683.

Preussmann, R., Druckrey, H., Ivankovic, S., and Hodenberg, A. V., 1969, Chemical structure and carcinogenicity of aliphatic hydrazo, azo, and azoxy compounds and of triazenes, potential *in vivo* alkylating agents, *Ann. N.Y. Acad. Sci.* **163:**697–716.

Reddy, B. S, Weisburger, J. H., and Wynder, E. L., 1974*a*, Effects of dietary fat level and dimethylhydrazine on fecal acid and neutral sterol excretion and colon carcinogenesis in rats, *J. Natl. Cancer Inst.* **52:**507–511.

Reddy, B. S., Weisburger, J. H., Narisawa, T., and Wynder, E. L., 1974*b*, Colon carcinogenesis in germ-free rats with 1,2-dimethylhydrazine and *N*-methyl-*N*′-nitro-*N*-nitrosoguanidine, *Cancer Res.* **34:**2368–2372.

Reddy, B. S., Narisawa, T., Wright, P., Vukusich, D., Weisburger, J. H., and Wynder, E. L., 1975*a*, Colon carcinogenesis with azoxymethane and dimethylhydrazine in germ-free rats, *Cancer Res.* **35:**287–290.

Reddy, B. S., Narisawa, T., Maronpot, R., Weisburger, J. H., and Wynder, E. L., 1975*b*, Animal models for the study of dietary factors and cancer of the large bowel, *Cancer Res.* **35:**3421–3426.

Rice, J. M., Joshi, S. R., Roller, P. P., and Wenk, M. L., 1975, Methyl (acetoxymethyl) nitrosamine: A new carcinogen highly specific for colon and small intestine (abstr.), *Proc. Am. Assoc. Cancer Res.* **16:**32.

Rogers, A. E., and Gildin, J., 1975, Effect of BCG on dimethylhydrazine induction of colon tumors in rats, *J. Natl. Cancer Inst.* **55:**385–391.

Rogers, A. E., and Newberne, P. M., 1975, Dietary effects on chemical carcinogenesis in animal models for colon and liver tumors, *Cancer Res.* **35:**3427–3431.

Schiff, L. J., 1975, Organ cultures of rat and hamster colon, *In Vitro* **11:**46–49.

Shank, R. C., and Magee, P. N., 1967, Similarities between the biochemical actions of cycasin and dimethylnitrosamine, *Biochem. J.* **105:**521–527.

Spatz, M., and Laqueur, G. L., 1967, Transplacental induction of tumors in Sprague-Dawley rats with crude cycad material, *J. Natl. Cancer Inst.* **38:**233–239.

Spatz, M., and Laqueur, G. L., 1968, Evidence for transplacental passage of the natural carcinogen cycasin and its aglycone, *Proc. Soc. Exp. Biol. Med.* **127:**281–286.

Springer, P., Springer, J., and Oehlert, W., 1970, Die Vorstufen des 1,2-Dimethylhydrazin-induzierten Dick- und Dünndarmcarcinoms der Ratte, *Ztschr. Krebsforsch.* **74:**236–240.

Thurnherr, N., Deschner, E. E., Stonehill, E. H., and Lipkin, M., 1973, Induction of adenocarcinomas of the colon in mice by weekly injections of 1,2-dimethylhydrazine, *Cancer Res.* **33:**940–945.

Van Den Berg, H. W., 1974, Alkaline sucrose gradient sedimentation studies of DNA from HeLa S_3 cells exposed to methyl methanesulphonate or methylazoxymethanol acetate, *Biochim. Biophys. Acta* **353:**215–226.

Ward, J. M., 1975, Dose response to a single injection of azoxymethane in rats: Induction of tumors in the gastrointestinal tract, auditory sebaceous glands, kidney, liver and preputial gland, *Vet. Pathol.* **12:**165–177.

Ward, J. M., Yamamoto, R. S., and Brown, C. A., 1973*a,* Pathology of intestinal neoplasms and other lesions in rats exposed to azoxymethane, *J. Natl. Cancer Inst.* **51:**1029–1039.

Ward, J. M., Yamamoto, R. S., Weisburger, J. H., and Benjamin, T., 1973*b,* Transplantation of chemically induced metastatic mucinous adenocarcinomas of the jejunum and colon in rats, *J. Natl. Cancer Inst.* **51:**1997–1999.

Ward, J. M., Weisburger, E. K., Benjamin, T., and Moss, R. A., 1974, Shift of organotropy of azoxy compounds—Replacement of methyl with an octyl group, *J. Natl. Cancer Inst.* **53:**1181–1185.

Ward, J. M., Sontag, J. M., Weisburger, E. K., and Brown, C. A., 1975, Effect of lifetime exposure to aflatoxin B_1 in rats, *J. Natl. Cancer Inst.* **55:**107–113.

Wattenberg, L. W., 1971, The role of the portal of entry in inhibition of tumorigenesis, in: *Progress in Experimental Tumor Research,* Vol. 14 (B. L. van Duuren, B. A. Rubin, and F. Homburger, eds.), pp. 89–104, Karger, Basel.

Wattenberg, L. W., 1974, Potential inhibitors of colon carcinogenesis, *Digest. Dis.* **19:**947–953.

Wattenberg, L. W., 1975, Inhibition of dimethylhydrazine-induced neoplasia of the large intestine by disulfiram, *J. Natl. Cancer Inst.* **54:**1005–1006.

Weisburger, J. H., 1971, Colon carcinogens: Their metabolism and mode of action, *Cancer* **28:**60–70.

Weisburger, J. H., 1972, Model studies on the etiology of colon cancer, in: *Topics in Chemical Carcinogenesis* (W. Nakahara, S. Takayama, T. Sugimura, and S. Odashima, eds.), pp. 159–174, University Park Press, Baltimore.

Weisburger, J. H., 1973, Chemical carcinogens and their mode of action in colonic neoplasia, *Dis. Colon Rectum* **16:**431–437.

Wiebecke, B., Krey, U., Löhrs, U., and Eder, M., 1973, Morphological and autoradiographical investigations on experimental carcinogenesis and polyp development in the intestinal tract of rats and mice, *Virchows Arch. Abt. A Pathol. Anat.* **360:**179–193.

Wittig, V. G., Wildner, G. P., and Ziebarth, D., 1971, Der Einfluss der Ingesta auf die Kanzerisierung des Rattendarms durch Dimethylhydrazin, *Arch. Geschwulstforsch.* **37:**105–115.

Wittkop, J. A., Prough, R. A., and Reed, D. J., 1969, Oxidative demethylation of *N*-methylhydrazines by rat liver microsomes, *Arch. Biochem. Biophys.* **134:**308–315.

Wynder, E. L., and Reddy, B., 1973, Studies of large-bowel cancer: Human leads to experimental application, *J. Natl. Cancer Inst.* **50:**1099–1106.

Zedeck, M. S., and Sternberg, S. S., 1974, A model system for studies of colon carcinogenesis: Tumor induction by a single injection of methylazoxymethanol acetate, *J. Natl. Cancer Inst.* **53:**1419–1421.

Zedeck, M. S., and Sternberg, S. S., 1975, Differential effects of methylazoxymethanol acetate (MAM) in rat colon and small intestine (abstr.), *Proc. Am. Assoc. Cancer Res.* **16:**32.

Zedeck, M. S., Sternberg, S. S., Poynter, R. W., and McGowan, J., 1970, Biochemical and pathological effects of methylazoxymethanol acetate, a potent carcinogen, *Cancer Res.* **30:**801–812.

15

Mathematical Models of Carcinogenesis and Tumor Growth in an Experimental Rat Colon Adenocarcinoma

Alain P. Maskens

1. Introduction

An accurate assessment of the growth behavior of cancers is of invaluable help in the understanding of their biological and clinical properties, as well as in the planning of appropriate therapies. Yet, in the important field of colorectal tumors, little such quantitative information is available, because of the inaccessibility of those lesions for direct serial measurements.

The development of chemical carcinogens with a highly specific colon activity in rodents (Druckrey *et al.*, 1967) paved the way for more detailed quantitation of colon cancer growth. Although direct serial measurements of individual tumors remain impossible in these models without modifying their natural environment and hence growth characteristics, their average proliferating pattern can at least be deduced from measurements obtained in serially sacrificed animals. On the other hand, such experimental systems where the schedule of drug administration and the rate of tumor yield and growth can be interrelated offer unique possibilities for better understanding the carcinogenesis mechanisms.

The mathematical treatment of such data is presented here. It proved helpful in devising models of carcinogenesis and growth pattern. It is stressed that the sole meaning of such models is to initiate and direct further biological testing. Suggestion is no demonstration.

Alain P. Maskens • Cancer Research Unit, Clinique Saint-Michel, B-1040 Brussels, Belgium.

2. *Experimental Design and Pathological Data*

2.1. *Colon Carcinogens*

Experimental colon cancer models became workable in 1967 with the introduction by Druckrey of two related compounds, 1,2-dimethylhydrazine (DMH) and azoxymethane (AOM). Under certain circumstances, both drugs exhibit a marked organotropism for the lower gut, and are potent carcinogens, a single dose being active in a fraction of the animals treated (Druckrey and Lange, 1972; Martin *et al.,* 1974). When repeated doses are given on a weekly basis, and the induction time is sufficient (16–24 weeks), 100% of the animals present with tumors. With increasing doses, the latency period is shortened. The lesions occur predominantly in the large bowel. In rats they appear as discrete tumors distributed in the ascending and descending colon, while in mice there is diffuse involvement of the distal colon and rectum. The most frequent neoplasm found is an adenocarcinoma (Druckrey *et al.,* 1967; Wiebecke *et al.,* 1969, 1973; Schauer *et al.,* 1969; Druckrey 1970; Martin *et al.,* 1973; Thurnherr *et al.,* 1973; Ward *et al.,* 1973*a;* Pozharisski and Klimashevski, 1974).

Although it is likely that DMH is mainly converted to AOM during its metabolic activation (Druckrey, 1970), the two drugs exhibit some differences in their respective activity. AOM is more toxic and less colon specific at similar doses. Indeed, while 21 mg DMH weekly is well tolerated, Druckrey (1970) reported that as little as 12 mg AOM weekly causes severe toxicity in rats. While a moderate dose of DMH (7–14 mg/kg weekly) produces almost exclusively colon tumors (Druckrey, 1970; Wiebecke *et al.,* 1973; Reddy *et al.,* 1974*a,b*), a comparable amount of AOM, 8 mg/kg weekly, induces a high proportion of duodenal tumors as well (Gennaro *et al.,* 1973; Nigro *et al.,* 1973; Ward *et al.,* 1973*a;* Chomcai *et al.,* 1974). Lower doses of AOM (6 mg) have a higher colon specificity; conversely, higher doses of DMH (21 mg) produce more small bowel cancers.

Besides dose, other factors have been shown to influence the carcinogenic activity of those compounds. Genetic susceptibility is suggested by a lower tumor production in BD II rats than in BD IX (Burdette, 1974). Age also plays a role, since differences in organotropism and tumor yield have been demonstrated after a single dose of AOM or DMH was given at various intervals after birth (Druckrey and Lange, 1972; Martin *et al.,* 1974). The bacterial as well as bile salts content of the gut likewise influences the colon tumor yield in DMH- or AOM-treated animals (Reddy *et al.,* 1974*a;* Chomcai *et al.,* 1974). Finally, dietary factors such as fat level and bulk can modify the activity of the carcinogen (Reddy *et al.,* 1974*b;* Ward *et al.,* 1973*b*).

2.2. *Animals and Treatments*

With the primary aim of obtaining a reproducible and specific animal model for quantitative studies on the growth of colon tumors, and taking into account the above properties of DMH and AOM, the following experimental regimen was adopted. Inbred male BD IX rats (Druckrey, 1971), maintained on a standard diet and water *ad libitum,* were used throughout the experiments. With exception of a control group of 26 rats, they were all given weekly subcutaneous injections of 9 mg DMH/kg [20 mg of the hydrochloride (DMH·HCl) provided by Schuchard, Munich, Germany]. The treatment was initiated between days 11 and 15 after birth and continued to the 24th week. The DMH·HCl was dissolved in 0.001 M EDTA and brought to pH 6.5 with sodium hydroxide. Pathology and volume measurement data from 80 animals distributed into four main experimental groups will be summarized in this report.

In group A, two treated animals were sacrificed together with controls at regular intervals from the third to the 40th week (26 control and 23 treated rats) in order to obtain preliminary information on the rate of tumor yield and growth. Three rats used for testing the tumor volume measurement technique were added to this group.

Group B consisted of 21 treated animals 33–40 weeks old serially sacrificed after a tritiated thymidine (TdR^{3}H) injection with the principal aim of constructing a labeled mitosis curve (which will be reported separately).

In group C, ten treated rats were sacrificed per group of two or three at three-week intervals between the 12th and 21st weeks to provide data on early (microscopic) pathological changes.

Group D consisted of 23 treated rats allowed to survive until natural death occurred, in order to obtain information on the maximal sizes reached by the tumors. Results from group A, B, and C experiments have been reported elsewhere (Maskens *et al.,* 1975; Maskens, 1976).

2.3. *Tumor Pathology*

Out of a total 275 macroscopic tumors (Fig. 1a) observed in this study, 261 were classified as adenocarcinomas, with local invasiveness through the muscularis mucosae demonstrated in 253 cases; 14 were signet ring cell infiltrating carcinomas.

2.3.1. *Adenocarcinomas*

A majority of the adenocarcinomas were found in the median portion of the colon, between the asending and descending segments (Fig. 1b). Two main and contrasting morphological types emerged (Fig. lc). One was a polypoid intraluminal growth, often with moderate invasion in the submucosal layer; the other infiltrated in depth to the serosa, had a marked tendency toward cyst formation, and eventually reached larger sizes than did the former. Metastases to the liver or lung occurred rarely (two cases in our experiments in animals more than 44 week old).

Macroscopic tumors were visible only after the 24th week. However, the microscopic analysis of serial sections of normal-appearing colon mucosa from rats sacrificed between the 12th and 21st weeks (group C animals) re-

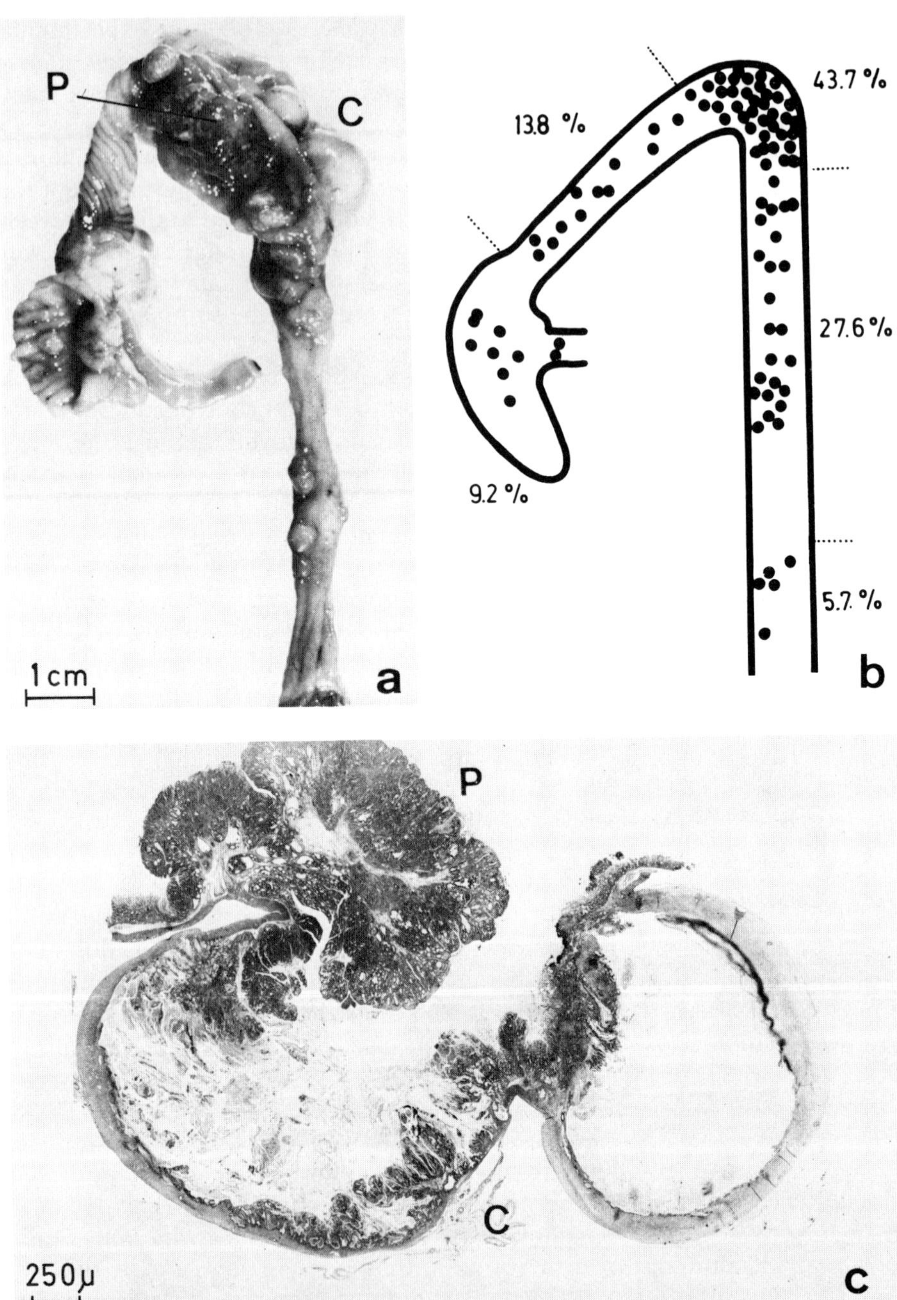

Fig. 1. (a) Macroscopic appearance of multiple colon tumors obtained in DMH-treated BD IX rats. (b) Distribution of the DMH-induced carcinomas (14 animals from group A experiment). (c) Histological preparation of tumors P and C in (a). Contrasting are the polypoid intraluminal growth on the one hand (P) and the in-depth infiltration with cyst formation on the other (C). Hematoxylin and eosin.

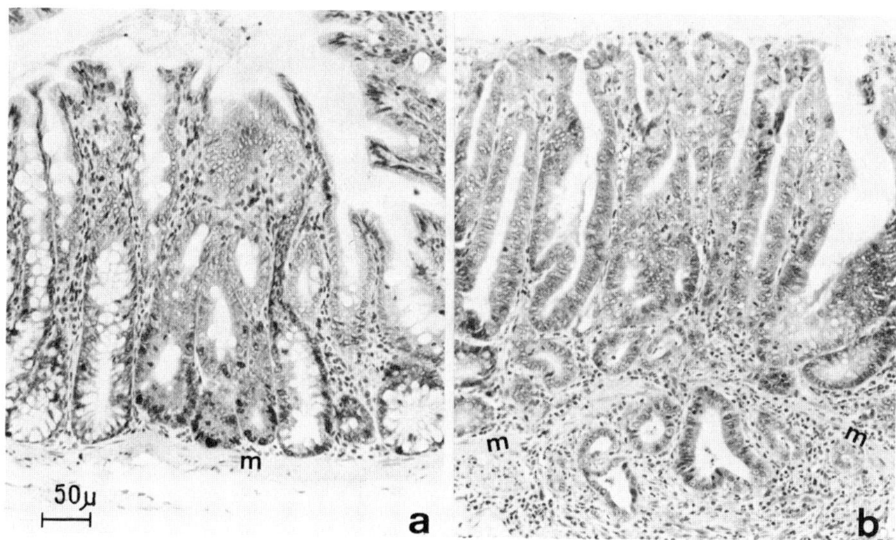

Fig. 2. (a) "Atypia" observed in flat colonic mucosa in a DMH-treated BD IX rat. Autoradiography after *in vivo* incorporation of tritiated thymidine. The radionuclide was given i.p. 40 min before sacrifice. Impaired cell differentiation and high thymidine uptake can be recognized. Hematoxylin and eosin. NTB_2 Kodak emulsion, exposure 8 weeks. (b) Microscopic adenocarcinoma observed in flat colonic mucosa in a DMH-treated BD IX rat, demonstrating early invasion of the submucosal spaces. m, Muscularis mucosae. Hematoxylin and eosin.

vealed atypical zones as early as the 12th week. These were characterized by an accumulation of undifferentiated cells with pleiomorphic nuclei and conspicuous nucleoli in the lower portion of some glandular crypts (Fig. 2a). From the 15th week on, characteristic carcinomatous changes could be observed: cellular atypias together with distorsion of the normal shape of the glands, and eventually invasion of the submucosa (Fig. 2b). It is stressed that no benign polyp–cancer sequence was observed in this material.

2.3.2. *Signet-Ring Cell Infiltrating Carcinomas*

The behavior of the 14 infiltrating carcinomas differed significantly from that of the adenocarcinomas. Their average size was larger; they predominated in the caecum and ascending colon. One such tumor was already visible in a 15-week-old rat. Adenocarcinomas only will therefore by considered in the following sections.

3. *Tumor Yield and Growth Pattern*

3.1. *Relationship between Tumor Volume, or Number, and Time*

Our preliminary approach to the problem of the relationship between tumor volume, or number, and time will be illustrated using data from group A animals. Since tumor shapes were variable and often irregular, a standard method was designed to estimate the volumes. Each tumor had its three main axes measured. The product of these axes multiplied by a coefficient of 0.69 was used as an approximation of the volume. This coefficient was obtained by regression analysis between the axes product and the weight (assuming a density equal to 1), in a control group of 21 tumors. It is intermediate between the coefficient for cylinders (0.79) and ellipsoids (0.52).

Based on the observation of the tumor sizes and number at the various times of sacrifice (Fig. 3), several deductions can be made. First, it is obvious that the number of tumors per animal increases with time in a nonlinear way. The simplest expression of this relationship is exponential (Fig. 4):

$$N_{(t)} = 0.089e^{0.0178t} \qquad r = 0.8302 \tag{1}$$

where N is the number of tumors per colon and t is the time in days from birth of the animal. An equally good fit is obtained using a quadratic fraction, which allows comparison with data computed in the carcinogenesis model to be described later in this chapter:

$$N_{(t)} = (-2.036 + 0.0190t)^2 \qquad r = 0.8063 \tag{2}$$

Second, tumor sizes also increase with time, as illustrated when the volume of the largest tumor present in each animal is plotted against time of sacrifice. An exponential-type growth is revealed whose rate can be obtained by regression analysis (Fig. 5):

$$V_{(t)} = 0.2385e^{0.0287t} \qquad r = 0.8251 \tag{3}$$

where V is tumor volume in mm^3 and t is time in days from birth. The corresponding doubling time is 24.2 days. Third, when several tumors are

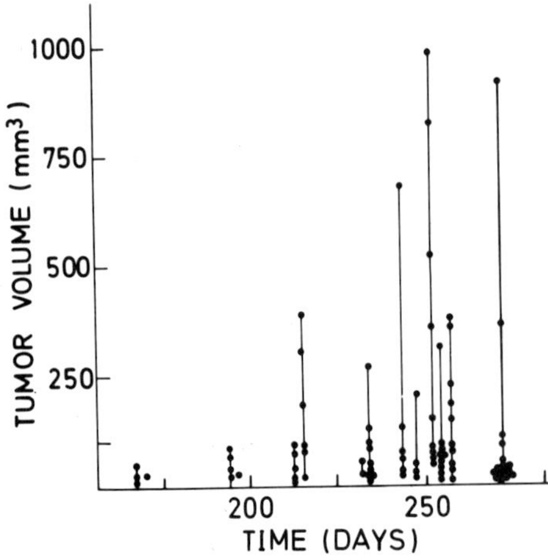

Fig. 3. Volume and number of adenocarcinomas obtained in DMH-treated BD IX rats sequentially sacrificed up to their 40th week (group A experiment). No macroscopic tumors were observed in animals sacrificed prior to their 24th week. Carcinomas from the same animal are linked by a vertical bar.

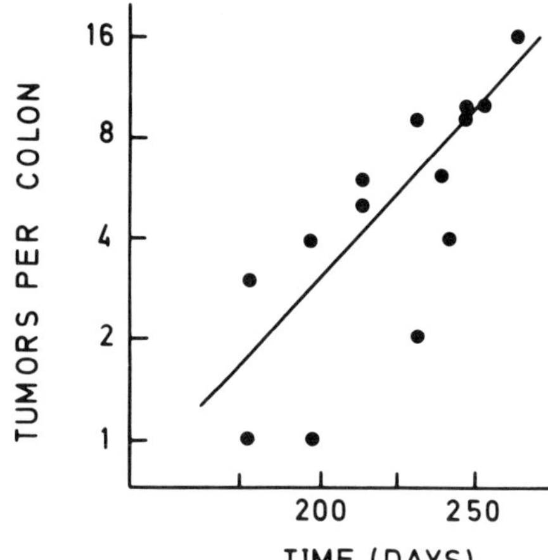

Fig. 4. Same experimental group as in Fig. 3. Number of adenocarcinomas per colon as a function of time of sacrifice (days from birth). Solid line, best-fitting exponential curve.

present in one colon, their sizes are not uniform but rather are graded. Since tumor volume and number are both positively correlated with time, one can postulate that, in the same animal, the largest tumor arose first, followed by the second largest tumor, and so forth. Accordingly, the exponential growth rates are computed for each set of homologous tumors (i.e., plotting the volume of the largest tumor in each animal vs. time of sacrifice, then the same for the second largest tumor, etc.). These exponential growth rates are quite comparable from one tumor group to the other, suggesting that different tumors in the same animal have quite similiar growth behaviors. Of interest also is the fact that the smallest tumors exhibit a somewhat faster growth rate (see Fig. 6).

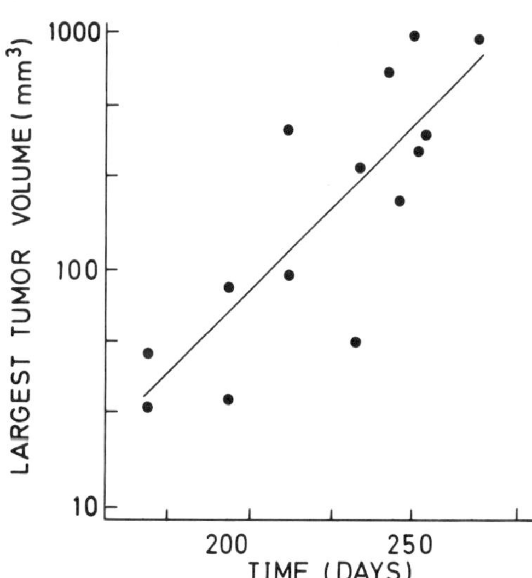

Fig. 5. Same experimental group as in Fig. 3. Exponential regression of the volume of the largest colon adenocarcinoma per animal vs. time of sacrifice.

3.2. The Gompertz Growth Curve

The possibility that smaller tumors grew more rapidly became evident when the volumes of the largest tumor per colon observed in the animals of the four experimental groups were plotted together (see Fig. 7). These include microscopic carcinomas observed at early stages (group C) as well as the largest sizes observed in the long-term survivors of group D, thereby extending the volume scale over 6 logarithmic units.

3.2.1. Development of the Best-Fitting Gompertz Curve

A Gompertz equation is used to describe this decay of growth rate of the tumors with increasing size:

$$V_{(t)} = V_{(0)} \cdot e^{(A/\alpha)(1-e^{-\alpha t})}$$

where $V_{(t)}$ is the tumor volume at time t, $V_{(0)}$ is the initial tumor volume, and A and α are specific constants. As such, it is a sigmoid curve with a maximum volume $= V_{(0)} \cdot e^{A/\alpha}$ and an inflection point at 37% of that maximum. In its logarithmic expression

$$\ln V_{(t)} = \ln V_{(0)} + \frac{A}{\alpha}(1 - e^{-\alpha t}) \quad (5)$$

it gives a curve whose slope exponentially decreases with time. The Gompertz curve that best fitted the observed data was generated using a method similar to that developed by Simpson-Herren and Lloyd (1970). Equation (5) may be expressed as $\ln V_{(t)} = a_0 + a_1 \nu$, where $a_0 = \ln V_{(0)} + A/\alpha$,$a_1 = -A/\alpha$, and $\nu = e^{-\alpha t}$. The parameters a_1 and a_0 are evaluated by the method of least squares for a given value of α, and the variance is calculated. The minimum value of this variance is obtained by an iterative procedure, giving the best α value. A and $V_{(0)}$ and then computed from $A = -\alpha \cdot a_1$ and $V_{(0)} = e^{(a0 + a1)}$.

The search for the best fit is time consuming and actually necessitates computer assistance, unless a good first approximation can be determined by some indirect method.* The curve that best fitted the experimental data was found for $\alpha = 0.0110$ (to the nearest 0.0005):

$$\ln V_{(t)} = -4.33 + \frac{0.155}{0.011}(1 - e^{-0.011t}) \quad (6)$$

*In the present case, this approximation was computed from the data in Fig. 6. Indeed, the exponential growth constants calculated for each set of homologous tumors can be considered the slope values of a hypothetical Gompertz curve at their respective median observation times. That slope is given by a derivative of equation (5) as expressed in equation (7). Its logarithm is a linear function of time: $\ln \{d[\ln V_{(t)}]/dt\} = \ln A - \alpha t$. Therefore, using a linear regression of the logarithm of these constants vs. their median observation time, an approximation of α can be computed.

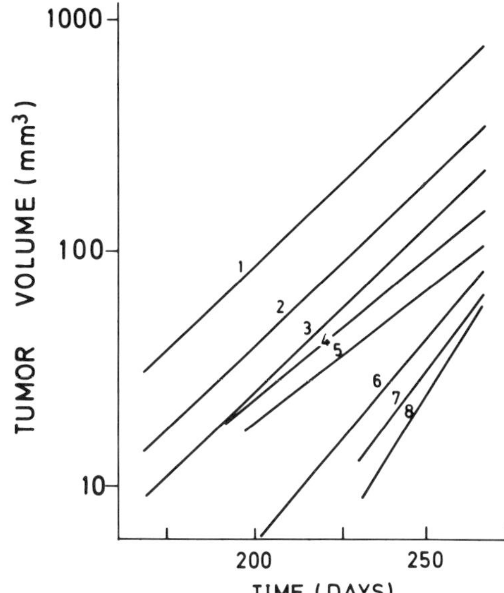

Fig. 6. Same experimental group as in Fig. 3. Exponential regressions obtained for the successive sets of homologous tumors. 1, Regression of the volume of the largest colon adenocarcinoma per animal vs. time of sacrifice (as shown in Fig. 5). 2,3, . . . , 8, Regression of the second, third, . . . , eighth largest tumor per animal.

where V is in mm^3, t is in days, and $t_{(0)}$ was arbitrarily set at 15 weeks after birth, when the earliest microscopic carcinomas can be observed ($r = 0.9146$). The fit of this Gompertz curve is significantly better than that of the corresponding best-fitting exponential ($r = 0.8395$).

3.2.2. *Implications of the Gompertz Function*

The extent to which the growth rate will decrease and the doubling time increase as tumors enlarge is illustrated in Table 1. The growth rate is calculated using the derivative of equation (5):

$$\frac{d[\ln V_{(t)}]}{dt} = A \cdot e^{-\alpha t} \tag{7}$$

It expresses the instantaneous exponential growth rate at a given time t. The corresponding instantaneous doubling time, $T_{d(t)}$ is obtained from $T_{d(t)} = (\ln 2)/A \cdot e^{\alpha t}$. Large tumors have a comparatively slow growth rate which varies little with time, mimicking a slow expotential growth. A slow exponential-type growth was also reported by Welin *et al.* (1963) for human colorectal tumors submitted to serial radiographic observations. This, however, cannot be extrapolated to small tumors, where, at least in this experimental model, the volume increase is fast, and the growth rate much more variable with size or time.

The first microscopic carcinomas were identified in 15-week-old rats. Their theoretical initial volume is 0.013 mm^3, or a small cluster of transformed crypts. If those tumors evolved from a single transformed cell, the

Table 1. Variation of the Exponential Growth Factor and Doubling Time According to Tumor Size in a DMH-Induced Rat Colon Carcinoma

Tumor volume (mm^3)	Exponential growth factor ($days^{-1}$)	Doubling time (days)
1×10^{-6}	0.2592	2.7
0.01	0.1579	4.4
0.1	0.1326	5.2
1.0	0.1073	6.5
10	0.0819	8.5
100	0.0566	12.2
1,000	0.0313	22.2
5,000	0.0136	51.1
10,000	0.0060	116.5

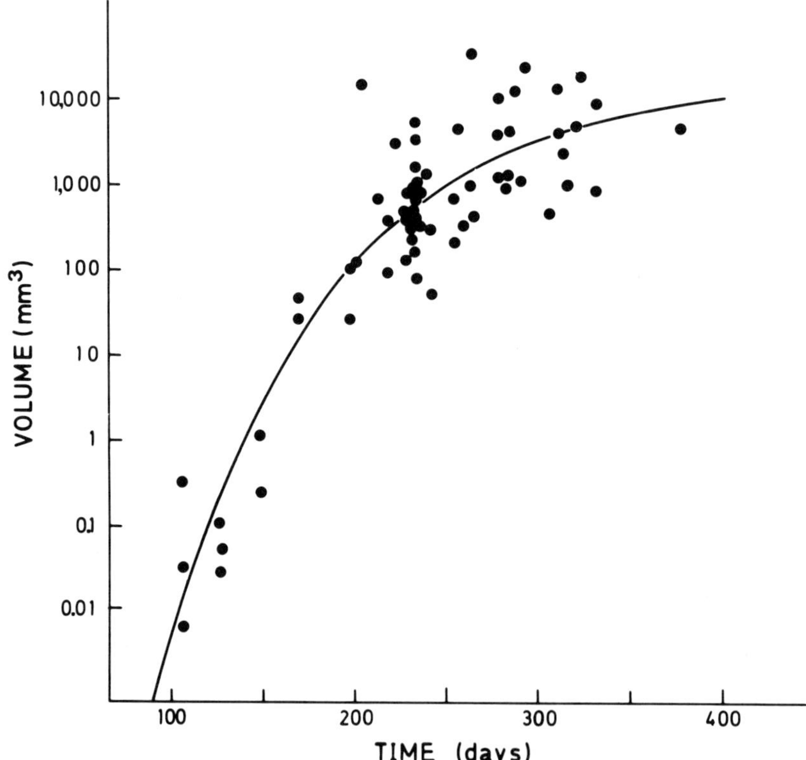

Fig. 7. Volume of the largest adenocarcinoma in the colon of DMH-treated rats vs. time of sacrifice. Microscopic tumors observed in younger animals (group C) are plotted together with the macroscopic measurements obtained in older animals (groups A, B, and D). The line represents the best-fitting Gompertz curve.

average period at which the first such transformation occurred can be predicted to be about 58 days after birth (or 47 days after the first DMH treatment) by extrapolating the curve to the volume of a single cell (10^{-6} mm^3). The corresponding theoretical doubling time at that stage (Table 1) should be 2.7 days, in accordance with available data on the cell cycle time of those tumors (Schauer *et al.,* 1971; Pozharisski and Klimashevski, 1974). The theoretical maximum volume, on the other hand, is 17,178 mm^3, well in the range of the largest tumors observed in this study (Fig. 7).

3.2.3. *Biological Meaning of the Gompertz Function*

After Laird (1964, 1969) used the Gompertz function to express the decaying growth rate of normal organisms and tumors, several human and experimental cancers have been fitted into this particular growth pattern (McCredie *et al.,* 1965; Frindel *et al.,* 1967; Simpson-Herren *et al.,* 1974). The exponential nature of this function is well adapted to the biological phenomenon it describes: a volume increment as a result of individual cell multiplication. This volume increment per unit of time therefore is a proportion of the volume as expressed by $dV/dt = KV$, which upon integration becomes $V_{(t)} = V_{(0)} \cdot e^{kt}$, where $k = d(\ln V)/dt$ is the exponential growth constant. In the simplest case of exponential growth, which consists of a system where all cells are actively replicating and no cell loss occurs, the tumor doubles its volume over the mean period needed for cells to reduplicate (or cell cycle time, T_c), and $k = \ln 2/T_c$. If only a fraction of the cells are proliferating—the so-called growth fraction, GF (Mendelsohn, 1960, 1962)—the exponential growth constant is reduced accordingly. For instance, if only 50% of the cells proliferate (GF of 0.5), then $k = (\ln 1.5)/T_c$. More generally, $k = [\ln(1 + \text{GF})]/T_c$. Finally, cell loss is a frequent feature in tumor biology (Steel, 1967). Again, it will contribute a decrease in the growth constant:

$$k = \frac{\ln (1 + \text{GF} - \text{CL})}{T_c} \tag{8}$$

where CL is fractional cell loss occurring during a period of time equivalent to T_c (this simplified formula implies that cell loss does not involve proliferating cells). Thus the exponential growth constant of a given tumor mainly depends on its mean cell cycle time, growth fraction, and degree of cell loss.

Experimental evidence has accumulated now that any of these three factors can vary during the expansion of a given tumor. In solid tumors, reduction in growth fraction and/or increasing cell loss has been clearly shown to accompany tumor growth (Killmann *et al.,* 1962; Frindel *et al.,* 1967; Hermens and Barendsen, 1969; Clifton and Yatvin, 1970; Griswold *et al.,* 1970; Huemer and Bickert, 1971; McCredie *et al.,* 1971; Cohen and Steel, 1972). In the present experimental colon carcinoma too, preliminary observations on tritiated thymidine incorporation indicate a lower labeling index in large vs. early lesions. In addition, increasing cell loss is quite likely to occur: necrotic zones are common in large lesions, and those tumors which grow within the intestinal wall and tend to form cysts where the necrotic material will be trapped reach larger sizes than do intraluminal carcinomas, which are probably more prone to continuous desquamation.

As a consequence of those modifications, the exponential growth factor of tumors will decrease with time. If this decay itself is exponential, as expressed in equation (7), the Gompertzian modification of the exponential model is fully justified.

Of interest also in a Gompertz function is the meaning of its extrapolated extreme values. When a newly transformed cancer cell, or a small group of transformed cells, starts proliferating, almost by definition the GF must be 1.0, and cell loss is to be limited, so that the doubling time must approach the value of the cell cycle time, as observed in this study. On the other hand, the concept of a maximum volume rather than an indefinite growth process is reasonable, at least in terms of vascularization and nutrient supply. It should be stressed, however, that these extrapolated extreme values are imprecise: 95% confidence limits of the mean maximum volume (sample mean 17.2 cm^3) are 11.4–25.9 cm^3; 95% confidence limits of the mean volume at the 58th day (sample mean 1×10^{-6} mm^3) are $0.3–2.8 \times 10^{-6}$ mm^3.

3.3. Other Growth Models

Although it is clear from the above data that a purely exponential model does not fit the growth properties of tumors observed over a long enough period, other mathematical expressions are available that describe a progressively decreasing exponential growth rate. Most interesting is the model introduced by Mendelsohn (1963) where the growth rate is proportional to a power of the volume:

$$dV/dt = kV^b \tag{9}$$

It has the advantage of being applicable to different modes of growth: for $b=0$, the growth is linear; for $b=1$, it is exponential; for $0 < b < 1$, a curve is obtained with upward convexity on a semilog diagram.

Upon integration, equation (9) becomes, for $b \neq 1$,

$$V^{1-b} = (1 - b)(kt + c) \tag{10}$$

Similarly to the Gompertz model, this is a three-constant function, and the best-fitting curve can be computed (Dethlefsen *et al.*, 1968) using an analogous principle: the constant b is given an empirical value, and the other two are obtained from a single regression analysis on the observed data. From equation (10), the $(1 - b)$ power of the volumes should indeed be a linear function of time. The analysis is reiterated for different values of b until the best measure of linearity is reached. The curve that best fitted our data is given by $V^{0.21} = 0.519 + 0.027t$.

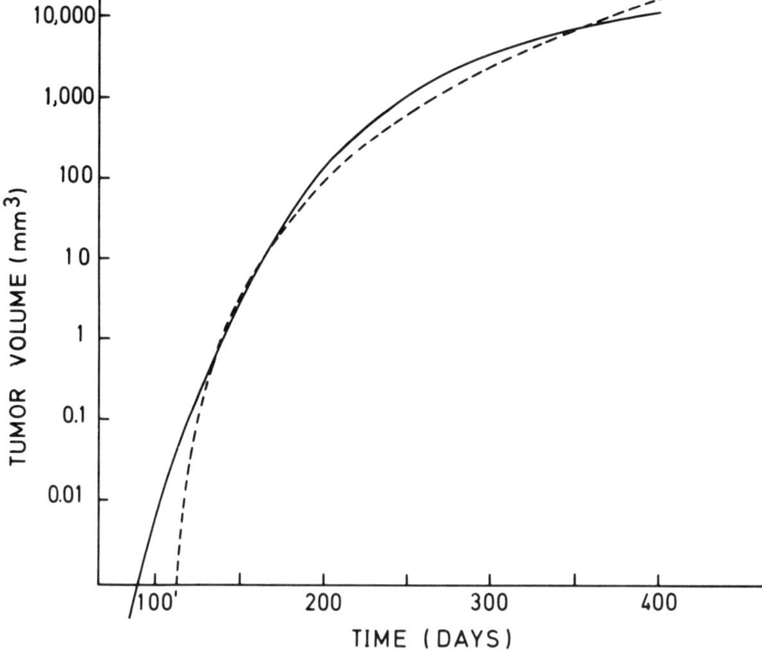

Fig. 8. Comparison between the best-fitting Gompertz curve (solid line) and power curve (dashed line).

When plotted on a semilog diagram, it closely approaches the best-fitting Gompertz curve (Fig. 8), with, however, a slightly poorer fit ($r = 0.8908$). It is therefore interesting to analyze the relationship between both models. As obtained from equation (9),

$$\ln \frac{dV}{dt} = \ln k + b \cdot \ln V \tag{11}$$

Therefore, data that fit the Mendelsohn model are characterized by a linear relationship between the logarithm of the instantaneous growth rate and the logarithm of the corresponding volume. When this test is applied to the Gompertz curve (Fig. 9), the linearity is well approximated over the range of observed tumor volumes; however, at the upper end of the observation the beginning of a sharp departure from linearity is present. It corresponds to this essential difference between the two systems: the growth rate asymptotically declines toward zero with time in the Gompertz function; in the Mendelsohn model, on the contrary, the growth rate will never decrease below a given minimal value. Another reason which made us prefer the Gompertz function is its exponential nature. By comparison, there is no clear relation between the mathematical expression of the power model and the underlying biological phenomenon.

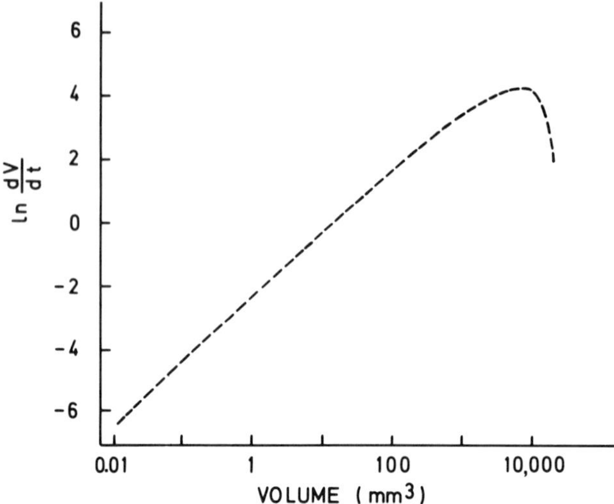

Fig. 9. Relation between the logarithm of the instantaneous growth rate computed from the Gompertz curve and the logarithm of the corresponding tumor volume. This relation approaches linearity over most of the observed volume range. For large tumor sizes, the Gompertz model implies a declining growth rate, and sharp departure from linearity is accordingly observed.

3.4. Individual Variations

Before closing this discussion of tumor growth models, it should be emphasized that they describe only the central tendency of the observed data. Individual variations are illustrated in Fig. 10, which shows the number of carcinomas per colon, and the volume of the largest tumor in 19 animals from group B, all sacrificed at the same age. The tumor number follows a Poisson distribution ($p > 0.50$) and the volumes are normally distributed ($p > 0.25$). Minor deviations can result from technical difficulties, mainly when tumor coalescence is occurring. The variation in tumor number can be an indication that the occurrence of new colon cancers in those DMH-treated rats follows a

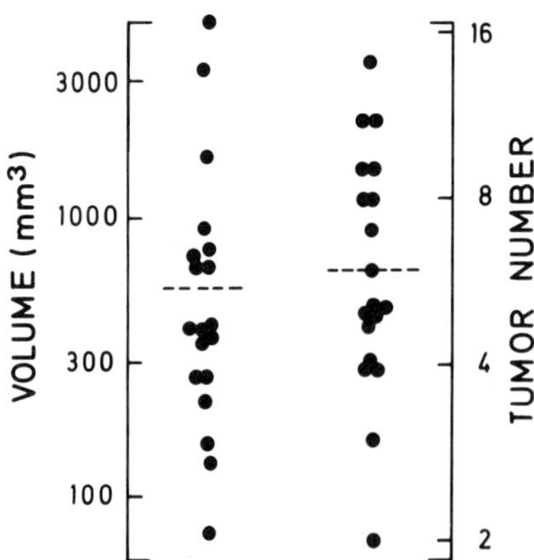

Fig. 10. Number of carcinomas and size of the largest carcinoma present in the colon of each of 19 DMH-treated BD IX rats sacrificed 31 weeks after initiation of the treatments. Dotted lines, respective means.

simple probability law. The variation in tumor size is more difficult to interpret, since it can be related both to the age and to the growth rate of a given tumor. Differences in the latter are likely to occur, as discussed before. Irregular growth within the same tumor is another possibility. These differences, however, which can become significant in large carcinomas, are probably minor in lesions of moderate size, in view of the limited divergences observed between the eight tumor sets of group A animals (Fig. 6).

4. A Model of Chemical Colon Carcinogenesis

4.1. Metabolic and Biochemical Properties of DMH and Related Compounds

Attempts to elucidate the final mechanism of colon carcinogenesis are converging from two directions. The first retrospectively analyzes the earliest tumor changes; it has been dealt with in the preceding section. The other traces the carcinogen from administration to its final target cell at the molecular level.

One possible metabolic pathway of DMH includes its oxidation to AOM, hydroxylation to methylazoxymethanol (MAM), and conjugation in the liver with glucuronic acid. Conjugated MAM is secreted in the bile to the gut, where it has to be regenerated before producing methyldiazonium (Fig. 11), which is thought to be the effective carcinogen (Druckrey, 1970, 1973; Weisburger, 1971; Fiala, 1975). Alternate possibilities include direct access of either glucuronated MAM (Pozharisski *et al.*, 1975) or other DMH metabolites to the gut via the blood circulation.

Methyldiazonium acts as an alkylating agent, resulting in methylation of nucleic acids in liver and colon of DMH-treated rats and mice (Hawks and Magee, 1974). MAM similarly methylates DNA and RNA (Matsumoto and

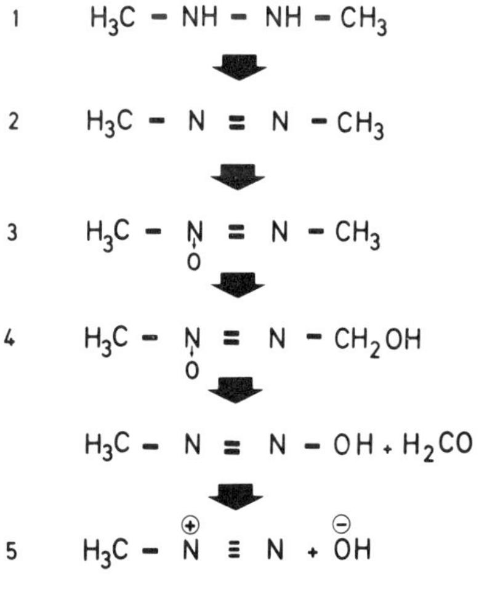

1 $H_3C - NH - NH - CH_3$

2 $H_3C - N = N - CH_3$

3 $H_3C - \underset{O}{\overset{\downarrow}{N}} = N - CH_3$

4 $H_3C - \underset{O}{\overset{\downarrow}{N}} = N - CH_2OH$

$H_3C - N = N - OH + H_2CO$

5 $H_3C - \overset{\oplus}{N} \equiv N + \overset{\ominus}{OH}$

Fig. 11. Metabolic activation of dimethylhydrazine. (1) Dimethylhydrazine. (2) Azomethane. (3) Azoxymethane. (4) Methylazoxymethanol. (5) Methyldiazonium. Modified from Druckrey (1970).

Higa, 1966; Shank and Magee, 1967). The latter compound also demonstrates potent mutagenic properties (Smith, 1966; Teas and Dyson, 1967).

In accordance with those known biochemical properties of DMH metabolites, we observed a severe nucleotoxic reaction in the colon mucosa within hours of DMH administration, as evidenced by karyorrhectic figures and decreased DNA synthesis (Maskens, 1976). Similar findings were demonstrated in both rats and mice by several authors (Zedeck *et al.*, 1970; Haase *et al.*, 1973; Hawks *et al.*, 1974). Extensive damage of rat intestinal DNA after DMH, followed by repair mechanisms, was in addition demonstrated by Kanagalingam and Balis (1975), using ultracentrifugation techniques with *in vivo* TdR^{3}H-labeled material.

In summary, DMH and related compounds do share most basic properties of chemical carcinogens. After metabolic activation, they produce electrophilic molecules capable of reacting with nucleic acids. They demonstrate a strong mutagenic activity. In target tissues, they induce nuclear damage and a temporary decrease in DNA synthesis activity, followed by a hyperplastic reaction. Tumors will eventually develop, after a dose-dependent latency period. (For reviews on chemical carcinogenesis, see Miller, 1970; Ryser, 1971; Heidelberg, 1973; Berenblum, 1974; Magee, 1974).

We therefore admitted as a first basis for the design of a carcinogenesis model that each DMH treatment, besides widespread unspecific reactions with nucleic acids and possibly other cell components in the colon mucosa, is capable of inducing permanent and transmissible changes in some cells that will ultimately lead to cancer transformation.

4.2. Multistep Theories of Carcinogenesis

In their attempt to correlate a mutational theory of carcinogenesis with the actual behavior of tumors induced by chemical or physical agents, several authors referred to the need for at least two consecutive changes in one single cell to achieve complete cancer transformation. A two-stage model was first proposed to explain the promoting action of some chemicals during skin carcinogenesis (Berenblum and Shubick, 1949). After Burch (1962) proposed that some childhood malignancies were compatible with multistage cancer transformations, the first mutational step being inherited through a parental germ cell, Knudson (1971, 1973) also proposed a convincing two-step model for embryonal tumors. It is based on the observation that hereditary retinoblastomas are often multiple and bilateral, as can be expected if a first mutation is affecting all retina cells, and that the only further requirement for tumor development is a second mutationlike event in any of those cells. Nonhereditary retinoblastomas, on the other hand, will require two consecutive somatic mutations in the same cell, a coincidence of very low probability which renders almost impossible the occurrence of multiple tumors in such cases, as confirmed by epidemiological observations.

Two-stage or multistage mutation models were also developed to explain the observation that cancer occurrence or cancer mortality rates in human are

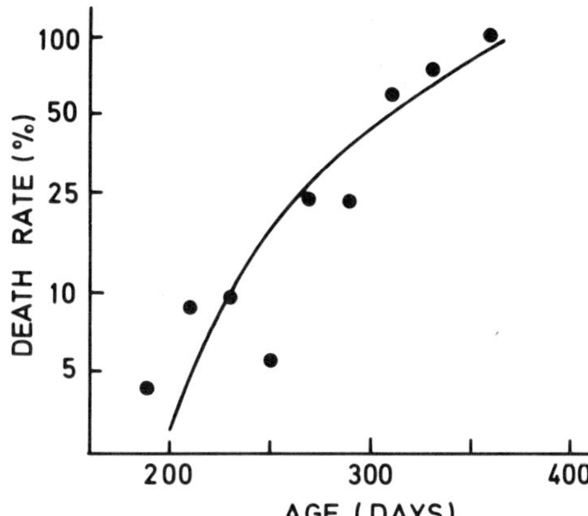

Fig. 12. Death rate (percent of survivors dying per period of time) in a group of 23 DMH-treated BD IX rats. Solid line, best-fitting quadratic curve. Ordinate, logarithmic scale.

a function of a power of time (Nordling, 1953; Stocks, 1953; Armitage and Doll, 1957; Fisher, 1958; Ashley, 1969). Under conditions of the continuous or repeated exposure to carcinogens, direct cancer transformation in one single step would indeed result in a linear increase of the tumor yield as a single function of time (provided that the carcinogen is rapidly metabolized and therefore does not accumulate as such).

In the present experimental system, we also turned to a model involving more than one step. Our data indeed also revealed a nonlinear relationship between time and death rate as well as tumor occurrence. The latter is described earlier in this chapter [see Fig. 4 and formulas (1) and (2)]. Mortality data were obtained using 23 DMH-treated rats allowed to die their natural death (group D experiments). The death rate (percent of survivors dying per period of time) exhibits a nonlinear relation with time, which can be approximated by an exponential or a quadratic function (Fig. 12). Although the mortality data can be greatly affected by variations in the growth rate of the induced carcinomas, data on tumor yield, on the other hand (Fig. 4), may be expected to roughly parallel the rate at which definitive cancer transformations do occur in those DMH-treated colons. A basic requirement of our model was therefore to allow for a cancer transformation rate comparable to the tumor increment with time actually observed. This was obtained in the following model, built on a two-step basis to take into account the short interval that separates the first DMH treatment (11th day) and the appearance of the first cancer cell capable of initiating cancer growth (58th day, as obtained by extrapolating the Gompertz growth curve).

4.3. A Two-Step Model for Experimental Colon Carcinogenesis

The model we propose is defined by the following properties:

1. DMH injections induce, among many unspecific changes, specific "mutationlike" events which render the affected cells ("pretransformed cells") prone to definitive cancer transformation.

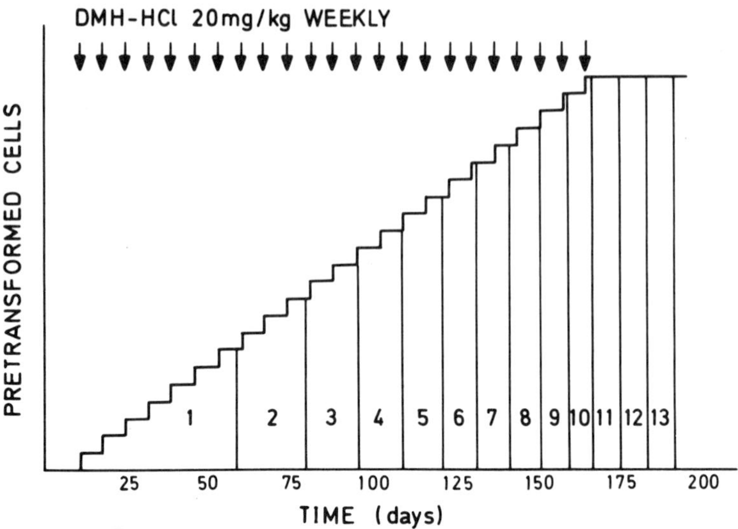

Fig. 13. A two-step model for DMH colon carcinogenesis. Each DMH treatment (arrows) induces an equal mean number of irreversibly "pretransformed" cells which accumulate with successive treatments ("stairs" line). These cells are at risk for a second transformation capable of initiating cancer growth. The surface areas numbered 1,2, . . . , 13 are all equal and represent each the probability of one such definitive transformation.

2. On the average, each treatment induces a similar number of "pretransformed cells" (N_p). Since the changes in those cells are irreversible and transmissible upon cell renewal, successive treatments will result in constant addition of new pretransformed cells (Fig. 13).
3. The probability that a second "mutational" event leading to full cancer transformation and growth initiation will occur in a pretransformed cell then depends on the total number of pretransformed cells and the time during which each of those cells is at risk. The number of precancer cells undergoing definitive cancer transformation (N_c) therefore is a function of N_p and time:

$$N_c = kN_p t \qquad (12)$$

Since N_p itself is proportional to time, N_c will be proportional to the square of time*:

$$N_c = (k't)^2 \qquad (13)$$

where N_c represents fully transformed cells, N_p represents pretransformed cells, t is the time from the first DMH treatment, and k and k' are constants.
4. Given that the first cancer transformation ($N_c = 1$) can be predicted to occur around the 47th day after the first DMH treatment, the constant

*In order to simplify the presentation of equations (12) and (13), a constant rather than intermittent increase of N_p has been assumed.

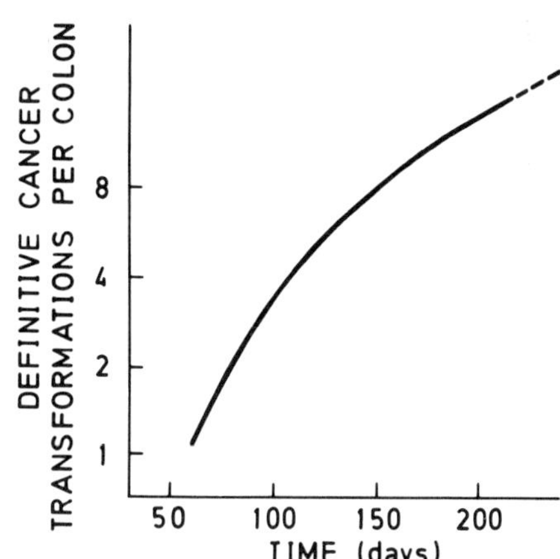

Fig. 14. Relation between the number of definitive cancer transformations and time in the colon of rats given weekly DMH treatments, as computed from the model in Fig. 13. Time, days from birth. Ordinate, logarithmic scale.

k' can be computed from (13), and the time of occurrence of the second, third, . . . transformed cell can be predicted:

$$N_c = (0.0212\, t)^2 \tag{14}$$

where t is expressed in days. This curve has a slope comparable to that observed for the mean increment of visible tumors [see formula (2)]. The full process is summarized in Fig. 15.

The author is well aware that this model clearly represents an oversimplification of several facts. What is the consequence of further treatment on pretransformed cells? What is the interference of immune mechanisms with pretransformed or transformed cells? Since the first treatments are given in growing animals, is their effectiveness equal or different? (The total number of cells exposed to DMH is lower but the affected cells will possibly have a larger progeny than cells from an adult colon.) Do pretransformed cells behave like normal cells in terms of cell renewal, or are they able to form growing clones at the expense of normal tissue? What is the nature of the changes involved in each step? These uncertainties, however, do not affect the concept itself of a two-step mechanism of carcinogenesis. The latter conversely provides a simple basis for further experimental testing of some of the above questions.

5. *Conclusions*

The biological behavior of rat colon adenocarcinomas induced by weekly treatments with DMH is characterized by three main properties:

1. These tumors are already truly invasive carcinomas when first recognized on microscopic examination of flat mucosa. Thus no benign polyp–cancer sequence is observed.
2. Their average growth pattern is best fitted by a Gompertz function.

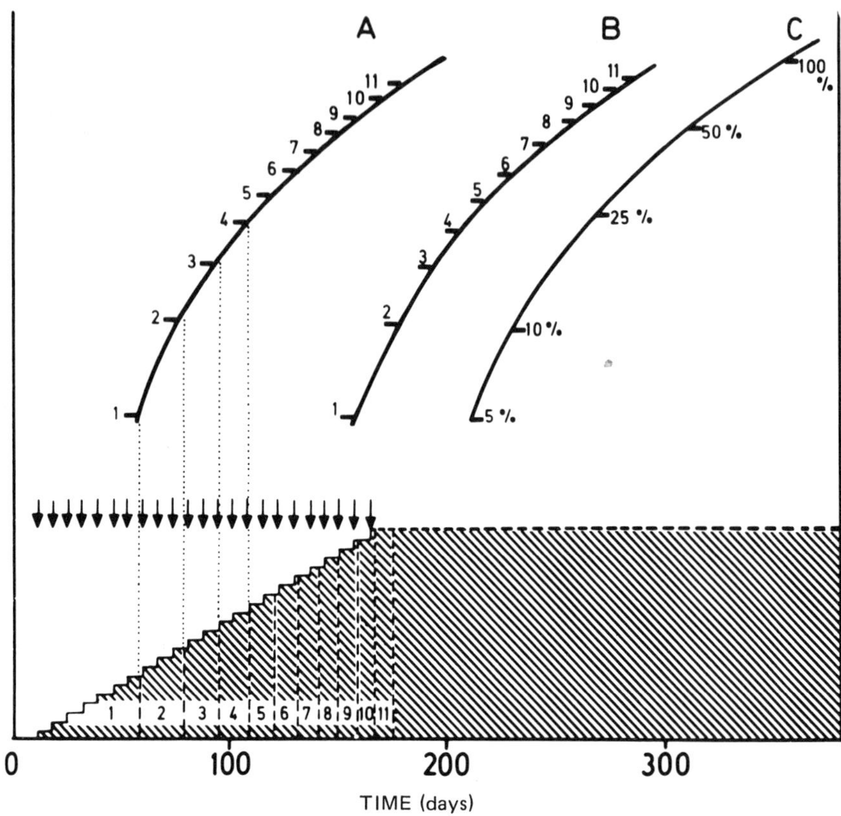

Fig. 15. Summary of the DMH colon cancer model. Weekly DMH treatments (arrows) induce the accumulation of "pretransformed cells," at risk for definitive cancer transformation. The latter occur after progressively smaller time intervals (A) as a result of this cumulative effect. About 102 days after the first definitive cancer transformation, the first macroscopic tumor can be observed. This delay corresponds to the time needed for a tumor to grow from one cell to a volume of 8 mm³ as computed from the Gompertz curve that best fits the experimental data. The number of macroscopic tumors per colon will thereafter increase (B) at a rate comparable to the cancer transformation rate (A). As tumors continue their growth in size and number, mortality will ensue with a rapidly increasing cumulative probability (C).

The doubling time is short in small lesions but will progressively increase as tumors enlarge.

3. The number of tumors per colon rises as a nonlinear function of time.

Based on the above findings, and bearing in mind the biochemical properties of DMH and related compounds, a two-step model of carcinogenesis is proposed. It implies that each DMH treatment induces a first stable and transmissible change in a number of colon epithelial cells, which thereafter will be at risk for a second mutationlike event responsible for initiating cancer growth.

Possible human implications of this model are several:

1. Although colorectal polyps are known to progress toward cancer with variable frequency according to histological type, this should in no way eliminate the possibility that some carcinomas arise *de novo* in flat mucosa.
2. The Compertz growth model implies that small and consequently most curable tumors represent an extremely brief stage as opposed to long-lasting, slowly growing large lesions. This could raise a serious challenge to the efforts aimed at early colon cancer detection.
3. A multistep mechanism of colon carcinogenesis implies that even minimal exposures to environmental carcinogens are of biological significance, since they could contribute to the accumulation of permanently modified cells susceptible to further malignant changes. Relevant to this last point is the growing evidence that carcinogenic *N*-nitroso compounds can arise in the gastrointestinal tract of man and other mammals from precursors widely present in man's environment. The ultimate carcinogen produced by metabolic activation of those compounds is probably identical to that of DMH (Druckrey, 1963; Preussmann, 1974).

Acknowledgments

The author wishes to thank Professor F. Meersseman, Dr. J. Haot, and Dr. J. Rahier for continued interest and discussion; Professor P. Baudhuin, Professor C. Deckers, Dr. M. Lipkin, and Dr. J. Fried for reviewing the manuscript; Mrs. R. M. Loits, Mrs. B. De Neuter-Maskens, and Mr. H. Withofs for skillful assistance; and Ms. F. Gennart for helpful secretarial assistance.

6. *References*

Armitage, P., and Doll R., 1954, The age distribution of cancer and a multi-stage theory of carcinogenesis, *Br. J. Cancer* **8:**1–12.

Armitage, P., and Doll R., 1957, A two-stage theory of carcinogenesis in relation to the age distribution of human cancer, *Br. J. Cancer* **11:**161–169.

Ashley, D. J. B., 1969, The two "hit" and multiple "hit" theories of carcinogenesis, *Br. J. Cancer* **23:**313.

Berenblum, I., 1974, Chemical carcinogenesis as a biological problem, in: *Frontiers in Biology,* Vol. 27, North-Holland, Amsterdam.

Berenblum, I., and Shubik, P., 1949, An experimental study of the initiating stage of carcinogenesis, and a re-examination of the somatic cell mutation theory of cancer, *Br. J. Cancer* **3:**109–118.

Burch, P. R. J., 1962, A biological principle and its converse some implications for Carcinogenesis, *Nature (London)* **195:**241–243.

Burdette, W., 1974, Colorectal carcinogenesis, *Cancer* **34:**872–877.

Chomcai, C., Bhadrachari, N., and Nigro, N. D., 1974, The effect of bile on the induction of experimental intestinal tumors in rats, *Colon Rectum* **17:**310–312.

Clifton, K. H., and Yatvin, M. B., 1970, Cell population growth and cell loss in the MTG-B mouse mammary carcinoma, *Cancer Res.* **30:**658–664.

Cohen, D., and Steel, G. G., 1972, Thymidine labelling studies in a transmissible veneral tumour of the dog, *Br. J. Cancer* **26**:413–419.

Dethlefsen, L., Prewitt, J., and Mendelsohn, M., 1968, Analysis of tumor growth curves, *J. Natl. Cancer Inst.* **40**:389–405.

Druckrey, H., 1970, Production of colonic carcinomas by 1, 2 dimethylhydrazines and azoxyalkanes, in: *Carcinoma of the Colon and Antecedent Epithelium* (W. J. Burdette, ed.), pp. 267–279, Thomas, Springfield, Ill.

Druckrey, H., 1971, Genotypes and phenotypes of ten inbred strains of BD-rats, *Arzneim.-Forsch. (Drug Res.)* **21**:1274–1278.

Druckrey, H., 1973, Specific carcinogenic and teratogenic effects of "indirect" alkylating methyl and ethyl compounds, and their dependency on stages of ontogenic developments, *Xenobiotica* **3**:271–303.

Druckrey, H., and Lange, A., 1972, Carcinogenicity of azoxymethane dependent on age in BD rats, *Fed. Proc.* **31**:1482–1484.

Druckrey, H., Preussman, R., Matzkies, F., and Ivankovic, S., 1967, Selektive Erzeugung von Darmkrebs bei Ratten durch 1, 2-Dimethylhydrazin, *Naturwissenchaften* **58**:285–286.

Fiala, E. G., 1975, Investigation into the metabolism and mode of action of the colon carcinogen 1,2-dimethylhydrazin, *Cancer* **36**:2407–2412.

Fisher, J. C., 1958, Multiple-mutation theory of carcinogenesis, *Nature (London)* **181**:651–652.

Frindel, E., Malaise, E., Alpen, E., and Tubiana, M., 1967, Kinetics of cell proliferation of an experimental tumor, *Cancer Res.* **27**:1122–1131.

Gennaro, A. R., Villanueva, R., Sukonthaman, Y., Vathanophas, and Rosemond, G. P., 1973, Chemical carcinogenesis in transposed intestinal segments, *Cancer Res.* **33**:536–541.

Griswold, D. P., Jr., Simpson-Herren, L., and Schabel, F. M., Jr., 1970, Altered sensitivity of a ramster plasmacytoma to cytosine arabinoside (NSC-63878), *Cancer Chemother. Rep.* **54**:337–340.

Haase, P., Cowen, D. M., Sr., Knowles, J. C., and Cooper, E. H., 1973, Evaluation of dimethylhydrazine induced tumors in mice as a model system for colorectal cancer, *Br. J. Cancer* **28**:530–543.

Hawks, A., and Magee, P., 1974, The alkylation of nucleic acids of rat and mouse *in vivo* by the carcinogen 1,2-dimethylhydrazine, *Br. J. Cancer* **30**:440–447.

Hawks, A., Hicks, R., Holsman, J., and Magee, P., 1974, Morphological and biochemical effects of 1,2-dimethylhydrazine and 1-methylhydrazine in rats and mice, *Br. J. Cancer* **30**:429–439.

Heidelberg, C., 1973, Current trends in chemical carcinogenesis, *Fed. Proc.* **32**:2154–2161.

Hermens, A. F., and Barendsen G. W., 1969, Changes of cell proliferation characteristics in a rat rhabdomyosarcoma before and after X-irradiation, *Eur. J. Cancer* **5**:173–189.

Huemer, R. P., and Bickert, C., 1971, Growth and differentiation of a transplantable plasmacytoma, *Oncology* **25**:439–445.

Kanagalingam, K., and Balis, A. E., 1975, *In vivo* repair of rat intestinal DNA damage by alkylating agents, *Cancer* **36**:2364–2372.

Killmann, S. A., Cronkite, E. P., Fliedner, T. M., and Bond, V. P., 1962, Cell proliferation in multiple myeloma studied with tritiated thymidine *in vivo, Lab. Invest.* **11**:845–851.

Knudson, A. G., 1971, Mutation and cancer: Statistical study of retinoblastoma, *Proc. Natl. Acad. Sci. USA* **68**:820–823.

Knudson, A. G., 1973, Mutation and human cancer, in: *Advances in Cancer Research,* Vol. 17 (G. Klein and S. Weinhouse, eds.), pp. 317–352, Academic Press, New York.

Laird, A., 1964, Dynamics of tumor growth, *Br. J. Cancer* **18**:490–502.

Laird, A., 1969, Dynamics of growth in tumors and in normal organisms, *Natl. Cancer Inst. Monogr.* **30**:15–28.

Magee, P. N., 1974, Molecular Mechanisms in chemical carcinogenesis, in: *Special Topics in Carcinogenesis* (E. Grundmann, ed.), pp. 2–8, Vol. 44 of *Recent Results in Cancer Research,* Springer-Verlag, New York.

Martin, M. S., Martin, F., Michiels, R., Bastien, H., Justrabo, E., Bordes, M., and Viry, B., 1973, An experimental model for cancer of the colon and rectum, *Digestion* **8**:22–34.

Martin, M. S., Martin, F., Justrabo, E., Knopf, J.-F., Bastien, H., and Knobel, S., 1974, Induction de cancers coliques chez le rat par injection unique de 1,2-dimethylhydrazine, *Biol. Gastroenterol.* **7:**37–42.

Maskens, A., 1976, Histogenesis and growth pattern of 1,2-dimethylhydrazine induced rat colon adenocarcinoma, *Cancer Res.* **36:**1585–1592.

Maskens, A., Meersseman, F., and Rahier, J., 1975, Growth rate of 1,2-dimethylhydrazine induced colon adenocarcinoma in rat (abstr.), *Proc. Am. Assoc. Cancer Res.* **16:**17.

Matsumoto, H., and Higa, H., 1966, Studies on methylazoxymethanol, the aglycone of cycasin: Methylation of nucleic acids *in vitro, Biochem. J.* **98:**20c–22c.

McCredie, J., Inch, W., Kruuv, J., and Watson, T., 1965, *Growth* **29:**331–347.

McCredie, J. A., Inch, W. R., and Sutherland, R. M., 1971, Differences in growth and morphology between the spontaneous C_3H mammary carcinoma in the mouse and its syngeneic transplants, *Cancer* **27:**635–642.

Mendelsohn, M., 1960, The growth fraction: A new concept applied to tumors, *Science* **132:**1496.

Mendelsohn, M., 1962, Autoradiographic analysis of cell proliferation in spontaneous breast cancer of C3H mouse. III. The growth fraction, *J. Natl. Cancer Inst.* **28:**1015–1029.

Mendelsohn, M., 1963, Cell proliferation and tumour growth, in: *Cell Proliferation* (L. F. Lamerton and R. J. M. Fry, eds.), pp. 190–210, Blackwell, London.

Miller, J. A., 1970, Carcinogenesis by chemicals: An overview, G. H. A. Clowes Memorial Lecture, *Cancer Res.* **30:**559–576.

Nigro, N. D., Bhadrachari, N., and Chomcai, C., 1973, A rat model for studying colonic cancer, *Dis. Colon Rectum* **16:**438–443.

Nordling, C. O., 1953, A new theory on the cancer inducing mechanism, *Br. J. Cancer* **7:**68–72.

Pozharisski, K., and Klimashevski, V., 1974, Comparative morphological and histoautoradiographic study of multiple experimental intestinal tumours, *Exp. Pathol.* **9:**88–98.

Pozharisski, K., Kapustin, Y., Likhachev, A., and Shaposhnikov, J., 1975, The mechanism of carcinogenic action of 1,2-dimethylhydrazine (SDMH) in rats, *Int. J. Cancer* **15:**673–683.

Preussmann, R., 1974, Formation of carcinogens from precursors occurring in the environment; new aspects of nitrosamine induced tumorigenesis, in: *Special Topics in Carcinogenesis* (E. Grundmann, ed.), pp. 9–15, Vol. 44 of *Recent Results in Cancer Research,* Springer-Verlag, New York.

Reddy, B., Weisburger, J., Narisawa, T., and Wynder, E., 1974*a,* Colon carcinogenesis in germ free rats with 1,2-dimethylhydrazine and *N*-methyl-*N'*-nitro-*N*-nitrosoguanidine, *Cancer Res.* **34:**2368–2372.

Reddy, B., Weisburger, J., and Wynder, E., 1974*b,* Effects of dietary fat level and dimethylhydrazine on fecal acid and neutral sterol excretion and colon carcinogenesis in rats, *J. Natl. Cancer Inst.* **52:**507–511.

Ryser, H. J. P., 1971, Chemical carcinogenesis, *N. Eng. J. Med.* **285:**721–734.

Schauer, A., Vollnagel, T., and Wildanger, F. 1969, Cancerisierung des Rattendarmes durch 1, 2-Dimethylhydrazine, *Ztschr. Ges. Exp. Med.* **150:**87–93.

Schauer, A., Kunze, E., and Boxler, K., 1971, Generationszeitzyklus 1,2-Dimethylhydrazin-induzierten Adenocarcinomen des Rattencolon, *Naturwissenschaften* **58:**221.

Shank, R. C., and Magee, P. N., 1967, Similarities between the biochemical actions of cycasin and dimethylnitrosamine, *Biochem. J.* **105:**521–527.

Simpson-Herren, L., and Lloyd, H., 1970, Kinetic parameters and growth curves for experimental tumor systems, *Cancer Chemother. Rep.* **54:**143–174.

Simpson-Herren, L., Sanford, A., and Holmquist, J., 1974, Cell population kinetics of transplanted and metastatic Lewis lung carcinoma, *Cell Tissue Kinet.* **7:**349–361.

Smith, D., 1966, Mutagenicity of cycasin aglycone (methylazoxymethanol), a naturally occurring carcinogen, *Science* **152:**1273–1274.

Springer, P., Springer, J., and Oehlert, W, 1970, Die Vorstufen des 1,2-Dimethylhydrazin-induzierten Dick- und Dundarmcarcinoms der Ratte, *Ztschr. Krebsforsch.* **74:**236–240.

Steel, G., 1967, Cell loss as a factor in the growth rate of human tumours, *Eur. J. Cancer* **3:**381–387.

Stocks, P., 1953, A study of the age curve for cancer of the stomach in connection with a theory of the cancer producing mechanism, *Br. J. Cancer* **7**:407–417.

Sullivan, P. W., and Salmon, S. E., 1972, Kinetics of tumor growth and regression in Ig G multiple myeloma. *J. Clin. Invest.* **51**:1697–1708.

Teas, J., and Dyson, J. G., 1967, Mutation in *Drosophila* by methylazoxymethanol, the aglycone of cycasin, *Proc. Soc. Exp. Biol. Med.* **125**:988–990.

Thurnherr, N., Deschner, E., Stonehill, E., and Lipkin, M., 1973, Introduction of adenocarcinomas of the colon in mice by weekly injections of 1,2-dimethylhydrazine, *Cancer Res.* **33**:940–945,

Ward, J. M., Yamamoto, R. S., and Brown, C. A., 1973*a*, Pathology of intestinal neoplasms and other lesions in rats exposed to azoxymethane, *J. Natl. Cancer Inst.* **51**:1029–1035.

Ward, J. M., Yamamoto, R. S., and Weisburger, J. H., 1973*b*, Cellulose dietary bulk and azoxymethane induced intestinal cancer, *J. Natl. Cancer Inst.* **51**:713–715.

Weisburger, J., 1971, Colon carcinogens: Their metabolism and mode of action, *Cancer* **28**:60–70.

Welin, S., Youker, J., and Spratt, J., 1963, The rates and patterns of growth of 375 tumors of the large intestine and rectum observed serially by double contrast enema study (Malmö technique), *Am. J. Roentgen Radium Ther. Nucl. Med.* **90**:673–687.

Wiebecke, B., Löhrs, U., Gimmy, J., and Eder, M., 1969, Erzeugung von Darmtumoren beim Mausen durch 1,2-Dimethylhydrazin, *Ztschr. Ges. Exp. Med.* **149**:277–278.

Wiebecke, B., Krey, U., Löhrs, U., and Eder, M., 1973, Morphological and autoradiographical investigations on experimental carcinogenesis and polyp development in the intestinal tract of rats and mice, *Virchows Arch. Pathol. Anat.* **360**:179–193.

Zedeck, M. S., Sternberg, S. S., Poynter, R. W., and McGowan, J., 1970, Biochemical and pathological effects of methylazoxymethanol acetate, a potent carcinogen, *Cancer Res.* **30**:801–812.

16

Development of Model Colorectal Cancer Systems for Pharmacological Research

John A. Double and Edward H. Cooper

1. Introduction and Scope

The success or failure of surgery to eliminate colorectal cancer depends on many factors. Essentially, they are hinged on whether the local lesion can be excised completely or whether the tumor is complicated by either overt metastases or occult micrometastases that are outside the confines of the portion of bowel that is resected. At present, the only hope of prolonged survival for patients with metastastic large bowel cancer is the use of other modalities of therapy in combination with surgery. Chemotherapy is the lynchpin of this strategy; preoperative radiotherapy may have an adjuvant role in carcinoma of the rectum and occasionally is a helpful palliative treatment of metastases in certain sites. As yet, the long-term benefits of immunotherapy are unknown, although there are enthusiasts for this novel approach. However, the immunostimulants available today are still a very crude way of effecting a biological cure of cancer.

Chemotherapy has two possible roles: (1) as an adjuvant in the hope that it may be able to eliminate micrometastases following removal of the primary lesion and (2) as definitive therapy of metastatic cancer. The latter can be in the form either of minimal residual disease not clinically detectable for several months after laparotomy or of more advanced and clinically apparent disease.

Compared to the various animal model systems that have been so useful in the research and development of leukemia chemotherapy and drug-

John A. Double and Edward H. Cooper • Department of Experimental Pathology and Cancer Research, School of Medicine, The University of Leeds, Leeds, England.

screening programs, there are relatively few animal model systems that reflect the problems likely to be encountered in planning chemotherapy for specific types of cancer and finding agents most likely to be effective.

Fortunately, in recent years several laboratories have developed methods of inducing bowel cancer in laboratory animals, and from these tumors a number of transplantable adenocarcinomas have been derived. At the same time, others have found ways of enabling human colon cancer to grow as xenografts in various animal hosts.

Although the study of primary cancers induced by chemicals in the large bowel of experimental animals is of fundamental importance, especially in identifying etiological factors in the disease, we propose to pay most attention to the transplantable colon cancers because we feel that it is from this research that results of more immediate relevance to clinical medicine will emerge.

2. *Induction of Experimental Colorectal Cancer*

The induction of chemical carcinogens of experimental colorectal cancer in animals is well documented, and there are several excellent reviews on the subject (Druckrey, 1972; Weisberger, 1971, 1973). Table 1 lists some of the agents that are used for the induction of experimental large bowel cancer. The reader with a knowledge of chemistry will observe that some of them have some connection with cycasin. It was probably the investigation of the carcinogenic properties of cycasin, a natural carcinogen occurring in the cycad nut, by Laqueur and his colleagues (Laqueur *et al.*, 1963, Laqueur, 1964) that laid the foundation of much of the research in this field, although it was probably Walpole *et al.* (1952), using 4-aminodiphenyl, who provided workers with the first reliable system for inducing colon cancer in animals.

The histopathology of the primary tumors in the bowel as well as the precancerous lesions that are associated with them has been well described (Ward *et al.*, 1973; Ward, 1974; Filipe, 1975; Martin *et al.*, 1973*a;* Haase *et al.*, 1973). In broad terms the induced colon cancers have many characteristics in common with adenocarcinoma of the colon and rectum in man with the

Table 1. Chemicals Known to Induce Colorectal Cancer in Experimental Animals

4-Aminobiphenyl
3,2′-Dimethyl-4-aminobiphenyl
Azomethane
Cycasin[a]
Methylazoxymethanol (MAM)[a]
1,2-Dimethylhydrazine[a]
Azoxymethane[a]
N-Methyl- or *N*-ethylnitrosourethane
N-Methyl-*N*′-nitro-*N*-nitrosoguanidine
Aflatoxin

[a]Cycasin derivatives and related compounds.

exception that metastases to local lymph nodes (the equivalent of a Dukes C tumor) are a rarity. Primary tumors can now be induced in a few species of laboratory animals; by far the greater number are in rats and mice, although there are a number of reports of tumors established in hamsters. The references to these papers can be found in the general reviews cited above. When the regime of the induction of cancer involves repeated administration of the carcinogen, the animals often exhibit a variety of pathological changes in organs other than the colon, as a result of the toxicity of the compound; in particular, the liver is very susceptible to damage (Ward *et al.*, 1973; Dixon *et al.*, 1975; Ward, 1974). Clearly these generalized disturbances of metabolism as a result of the side effects of the carcinogens are a very considerable restraint to the use of primary tumors to study the mode of action of chemotherapeutic compounds. Furthermore, from a purely clinical point of view, it is very unlikely that chemotherapy could ever be substituted for surgery in the management of the primary tumor, as it is essential for the patient's health to remove it whenever possible even though there may be metastatic cancer present at the time of laparotomy. On the other hand, such primary tumors may be important if they can be adquately localized and measured to study the effects of radiotherapy. Identification of colonic tumors in animals, without laparotomy, is often difficult; in our experience, rats with tumors of the colon induced by dimethyhydrazine (Dixon *et al.*, 1975) frequently exhibit rectal bleeding, and some other investigators advise miniaturized barium enemas to study the behavior of tumors in rats (Steele *et al.*, 1975). Finally, unlike the human tumor which is usually unifocal except in rare conditions such as multiple polyposis, multifocal tumors in the bowel of the experimental animal are the rule rather than the exception. It is clear, therefore, that if the therapy of large bowel cancer is to be studied under controlled conditions a consistent transplantable tumor system is required whose characteristics must be defined precisely.

In principle, there are two basic systems available: (1) a system of human tumor xenografts, i.e., a line of human colorectal cancer that can be transplanted serially into immunologically incompetent hosts or immunologically privileged sites in an immunocompetent animal, and (2) syngeneic systems developed from primary carcinogen-induced tumors in the colon of experimental animals. The contribution of xenografts to experimental chemotherapy has been reviewed by Double (1975), and certain points of detail will be discussed later. To date, there are only a few syngeneic transplantable models for colorectal cancer and they are listed in Table 2. In general, we can make some broad statements about their properties. The doubling time varies from 1.7 to 30 days, average 4–5 days. Their labeling index is between 12% and 25%, and in the few tumors where it has been identified the growth fraction is 80–90%. It will be seen that these tumors tend to lie in the intermediate range as far as their general growth characteristics are concerned (Tubiana and Malaise, 1976).

There is a general paucity of information about the detailed characteristics of these tumors as compared to the favorites such as the Lewis lung

Table 2. Syngeneic Lines of Adenocarcinomas of the Colon in Experimental Animals

Animal	Inducing agent	Reference
NMRI mice	1,2-Dimethylhydrazine	Double *et al.* (1975)
Balb C mice	*N*-Methyl-*N*-nitrosourethane	Corbett *et al.* (1975*b*)
C57 mice	1,2-Dimethylhydrazine	Corbett *et al.* (1975*b*)
Balb C mice	1,2-Dimethylhydrazine	Corbett *et al.* (1975*b*)
Buffalo rat	1,2-Dimethylhydrazine	McCall and Cole (1974)
Fischer rat	1,2-Dimethylhydrazine	Ward *et al.* (1973)
ACI/N rat	*N*-Methyl-*N'*-nitro-*N*-nitrosoguanidine	Goto *et al.* (1975)
BD IX rat	1,2-Dimethylhydrazine	Martin *et al.* (1973*a*)
Golden hamster	Spontaneous? after testerosterone and cortisone treatment	Kirkman and Chesterman (1972)

carcinoma and the Harding-Passey melanoma that have a long pedigree and have been studied on a comparatively vast scale in many laboratories throughout the world, but this is purely a reflection of the comparative novelty of the colon cancer models.

3. Uses of Model Colorectal Cancer Systems

There are many ways in which a reliable animal model colorectal cancer could be used. One of the most obvious is the screening of compounds for their specificity against adenocarcinomas arising from the colonic epithelium. However, even if a model tumor were shown to be reasonably disease specific with respect to its chemosensitivity—in other words, to reflect the situation in man—its suitability as a screening system would not necessarily be assured. The model must also have the right host–tumor combination to make it usable in a chemotherapy screening system.

The protocols for screening chemical agents and natural products against animal tumors have been documented by Geran *et al.* (1972). Although these criteria strictly apply to established tumor models, any new model would eventually have to comply with the general principles that underlie modern drug-screening practice, even though it may have specific properties that make its results applicable only to a particular class of tumors in man. Initially

Table 3. Properties Required by an Animal Model System in Experimental Cancer Chemotherapy Studies[a]

1. Bacteriological sterility
2. Growth stability
   a. Consistent volume doubling time for solid tumors
   b. Consistent median survival time for ascities tumors
3. No histocompatability problems—"no takes" should be less than 5%
4. No excessive death from tumor before assessment time
5. Consistent response to positive control compounds

[a]From Geran *et al.* (1972).

it is possible that less strict criteria may be acceptable, but there are minimum standards that must not be lowered—in particular, it is essential that the model provide an objective end point where the efficacy of treatment is assessed. A list of these criteria is given in Table 3.

The MAC tumor system (*M*ouse *A*denocarcinoma of the *C*olon) developed in our laboratory fulfils the basic criteria (Double *et al.*, 1975; Ball and Double, 1975; Double and Ball, 1975*a, b*). The various tumors lines are bacteriologically sterile, the tumors have stable growth rates, the take rate for

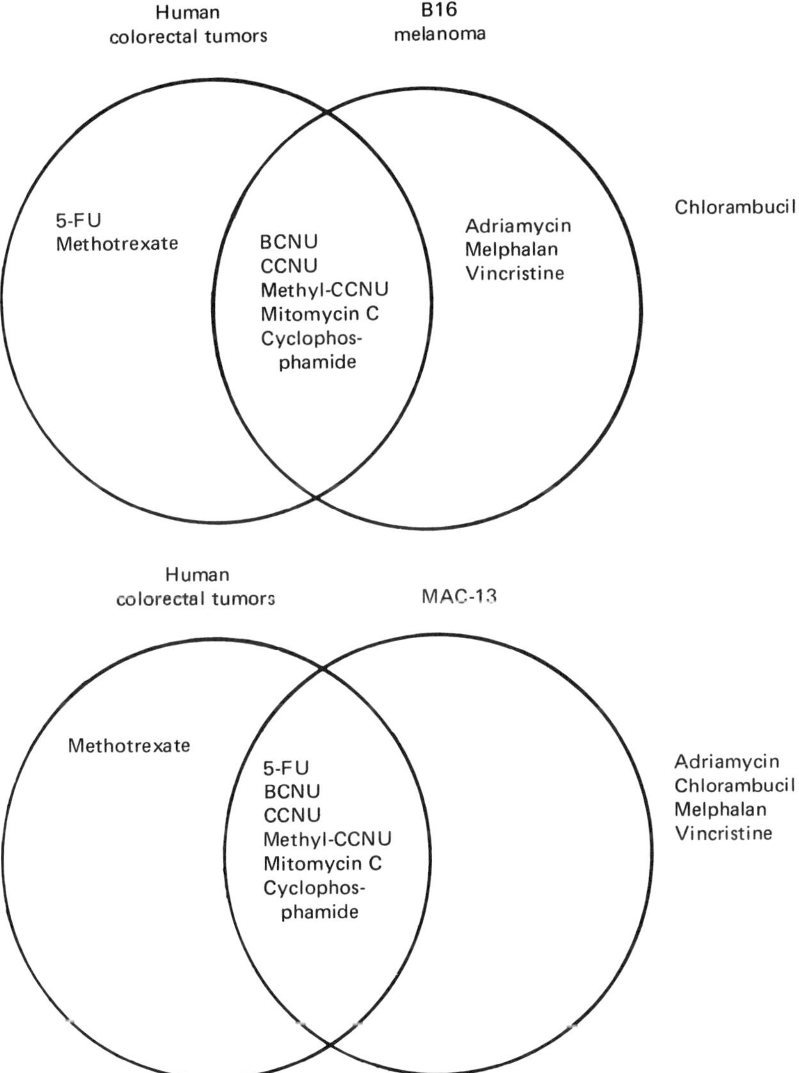

Fig. 1. Predictive efficiency of the B16 melanoma and MAC-13 for agents against human colorectal cancer. Each tumor is represented by a circle, and the drugs that show activity are placed within the circle.

both the solid and ascites tumors is greater than 95%, there do not appear to be any histocompatibility problems, and their spectrum of sensitivity shows good agreement with the response rates for standard therapeutic agents against human colorectal cancer. Figure 1 shows diagrammatically the chemotherapeutic sensitivity of line MAC-13 to 11 standard agents. The failure to respond to methotrexate should not be regarded as a serious drawback since clinically it is still equivocal whether this compound (Carter and Soper, 1974) has any beneficial activity. In practical terms, the MAC system is easy to handle; various tumor lines grow readily from subcutaneous implants of trocar fragments. The fragments are also viable after storage in liquid nitrogen. With experience a series of tumors can be grown up, from trocar implants, that will have only a threefold variation in size between the smallest and the largest tumor at the beginning of a drug-testing experiment; such a variation does not interfere with the statistical analysis of drug response. Detailed results of 11 standard agents against the MAC-13 line are shown in Tables 4 and 5. It can be seen that although there are several clearly positive antitumor effects, these are obtained only at a dose level close to the maximum tolerated dose, indicating the general insensitivity of the MAC lines to chemotherapy. This dose and drug spectrum, in terms of the models' clinical relevance, is encouraging, as it is well known that one of the disappointing features of human colonic cancer, in common with other types of adenocarcinoma, is its relative insensitivity to chemotherapy. With the exception of the model developed by Corbett and Griswold at the Southern Research Institue in Alabama (Corbett *et al.,* 1975*a,b;* Griswold and Corbett, 1975), the chemotherapeutic sensitivities of other model systems do not appear to have been well documented. The results of these studies are summarized in Table 6. Once again this system shows a good correlation with the clinical evaluation of the standard agents, and the results are comparable to those attained using the MAC system. Both systems seem to be useful tools for pharmacological research. Combination chemotherapy, drug scheduling, and surgical adjuvant therapy are typical problems in which this model may help to move from an empirical to a scientific approach. A combined project between Dr. L. van Putten's group in Rijswijk, Holland, and the Leeds team is running at present. The Dutch collaborators are using the model systems obtained from the Southern Research Institute. Corbett *et al.* (1975*a*) have reported that combinations of nitrosoureas and fluorinated pyrimidines are highly active against these mouse colon tumors and are at least moderately potentiating, and the high curative potential of two of the combinations (methyl CCNU plus 5FU, BCNU plus 5FUdR) makes them attractive regimes for adjuvant trials to be used after "curative" surgery in man. Both van Putten's group and our own have been able to confirm Corbett's observation, which is another factor showing how the mouse model tends to mirror at least some aspects of the disease in man.

At present there do not appear to be data available on the chemotherapeutic sensitivities of any of the model systems in rats; this may be

Table 4. Chemotherapy Results for MAC-13

Drug	Schedule	Vehicle	Dose (mg/kg)	Fraction LD_{10}	Number of survivors/ number of animals treated	T/C (%)	Inhibition (%)
5FU	Single	Saline	320	—	2/8	—	—
			214	1.0	7/8	34[a]	66[a]
			142	0.66	8/8	39[a]	61[a]
			60	—	0/8	—	—
	qd × 5	Saline	40	0.91	8/8	54	46
			27	0.61	8/8	69	31
Cyclophosphamide	Single	Saline	450	0.82	7/7	—	—
			300	0.54	7/7	18[b]	83[b]
			300	0.36	7/7	33[a]	67[a]
Methotrexate	qd × 5	Saline	6.0	—	4/8	—	—
			4.0	0.95	7/8	89	11
			2.7	0.64	8/8	104	0
BCNU	Single	10% ethanol, peanut oil	90	—	1/8	—	—
			60	0.85	8/8	29[a]	71[a]
			40	0.57	8/8	56	44
CCNU	Single	10% ethanol, peanut oil	90	—	1/8	—	—
			60	1.0	7/8	4[b]	96[b]
			40	0.67	8/8	2[b]	98[b]
Methyl CCNU	Single	10% ethanol, peanut oil	40	0.95	8/8	—	—
			27	0.64	8/8	21[a]	79[a]
			18	0.43	8/8	61	39
Mitomycin C	Single	Saline	10	—	0/8	—	—
			6.7	0.96	8/8	25[a]	75[a]
Adriamycin	Single	Saline	9	0.82	7/7	—	—
			6	0.55	7/7	88	12
			4	0.37	7/7	120	0
Melphalan	Single	Propylene glycol buffer	12	0.8	7/7	—	—
			8	0.53	7/7	45	55
			5.6	0.37	7/7	79	21
Chlorambucil	Single	10% ethanol, peanut oil	45	—	3/6	—	—
			30	0.79	6/6	48	52
Vincristine	Single	Saline	4.0	—	1/8	—	—
			2.7	0.84	8/8	44	56
			1.8	0.56	8/8	87	13

[a]Significant tumor inhibition by analysis of variance at $0.05 > p > 0.01$.
[b]Significant inhibition at $p < 0.01$.

because the rat is less well suited to chemotherapeutic studies as the cost per animal and the space needed to keep a large animal production line and test system are much greater than for mice, although from a biochemical standpoint and as a model for immunological studies, the rat tumors may prove to be extremely valuable. An important series of colon tumor lines in rats has been developed by the Martins (Martin *et al.*, 1973*a,b*). Some of them can be grown in tissue culture as monolayers and will produce solid adenocarcinoma when injected into a recipient rat.

Immunological studies on colorectal tumors in the mouse models have not been reported to date. This is probably a reflection of the technical diffi-

Table 5. Chemotherapy Results for MAC-15

Drug	Schedule	Vehicle	Dose (mg/kg)	Fraction LD_{10}	Number of survivors/ number of animals treated	T/C (%)	Inhibition (%)
5FU	Single	Saline	320	—	3/8	—	—
			214	1.0	6/8	37[a]	63[a]
			142	0.66	8/8	80	20
			45	1.0	5/7	62	38
	qd × 5	Saline	30	0.68	7/7	102	0
			20	0.46	7/7	108	0
Cyclophosphamide	Single	Saline	600	—	6/8	—	—
			400	0.73	8/8	14[b]	86[b]
			266	0.48	8/8	24[b]	76[b]
Methotrexate	qd × 5	Saline	6.0	—	3/8	—	—
			4.0	0.95	8/8	68	32
			3.0	0.71	8/8	75	25
BCNU	Single	10% ethanol,	80	—	1/8	—	—
		peanut oil	56	0.80	8/8	57	43
CCNU	Single	10% ethanol,	60	1.0	7/8	—	—
		peanut oil	40	0.67	8/8	13[b]	87[b]
			27	0.45	8/8	43[b]	57[b]
Methyl CCNU	Single	10% ethanol,	45	—	1/8	—	—
		peanut oil	30	0.71	8/8	34[b]	66[b]
			20	0.48	8/8	45[b]	55[b]
Mitomycin C	Single	Saline	10	—	3/8	—	—
			6.6	0.94	8/8	44[a]	56[a]
Adriamycin	Single	Saline	12	—	8/8	—	—
			8	0.73	8/8	76	24
			5.3	0.48	8/8	80	20
Melphalan	Single	Propylene	18	—	2/7	—	—
		glycol	12	0.80	7/7	81	19
		buffer	8	0.44	7/7	94	16
Chlorambucil	Single	10% ethanol,	45	—	7/8	—	—
		peanut oil	30	0.71	8/8	50[a]	50[a]
			20	0.48	8/8	62	48
Vincristine	Single	Saline	4.0	—	1/8	—	—
			2.6	0.81	8/8	107	0
			1.8	0.43	8/8	86	14

[a]Significant tumor inhibition by analysis of variance at $0.05 > p > 0.01$.
[b]Significant inhibition at $p < 0.01$.

culties involved in working with the very small amount of material produced in mice. The rat, being larger, is more suited to such studies, and various basic immunological investigations have been carried out. In broad terms it seems that the model systems investigated have features in common with the human disease.

Cross-reacting tumor-specific surface antigens have been demonstrated by Steele and Sjögren (1974) using *in vitro* microtoxicity assays among colon carcinomas induced by three separate chemical carcinogens in two different rat strains. More recently, they have shown (Sjögren and Steele, 1975) that their rat model has many close similarities to the currently known immunological features of human colorectal cancer. The model has common antigens

Table 6. Chemotherapy Data of Corbett et al.[a] *and Clinical Correlation*[b]

Agent	Clinical activity in colorectal cancer	Antitumor activity per tumor line		
		No. 26	No. 36	No. 38
CCCNU-trans	NE	+	+	+
MeCCNU	+	+	+	+
BCNU	+	+	+	NE
5FUdR	NE	+	−	+
Cyclophosphamide	+	+	+	+
Mitomycin C	+	+	+	+
Hexamethylmelamine	NE	−	NE	−
Dibromodulcitol	−	+	+	+
Adriamycin	−	+	−	+
Amethopterin	NE	−	−	−
Vinblastine	NE	NE	+	+
5FU	+	NE	+	+
PalmO-araC	NE	NE	NE	+
Dianhydrogalactitol	NE	NE	NE	+
Vincristine	−	NE	NE	−
Actinomycin D	−	NE	NE	+

[a]Corbett *et al.* (1975*a,b*) and Griswold and Corbett (1975).
[b]+, Antitumor activity; −, no antitumor activity; NE, not evaluated or not determined.

with tissue-type specificity, and it expresses immunogenic gut-specific embryonal antigens. Cell-mediated immunity can be demonstrated in tumor-bearing rats, and their sera are capable of blocking the lymphocyte effect specifically. Finally there is a rapid disappearance of the serum blocking activity after tumor excision. The presence of common membrane antigens in rat colon carcinomas has also been demonstrated by Martin *et al.* (1975, *a,b*) using an *in vivo* adsorbed rabbit antiserum against the tumor cells. An indication that the common tumor antigens were probably of embryonal origin was given as these sera also recognized a membrane antigen in the fetal gut.

Chemotherapy of xenografts of human tumors has in many instances been studied with enthusiasm rather than with the precision that is now the accepted practice of standard protocols for chemotherapy screening in animals, but this is the main a reflection of the type of investigator who has become interested in this system. In theory, a xenograft should provide a far better model system for testing drugs against a human cancer, for, after all, the tumor itself is of human origin. However, although the histological appearance of the transplantable tumor has many characteristics resembling the primary tumor from which it was derived, it is highly probable that there have been subtle adaptations as a result of growing in a foreign environment. In particular, there is always the possibility that cells of host origin will as time progresses form an intrinsic part especially of the supporting elements of the tumor, and there is always the possibility that some form of hybridization could ensue. The studies of Tubiana and Malaise (1976) have shown the immense variation in the growth characteristics of human tumors; in broad terms, adenocarcinomas tend to be the slower-growing cancers whose doubling times are usually to be counted in weeks rather than days. The growth fraction is usually low, but can vary enormously; likewise, the cell loss factor tends to be high, especially in the poorly differentiated tumors. It would appear that when human tumors are transplanted in immunodepressed animals the doubling time is considerably shortened. The direct extrapolation from the xenograft to man is probably unwise despite the fact that the tumor is of human origin. Although it would be exacting to use a xenograft to follow precisely the general protocols for chemotherapy screening described by Geran *et al.* (1972), investigators should attempt to adopt well-defined criteria when assessing therapeutic effects in this system. Procedures should be included such as randomization of the animals into treatment groups, use of dose–response curves that include a toxic dose (because unless the treated animals receive a maximum tolerated dose it is impossible to describe negative effects), and inclusion of the appropriate control in which the drug solvent is administered alone. This mode of antitumor effect should be based on a clearly defined objective end point, such as tumor weight at a standard time or survival time. From the literature it is not possible to judge to what extent such procedures have been adopted, as all too frequently the vital data which give the key to this question are missing from the paper.

It appears that xenografts of human colon cancer grow more readily than those of most of the tumor types; as yet, there is no explanation for this phenomenon. Perhaps one of the best-established xenografts is the system developed by Goldenberg and his colleagues (Goldenberg and Hansen, 1972; Goldenberg *et al.,* 1974), who have been able to propagate human colon cancer in the cheek pouch of unconditioned hamsters for as long as 3 years. These tumors have retained their morphology as well as the production of carcinoembryonic antigen which has complete identity with human CEA. Rygaard and Povlsen (1969) and Povlsen and Rygaard (1971) established several lines of human colorectal cancer in nude mice and demonstrated that their chemotherapeutic response to standard agents is in broad agreement with the documented clinical evaluation of the agents. Giovanella *et al.* (1974) have reported the results of extensive chemotherapy studies in a nude mouse system, and this system seems to be of value both in the field of screening new agents and as a tool for chemotherapy studies. A theoretically attractive feature of the xenograft system is that it should be possible to determine the spectrum of chemosensitivity in a given individual. However, the time required to grow sufficient tumors to an adequate size to make an assessment of their chemosensitivities would be several months, and this in many instances would be far too long. Nevertheless, it is highly probable that for some who seek immortality this personalized service may be attractive whatever the cost. Finally, before we leave the subject of xenografts, it must be borne in mind that although the tumor is of human origin, its host is of a completely different species, hence the pharmacokinetic behavior of the injected compounds could be quite different from what occurs in man.

Eventually the cost effectiveness of the various systems, i.e., syngeneic tumors in mice and rats or xenograft systems, needs to be taken into account, because drug-screening programs are extremely expensive, with the labor charge being one of the major items of expenditure. Looked at in these terms, the xenografts emerge as the most expensive. Nude mice are fragile creatures and require highly specialized husbandry. Immunodeprived mice are costly to produce in terms of labor and time, and again often require specialized protected environments in the animal house. The hamster cheek pouch system is also labor intensive as even routine examination of the graft requires anesthetizing the animal. It could be argued that these disadvantages are outweighed by the fact that one has a model composed of tumor of human origin, but in the face of continually rising costs this argument may falter, and such systems may have to be reserved for specialized types of research where the particular characteristics of the xenograft have unique advantages that are not present in the cheapter standard mouse or rat model, e.g., the production of CEA by the GW39 tumor line (Goldenberg and Hansen, 1972; Goldenberg *et al.*, 1974).

The experimentalist is well aware of the deficiencies in the model systems. Obviously the major biological difference between the behavior of solid tumors in rats and mice and that of solid tumors in man is that with few exceptions (Lewis lung carccinoma) dissemination is a late event in the evolution of the tumor. To a certain extent, it can be overcome by producing various forms of artificial metastases. In our own laboratory, we have developed an ascitic form of one of our tumor lines designated MAC -15/A. The tumor has been shown to have the same spectrum of chemosensitivity as the solid tumor from which it arose and therefore could have considerable potential as a system for chemotherapy screening. Subcutaneous inoculation of the ascites cells produces a solid, poorly differentiated adenocarcinoma of similar appearance to the solid deposits found in the peritoneum of a mouse with malignant ascites. This model would appear to have two applications to the study of metastastic cancer and subsequent treatment by chemotherapy. Intravenous inoculation of ascites tumor cells can be used to produce microtumors in the lungs, and we are attempting to develop this as a system to imitate the behavior of tumors growing in the parenchyma of distant organs. The blood of animals bearing solid tumors produced by these subcutaneous inoculations of ascites cells has been shown to contain viable tumor cells. If such animals are left untreated, metastases will occur in various organs, including the liver and lung.

4. Conclusion

It now looks as though some of these model systems can hold out real promise of offering the experimentalist new tools for studying the therapy of large bowel cancer. Perhaps one of the most interesting aspects is the potential value of a colon cancer model as a secondary screen for new agents with a high trophism for differentiated adenocarcinoma. The present method of moving from standard screens via toxicity trials to phase I studies in advanced cancer in man hardly seems the best way to test the compound under optimal conditions. However, ethical restraints preclude any other method. Likewise, the time factor in working out the best combination of drug dose and timing using randomized clinical trials is extremely long. This is due to the slow rate of progression of the disease and its intrinsic heterogeneity in its proliferative behavior in man (Tubiana and Malaise, 1976). Here then is the challenge: can the model help to find the right compounds and suggest a strategy that is best suited to the behavior of adenocarcinomas?

5. References

Ball, C. R., and Double, J. A., 1975, Transplantable colon tumors as chemotherapy screening models, *Cancer* **36:**2437–2440.

Carter, S. K., 1976, Large bowel cancer—The current status of treatment, *J. Natl. Cancer Inst.* **56(1):**3–10.

Carter, S. K., and Soper, W. T., 1974, Integration of chemotherapy into combined modality treatment of solid tumors. 1. The overall strategy, *Cancer Treat. Rev.* **2:**1–13.

Corbett, T. H., Griswold, D. P., Jr., Roberts, B. J., Peckham, J. C., and Schabel, F. J., Jr., 1975*a,* Tumor induction relationships in the development of transplantable cancers of the colon in mice for chemotherapy assays, with a note on carcinogen structure, *Cancer Res.* **35:**2434–2439.

Corbett, T. H., Griswold, D. P., Jr., Roberts, B. J., Peckham, J., and Schabel, F. M. J, 1975*b,* A mouse colon-tumor model for experimental therapy, *Cancer Chemother. Rep. Part 2* **5(1):**169–186.

Detre, S. I., Davies, A. J. S., and Connors, T. A., 1975, New models for cancer chemotherapy, *Cancer Chemother. Rep. Part 2* **5(1):**133–143.

Dixon, M. F., Cowen, D. M., and Cooper, E. H., 1975, Chronic hepatotoxicity and intestinal bleeding in 1, 2-dimethylhydrazine carcinogens in rats and mice, *Biomedicine* **23:**247–252.

Double, J. A., 1975, Human tumor xenografts, *Biomedicine* **22:**461–465.

Double, J. A., and BAll, C. R., 1975*a,* Chemotherapy of transplantable colon tumors in mice, in: *Chemotherapy,* Vol. 7: *Cancer Chemotherapy I,* Plenum, New York.

Double, J. A., and Ball, C. R., 1975*b,* Chemotherapy of transplantable adenocarcinomas of the colon in mice, *Cancer Chemother. Rep.* **59(6):**1083–1089.

Double, J. A., Ball, C. R., and Cowen, P. N., 1975, Transplantation of adenocarcinomas of the colon in mice, *J. Natl. Cancer Inst.* **54(1):**271–275.

Druckrey, H., 1972, Organospecific carcinogenesis in the digestive tract, in: *Topics in Chemical Carcinogenesis* (W. Wakahara, S. Takayama, T. Sugimara, and S. Odushima, eds.), pp. 73–120, Tokyo University Press, Tokyo.

Filipe, M. I., 1975, Mucous secretion in rat colonic mucosa during carcinogenesis induced by dimethylhydrazine: A morphological and histochemical study, *Br. J. Cancer* **32:**60–77.

Geran, R. I., Greenberg, N. H., MacDonald, M. M., Schumacher, A. M., and Abbot, B. J., 1972, Protocols for screening chemical agents and natural products against animal tumor and other biological systems (third edition), *Cancer Chemother. Rep. Part 3* **3(2).**

Giovanella, B. C., 1974, Testing of chemotherapeutic agents on individual human solid tumors transplanted in "nude" mice, in: *UICC Workshop on New Animal Models for Chemotherapy of Human Solid Tumors*(E. Mihich, D. J. R. Laurence, D. M. Laurence, and S. Eckhardt, eds.), p. 29, UICC Technical Report Series, Vol. 15.

Giovanella, B. C., Stelhein, J. S. and Williams, L. J., Jr., 1974, Hetero transplantation of human malignant tumors in "nude" thymusless mice. II. Malignant tumors induced by injection of cell cultures derived from human solid tumors, *J. Natl. Cancer Inst.* **52:**921–927.

Goldenberg, D. M., 1974, Human tumors in the hamster cheek pouch, in: *UICC Workshop of New Animal Models for Chemotheraphy of Human Solid Tumors* (E. Mihich, D. J. R. Laurence, D. M. Laurence, and S. Eckhardt, eds.), p. 18, UICC Technical Report Series, Vol. 15.

Goldenberg, D. M., and Hansen, H. J., 1972, Carcinoembryonic antigen present in human colonic neoplasms serially propagated in hamsters, *Science* **175:**1117–118.

Goldenberg, D. M., Bhan, R. D., and Pavia, R. A., 1970, Retention of human properties by a xenografted human colonic tumor, G. W. 77, propagated in unconditioned hamsters, *Proc. Soc. Exp. Biol. Med.* **135:**657–659.

Goldenberg, D. M., Preston, D. F., Primus, F. J., and Hansen, H. J., 1974, Photoscan localisation of G. W.-39 tumors in hamsters using radio labelled anticarcinoembryonic antigen immunoglobulin G, *Cancer Res.* **34:**1–9.

Goto, K., Kurokawa, Y., Hayashi, J., and Sato, H., 1975, Transplantable adenocarcinomas from colo-rectal tumors induced by infusion of *N*-methyl-*N*-nitro-*N*-nitrosoguanidine in AC1/N rats, *Gann* **66:**84–93.

Griswold, D. P., and Corbett, T. H., 1975, A colon tumor model for anticancer agent evaluation, *Cancer* **36:**2441–2444.

Haase, P., Cowen, D. M., and Knowles, J. C., 1973, Evaluation of dimethyl hydrazine induced tumors in mice as a model system for colorectal cancer, *Br. J. Cancer* **28:**530.

Kirkman, H., and Chesterman, F. C., 1972, Additional data on transplanted tumors of the golden hamster, *Progr. Exp. Tumor Res.* **16:**580–62.

Laqueur, G. L., 1964, Carcinogenic effects of cycad meal and cycasin, methylazoxymethanol-glycoside in rats and effects of cycasin in germ free rats, *Fed. Proc.* **23:**1386.

Laqueur, G. L., 1970, Contribution of intestinal macroflora and microflora to carcinogenesis, in: *Carcinoma of the Colon and Antecedent Epithelium* (W. J. Burdette, ed.), pp. 305–313, Thomas, Springfield, Ill.

Laqueur, G. L., Michelsen, O., Whiting, M. G., and Kunland, L. T., 1963 Carcinogenic properties of nuts from cycas circinals, *J. Natl. Cancer Inst.* **31:**919–933.

Martin, M. S., Martin, F., Michiels, R., Bastien, H., Justarbo, E., Bordes, M., and Virg. B., 1973*a,* An experimental model for cancer of the colon and rectum, *Digestion* **8:**22–34.

Martin, M. S., Bastien, H., Martin, F., Michiels, R., Martin, M. R., and Justarbo, E., 1973*b,* Transplantation of intestinal carcinoma in inbred rats, *Biomedicine* **19:**555–558.

Martin, F., Martin, M. S., Bordes, M., and Knobel, S., 1975*a,* Antigens associated with chemically induced intestinal carcinomas of rats, *Int. J. Cancer* **15:**144–151.

Martin, F., Knobel, S., Martin, M., and Bordes, M., 1975*b,* A carcino-fetal antigen located on the membrane of cells from rat intestinal carcinoma in culture, *Cancer Res.* **35:**333–336.

McCall, D. C., and Cole, J. W., 1974, Transplantation of chemically induced adenocarcinomas of the colon in an inbred strain of rats, *Cancer* **4:**1021–1026.

Povlsen, C. O., and Rygaard, J., 1971, Heterotransplantation of human adenocarcinomas of the colon and rectum to the mouse mutant nude: A study of nine consecutive transplantations, *Acta Pathol. Microbiol. Scand.* **79:**159.

Rygaard, J., and Povlsen, C. O., 1969, Heterotransplantation of human malignant tumors to "nude" mice, *Acta Pathol. Microbiol. Scand.* **77:**758.

Sjögren, H. O., and Steele, G., 1975, The immunology of large bowel carcinoma in a rat model, *Cancer* **36:**2469–2471.

Steele, G., Jr., and Sjögren, H. O., 1974, Cross-reacting tumor-associated antigen(s) among chemically induced rat colon carcinomas, *Cancer Res.* **34:**1801–1907.

Steele, G., Jr., Sjögren, H. O., and Rosengren, J. E., 1975, Sequential studies of serum blocking activities in rats bearing chemically induced primary bowel tumors, *J. Natl. Cancer Inst.* **54(4):**959–967.

Tubiana, M., and Malaise, E. P., 1976, Growth rate and cell kinetics in human tumors: Some prognostic and therapeutic implications, in: *Scientific Foundations of Oncology* (T. Symington and R. L. Carter, eds.), pp. 126–135, Heinemann Medical Books, London.

Walpole, A. L., Williams, M. H. C., and Roberts, D. C., 1952, The carcinogenic action of 4-aminodiphenyl, *Br. J. Ind. Med.* **9**:255–263.

Ward, J. M., 1974, Morphogenesis of chemically induced neoplasms of the colon and small intestine in rats, *Lab. Invest.* **30(4)**:505–513.

Ward, J. M., Yamamoto, R. S., and Brown, C. A., 1973, Pathology of intestinal neoplasms and other lesions in rats exposed to azoxymethane, *J. Natl. Cancer Inst.* **51**:1029–1039.

Weisburger, J. H., 1971, Colon carcinogens: Their metabolism and mode of action, *Cancer* **28**:60–70.

Weisburger, J. H., 1973, Chemical carcinogenesis in the gastrointestinal tract, in: *Seventh National Cancer Conference Proceedings,* pp. 465–473.

17

Use of Experimental Models in the Study of Approaches to Treatment of Colorectal Cancer

Daniel P. Griswold, Jr., and Thomas H. Corbett

1. Introduction

Animal tumors have been widely used as models in studies of the etiology, behavior, and treatment of cancer of man. It is the last consideration that is of concern here, i.e., the development of optimal approaches to therapy through the use of experimental models. Many questions of the clinical oncologist cannot be answered from therapeutic trials in man because of the limitations imposed by ethics that preclude the use of certain controls and assay procedures. If, then, a totally empirical approach is to be avoided, the answers to those questions must come through the use of likely relevant animal tumors. Yet relevancy can often be determined only in retrospect. Nevertheless, experimentalists as well as clinicians have already recognized the need for better tumor models. It is hoped that their use will lead to improved therapeutic results as well as a better understanding of the nature of cancer growth and spread.

2. The Problem

It seems paradoxical that the greatest improvements in 5-year survival rates have been noted among the less common cancers (Silverberg and Holeb, 1975), In contrast, 5-year survival rates of patients with the most commonly

Daniel P. Griswold, Jr., and Thomas H. Corbett • Southern Research Institute, Birmingham, Alabama 35205.

occurring cancers, those of lung, colon–rectum, and breast, were not observed to change significantly over the 20-year period 1950–1969. Why has this difference occurred? There may be several reasons. It is apparent that greater emphasis was placed on treatment of those cancers that were subsequently found to be most responsive (Sherlock, 1974), resulting in earlier diagnosis, shorter time interval between diagnosis and treatment, and greater use of systemic therapy, particularly chemotherapy. Moreover, as Zubrod (1972) has noted, the greatest improvements have been observed in ten cancers which, in common, share the characteristic of rapid growth. Ironically, those animal tumor models used for the selection of clinical chemotherapeutic agents also were noted for the characteristic of rapid growth, the L1210 leukemia being the most widely used animal tumor "screening" model.

The trend in emphasis, however, is changing. The need to improve survival rates of patients with, say, large bowel cancer is well recognized, and the urgency has been made apparent by the development of national, goal-oriented programs directed at the eradication of specific high-risk cancers. Horton *et al.* (1974) only recently made an appeal to the scientific community encouraging the use of animal tumor models for the development of improved therapeutic regimens and for intensified clinical trials.

3. Animal Tumor Models

Triolo (1964) in his excellent review on the foundations of cancer research pointed to Novinsky as the one to whom credit must be given for the first successful tumor transplantation. Describing that work of the latter half of the nineteenth century, Triolo went on to credit Leo Loeb and Carl O. Jensen for establishment of the first rodent tumor lines during the period 1901–1903. Since that time, hundreds of tumor lines, *in vivo* and *in vitro,* have been established. Many of those have been considered as models for one or more cancers of man. But as Schabel (1975*a*) has stated, "It should be pointed out and emphasized that, at this time, direct positive correlation between any experimental tumor system and any specific histologic type of human cancer has not been clearly shown." In fact, similarity of morphology of tumors of man and animal as a basis for likely similar behavior and response to therapy is a moot question.

Animal tumor models, of course, have been useful in the development of cancer therapy. In chemotherapy, for example, they have been useful in two distinct ways. Used as screens, animal tumors have selected close to 50 natural or synthetic chemicals subsequently found to have activity against one or more cancers of man. Of equal importance, the use of animal tumors in laboratory research (using tumors of peculiar characteristics to answer specific questions) has provided the means for the development of biological and therapeutic principles which have far-ranging application, many having already been found valid in human cancer. Schabel (1975*a*), in his elegant paper on "Concepts for Systemic Treatment of Micrometastases," noted that "general principles appear to be broadly valid in biology and, I believe, physicians will be well advised to consider reproducible observations in animals as likely indications of principles applicable to human disease, and therapeutic responses in animals as probably useful indicators of response in man." It is now well recognized that therapeutic concepts and principles from animal tumor studies have found application in the treatment of leukemias and lymphomas of man. The question must be asked now: will any of these concepts apply to the treatment of solid tumors of man, or is colorectal cancer so different that none of these concepts applies to its treatment?

3.1. *Specific Tumor Models*

The principles and concepts alluded to were derived from studies of a wide variety of experimental tumors *in vitro* and *in vivo,* the latter ranging from dispersed cell populations of rapid growth and marked chemotherapeutic sensitivity to relatively slow-growing, solid tumors with little if any observable therapeutic sensitivity. It subsequently became apparent to experimentalists and clinicians alike that animal tumor models more akin in known characteristics to solid tumors of man were both desirable and needed. This need was most lucidly pointed out with the emergence of tumor cell population kinetic studies. Although many other factors, including biochemical and pharmacological ones, may bear on the basic response differences of various tumor types, it was the difference in growth characteristics that was most widely recognized and acclaimed.

To further clarify the problem it must be recognized that the cytotoxic anticancer agents exert their toxicity by means of interaction with tumor cells whose sensitivity is dependent on the phase of the cell cycle as well as characteristics of the drug. Since the extent of the differential cytotoxicity to normal and tumor cell populations determines a drug's usefulness, it is evident that differences in growth characteristics of those cell populations may determine the potential usefulness of a drug as an anticancer agent. The importance of cell population kinetics to chemotherapy is made clear by an analysis (Skipper, 1968, 1971) of data that resulted from *in vitro* drug exposure of a wide variety of cell types, both normal and neoplastic, to anticancer agents of several classes. Those data showed that when cell populations were adapted to log-phase growth and were rapidly dividing, they all became about equally sensitive to all of the agents used. Bruce *et al.* (1966), using a spleen colony assay, demonstrated the effect that cell population kinetics of bone marrow stem cells and lymphoma cells had on determination of the cytotoxic differential exhibited by an agent. The rapidly proliferating lymphoma cells were more sensitive to certain types of agents than were the "steady-state" or "resting" bone marrow stem cells. That work led to a classification of chemotherapeutic agents as cell-cycle stage specific, cell-cycle specific, or nonspecific. Those observations were further refined by *in vitro* studies which demonstrated the concentration dependence or time-of-exposure dependence of specific agents (Wilkoff *et al.,* 1967). Most importantly, those studies helped explain the reason for failure of certain classes of anticancer agents to demonstrate effectiveness against low-growth-fraction cell populations, a characteristic of solid tumors.

At least one problem in tumor modeling then became apparent. It is depicted by the contrasting kinetic parameters of L1210 leukemia and B16 melanoma (Skipper and Schabel, 1973). The former, when implanted intraperitoneally, is for a while a dispersed cell population of rapid growth (volume doubling time, T_d, of about 0.5 day) and a pulse-labeling index of 65%. It is, quite understandably, markedly sensitive to 1-β-D-arabinofuranosylcytosine (araC), an S-phase-specific agent. The T_d of B16 ranges from about 1.0 day, when first detectable, to near infinity during the latter part of its asymptotic growth. Coincidentally, it has a pulse-labeling index of only 23%. This tumor is poorly responsive to araC even under presumably optimal conditions of exposure. This kinetic picture seems to characterize solid tumor growth as understood today, the kinetic parameters being influenced by tumor architecture and vascularity (Tannock and Steel, 1969; van Putten and Lelieveld, 1970). In brief, solid tumors during growth exhibit an increasing volume doubling time which may be dependent on an increasing generation time of the proliferating pool, a declining growth fraction, or increasing cell loss, or any combination of these (Baserga, 1965; Mendelsohn, 1969; Steel, 1967).

Yet even tumors of similar growth characteristics often fail to respond to chemotherapy in an identical manner. Such varied responses indicate the importance of other characteristics, subtle and less well understood, and point to the need for a variety of tumor models. Fortnér *et al.* (1961) recognized this need when they developed a series of transplantable tumors of different sites of origin in the hamster. Solid tumors of mice that have been of considerable interest include, but are not limited to, the B16 melanoma (Griswold, 1972), the spontaneous breast tumor of C3H mice (Sandberg and Goldin, 1971) or of $CD8F_1$ (Balb/c × DBA/8) mice (Martin *et al.*, 1970), the Lewis lung carcinoma (Karrer *et al.*, 1967; Mayo *et al.*, 1972), and the Ridgway osteogenic sarcoma (Schabel, 1975*b*). Although they vary somewhat in growth characteristics and markedly in response to treatment, all are solid tumors, and the variability adds to their usefulness as attempts are made to understand the basis for that variability. More recently, efforts have been extended by other investigators to develop animal models of specific tumor types, including colorectal cancer (Corbett *et al.*, 1975*a*; Double *et al.*, 1975). Such models, if useful in therapeutic regimen design, will add to the armamentarium of solid tumor models.

3.2. Development of a Colon Tumor Model

At the beginning of our efforts to obtain a suitable colon tumor model for chemotherapy studies, only two transplantable colon tumors were available, both in rats (Narisawa *et al.*, 1971; McCall and Cole, 1974). Because of the quantities of drugs available and the expense, we decided to attempt colon tumor induction and transplantation in mice. This work is described elsewhere in detail (Corbett *et al.*, 1975*a*). Colon tumor induction in experimental animals and humans is probably similar (Weisburger, 1971). These tumors are not spontaneous in origin but instead require chemical carcinogen induction (Weisburger, 1971; Howeld, 1975). In the case of man, it is generally agreed that the chemicals are probably in the diet (Weisburger, 1971; Howeld, 1975), and we believe that these chemicals are naturally occurring in one or more common foodstuffs rather than additives to the foods. Colon tumor induction in experimental animals dates to 1964, when cycasin (a naturally occurring chemical isolated from cycad nuts) was fed to rats (Laqueur, 1965). The compound induced tumors of the liver and kidney and, most impressively, in the colon. Since that time, colon tumors have been induced in many strains of rats and mice with chemicals that have molecular similarities to cycasin (Narisawa *et al.*, 1971; McCall and Cole, 1974; Corbett *et al.*, 1975*a*; Thurnherr *et al.*, 1973; Double *et al.*, 1975). All of the effective colon carcinogens contain a N-N-CH_3 grouping. We have proposed that the naturally occurring colon carcinogens in our foodstuffs may likewise have this characteristic structure.

Beginning with over 1000 mice, we induced and transplanted 82 colon tumors in inbred strains of mice. Four of these tumors survived transplant and are now in serial passage (colon tumors No. 26, 36, 38, 51). Colon tumor No. 26 is the only undifferentiated colon tumor that was obtained, and as such offers the poorest histological correlation with human colon tumors. Yet it is the most invasive and metastatic of the four tumors. It metastasizes mainly to the liver if implanted intraperitoneally and mainly to the lungs if implanted subcutaneously. Metastatic foci have also been observed in the kidneys, adrenals, and ovaries. A graphic illustration of the relationship among tumor growth, rate of metastasis, and host lethality may be seen in Fig. 1. Because this tumor has high metastatic potential, it is most suitable for surgery-chemotherapy adjuvant trials.

Colon tumor No. 36 is a well-differentiated adenocarcinoma and is the slowest growing, least metastatic, and least invasive of the four tumors. Colon tumor No. 38 is a well-differentiated adenocarcinoma. Following subcutaneous implantation it metastasizes to the lungs in 30–70% of the mice. If implanted intraperitoneally, it metastasizes mainly to the liver. Colon tumor No. 51 is a mucus-producing carcinoma with considerable connective tissue architecture. It metastasizes from a subcutaneous site to the lungs in nearly 100% of the mice, and may be suitable for surgery-chemotherapy adjuvant experimentation. However, because it invades the overlying skin and ulcerates quickly to the surface, accurate tumor measurements cannot be obtained with tumors over 800 mg in size. For this reason, minimal use has been made of this tumor.

The major demand of a tumor model is that it predict therapeutic responses in man. The determination of correlative drug sensitivities between these mouse colon tumors and human colon tumors was a critical step toward assessing their utility as predictive models. In addition to drug response correlations, an ideal model should have biological properties similar to those of

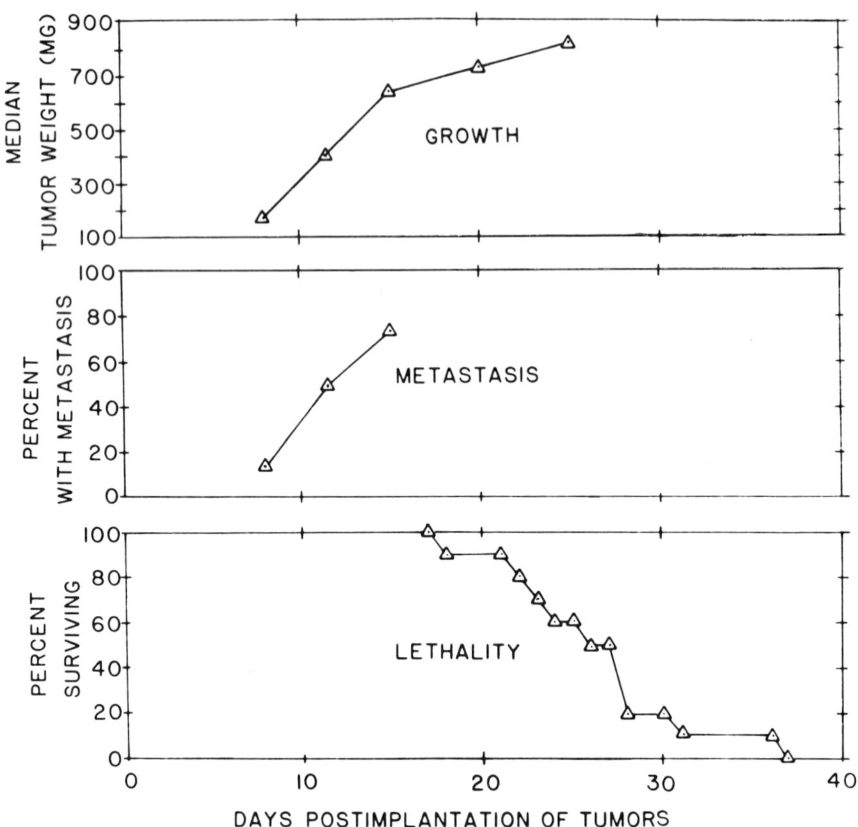

Fig. 1. Tumor growth, metastasis, and host mortality after subcutaneous implantation of a mouse colon tumor. Metastasis was determined only at autopsy by direct visual examination.

human colon tumors. It is, of course, obvious that no two human colon tumors and no two mouse colon tumors are exactly alike. Nonetheless, all of the tumors of this type are "solid" in nature and should have growth, cell kinetic, vascular, and architectural patterns common among all malignant solid tumors. These similarities alone, because of their influence on the distribution and efficacy of drugs, should make these mouse colon tumors better predictors for the human disease than experimental leukemias. Certainly the responses of human leukemias have not predicted optimum therapies for the major solid malignancies in humans (breast, colon, lung) any more than the experimental mouse leukemias have predicted for the response of these same malignancies in the mouse.

In addition to the properties of growth, cell kinetics, vascularity, and solid architecture, one or more of the four mouse colon tumors have the properties of metastasis, invasiveness, mucus production, and histological type that are similar to those of many human colon tumors. These similarities, in addition to common carcinogen induction and correlative drug sensitivities with human colon tumors, strengthen the utility of these mouse colon tumors as predictive models for the human disease.

4. General Therapeutic Concepts

How, then, may these specific, solid tumor models be used? As earlier mentioned, a number of concepts and principles have been developed with the view of improving therapeutic regimen design. Some appear to be broadly applicable to tumors of a variety of types and require no further confirmation. Others may be valid only under peculiar conditions and may not be generally applicable. Thus it seems pertinent to use the most relevant models in attempts to validate current concepts and to develop new ones. It is beyond the scope of this endeavor to consider the detailed background of each potentially useful concept or the historical development of cancer treatment.* Yet there are several clinically related questions that may be addressed, using the more pertinent solid tumors of animals as model systems.

4.1. Clinical Questions

Among questions most frequently asked are those that bear on the timing of treatment, modality and agent selection, dose regimen selection, and intensity of treatment. These are discussed below in light of currently available knowledge. But before those questions are specifically addressed, some discussion is in order in regard to the similarity or dissimilarity of quantitative measures used by experimentalists and clinicians.

Correlation of animal and human therapeutic trial results presupposes the use of equivalent end points for a meaningful interpretation of results and translation of methods. Quantitative end points commonly used for the evaluation of therapeutic results include percent responders, i.e., those patients whose tumor volume regresses by 50% or more, increased patient survival time, and duration of tumor remission. Each of these must be considered only an indirect measure of the ultimate quantitative goal: the number of surviving tumor cells that retain proliferative integrity. They are intermediate end points. Without precise calculations based on accurate knowledge of growth, regression, and recurrence characteristics of the particular tumor in question, those intermediate end points may yield misleading measures of the numbers of cells killed and surviving.

The measurement percent responders can be particularly misleading. Percent responders is a measure of the spectrum of an agent's activity, not the number or percent of tumor cells killed. Tumor mass or volume regression is dependent on lysis and loss of dead cells, the continued proliferation of live

*Some of the more basic biological concepts that bear on cancer treatment have been listed and discussed by Skipper (1971, 1973), and Skipper *et al.* (1964), Schabel (1975*a*), Griswold *et al.* (1968), Fowler (1966), Mayo *et al.* (1972), and Van Putten (1974).

cells, and any accompanying stromal changes (Wilcox *et al.*, 1965). The extent of regression varies widely for tumors of different types (Griswold, 1975). The duration of the response, on the other hand, may be used as an indication of the fraction of a tumor cell population surviving therapy if the growth rate of the tumor is known and if the measurement is made after all therapy has been discontinued. Even then, it is not a precise measure, but it is a useful indicator.

4.2. *Timing of Treatment*

It is now well recognized that prognosis is dependent to a great extent on the size of the primary tumor and metastatic outgrowth at diagnosis. Early diagnosis favors good prognosis. It must additionally be recognized that there are limitations to the curative potential achievable by surgery or by chemotherapy. As earlier noted, 5- and 10-year survival figures for patients with colorectal cancer clearly indicate that little improvement in surgical cure rates has been observed in the 20-year period 1950–1969. The reason behind this fact is made apparent by experimental results which have shown that (1) host survival time is directly related to size of the tumor cell population, (2) the extent of metastasis is directly related to primary tumor size, and (3) curability is therefore a function of the size of the primary tumor at the time of surgical excision (Table 1). Similarly, chemotherapeutic curability is limited by the size of the tumor cell population at the initiation of treatment. The data in Table 2 demonstrate this point in an oversimplified manner. While it is plain that tumor size is the major limiting factor to curability, many other considerations are involved. Skipper and Schabel (1973) have reviewed the cytokinetic aspects and no further attempt will be made here.

The importance of timing of treatment cannot be overemphasized. While it is understood that surgical cure is limited by tumor invasion and metastasis

Table 1. Surgical Curability as a Function of Tumor Size

Experimental tumor	Tumor size at surgery (g)	Tumor-free survivors: Number/total	Tumor-free survivors: Percent	References
Lewis lung carcinoma	0.06	6/20	30	Mayo *et al.* (1972)
	0.10	8/20	40	
	0.35	0/20	0	
C3H breast carcinoma	0.10–0.20	25/44	57	Griswold (1975)
	0.25–0.30	13/45	29	
	0.50–0.70	1/44	2	
Colon carcinoma	0.15–0.25	24/29	83	Corbett *et al.* (1975*b*)
	0.35–0.55	15/31	48	
	0.65–0.85	8/32	25	

Table 2. Chemotherapeutic Curability as a Function of Tumor Size[a]

Experimental tumor (chemotherapy)	Tumor size at initiation of treatment (number of cells or g)	Tumor-free survivors		References
		Number/total	Percent	
B16 melanoma	10^3	9/10	90	Griswold (1975)
(MeCCNU + cyclophosphamide)	10^5	4/10	40	
	10^7	0/10	0	
C3H breast carcinoma	10^3	9/10	90	Griswold and Corbett (1976)
(MeCCNU)	10^5	6/10	60	
	10^7	6/10	0	
Lewis lung carcinoma	0.4	27/40	68	Mayo *et al.* (1972)
(MeCCNU + cyclophosphamide)	1.0	5/20	20	
	2.0	0/18	0	

[a] All tumors were implanted s.c. The dose and regimen for each tumor type were the same for all tumor sizes.

(thus the time in the tumor age at which surgery is employed is critical), it must be equally understood that the efficacy of present-day systemic therapy is limited by the tumor population size and responsiveness. These facts point to the need for sophisticated and precise staging to improve cure rates.

4.3. Modality and Agent Selection

Moertel (1973) has stated that "the only universally accepted curative treatment for invasive adenocarcinoma of the large bowel, regardless of location or degree of invasion, is radical surgical excision." Cure under those circumstances, of course, is dependent on early diagnosis and treatment. In the treatment of more advanced disease, beyond surgical curative potential, neither radiation nor chemicals have been found markedly curative, and their role has been ascribed, by default, to *palliative* therapy. Moertel went on to show that 5-fluorouracil (5FU), the most widely used chemotherapeutic agent in the treatment of large bowel cancer to date, has failed to provide a significant increase in patient survival at the 36-month time period following diagnosis. The median survival time of 5FU responders, however, was 10 months longer than that of 5FU nonresponders or untreated patients. This fact alone should be viewed as encouraging rather than as defeat. It must be remembered that the response was to a single agent, and the progress observed, although minimal, may be thought of as a forward step on which to build.

A review (Wasserman *et al.*, 1974) of chemotherapeutic agent activity against colon cancer indicated only two agents as actives, 5FU and mitomycin C. Five others were categorized as having some evidence of activity, while 23 agents were considered inactive or inadequately evaluated. On the face of it, this is a disturbing view of the future of chemotherapy. But it must be recognized that response of colorectal cancer in man, when less than curative, is difficult to measure. A review of the results of 5FU therapy of large bowel cancer by 21 investigators showed objective response rates that varied from 8% to 85% (Moertel, 1973). Two possible reasons for such a wide range become immediately apparent. One is the basis of the response measurement and the other is related to the heterogeneity of individual tumors, even when of the same morphological type, site, grade, etc. A third reason, differing therapeutic regimens, will be discussed later.

Tumor heterogeneity, in terms of chemotherapeutic response, can be demonstrated from animal tumor studies. The data in Table 3 show the extreme variability in response of experimental colon and breast tumors to identical regimens of treatment with each of several commonly used chemotherapeutic agents. Each tumor line was derived from a single, spontaneous mammary carcinoma of C3H mice or a single, chemically induced colon carcinoma. None of those tumor lines responded in an identical fashion to chemotherapy. Even more perplexing are observations that tumors, each initiated from a fragment implant derived from a single, common donor tumor, failed to respond in the same manner to identical treatment (Fig. 2). In

Table 3. Arbitrary Response Rating of Experimental Tumors of Breast and Colon to Selected Anticancer Agents[a]

	Breast tumor line				Colon tumor line		
Agent	04/a	15/c	16/c	44	26	36	38
Cyclophosphamide	+++	+++	+++	+++	++	+++	+++
L-Sarcolysin	+++	−	++	+			
Mitomycin C					+	+++	++
Adriamycin	+++	++	+++	+	++	±	++
5FU	+++	+++	++	−	+	++	+++
Vincristine	+++	−	++	−			
Vinblastine					−	++	++

[a]Each tumor line was derived from a separate spontaneous mammary tumor of a C3H mouse or from a chemically induced colon tumor of a mouse. For agent evaluation, tumor fragments were implanted s.c. into mice which were then treated with LD_{10} doses and fractions thereof, using a variety of treatment schedules. For this comparison, optimal treatment schedule results are shown.

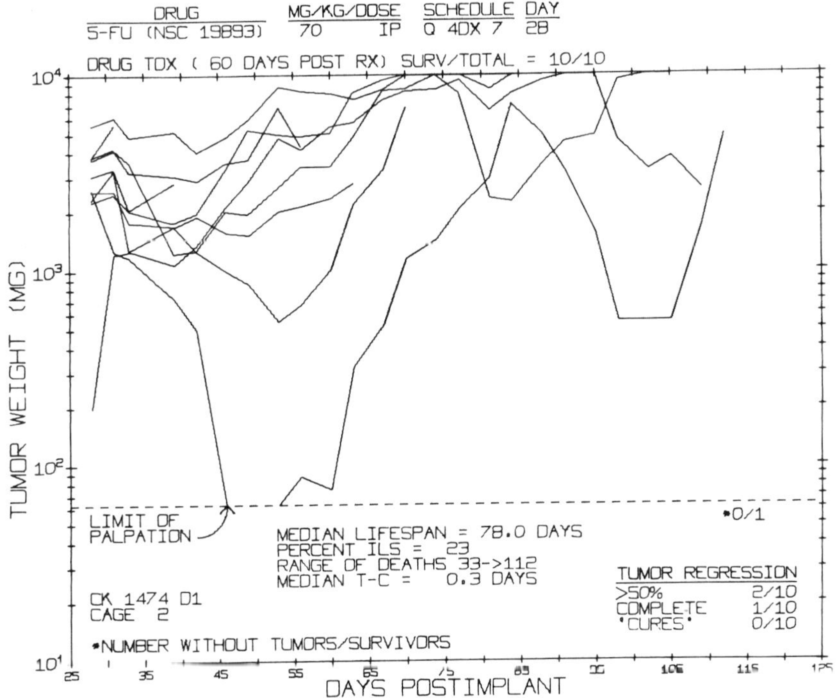

Fig. 2. Observations on the varied response of subcutaneously implanted colon tumors of mice to 5-fluorouracil. All tumor implants were derived from a common donor.

spite of direct, common ancestry, the chemotherapeutic responses ranged from temporary growth stasis to complete regression.

It is now obvious that such wide variations in response cannot be entirely attributed to cytokinetic differences, although they undoubtedly play a part. Biochemical and pharmacological factors are most certainly involved but are poorly understood. Nevertheless, response variation is a real problem in tumors of both animals and man. It deserves serious study, for it logically follows that unpredictable response makes difficult the selection of single chemotherapeutic agents for clinical trial and, moreover, may confuse the interpretation of results of combination-agent trials. The latter point is made apparent from the data in Table 4. When breast tumors of mice were treated with either of two single agents or the combination, the percent responder's value was simply an additive effect from the two individual drugs. The similarity of other measurement end points makes it clear that, in this instance, the effectiveness of the combination treatment was an increased spectrum of activity, not an increased cell kill.

It would be unfair to imply that single agents have not been effective in a curative sense. However, this appears to be the exception rather than the rule. The two notable exceptions are choriocarcinoma (Hertz *et al.,* 1961) and Burkitt's lymphoma (Morrow *et al.*, 1967). And projections of enhanced cure rates are now being made from surgical-adjuvant trial results with osteosarcomas (Cortes *et al.*, 1974; Jaffe *et al.*, 1974) and cancer of the breast (Fisher *et al.*, 1975) where single agents were employed as the adjuvants.

In any event, the more often discouraging results from single-agent chemotherapy naturally made the potential of combination-agent chemotherapy more attractive. DeVita *et al.* (1974) have traced the progression, using as examles acute lymphatic leukemia of children, breast cancer, and Hodgkin's disease. In the first disease, for example, moving from single agents to as many as four drugs in combination, he showed that the percent of complete bone marrow remissions was increased from as little as 22% to 100% with concomitant increases in duration of response and survival time. In discussing the response of Hodgkin's disease patients to the MOPP program, DeVita noted that "As with acute leukemia studies, intensive treatment

Table 4. Response to Chemotherapy of First Generation Transplants of $CD8F_1$ Mammary Adenocarcinomas

Treatment[a]	Toxicity control mortality	Percent ILS	Percent responders	Response duration (days)
L-Sarcolysin (8.0 mg/kg/dose)	1/10	33	30	36
Adriamycin (6.0 mg/kg/dose)	0/10	70	40	51
L-Sarcolysin (5.4 mg/kg/dose) + adriamycin (4.0 mg/kg/dose)	1/10	45	70	46
L-Sarcolysin (5.4 mg/kg/dose) + adriamycin (2.6 mg/kg/dose)	0/10	64	60	49

[a]Tumor fragments were implanted s.c. All treatment was q7d × 5, beginning 2 days after tumor implantation.

schedules for lymphomas are often given over periods of time longer than with the use of single drugs. However, the time free of evidence of disease following cessation of therapy after combination drug therapy has far exceeded the duration of remissions achieved with single drugs even when drug maintenance therapy is given." That was a most important observation, not only because it points to the advantages of combination agent therapy but also because, as mentioned earlier, the time interval between last treatment and evidence of tumor recurrence may be used as a direct, quantitative measure of the number of tumor cells surviving therapy.

One cannot now question the advantages of combination-agent chemotherapy. It has been proven an efficacious treatment in leukemias, lymphomas, and solid tumors as well. But the problem of agent selection remains. On what basis may clinical oncologists select agents for combination use? If the basis for selection is proven single-agent activity, then the future is dismal in certain types of cancer. Moertel (1975) has painted a bleak picture for single-agent chemotherapy of colorectal cancer, showing that 2-month objective response rates for 27 agents ranged from 0% (11 agents) to only 22% (one agent). Should all of these agents be dismissed from consideration for use in combinations? Experimental evidence indicates the answer to be no. There are several reasons.

As Wilcox *et al.* (1965) noted, tumor mass regression does not adequately measure percent cell kill. It has been shown that as much as 99.95% cell kill may result from treatment that gives a response rate of only 6% (Griswold, 1975). Further, Steel and Adams (1975) and Shipley *et al.* (1975) have shown that small tumors are more responsive than large tumors to chemotherapy or to radiation. Finally, until exhaustive, well-controlled clinical trials are undertaken, there can be no assurance that treatment discounted as negative was given in an optimal manner. Agents with limited activity in advanced disease or when used alone may be useful in combinations or in early disease. A case in point is that of the urea, 1-(2-chloroethyl)-3-(4-methylcyclohexyl)-1-nitroso-*trans*-(MeCCNU). Two- or three-drug combinations that included MeCCNU, a marginally effective agent against colorectal cancer of man, were shown to be more effective than any of the single agents—both clinically (Moertel *et al.*, 1975) and experimentally (Fig. 3).

Multiple modality therapy, although championed for years by a few, has now become acceptable in clinical practice. The advantage gained by following surgical *debulking* of the tumor burden with systemic therapy is obvious and has been so well documented that it requires no further proof. The utility may be demonstrated by a simple example (see Fig. 5). Most importantly, the use of surgical-adjuvant techniques in experimental *in vivo* settings with relevant tumor models offers the promise of providing a means of selection of agents with activity against metastatic foci. Cyclophosphamide, an agent of only modest activity against our colon tumor No. 26 when treatment was started early (Table 3), was almost totally ineffective against advanced, about 800 mg, tumors but was curative in 40% of mice whose primary tumors were surgically removed prior to chemotherapy (Fig. 4). That is but one example of a marginally useful agent being made markedly effective by employment in a combined modality approach.

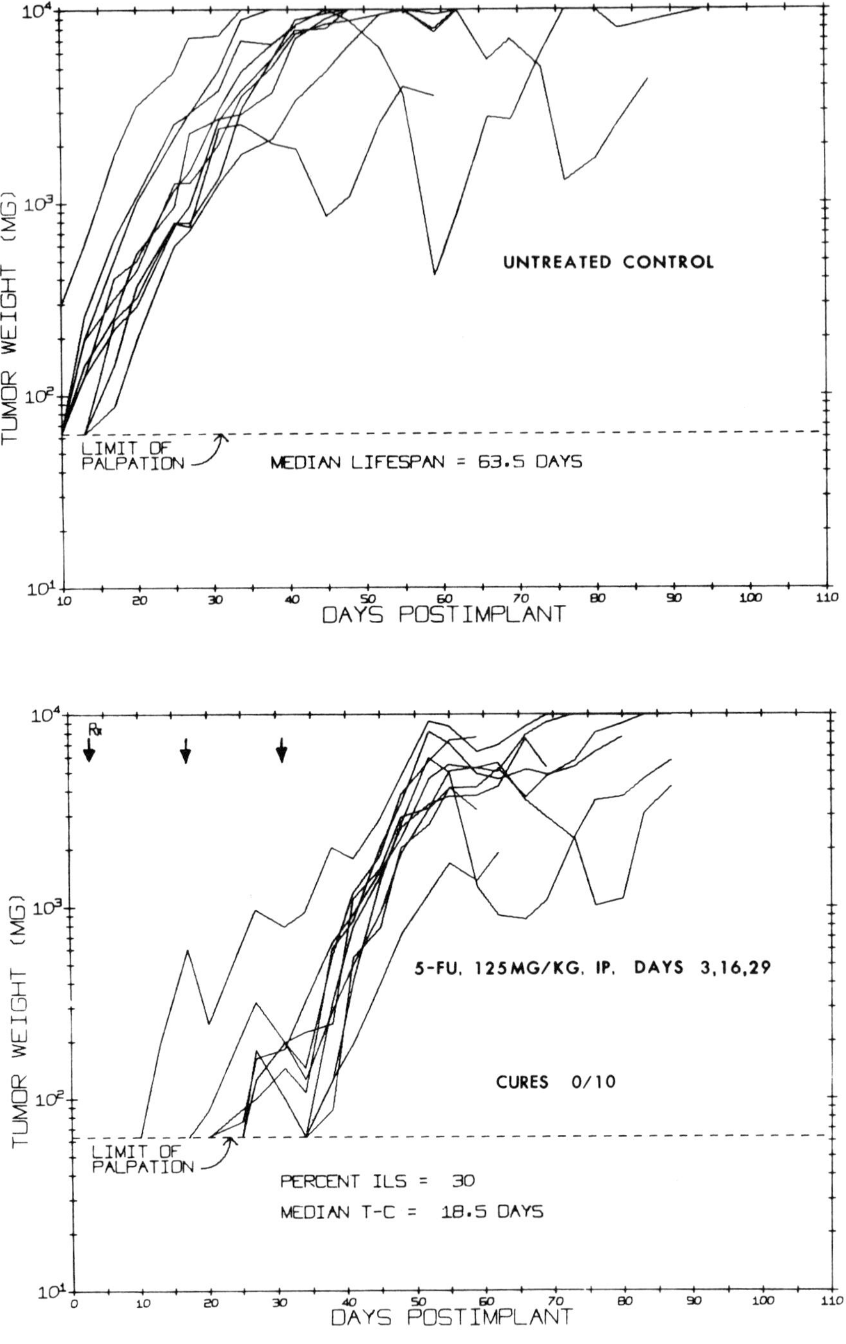

Fig. 3. Improved response of subcutaneously implanted colon tumors of mice to combination chemotherapy.

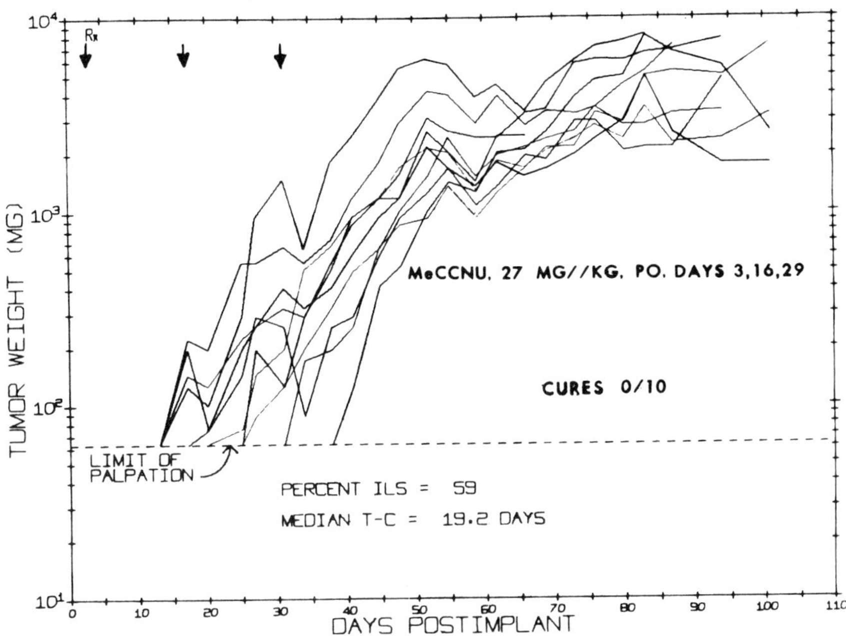

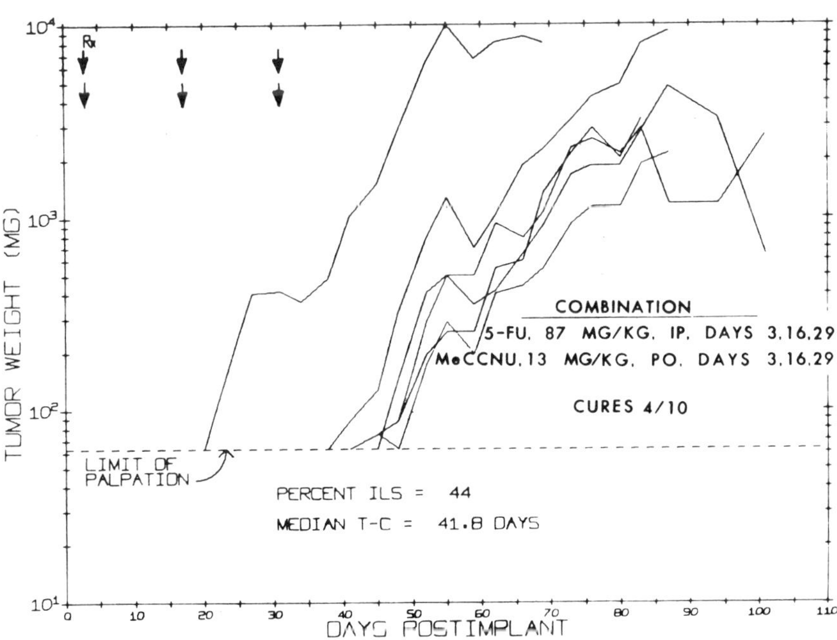

Fig. 3. (*continued*)

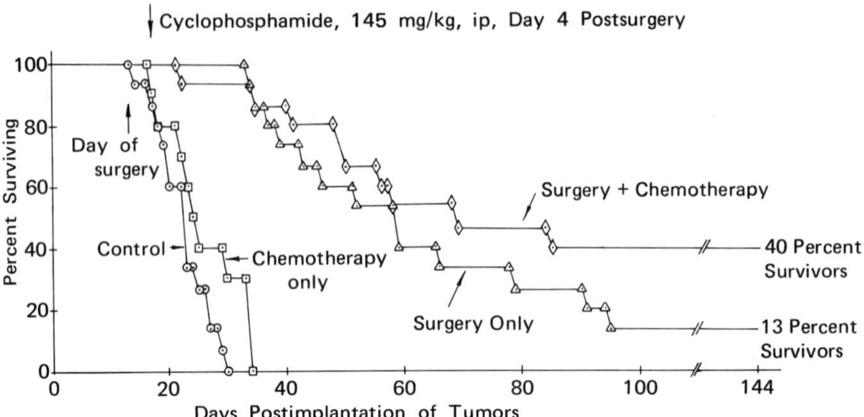

Fig. 4. Improved response of subcutaneously implanted colon tumors of mice to combination modality therapy. Tumors were 600–1000 mg on the day of surgical excision.

4.4. Dose Regimen Selection

Goldin *et al.* (1956) showed the importance of treatment schedule on the effectiveness of amethopterin against a mouse leukemia. Skipper *et al.* (1964) later laid the foundation for dosage schedule exploitation. Agent, dosage, and regimen selection have since been given more consideration* than, perhaps, any other single aspect of cancer chemotherapy. Yet dose regimen selection remains a problem because of a lack of knowledge of drug mechanism of action and the changing and poorly understood cell kinetics and biochemical parameters of tumor and normal tissues. An approach to this question on an empirical basis, as is most often done, is hampered by the logistics involved. Nevertheless, in spite of our lack of complete understanding, successes, in terms of cure, have been achieved.

The importance of proper dose regimen selection is illustrated in Fig. 5, which shows the idealized response of the solid, subcutaneously implanted B16 melanoma to each of three dose regimens of cyclophosphamide. These data clearly show the superiority of one treatment, although all three were approximately equitoxic to the hosts, and although the intermediate end points, duration of tumor response and host life span, indicated equivalent antitumor activity. The point must be made that treatment to toxicity does not ensure optimal therapeutic activity.

5. The Future

Progress in the future would seem to rest on the development of improved means for selection of modality, agent, and dose regimen. The suc-

*It would be impossible to consider here all available references to this point. A few pertinent references, whose bibliographies allow further reading, are Skipper (1968), Skipper *et al.* (1970), Schabel (1969), van Putten (1974), Valeriote and van Putten (1975), and Wheeler and Simpson-Herren (1973).

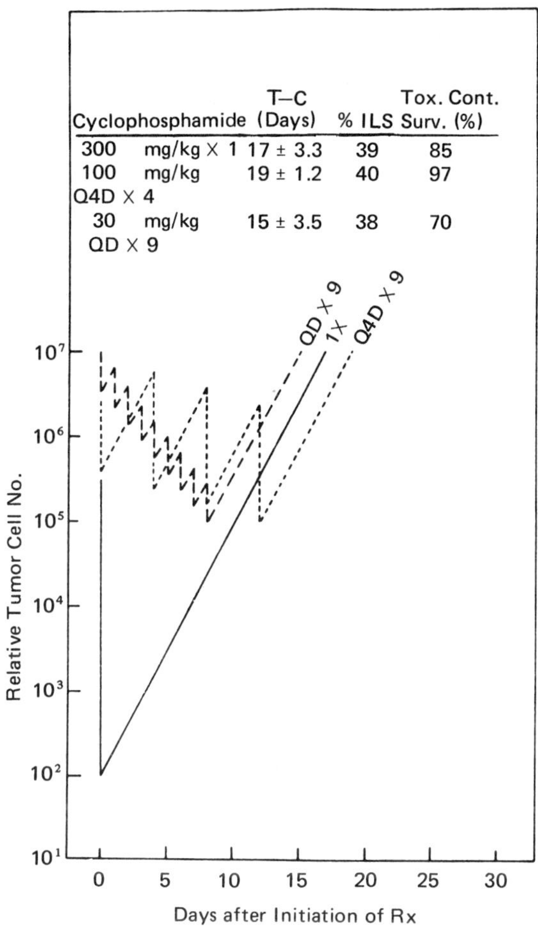

Fig. 5. Idealized response of subcutaneously implanted B16 melanoma to three different schedules of treatment with cyclophosphamide.

cessful employment and timing of the various modalities, surgery, radiation, chemotherapy, and immunotherapy, will depend on better understanding of biochemical, pharmacological, toxicological, and kinetic parameters. Specific problem areas include predetermination of normal tissue toxicity, potential carcinogenicity, and tumor-host immunological status. Limitations of therapy imposed by normal tissue responses must be recognized so that therapies may be utilized to the fullest extent without incurring objectionable (and often lethal) side effects. The development of specific drug resistance as well as pharmacological and anatomical tumor cell sanctuaries remains a real or potential problem.

Systemic cancer therapy, today, is limited by some if not all of the poorly understood problems mentioned above. It is to be hoped that through the development and use of better animal tumor models many of these questions can be addressed with a view toward translation of likely useful concepts, so derived, to the treatment of cancer in man.

ACKNOWLEDGMENTS

Research reported in this paper was supported in part through Grant CA 17303, National Large Bowel Cancer Project, National Cancer Institute, and Contract NO1-CM-43756, National Cancer Institute.

6. References

Baserga, R., 1965, The relationship of the cell cycle to tumor growth and control of cell division: A review, *Cancer Res.* **25:**581–595.

Bruce, W. R., Meeker, B. E., and Valeriote, F. A., 1966, Comparison of the sensitivity of normal hematopoietic and transplanted lymphoma colony-forming cells to chemotherapeutic agents, *J. Natl. Cancer Inst.* **37:**233–245.

Corbett, T. H., Griswold, D. P., Roberts, B. J., Peckham, J. C., and Schabel, F. M., Jr., 1975*a*, Tumor induction relationships in development of transplantable cancers of the colon in mice for chemotherapy assays, with a note on carcinogen structure, *Cancer Res.* **35:**2434–2439.

Corbett, T. H., Griswold, D. P., Roberts, B. J., Peckham, J., and Schabel, F. M., Jr., 1975*b*, A mouse colon tumor model for experimental therapy, *Cancer Chemother. Rep.* **5**(2)**:**169–186.

Cortes, E. P., Holland, J. F., Wang, J. J., Sinks, L. F., Blom, J., Hansjurg, S., Bank, A., and Glidewell, O., 1974, Amputation and adriamycin in primary osterosarcoma, *N. Eng. J. Med.* **291:**998–1000.

DeVita, V. T., Young, R. C., and Canellos, G. P., 1974, Combination versus single agent chemotherapy: A review of the basis for selection of drug treatment of cancer, *Cancer (Philadelphia)* **35:**98–110.

Double, J. A., Ball, C. R., and Cowen, P. N., 1975, Transplantation of adenocarcinomas of the colon in mice, *J. Natl. Cancer Inst.* **54:**271–275.

Fisher, B., Carbone, P., Economou, S. G., Frelick, R., Glass, A., Lerner, H., Redmond, C., Zelen, M., Band, P., Katrych, D. L., Wolmark, W., and Fisher, E. R., 1975, L-Phenylalanine mustard (L-PAM) in the management of primary breast cancer, a report of early findings, *N. Eng. J. Med.* **292:**117–122.

Fortnér, J. G., Mahy, A. G., Schrodt, G. R., and Cotran, R. S., 1961, Transplantable tumors of the Syrian (golden) hamster. Parts I and II, *Cancer Res.* **21:**161–234.

Fowler, J. F., 1966, Radiation biology as applied to radiotherapy, in: *Current Topics in Radiation Research* (M. Ebert and A. Howard, eds.), pp. 303–364, North-Holland, Amsterdam.

Goldin, A., Venditti, J. M., Humphreys, S. R., and Mantel, N., 1956, Modification of treatment schedules in the management of advanced mouse leukemia with amethopterin, *J. Natl. Cancer Inst.* **17:**203–212.

Griswold, D. P., 1972, Consideration of the subcutaneously implanted B16 melanoma as a screening model for potential anticancer agents, *Cancer Chemother. Rep. Part 2* **3:**315–324.

Griswold, D. P., Jr., 1975, The potential for murine tumor models in surgical adjuvant chemotherapy, *Cancer Chemother. Rep.* **5**(2)**:**187–204.

Griswold, D. P., and Corbett, T. H., 1976, Breast tumor modeling for prognosis and treatment, in: *Recent Results in Cancer Research,* Vol. 57, pp. 42–58, Springer Verlag, Berlin.

Griswold, D. P., Schabel, F. M., Wilcox, W. S., Simpson-Herren, L., and Skipper, H. E., 1968, Success and failure in the treatment of solid tumors. I. Effects of cyclophosphamide (NSC 26271) on primary and metastatic plasmacytoma in the hamster, *Cancer Chemother. Rep.* **52:**345–387.

Hertz, R., Lewis, J., and Lippset, M., 1961, Five years experience with the chemotherapy of metastatic choriocarcinoma and related tropoblastic tumors in women, *Am. J. Obstet. Gynecol.* **82:**631.

Horton, J., Hacker, B., Cunningham, T. J., and Sponzo, R. W., 1974, The chemotherapy of large-bowel cancer: Present status and future prospects, *Digest. Dis.* **19:**1040–1046.

Howeld, M. A., 1975, Diet as an etiological factor in the development of cancers of the colon and rectum, *J. Chron. Dis.* **28:**67–80.

Jaffe, N., Frei, E., Traggis, D., and Bishop, Y., 1974, Adjuvant methotrexate and citrovorum-factor treatment of osteogenic sarcoma, *N. Eng. J. Med.* **291**:994–997.

Karrer, K., Humphreys, S. R., and Goldin, A., 1967, An experimental model for studying factors which influence metastases of malignant tumors, *Int. J. Cancer* **2**:213–223.

Laquer, G. L., 1965, The induction of intestinal neoplasms in rats with the glycoside of cycasin and its aglycone, *Arch. Pathol. Anat.* **340**:151–163.

Martin, D. S., Hayworth, P. E., and Fugmann, R. A., 1970, Enhanced cures of spontaneous murine mammary tumors with surgery, combination chemotherapy and immunotherapy, *Cancer Res.* **30**:709–716.

Mayo, J. G., Laster, W. R., Andrews, C. M., and Schabel, F. M., Jr., 1972, Success and failure in the treatment of solid tumors. III. "Cure" of metastatic Lewis lung carcinoma with methyl-CCNU (NSC 95441) and surgery-chemotherapy, *Cancer Chemother. Rep. Part I* **56**:183–195.

McCall, D. C., and Cole, J. W. 1974, Transplantation of chemically induced adenocarcinomas of the colon in an inbred strain of rats, *Cancer (Philadelphia)* **33**:1021–1026.

Mendelsohn, M. L., 1960, The growth fraction: A new concept applied to tumors, *Science* **132**:1496.

Moertel, C. G., 1973, Alimentary tract cancer XXIV-12: Large bowel, in: *Cancer Medicine* (J. F. Holland and E. Frei, III, eds.), p. 1615, Lea and Febiger, Philadelphia.

Moertel, C. G., 1975, Clinical management of advanced gastrointestinal cancer, *Cancer (Philadelphia)* **36**:675–682.

Moertel, C. G., Schutt, A. J., Hahn, R. G., and Reitemeir, R. J., 1975, Therapy of advanced colo-rectal cancer with a combination of 5-fluorouracil, methyl-1,3 *cis*(2-chloroethyl)-1-nitrosourea, and vincristine, *J. Natl. Cancer Inst.* **54**:69–71.

Morrow, R. H., Pike, M. C., and Kisule, A., 1967, Survival of Burkett's lymphoma patients in Mulago Hospital, Uganda, *Br. Med. J.* **4**:323.

Narisawa, T., Sato, T., Hayakawa, M., Sakuma, A., and Nakano, H., 1971, Carcinoma of the colon and rectum of rats by rectal infusion of *N*-methyl-N'-nitro-N-nitrosoguanidine, *Gann* **62**:231–234.

Sandberg, J., and Goldin, A., 1971, Use of first generation transplants of a slow growing solid tumor for the evaluation of new cancer chemotherapeutic agents, *Cancer Chemother. Rep. Part I* **55**:233–238.

Schabel, F. M., Jr., 1969, The use of tumor growth kinetics in planning "curative" chemotherapy of advanced solid tumors, *Cancer Res.* **29**:2384–2389.

Schabel, F. M., Jr., 1975*a*, Concepts for systemic treatment of micrometastases, *Cancer (Philadelphia)* **35**:15–24.

Schabel, F. M., Jr., 1975*b*, Animal models as predictive systems, in: *Cancer Chemotherapy*, pp. 323–355, Year Book Medical Publishers, Chicago.

Sherlock, P., 1974, The gastroenterologist and gastrointestinal cancer, *Digest. Dis.* **19**:933–934.

Shipley, W. U., Stanley, J. A., and Steel, G. G., 1975, Tumor size dependency in the radiation response of the Lewis lung carcinoma, *Cancer Res.* **35**:2488–2493.

Silverberg, E., and Holeb, A. I., 1975, Major trends in cancer: 25-year survey, *CA Cancer J. Clin.* **25**:2–21.

Skipper, H. E., 1968, Biochemical, biological, pharmacologic, toxicologic, kinetic and clinical (subhuman and human) relationships, *Cancer (Philadelphia)* **21**:600–610.

Skipper, H. E., 1971, Kinetics of mammary tumor cell growth and implications for therapy, *Cancer (Philadelphia)* **28**:1479–1499.

Skipper, H. E., 1973, Successes and failures at the preclinical level; where now? in: *Seventh National Cancer Conference Proceedings*, American Cancer Society.

Skipper, H. E., and Schabel, F. M., Jr., 1973, Quantitative and Cytokinetic studies in experimental tumor models, in: *Cancer Medicine* (J. F. Holland and E. Frei, III, eds.), Lea and Febiger, Philadelphia.

Skipper, H. E., Schabel, F. M., Jr., and Wilcox, W. S., 1964, On the criteria and kinetics associated with "curability" of experimental leukemia, *Cancer Chemother. Rep.* **35**:1–111.

Skipper, H. E., Schabel, F. M., Jr., Mellett, L. B., Montgomery, J. A., Wilkoff, L. J., Lloyd, H. H., and Brockman, R. W., 1970, Implications of biochemical cytokinetic pharmacologic and toxicologic relationships in the design of optimal therapeutic schedules, *Cancer Chemother. Rep. Part 1* **54:**431–450.

Steel, G. G., 1967, Cell loss as a factor in the growth rate of human tumors, *Eur. J. Cancer* **3:**381–387.

Steel, G. G., and Adams, K., 1975, Stem-cell survival and tumor control in Lewis lung carcinoma, *Cancer Res.* **35:**1530–1535.

Tannock, I. F., and Steel, G. G., 1969, Quantitative techniques for study of the anatomy and function of small blood vessels in tumors, *J. Natl. Cancer Inst.* **42:**771–782.

Thurnherr, N., Deschner, E. E., Stonehill, E. H., and Lipkin, M., 1973, Induction of adenocarcinomas of the colon in mice by weekly injections of 1,2-dimethylhydrazine, *Cancer Res.* **33:**940–945.

Triolo, V. A., 1964, Nineteenth century foundations of cancer research—origins of experimental research, *Cancer Res.* **24:**4–27.

Valeriote, F. A., and Van Putten, L. M., 1975, Proliferation-dependent cytotoxicity of anticancer agents: A review, *Cancer Res.* **35:**2619–2630.

Van Putten, L. M., 1974, Are cell kinetic data relevant for the design of tumour chemotherapy schedules? *Cell Tissue Kinet.* **7:**493–504.

Van Putten, L. M., and Lelieveld, P., 1970, Factors determining cell killing by chemotherapeutic agents *in vivo.* I. Cyclophosphamide, *Eur. J. Cancer* **6:**313–321.

Wasserman, T. H., Comis, R. L., Handelsman, H., Penta, J. S., Slavik, M., Soper, W. T., and Carter, S. K., 1974, Tabular overview of cancer chemotherapy of solid tumors, in: *Report of the Division of Cancer Treatment NCI, 1974,* Vol. 2: *Program Logic and Scientific Reports,* DHEW, NIH, Bethesda, Md.

Weisburger, J. H., 1971, Colon carcinogens: Their metabolism and mode of action, *Cancer (Philadelphia)* **28:**60–70.

Wheeler, G. P., and Simpson-Herren, L., 1973, Effects of purines, pyrimidines, nucleosides, and chemically related compounds on the cell cycle, in: *Drugs and the Cell Cycle* (A. M. Zimmerman, G. M. Padilla, and I. L. Cameron, eds.), Academic Press, New York.

Wilcox, W. S., Griswold, D. P., Laster, W. R., Schabel, F. M., Jr., and Skipper, H. E., 1965, Experimental evaluation of potential anticancer agents. XVII. Kinetics of growth and regression after treatment of certain solid tumors, *Cancer Chemother. Rep.* **47:**27–39.

Wilkoff, L. J., Wilcox, W. S., Burdeshaw, J. A., Dixon, G. J., and Dulmadge, E. A., 1967, Effect of antimetabolites on kinetic behavior of proliferating cultured L1210 leukemia cells, *J. Natl. Cancer Inst.* **39:**965–976.

Zubrod, G. G., 1972, Chemical control of cancer, *Proc. Natl. Acad. Sci. USA* **69:**1042–1047.

IV

Future Directions in Early Detection and Diagnosis

18

Early Diagnosis and Detection of Colorectal Cancer in High-Risk Population Groups

Martin Lipkin, Paul Sherlock, and Sidney J. Winawer

1. Introduction

Cancer of the colon and rectum is presently responsible for about 15% of all malignant neoplasms found in the United States. It now exceeds the frequency of lung cancer when male and female rates of occurrence are combined. The American Cancer Society predicted 100,000 new colorectal cancer cases in 1976; of these, 70,000 were expected to be colon and 30,000 rectal in origin (Silverberg and Holleb, 1975), with a total of 50,000 deaths. It is obvious that colorectal cancer poses a major problem in the United States as well as many other countries. Detection and diagnosis when the disease is at an earlier stage could result in earlier treatment and improvement in survival.

Current research has shown improvement in the elucidation of predisposing factors that are associated with colon cancer and in the identification of early changes within colonic cells that identify increased susceptibility to neoplasia. This chapter will discuss these means of identification, their association with the early diagnosis of neoplasia, and the possibilities they offer in improving the early detection and prevention of malignancy. The identification of inherited and environmental factors in the genesis of colorectal cancer will be considered together with leads they provide for early detection.

Martin Lipkin, Paul Sherlock, and Sidney J. Winawer • Memorial Sloan-Kettering Cancer Center, New York, New York 10021.

2. Diseases in Which Inherited Factors Increase the Risk of Colon Cancer

Current evidence indicates that environmental elements have an important role in the development of colorectal cancer. However, genetic susceptibility has a major role in certain diseases that predispose to colon cancer. Recent findings also have suggested that inherited factors may have a greater role than generally believed in the development of the disease. Thus a significant fraction of colorectal cancer patients show a risk that is greater than expected in the general population (Moertel *et al.*, 1958). Individuals under age 40 who develop colorectal cancer have been reported more likely to have a family history of colon cancer than those over age 40 (Wynder and Shigematsu, 1967). Furthermore, it has been noted that the age at onset of colonic cancer is significantly earlier in relatives of patients with multiple primary colonic malignancies than in the general population (Moertel *et al.*, 1958).

The disease entity of hereditary adenocarcinomatosis has been described, believed to be inherited as an autosomal dominant with 90% penetrance Anderson, 1969). The concept of "cancer families" also has been developed to describe familial aggregates showing a striking incidence of malignancy at multiple anatomical sites including colon, as well as multiple primary neoplasms and an early age at onset (Fraumeni, 1973; Lynch, 1967). The neoplasms in these families which appear to be influenced by genetic predisposition affect diverse organs, e.g., colon and endometrium.

With the exception of the well-known inherited disease adenomatosis of the colon and rectum (ACR, familial polyposis), efforts to indicate a single-gene difference in colonic carcinomas with a genetic basis have largely been unsuccessful. Genetic studies in cancer families have shown neither excessive consanguinity nor the presence of an identifiable single recessive gene. Duffy blood groups have been linked to the gene for ACR susceptibility, but linkage studies have not been successful in other premalignant colonic states (Veale, 1965). Hyperploidy principally characterizes the chromosomal abnormalities in adenomatous polyps and colon carcinoma in ACR, although pseudodiploids have also been identified (Enterline and Arvan, 1967; Mitelman *et al.*, 1974). Atypical adenomas have shown both greater hyperploidy and more numerous abnormal chromosomes including those of C and D groups.

To date, no chromosomal entity can be cited as a useful diagnostic or prognostic marker for colon carcinoma which is comparable to the Philadelphia chromosome (an indicator of chronic granulocytic leukemia). It has been proposed that individuals with hereditary predisposition to neoplasia carry a germinal mutation and acquire another somatic mutation leading to cancer, while individuals with nonhereditary cancers are believed to acquire additional somatic mutations having a later age at onset than hereditary cancer (Knudsen *et al.*, 1973). An important concept relates to the possibility that interactions between environmental and inherited factors contribute to the evolution of neoplasia (Fraumeni, 1973; Knudsen, 1976; Lipkin, 1975).

In ACR, associated with innumerable colonic polyps, it has been possible to estimate population frequency, relative fitness, and mutation rate. It is one of the few genetic disorders associated with malignancy offering as many data of this type, enabling a fairly accurate gross description of the premalignant phase of the disease. Three different studies have estimated disease frequency in the population based on the clinical expression of the disease: 1 in 8300 in Michigan (Reed and Neel, 1955), 1 in 23,750 at St. Mark's Hospital in London (Veale, 1965), and 1 in 7150 in Kentucky (Pierce, 1968). A penetrance rate of approximately 80% with an autosomal dominant mode of inheritance has been well established. Fewer cases have resulted because of this incomplete penetrance.

The presence of hundreds to thousands of adenomatous polyps characterizes the classically recognized form of the disease. These may carpet the entire colon and rectum, with the rectum showing denser adenomatosis. Sessile and pedunculated adenomatous and villous tumors are usually seen.

In the past, estimates have indicated that two-thirds of patients when first seen with adenomatosis will show evidence of cancer; by 37 years of age, over 50% will develop adenocarcinoma. The average age in ACR for diagnosis has been 25 years, while cancer in polyposis patients is usually diagnosed at a later age. This is about 30 years earlier than average figures for cancer without adenomatosis. Patients usually manifest multiple cancers, and approximately 50% of colectomy specimens show two or more cancers, (Morson and Bussey, 1970). The duration of the phase of adenomatosis before cancer is between 5 and 15 years. Cancers also have been reported in patients with adenomatosis who were less than 20 years old. The usual pattern for adenoma formation is generally after puberty and extends to the age of 40 and above. However, the onset of polyposis rarely occurs above the age of 40.

Individuals who are examined because they have a relative with adenomatosis are usually diagnosed as having the disease without cancer at a much earlier age than those seeking medical advice because of adenoma symptoms. The identification of individuals on the basis of the former results in the development of fewer malignancies, because of earlier age at investigation and treatment. It is well established that inherited adenomatosis is a premalignant disorder and that almost all patients develop colon carcinoma by age of 50 unless a colectomy is performed.

Gardner's syndrome is another autosomal dominant disorder showing a high degree of penetrance. Adenomatous polyps of the colon, and occasionally the small intestine, are formed, and there is a propensity for adenocarcinoma development within the polyps. Other characterizing features include sebaceous cysts, epidermoid cysts, desmoid tumors (following surgical treatment), fibromas, and facial bone osteomas. These conditions may be associated in various combinations. Abnormal dentition and carcinomas of the thyroid, ampulla of Vater, duodenum, and adrenal gland are other conditions associated with Gardner's syndrome. Variants of this syndrome can include the Turcot syndrome (polyposis coli associated with tumors of the CNS) and the Oldfield syndrome (extensive familial sebaceous cysts, polyposis coli, and adenocarcinoma).

One in seven cases of inherited ACR have been estimated to be the Gardner type. Frequency estimates in the population are approximately 1 in 14,025. The adenomatosis and other stigmata can be due to a single gene, although it is possible that additional genes are involved. It is interesting to note that some individuals with Gardner's syndrome are refractory with respect to the phosphaturic effect of parathyroid extract on the renal tubule (Trygstad *et al.*, 1968).

A third autosomal dominant inheritance with variable expression is the Peutz-Jeghers syndrome. It is characterized by melanin pigmentation of the buccal mucosa, lips, face, fingers, toes, vagina, and anus. Polyps of the gastrointestinal tract, specifically the small intestine, are found; about one-third are in the colon and rectum. The polyps, however, are hamartomas rather than adenomas (Moertel *et al.*, 1966). This disorder appears to have little malignant expression when compared to ACR or Gardner's syndrome. Nevertheless, some associated stomach and duodenal carcinomas have been reported (Dodds et al., 1972).

One or more adenomas are present in 5–10% of individuals in the general population. One or more colorectal adenomas can be associated with adenocarcinoma development. Kindreds have also been reported showing an association of single and multiple polyps with adenocarcinoma, a link that appears to be genetically influenced. One kindred study showed that 45% of the adult members of one generation had solitary adenomas and that adenomas occurred in multiple generations (Woolf *et al.*, 1955). This family also had a high incidence of colon carcinoma. An autosomal dominant mode of inheritance is reinforced by these observations.

Another inherited disorder is juvenile polyposis of the colon. These polyps are hamartomas and are not viewed as having malignant potential. Relatives of these juveniles do, however, express an increased occurrence of adenomas and colorectal adenocarcinoma (Lynch and Krush, 1967), and individuals with juvenile polyps may themselves develop true adenomas and cancer later in life.

3. Contribution of Environmental Factors Increasing the Risk of Colon Cancer

That environment has a role in the development of colorectal cancer in the general population has been well established. Numerous studies have shown a strong correlation between geographical, economic, and dietary exposure and cancer development. These are described in Chapter 9 of this volume, and only brief comments are made here.

Within the United States, past studies have shown the following patterns of colorectal cancer incidence: northern states greater than southern; urban greater than rural; Jewish greater than non-Jewish; white greater than black. These patterns are now decreasing, mainly because of migrational shifts into urban regions (especially noted in white-black differences) (Berg, 1973; Haenszel and Correa, 1971; Bolt, 1971; Wynder and Shigematsu, 1967).

Global geographical patterns show a generally higher incidence of colonic cancer in the developed countries. South America, Africa, and Asia generally show lower rates. The United States has one of the highest rates in the world. This distribution suggests a correlation with the level of economic development, although environmental factors influencing colon cancer development are still unknown. With Japanese migrating to Hawaii and Puerto Ricans migrating to the U.S. mainland, individuals usually assume the cancer risk pattern of the adopted area within a few generations. It has been of longstanding interest that colon and stomach cancer show a negative correlation. With the present exception of asbestos workers, there does not appear to be a specific relationship between occupation and the disease. However, there is a positive correlation of economic development, general nutritional patterns, fat and protein consumption, and arteriosclerotic heart disease to the incidence of colon cancer (Berg, 1973; Haenszel and Correa, 1971; Wynder and Shigematsu, 1967).

The most convincing epidemiological data correlating worldwide colonic cancer distribution are related to those societies whose diets are rich in fat and animal protein. Again the United States shows a much higher incidence of the disease than, for example, Japan, where there has been one-fourth the consumption of fat and animal protein. The observed difference in geographical distributions could also be related to dietary factors which control the composition of gut microbial flora, an area under intensive investigation at this time. It has been postulated that variation in microbe populations might possibly produce carcinogens from intestinal secretions or food. Greater population densities of the microbes *Bacteroides* and *Clostridium* with fewer lactobacilli and streptococci (Aries *et al.*, 1969) were initially reported in some populations with a high colon cancer rate, together with a higher ratio of anaerobic to aerobic bacteria in the feces (Hill *et al*, 1971; Hill, 1975); however, more recent work has questioned this. If developed in a satisfactory way, identification of critical microbial organisms or microbial products in susceptible individuals might aid detection programs. More recently, the detection of mutagenic activity in human feces, its possible suppression, and the anticipated identification of causative factors, offer new leads to our understanding of environmental and genetic interrelationships (Land and Bruce, 1968).

4. *Identification of Increased Susceptibility to Colon Cancer in High-Risk Population Groups*

4.1. *Before the Development of Neoplasms*

4.1.1. *Abnormal Colon Cell Identification: Biopsies and Colonic Cell Washings*

As noted in Chapter 1 of this volume, cell proliferation studies in man and other mammalian species have shown that an overall steady-state condition is reached in the gastrointestinal mucosa resulting from the kinetics of cell birth, migration, and extrusion (i.e., rate of cell loss equals rate of cell production). The location of normal proliferating, mature and abnormal cells has been demonstrated (Messier and Leblond, 1960; Deschner *et al.*, 1963; Deschner and Lipkin, 1970; Lipkin, 1973; Lipkin and Deschner, 1968; Lipkin *et al.*, 1963). Proliferative abnormalities developing in mucosa believed to be normal, in diseased colon, and during the induction of tumors in rodents have all been defined in terms of their spatial boundaries in the epithelial lining of the gastrointestinal tract. In some cases, subtle and early changes that have eluded conventional examinations have now been detected (Deschner and Lipkin, 1970; Lipkin, 1974; Lohrs *et al.*, 1969; Springer *et al.*, 1970; Thurnherr *et al.*, 1973; Wiebecke *et al.*, 1973).

In inherited adenomatosis of the colon and rectum, progressive phases of abnormal growth appear in colonic epithelial cells. In subjects with ACR, patches of flat mucosa can be detected having colonic epithelial cells that fail to repress DNA synthesis during migration to the surface of the mucosa (Deschner and Lipkin, 1970; Deschner *et al.*, 1966). This finding has been observed in normal-appearing colonic epithelial cells of subjects with ACR before the cells begin to accumulate as polyps. It has been noted in 85% of random biopsy specimens.

In inherited adenomatosis, colonic epithelial cells develop additional properties. Cells that fail to undergo normal maturation with repression of

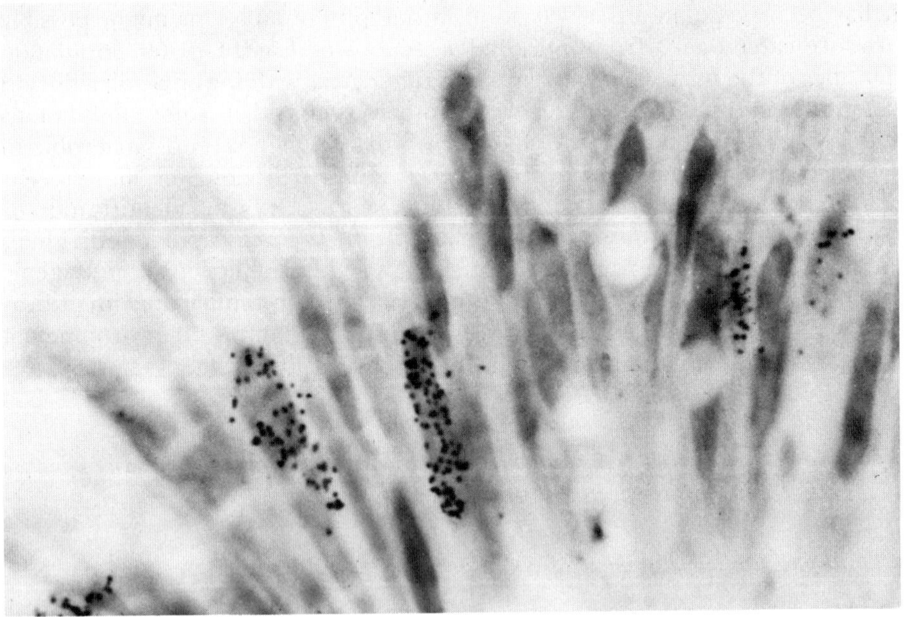

Fig. 1. Example of incorporation of tritiated thymidine into epithelial cells of an expanding adenomatous polyp, after injection of thymidine into a subject with inherited ACR and metastatic malignancy. (From Lipkin, 1977.)

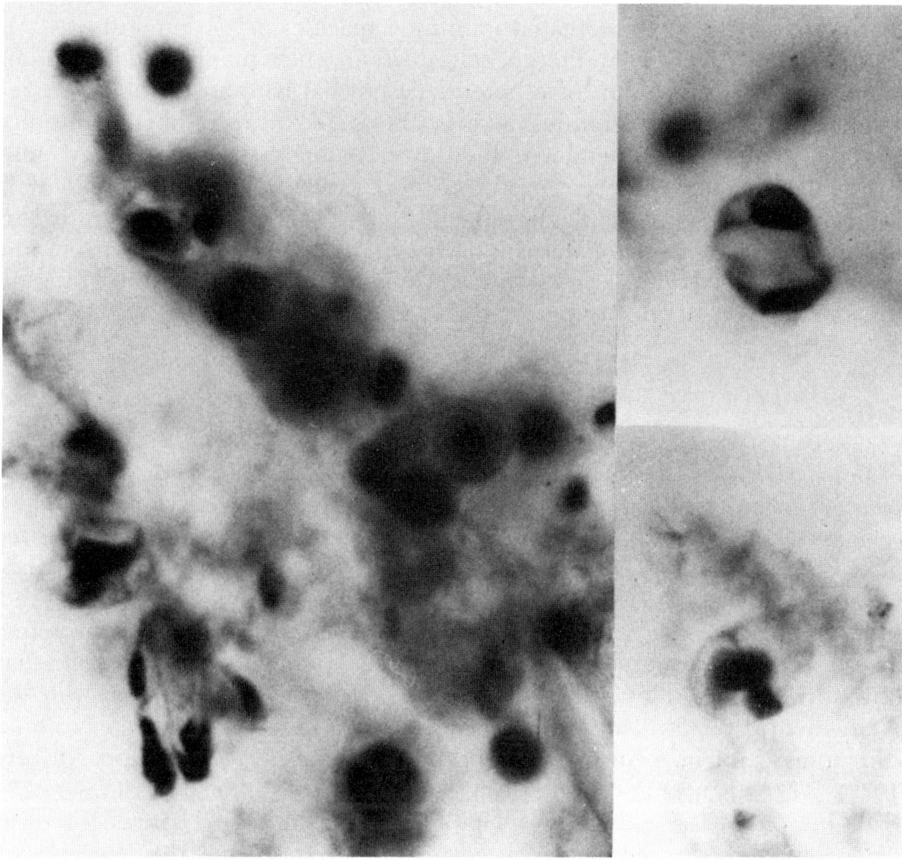

Fig. 2. Cytological specimen from washings removed by pulsatile lavage from colon of subject with inherited ACR. Cells suspected to be adenocarcinoma were observed and were later found in a specimen of mucosa. (From Lipkin, 1977.)

proliferative activity also acquire altered morphological characteristics identified pathologically as "adenomatous" (Lipkin, 1977) (Fig. 1). These cells accumulate in the colonic mucosa and form tubular or villous structures initiating the formation of adenomas. Carcinomas develop with increasing frequency as these adenomatous excrescences enlarge and as they develop villous components. All of these cellular abnormalities have been found with high frequency in colonic biopsies and in washings containing colonic cells (Deschner *et al.*, 1975) in the high-risk group with ACR (Fig. 2).

4.1.2. *Immunological Studies*

An immunological abnormality has now been detected in individuals at increased risk of colon cancer. When cancer-free individuals from families predisposed to colon cancer (without classic ACR) were studied to determine the nature of their cell-mediated immune capacities, 44% demonstrated an apparent perturbation of adherent cell function, which manifested itself as an inappropriate suppression of a potentially normal lymphocyte ability to respond to an allogeneic stimulus. This *in vitro* defect in recognitive immunity was the same defect demonstrated in individuals with established malignancies. Patients with recognized Gardner's syndrome also showed the deficit of recognitive immunity (Berlinger *et al.*, 1977). These studies are also being extended to additional series of disorders leading to colon cancer, and offer the possibility of new immunological means of early detection of highly susceptible population groups.

4.1.3. *Nuclear Protein Studies*

Recent studies have described changes in nuclear proteins of colonic cells, of potential interest in the early detection of malignancy. Characteristic complements of nuclear nonhistone proteins can be isolated from normal colonic cells and from tumors. After isolation of nuclei, differences in density, size, nonhistone protein-to-DNA ratio, and DNA synthetic activity were found. Different nuclear classes isolated from 1,2-dimethylhydrazine-induced tumors contained characteristic complements of nonhistone nuclear proteins. These were not prominent in normal colonic epithelial nuclei, in epithelial cells surrounding the tumors, or in nuclei of animals not treated with dimethylhydrazine. Similar nuclear proteins were detected in human colonic carcinomas and in a human colon carcinoma cell line (Boffa and Allfrey, 1976). The identification and selective accumulation of such proteins in colonic tumor nuclei, and the development of analytical procedures for their detection in single cells, offer a new approach to the early detection of molecular events associated with malignancy in man.

4.1.4. *Enzyme Studies*

It has also been shown that the development of neoplasia is associated with changes in enzyme composition of colonic cells. Thus the nucleotide precursor enzyme thymidine kinase has been shown to be elevated in neoplastic colonic lesions (Troncale *et al.*, 1971; Salser and Balis, 1973). After administration of the colonic carcinogen 1,2-dimethylhydrazine, thymidine kinase was shown to be altered both quantitatively and qualitatively. The tumor enzyme had many fetal-like properites. Long-term treatment with DMH led to changes in thymidine kinase reminiscent of the fetal enzyme. Treatment with DMH also resulted in a large increase in ornithine decarboxylase in colon but not in liver, whereas the liver carcinogen acetylaminofluorene induced a marked increase in liver but not in colon (Ball *et al.*, 1976; Salser and Balis, 1973). The contribution of these changes in enzyme activity to the early identification of cellular abnormalities associated with neoplasia is now being analyzed.

4.1.5. *Studies of Cutaneous Cells*

Recent studies have also indicated that phenotypic expressions of the disease inherited adenomatosis may extend to cutaneous cells. It has been reported that cutaneous fibroblasts derived from individuals with ACR have shown larger regions of criss-cross arrays and random orientation than those from normal subjects. Initial experiments on serum requirement and exposure to Kirsten murine sarcoma virus also have suggested differences in cutaneous fibroblasts from individuals with ACR (Pfeffer and Kopelovich, 1977). These observations are now being extended to include analysis of additional families with various patterns of inherited polyposis and colon cancer, to determine the specificity of the findings. A recent study of the protein action in the cytoskeletal structure of cutaneous fibroblasts (Kopelovich *et al.*, 1977) and heteroploidy in cutaneous epidermal cells (Danes, 1977) offer promising leads to early detection of familial polyposis and Gardner's syndrome.

4.1.6. *Fecal Content Examination*

Important work is in progress to identify abnormal constituents of fecal contents, and to examine their potential carcinogenic activity in colon cells. It was recently reported that fecal contents of individuals with ACR (Table 1) and about one-fourth of individuals in the general population include increased amounts of undegraded cholesterol (Draser *et al.*, 1975; Reddy *et al.*, 1976; Hackman *et al.*, 1976; Watne *et al.*, 1975).

As previously noted, colon cancer occurs in the general population in geographical regions where there is high fat or animal protein consumption. Various investigators have looked for stool markers which might denote increased risk (Hill, 1975; Hill *et al.*, 1971; Weisburger, 1973). These include bacterial enzymes and metabolic breakdown products which might be associated with the formation of carcinogenic compounds. Species of clostridia

Table 1. Fecal Neutral Sterols in Patients with Familial Polyposis, Relatives of Patients, and Controls Consuming a Mixed Western Diet[a]

Neutral sterols	Patients with familial polyposis (8)	Relatives of patients (controls) (10)	Controls (17)
		mg/g dry feces	
Cholesterol	11.9 ± 1.4*[,b]	1.5 ± 0.43†	1.2 ± 0.3†
Coprostanol	2.2 ± 1.23*	13.4 ± 2.46†	14.7 ± 1.7†
Coprostanone	0.5 ± 0.22*	2.5 ± 0.58†	2.1 ± 0.4†
Total	14.6 ± 1.39*	17.4 ± 2.84*	18.0 ± 1.8*

[a]From Reddy *et al.*, (1976).
[b]Averages ± SEM; averages for each compound not sharing a common superscript symbol (*, †) are significantly different, $p < 0.05$.

known to dehydrogenate steroids into compounds with structures similar to those of carcinogens have been under study. Weisburger has noted four mechanisms by which bacteria could be involved in colon carcinogenesis. These include (1) metabolization of dietary components into carcinogens (i.e., bile acids), (2) host metabolite conversion into carcinogens (i.e., nitrates and 2-amines into tryptophan and nitrosamine), (3) formation of carcinogenic or cocarcinogenic metabolic by-products, and (4) intrinsic bacterial carcinogenic compound activation by autolysis.

The well-established role that intestinal bacteria play in modifying intraluminal metabolites offers a fertile area of continued investigation. The bile acids and their bacterial conversion products, compounds with structural similarity to potent carcinogens, are of interest in this regard, and the newer work on fecal mutagens referred to above is particularly relevant.

4.2. *Identification of Increased Susceptibility after the Development of Neoplasms*

Numerous diagnostic approaches are available to determine the early development of benign and malignant colonic neoplasms. Each has specific advantages and limitations. They are described below.

4.2.1. *Occult Blood*

Although most colon cancers bleed, a random stool test on an unmodified diet has very limited utility, as there are many false-negative and false-positive reactions. False-positive reactions can be moderately reduced by a meat-restricted diet. The impregnated guaiac slide (Hemoccult) provides an adequate commercially prepared slide and stabilized reagent. Its decreased sensitivity offers fewer false-positive tests than the standard guaiac test. This test has its greatest utility in screening for colonic disease only when it is properly used. This requires patient cooperation to obtain two daily slides for 3 days on a meat-free high-bulk diet. The method has been shown to detect colon cancers in asymptomatic individuals at any early pathological stage. It shows low false negatives and an estimated 1% false positives. Excessive intake of vitamin C and delay in testing of the slides may result in false negativity.

Table 2. Significant Lesions Detected by Fecal Occult Blood Testing in One Series[a]

	Number of patients
Neoplastic lesions	
Cancer	7
Adenomas	23
	30 (54%)
Nonneoplastic lesions	
Hyperplastic polyps	9
Other	26 (46%)

[a]Fifty-six patients with positive Hemoccult slide tests. From Winawer *et al.* (1977*a*).

Table 3. Application of Fecal Occult Blood Test: Cancers Detected in Screened Asymptomatic Patients and Control Patients[a]

Group	Number of cancers localized[b]
Screened	6/7 (86%)
Control	4/8 (50%)

[a]From Winawer *et al.* (1977*a*).
[b]*In situ,* Dukes's A and B.

Studies by Gregor and others have shown the test to be relatively consistent in the detection of localized colon cancers (Gregor, 1967). Hemoccult-positive patients also have a high percentage of polyps found by others tests including colonoscopy and air-contrast barium enema (Winawer *et al.,* 1976).

This test offers the asymptomatic patient, without underlying disease (i.e., familial polyposis syndrome or ulcerative colitis), a simple screen for identifying an independent source of bleeding (Tables 2 and 3). The reduced sensitivity of the test, however, may fail to identify occult bleeding in the upper gastrointestinal tract due to an in-transit loss of peroxidase activity (Ostrow *et al.*, 1973). Individuals with a positive test who manifest no colon pathology should be examined for upper gastrointestinal and small bowel disorders. Further investigations are still needed to thoroughly evaluate this method's utility and application for mass screening programs.

4.2.2. *Proctosigmoidoscopy*

The value of proctosigmoidoscopy in the early detection of colon cancer in asymptomatic individuals has been well established (Hertz *et al.*, 1960). Estimates indicate that proctoscopy can detect invasive carcinoma in patients initially examined, over age 40, at the rate of 1 in 667 (Moertel *et al.*, 1966). Approximately 55% of colon cancer occurs within the 25-cm sigmoidoscope range. The Preventive Medicine Institute–Strang Clinic has had relatively good success in detecting colon cancers in the tens of thousands of patients it has examined. It has close to a 90% survival rate, over a 15-year follow-up, on 50 patients in which cancers were initially diagnosed by proctosigmoidoscopic examination (Bolt, 1971; Hertz *et al.*, 1960; Wilson *et al.*, 1955).

Proctosigmoidoscopy also has significant value in the detection of adenomatous polyps, which are much more commonly found than cancer. Several studies have shown the occurrence of polyps in patients over age 40 to vary between 4.7% and 9.7% (Bolt, 1971; Hertz *et al.*, 1960; Moertel, *et al.*, 1966; Wilson *et al.*, 1955). Removal of adenomatous polyps as well as villous adenomas has been shown to decrease rectosigmoid cancer incidence (Gilbertsen, 1974).

4.2.3. *Barium Enema*

Although too costly and time consuming for routine screening tests, barium enemas do provide an important technique for the investigation of the symptomatic patient or those at high risk. Its value, however, is often variable because of poor patient preparation or air-contrast technique omission. Faulty air-contrast preparations often miss as much as 40% of polypoid lesions and 20% of carcinomas (Miller, 1974; Williams *et al.*, 1974). Air-contrast studies should precede colonscopic examinations, as blind areas are present on colonscopic examination (i.e., rectosigmoid, splenic and hepatic flexures, caecum). The assessment of extramural and mucosal disease following colon resection should include combined radiological-endoscopic techniques.

4.2.4. *Colonoscopy*

Colonoscopy has revolutionized diagnostic and therapeutic procedures by extending the routine endoscopic observation to include the entire colon. It enables the visualization of polyps and cancers which often elude barium enemas and clarifies the results of negative or positive enemas. Colonoscopy can play a useful role in postoperative colon evaluation, polyposis diagnosis, and selected assessment of inflammatory bowel disease. Colonoscopy has limitations in this instance, and biopsy combined with cytological tests increases the diagnostic potential of the examination. The caecum is reached by experienced colonoscopists in only about 90% of instances, and this represents a limitation of the technique. Previous pelvic surgery, radiation, diverticulitis, and strictures or tumors also are limiting factors. One study has shown an overall morbidity rate of 0.4% (Berci *et al.*, 1974).

4.2.5. *Colonic Cytology*

Cytological lavage studies of the upper gastrointestinal tract and colon offer diagnostic procedures for cancer detection. However, colon lavage has remained an unpopular technique because of the unattractiveness of working with stool-contaminated material and the lack of sufficiently trained technical personnel. Numerous methods have been developed; one involves a pulsatile instrument which is used through either a sigmoidoscope or a colonoscope, thereby taking advantage of a prepared bowel (Katz *et al.*, 1972). The technique probably has its greatest advantage in ulcerative colitis or familial polyposis. When specific lesions are present, the diagnostic yield of biopsy is increased by the use of brush cytology. Brush smears also offer the advantage in their ease of preparation and screening. Lavage is best suited in patients with diffuse premalignant lesions, strictures, and inaccessible areas of the bowel due to fixation by radiation, adhesion, or diverticulitis.

4.2.6. *Tumor-Related Antigens*

Carcinoembryonic antigen (CEA) in blood has been used as an indicator for the diagnosis and management of colon malignancy. Radioimmunoassay is used to detect nanogram quantities of the antigen (Fleisher *et al.*, 1973; LoGerfo *et al.*, 1971; Martin and Martin, 1970; Moore *et al.*, 1971; Reynoso *et al.*, 1972; Thomson *et al.*, 1969). However, the method has mainly been of interest in following individuals for recurrence after cancer resection, rather than in routine screening (Reynoso *et al.*, 1972; Sorokin *et al.*, 1974; Winawer *et al.*, 1977*b*). It has been disappointing as a method for early detection since CEA often is not elevated in early cancers of the colon and elevation may be present in many benign diseases such as cirrhosis, pancreatitis, and inflammatory bowel disease, and in heavy smokers.

5. *Early Detection of Colon Cancer Utilizing Indices of Increased Risk*

The findings described herein have provided a basis for the early identification of abnormal stages of development of colonic epithelial cells, physiological and environmental factors that are associated and that may influence the development of neoplasia, and individuals and population groups at increased risk. It now appears possible to identify individuals in some of the high-risk groups before the appearance of overt disease, as well as after the appearance of neoplasms. Classification of individuals and population groups on the basis of the findings described can also be carried out (Lipkin, 1977). New classifications of this type are leading to the identification of heightened degrees of susceptibility, and are attempting to predict the evolution of stages of disease. Related improvements in laboratory analysis and instrumentation are also being applied to high-risk population segments on a larger scale than heretofore for the identification of early disease.

Future programs designed to improve the early diagnosis and detection of colon cancer will continue to require systematic identification of segments in the general population who are at greatest risk, on the basis of phenotypic abnormalities appearing before the development of overt neoplasia, as well as after its appearance. Classification of individuals and population aggregates who are at greatest potential risk on the basis of early identification of these abnormalities, and analysis of the contributions of physiological and environmental elements to the progression of disease, will result in more comprehensive approaches to diagnosis and detection than have been carried out in the past. With identification of early findings in population groups, studies designed to prevent the evolution of malignancy in these individuals at high risk are also being considered at the present time.

Acknowledgments

The authors' original work reported in this chapter was carried out in the Laboratory of Gastrointestinal Research of the Sloan-Kettering Institute, and the Gastroenterology Service of the Department of Medicine, Memorial Sloan-Kettering Cancer Center, and was aided by Contract 1-CP-43366 and Grants 08748 and CA15429 from the National Cancer Institute, Department of Health, Education and Welfare.

6. References

Anderson, E. E., 1969, Genetic varieties of neoplasia, in: *Genetic Concepts and Neoplasia,* University of Texas, M. D. Anderson Hospital and Tumor Institute at Houston: [23rd Annual] Symposium on Fundamental Cancer Research, Williams and Wilkins, Baltimore.

Aries, V., Crowther, J. S., Drasar, B. S., Hill, M. J., and Williams, R. E. O., 1969, Bacteria and the etiology of cancer of the large bowel, *Gut* **10:**334–335.

Ball, W. J., Salser, J. S., and Balis, M. E., 1976, Biochemical changes in preneoplastic rodent intestines, *Cancer Res.* **36:**2686–2689.

Berci, G., Ranish, J. F., Schapiro, M., and Corlin, R., 1974, Complications of colonoscopy and polypectomy: Report of the Southern California Society for Gastrointestinal Endoscopy, *Gastroenterology* **67:**584–585.

Berg, J. S., 1973, Geographic pathology of colon cancer, in: *Proceedings of the Second Conference on Cancer of the Colon and Rectum,* American Cancer Society, Bar Harbor, Fla., September 27–29.

Berlinger, N. T., Lopez, C., Vogel, J., Lipkin, M., and Good, R. A., 1977, Defective recognitive immunity in family aggregates of colon carcinoma, *J. Clin. Invest.* **59:**761–769.

Boffa, L. C., and Allfrey, V. G., 1976, Characteristic complements of nuclear non-histone proteins in colonic epithelial tumors, *Cancer Res.* **36:**2678–2685.

Bolt, R. J., 1971, Sigmoidoscopy in detection and diagnosis in the asymptomatic individual, *Cancer* **28:**121.

Danes, B., 1977, Brief communication: The Gardner syndrome: a family study in cell culture, *J. Natl. Cancer Inst.* **58:**771.

Deschner, E., and Lipkin, M., 1970, Study of human rectal epithelial cells *in vitro.* III. RNA, protein and DNA synthesis in polyps and adjacent mucosa, *J. Natl. Cancer Inst.* **44:**175–185.

Deschner, E. E., Lewis, C. M., and Lipkin, M., 1963, *In vitro* study of human epithelial cells. I. Atypical zone of H^3 thymidine incorporation in mucosa of multiple polyposis, *J. Clin. Invest.* **42:**1922–1928.

Deschner, E., Lipkin, M., and Solomon, C., 1966, *In vitro* study of human epithelial cells. II. H^3 thymidine incorporation into polyps and adjacent mucosa. *J. Natl. Cancer Inst.* **36:**849–857.

Deschner, E. E., Long, F. C., and Katz, S., 1975, The detection of aberrant DNA synthesis in a member of a high risk cancer family, *Am. J. Digest. Dis.* **20:**418–424.

Dodds, W. J., Schulte, W. J., Henley, G. T., and Hogan, W. J., 1972, Peutz-Jeghers syndrome and gastrointestinal malignancy, *Am. J. Roentgenol.* **115:**374–377.

Drasar, B. S., Bone, E. S., Hill, M. J., and Marks, C. G., 1975, Colon cancer and bacterial metabolism in familial polyposis, *Gut* **16:**824–825.

Enterline, H. T., and Arvan, D. A., 1967, Chromosome constitution of adenoma and adenocarcinoma of the colon, *Cancer* **20:**1746–1759.

Fleisher, M., Besenfelder, E., Schwartz, M. K., and Oettgen, H. F., 1973, Evolution of three CEA assays, *Proc. Am. Assoc. Cancer Res.* **14:**68.

Fraumeni, J. F., Jr., 1973, Genetic factors in: *Cancer Medicine* (J. F. Holland and E. Frei, eds.), pp. 7–15, Lea and Febinger, Philadelphia.

Gilbertsen, V., 1974, Proctosigmoidoscopy and polypectomy in reducing the incidence of rectal cancer, *Cancer* **34:**936–939.

Gregor, D. H., 1967, Diagnosis of large bowel cancer in the asymptomatic patient, *J. Am. Med. Assoc.* **201:**943–945.

Hackman, A. S., Wilkins, T. D., Finegold. S. M., and Sutter, V. L., 1976, Faecal cholesterol conversion and polyp status, *Lancet* **1:**252.

Haenszel, W., and Correa, P., 1971, Cancer of the colon and rectum and adenomatous polyps: A review of epidemiologic findings, *Cancer* **28:**14.

Hertz, R. E., Deddish, M. R., and Day, E., 1960, Value of periodic examination in detecting cancer of the rectum and colon, *Postgrad. Med.* **27:**290–294.

Hill, M. J., 1975. Role of colon anaerobes in metabolism of bile acids and steroids and its reaction to colon cancer, *Cancer* **36:**2387–2400.

Hill, M. J., Drasar, B. S., Aries, V., Crowther, J. S., Hawksworth, G., and Williams, R. E. O., 1971, Bacteria and the etiology of cancer of the large bowel, *Lancet* **2:**95.

Katz, S., Sherlock, P., and Winawer, S. J., 1972, Rectocolonic exfoliative cytology, *Am. J. Digest. Dist.* **17:**1109–116.

Knudsen, A. G., Jr., 1976, in: *Proceedings of the 11th Canadian Cancer Conference,* Toronto, pp. 93–103.

Knudsen, A. G., Jr., *et al.,* 1973, Heredity and cancer in man, in: *Progress in Medical Genetics* (A. G. Steinberg and A. G. Bearn, eds.) (Grune and Stratton, New York.)

Kopelovich, L., Coulon, S., and Pollack, R., 1977, Defective organization of actin in cultured skin fibroblasts from patients with inherited adenocarcinoma, *Proc. Natl. Acad. Sci. USA* **74:**3019–3022.

Land, P. C., and Bruce, W. R., 1978, Fecal mutagens: a possible relationship with colorectal cancer, *Proc. Amer. Assoc. Cancer Res.* **19:**167(abst.).

Lipkin, M., 1973, Proliferation and differentiation of gastrointestinal cells, *Physiol. Rev.* **53:**891–915.

Lipkin, M., 1974, Phase I and phase II proliferative lesions of colonic epithelial cells in diseases leading to colonic cancer, *Cancer* **34:**878–888.

Lipkin, M., 1975, Biology of large bowel cancer, *Cancer* **36:**2319–2324.

Lipkin, M., 1977, Growth kinetics of normal and premalignant gastrointestinal epithelium, in: *Growth Kinetics and Biochemical Regulation of Normal and Malignant Cells,* [29th Annual] Symposium on Fundamental Cancer Research, Williams and Wilkins, Baltimore.

Lipkin, M., and Deschner, E., 1968, Comparative analysis of cell proliferation in the gastrointestinal tract of newborn hamster, *Exp. Cell Res.* **49:**1–12.

Lipkin, M., Bell, B., and Sherlock, P., 1963, Cell proliferation kinetics in the gastrointestinal tract of man. I. Cell renewal in colon and rectum, *J. Clin. Invest.* **42:**767–776.

LoGerfo, P., Krupey, J., and Hansen, H. J., 1971, Demonstration of a common neoplastic antigen: Assay using zirconyl gel, *N. Eng. J. Med.* **285:**138.

Lohrs, U., Wiebecke, B., and Edgar, M., 1969, Morphologische and autoradiographische Untersuchung der Darmschleim-hautveranderringen nach einmaliger Injektion von 1,2-Dimethylhydrazin, *Ztschr. Ges. Exp. Med.* **151:**297–307.

Lynch, H. T., 1967, Hereditary factors in carcinoma, in: *Recent Results in Cancer Research,* Vol. 12, pp. 67–85, Springer-Verlag, New York.

Lynch, H. T., and Krush, A. J., 1967, Heredity and adenocarcinoma of the colon, *Gastroenterology* **53:**517–527.

Martin, F., and Martin, M. S., 1970, Demonstration of antigens related to colonic cancer in the human digestive system, *Cancer* **6:**352.

Messier, B., and Leblond, C. P., 1960, Cell proliferation and migration as revealed by radioautography after injection of thymidine-H^3 into rats and mice, *Am. J. Anat.* **106:**247–254.

Miller, R. E., 1974, Detection of colon carcinoma and the barium enema, *Am. Med. Assoc.* **230:**1195.

Mitelman, F., Mark, J., Nilsson, D. G., Deucker, H., Norryd, C., and Tranberg, K.G., 1974, Chromosome banding pattern in human colonic polyps, *Hereditas* **78:**63–68.

Moertel, C. G., Bargen, J. A., and Dockerty, M. B., 1958, Multiple carcinomas of the large intestine: A review of the literature and a study of 261 cases, *Gastroenterology* **34:**285.

Moertel, C. G., Hill, J. R., and Dockerty, M. B., 1966, The routine proctoscopic examination: A second look, *Mayo Clin. Proc.* **41:**368–374.

Moore, T. L., Kupchik, H. Z., Marcon, N., and Zamcheck, N., 1971, Carcinoembryonic antigen assay in cancer of the colon and pancreas and other digestive disorders, *Am. J. Digest. Dis.* **16:**1.

Morson, B. C., and Bussey, H. J. R., 1970, Predisposing causes of intestinal cancer, in: *Current Problems in Surgery* (M. Ravitch, ed.), Year Book Medical Publishers, Chicago.

Ostrow, J. D., Mulvaney, C. A., Hansel, J. R., and Rhodes, R. S., 1973, Sensitivity and reproducibility of chemical tests for fecal occult blood with an emphasis on false-positive reactions, *Digest Dis.* **18:**930–940.

Pfeffer, L. M., and Kopelovich, L., 1977, Differential genetic susceptibility of cultured human skin fibroblasts to transformation by KiMSV, *Cell* **10:**313–320.

Pierce, E. R., 1968, Some genetic aspects of familial polyposis of the colon in a kindred of 1422 members, *Dis. Colon Rectum* **11**:321.

Reddy, B. S., Mastromarino, A., and Wynder, E. L., 1975, Further leads on metabolic epidemiology of large bowel cancer, *Cancer Res.* **35**:3403–3406.

Reddy, B. S., Mastromarino, A., Gustafson, C., Lipkin, M., and Wynder, E. L., 1976, Fecal bile acids and neutral sterols in patients with familial polyposis, *Cancer* **38**:1694–1698.

Reed, T. E., and Neel, J. W., 1955, A genetic study of multiple polyposis of the colon, *Am. J. Hum. Genet.* **7**:236.

Reynoso, G., Chu, T. M., Holyoke, D., Cohen, E., Valensuela, L. A., Nemoto, T., Wang, J. J., Chuang, J., Guinan, P., and Murphy, G. P., 1972, Carcinoembryonic antigen in patients with different cancers. *J. Am. Med. Assoc.* **220**:361.

Salser, J. S., and Balis, M. E., 1973, Distribution and regulation of deoxythymidine kinase activity in differentiating cells of mammalian intestines, *Cancer Res.* **33**:1889–1897.

Silverberg, E., and Holleb, A., 1975, Cancer statistics, 1975, *CA Cancer J. Clin.* **25**:8–22.

Sorokin, J. J., Sugarbaker, P. H., Zamcheck, N., Pisick, M., Kupchik, H. Z., and Moore, F. D., 1974, Serial CEA assays: Use in detection of recurrence following resection of colon cancer, *J. Am. Med. Assoc.* **228**:49–53.

Springer, P., Springer, J., and Oehlert, W., 1970, Early stages of DMH induced carcinoma of the small and large intestine of the rat, *Ztschr. Krebsforsch.* **74**:236–240.

Thomson, D., Krupey, J., Freedman, S., and Gold, P., 1969, The radioimmunoassay of circulating carcinoembryonic antigen of the human digestive system, *Proc. Natl. Acad. Sci. USA* **64**:161.

Thurnherr, N., Deschner, E., Stonehill, E., and Lipkin, M., 1973, Induction of adenocarcinomas of the colon in mice by weekly injections of 1,2-dimethylhydrazine, *Cancer Res.* **33**:940–945.

Troncale, F., Hertz, R., and Lipkin, M., 1971, Nucleic acid metabolism in proliferating and differentiating cells of man and neoplastic lesions of the colon, *Cancer* **31**:463–467.

Trygstad, C. W., Zisman, E., Witkop, C. J., and Bartter, F. C., 1968, Resistance to parathyroid extract in Gardner's syndrome, *J. Clin. Endocrinol.* **28**:1153–1159.

Veale, A. M. O., 1965, *Intestinal Polyposis,* Cambridge University Press, London.

Watne, A. L., Lai, H. L., Mance, T., and Core, S., 1975, Fecal steroids and bacterial flora in polyposis coli patients, in: *Society for Surgery of the Alimentary Tract,* San Antonio, Texas, May.

Weisburger, J., 1973, *Proceedings of the 7th Cancer Conference,* Lippincott, Philadelphia.

Wiebecke, B., Krey, U., Lohrs, U., and Eder, M., 1973, Morphological and autoradiographical investigations on experimental carcinogenesis and polyp development in the intestinal tract of rats and mice, *Virchows Arch. Pathol. Anat.* **360**:179–193.

Williams, C. B., Hunt, R. H., Loose, H., Riddel, R. H., Sakai, Y., and Swarbrick, E. T., 1974, Colonscopy in the management of colon polyps, *Br. J. Surg.* **61**:673.

Wilson, G. S., Dale, E. H., and Brines, O. A., 1955, An evaluation of polyps detected in 20,847 routine sigmoidoscope examinations, *Am. J. Surg.* **90**:834.

Winawer, S. J., Miller, D. G., Schottenfeld, D., Leidner, S. D., Sherlock, P., Befler, B., and Stearns, M. W., Jr., 1977*a,* Feasibility of fecal occult blood testing for detection of colorectal neoplasia, *Cancer* **40**:2616–2619.

Winawer, S. J., Fleischer, M., Green, S., Bhargava, D., Leidner, S. D., Boyle, C., Sherlock, P., and Schwartz, M. K., 1977*b,* Carcinoembryonic antigen in colonic lavage, *Gastroenterology* **73**:719–722.

Woolf, C. M., Richards, R. C., and Gardner, E. J., 1955, Occasional discrete polyps of colon and rectum showing inherited tendency in kindred, *Cancer* **8**:403–408.

Wynder, E. L., and Shigematsu, T., 1967, Environmental factors of cancer of the colon and rectum, *Cancer* **20**:1520.

19

Logic and Logistics of Monitoring Large Bowel Cancer

Edward H. Cooper and A. Munro Neville

1. Introduction

There is still a general dissatisfaction with the results of surgery for the treatment of large bowel cancer; the overall 5-year survival rate for resectable tumors is approximately 40% (Rhoads, 1975; Silverberg and Hollet, 1974). This survival rate has remained static for many years in major hospitals with extensive experience in this disease. Chemotherapy has had a limited success so far; many adenocarcinomas of the bowel have been shown to be relatively resistant to the drugs available, although short-term palliation is not too difficult to obtain, the more recent forms of combination chemotherapy perhaps giving ground for cautious optimism (Carter, 1976). Nevertheless, it looks as if for the next few years we must place our hopes in chemotherapy to aid surgery. The problem then is to find the right combination of drugs, dose, and timing to suit the individual patient and his particular tumor. Current knowledge suggests that chemotherapy will have the best chance of being effective when the tumor load is small. This in turn has created a greater demand for aids to identify patients with a high risk of recurrence after surgery and systems to monitor the patient after excision of a primary tumor of the large bowel, as well as helping to assess the response of a tumor to therapy.

It was in this somewhat pessimistic climate—the belief that surgery had nothing new to contribute to the cure of large bowel cancer—that the discovery of carcinoembryonic antigen (CEA) was made by Gold and Freedman (1965). At first it was hoped and indeed believed by some that this test for a

Edward H. Cooper and A. Munro Neville • Department of Cancer Research, University of Leeds, and the Ludwig Institute for Cancer Research, in conjunction with the Royal Marsden Hospital, London SW3 6JB, England.

tumor marker substance could turn the tide by providing a way of finding early asymptomatic primary colorectal cancers, and such patients should have a good prognosis. Alas, this expectation has not been realized, although the CEA test has been shown, when used and interpreted correctly, to be capable of providing the clinician with valuable information to help with the management of the patient. The past 10 years has seen an immense resurgence of interest in cancer therapy. The medicopolitical pressures have resulted in cancer having a high priority for treatment and research in Western society. The advent of the CEA test has brought the laboratory workers into a much closer relation with the surgeons and chemotherapists, and the trial and error of these past few years has resulted in a better understanding of the way laboratory tests should be employed and how in no way they should be a substitute for clinical acumen. Tests can provide the clinician with information that intervention may be required; only the clinician is responsible for the decision whether to intervene and what form of intervention is appropriate. The laboratory scientist is responsible for assuring the accuracy of the measurements. It could be argued that the responsibility of the laboratory ends once it is certain that the results are provided with the assurance of a high standard of quality control. We feel that while the search for ideal cancer monitoring systems is still in progress a clear understanding of the clinical problem and the limitations of laboratory tests is required to avoid misunderstanding and discrediting the tests due to their use under inappropriate circumstances.

During the past few years the authors have been involved in clinical evaluation of the CEA test as part of a national program supported by the Medical Research Council and Department of Health and Social Security. Our views on the clinical-laboratory interface have come from discussions with surgeons who practice both in the large hospitals with units specializing in gastrointestinal surgery and in community hospitals where the treatment of large bowel cancer is an integral part of the work of the general surgeon; numerically the latter provide the major share of primary care for the disease on a nationwide basis.

When a new cancer test appears, it has to be evaluated rigorously before its right place in medical practice can be defined. In looking over the history of the CEA test, it can be seen to have involved a considerable investment of resources and money by governments and industry. Consequently, there are bound to be strong advocates whose judgment may have been clouded by a desire to demonstrate that every idea, however trivial, is a boon to surgeons; no wonder that many experienced surgeons are still skeptical of how new knowledge can help them improve the results of treatment. It is interesting to note that the majority of articles about CEA, in the context of bowel cancer, have been written by pathologists and laboratory scientists and not surgeons. This has tended to obscure some well-established facts about the behavior of large bowel cancer that were identified by surgeons, histopathologists, and chemical pathologists on both sides of the Atlantic 40 years ago. Now would seem an appropriate moment to try to make a synthesis of these various bits of information both old and new to plot a course of action suitable for the practice of modern medicine.

Before dealing with the laboratory tests, it is necessary to establish firmly the framework of clinical conditions under which they are likely to be used. Once a diagnosis of large bowel cancer has been made or considered to be highly probable, the findings at laparotomy provide the key point of departure on which all future judgement is based. At laparotomy the patients can broadly be divided into two groups:

1. Those in whom there is reason to believe the surgery may have been curative.
2. Those in whom it was not possible to excise all the cancer.

In the first group careful histopathological examination of the excised specimen can define the probability of the treatment's being successful. In general terms it is reduced in proportion to the extent of spread through the bowel wall and to the local lymph nodes in the excised portion of mesentery. It is important to bear in mind that a large Dukes's B tumor that penetrates the serosa may carry just as high a risk of local recurrence as a Dukes's C lesion (Table 1). However, despite the powerful discriminant effect of Dukes's classification and the increased weighting for a bad prognosis if the tumor is poorly differentiated histologically, it is still not possible to be sure how an *individual patient* with a Dukes's B or C lesion will fare after excision of the primary tumor.

In the second group the amount of residual tumor that remains after surgery varies greatly from a few lesions just visible on the surface of the peritoneum or liver to massive spread that precludes any form of surgical resection excision. For convenience these patients can be subdivided into two subsets:

a. Minimal residual disease in which lesions cannot be detected clinically after closing of the abdomen.

Table 1. Prognosis in Rectal Cancer According to Local Spread

Classification	Number of cases	Corrected 5-year survival rate (%)
Dukes's B[a]		
Slight extrarectal spread[b]	266	89.7
Moderate extrarectal spread[c]	109	80.0
Extensive extrarectal spread[d]	148	57.0
Dukes's C		
C_1	680	40.9
C_2	282	13.6

[a]From Dukes (1960).
[b]Commencing to invade (slight).
[c]Well-established in mesentery.
[d]Deeply invasive, possibly into neighboring organs (extensive).

b. Advanced residual disease in which lesions can be detected on clinical examination after the wound has been closed (indicator lesions).

Clearly, the more carefully the abdomen is examined at laparotomy and the excised specimen studied, the more accurate will be the surgeon's assessment of the patient's prognosis. For a detailed discussion of the stratification of colorectal cancer, the reader is referred to Gérard's (1975) summary of this complex subject. The observations of Botsford *et al.* (1971) illustrate the distribution of lesions in the incurable group. They observed in 60 cases of colorectal tumors at operation that 39 involved liver metastases, 13 with extensive local spread, 11 of which were rectal tumours. Unfortunately, these fundamental staging procedures are not standard practice in all hospitals, which is a disadvantage if the patient should require referral elsewhere at a later stage in the evolution of the cancer. Dukes's (1932) classification as it was written originally did not take into account the surgeons' evidence of what was seen outside the confines of the excised specimen. In the Astler–Coller (1954) modification of the Dukes's classification a class D has been added to cover lesions that have spread beyond the confines of the excised specimen. While this device is useful in a practical sense and is in common use in North America, it can lead to confusion in comparison of data from British and Scandinavian sources in which Dukes's original classification is more often used. In addition to macroscopic and microscopic examination of the abdomen and the tumor, the surgeon will have information such as the appearance of the chest X-ray and possibly the results of routine liver function tests and liver scan, although the last is rarely requested as a routine preoperative measure in British surgical practice. Clearly it is the patients for whom it is hoped that surgery has been curative who present the greatest uncertainty as to the eventual outcome. The patients' fate hinges on whether the lesion was complicated by metastases too small for detection by inspection or routine investigations. Usually the answer to this question will become apparent within 2 years of excision of the primary, although the apparently disease-free interval can be as long as 5 years or more. The general information available shortly after surgery is summarized in Table 2.

Table 2. Information after Laparotomy

1. Preoperative	Routine biochemical assessment (multiphasic profile)
	Routine hematological assessment
	CEA level
	Chest X-ray (liver scan)
2. Surgical observations	Evidence of spread beyond excised specimen
3. Histopathological observations	Staging and tumor grading
	Biopsy material of suspected metastatic spread

2. *Laboratory Tests*

Laboratory-based measurements can help the clinician in three major areas of management of large bowel cancer:

1. Earlier detection of recurrences and metastases.
2. Evaluation of the effects of therapy on recurrence of a metastatic cancer.
3. Assistance in the assessment of the prognosis of the patient undergoing "curative surgery."

To these may be added in a far more tentative fashion the attempted prediction of the types of chemotherapeutic compounds effective for the patient's tumor, in the hope of exploiting differences intrinsic in the particular cancer.

It will be shown that CEA tests play a key role for the first three of these monitoring and assessment functions and that the information can be enhanced if CEA is considered in conjunction with other biochemical parameters. On the other hand, there is no evidence that the level of CEA has any real part to play in establishing the primary diagnosis of large bowel cancer or in its differential diagnosis (Laurence and Neville, 1972; Neville and Cooper, 1976). Many of the inflammatory diseases of the large bowel such as ulcerative colitis, Crohn's disease, and diverticulitis can imitate the changes found in the sera in large bowel cancer (Laurence *et al.*, 1972; Booth *et al.*, 1974 *a,b*). Likewise, primary cancers of the large intestine are not invariably associated with an elevation of the level of CEA in the blood. Experience over the past decade has demonstrated that for a variety of reasons population screening using the plasma CEA level as an indicator to detect asymptomatic early large bowel cancer is scientifically unsound and impractical. It would place an intolerable burden on medical resources as well as arousing both unnecessary fear in subjects with borderline results and, worse false confidence in true victims of the disease which could lead to a prolongation of the delay until diagnosis (Galen, 1975). To fulfill the requirements of a monitoring system, the test must be capable of distinguishing the signals of events due to the progress of the cancer from background noise. This is often a severe criterion as the population with large bowel cancer has a median age of about 68 years a time of life when many degenerative phenomena are a part of the general decline of health that is associated with old age. It is important that the frequency of testing should not become an undue burden to the patient in proportion to the probable benefit it may afford. Academic curiosity sometimes involves the patient quite unnecessarily in tedious investigations that will at best only add another confirmation of facts that are well known. If the clinician favors an aggressive treatment policy which will involve many nice points of judgment, be it chemotherapy or even second-look surgery on the basis of the evidence of recurrence provided by the monitoring tests, then the frequency of these tests should be about every 2–3 months, especially during the first 2 years after resection of the primary tumor. On the other hand, some surgeons prefer to take a more conservative view and reserve treatment for the palliation of symptoms; this approach makes the necessity for monitoring far less pressing. The general surgical practice, at least in the United Kingdom, of reviewing patients after resection of a large bowel cancer at fairly long intervals after the end of the first year might be put on to a more rational basis if it were associated with appropriate biochemical monitoring. However, the logistics and cost effectiveness of a nationwide monitoring system would be such that it would probably be wiser to restrict its use to patients for whom earlier discovery of metastatic cancer and appropriate therapy are believed to confer prolongation of useful life or relief from troublesome complications. At the time of writing of this chapter there is good evidence that tests can provide the clinician with advanced warning of metastases, but so far there is no firm experience as to how this can be best used in the patients' interest.

3. Carcinoembryonic Antigen in the Surveillance of Colorectal Cancer

Several different CEA assay systems have been devised and tried in Europe and North America, the precise CEA values depending on the type of radioimmunoassay employed; one of them being brought into more widespread use in the United States is marketed and advertised by the Hoffmann-La Roche Company. In the United Kingdom the MRC-DHSS trial has used a modification of the Egan *et al.* (1972) assay; the details of this technique, as run in our laboratory in London, have been described by Laurence *et al.* (1972). The CEA levels reported by this test are higher than those of the commercial system. Despite the technical differences of the assays, there is broad clinical agreement using either of these assays or other forms of CEA assay that sequential measurement of the plasma CEA level after an apparently successful resection of a large bowel cancer can provide an early warning of recurrence (Booth *et al.*, 1974*b*; Mach *et al.*, 1974; Mackay *et al.*, 1974; Sorokin *et al.*, 1974; Turner, 1975). The duration of the lead time is in part a reflection of the frequency of the measurements, the extent to which an asymptomatic postoperative patient is examined at the follow-up clinic, the experience and interest of the clinician, as well as the use of procedures such as liver scan and chest X-ray. Tables 3 and 4 show the frequency of early warning given by our assay system. A plasma CEA value of 40 ng/ml was considered to indicate recurrence or metastases; the mean normal value for our assay is 15 ng/ml. The reason for choosing this relatively high value compared to the mean was to reduce the incidence of false positives. The sequential measurements were analyzed iteratively to find a value at which there was a probability of 0.95 of the subsequent value being elevated and the false positives virtually eliminated. It is admitted this approach may reduce the lead time, but the clinicians will not be helped if the advice from the laboratory is hedged with uncertainty—especially if it is to be the starting point of extensive investigations or potentially dangerous treatment in a fit patient. The population was aged 35–95 years, median 68 years, and the

Table 3. Monitoring of Colorectal Carcinoma[a]

Clinical condition	Plasma CEA	Number of patients: Colon	Rectum	Total
No evidence of recurrence	Normal	250	273	525
	Rising	23	31	54
Recurrent tumor	Normal	34	32	66
	Antecedent rise	14	23	37
	Synchronous rise[b]	41	48	89
	At operation or first observation[b]	(38)	(43)	
	Other time[b]	(3)	(5)	
Totals		362	409	771

[a]These results are based on measurements of CEA made at Chester Beatty Institute as part of the current MRC assessment of CEA analysis in June 1976).
[b]The majority of these patients had metastatic tumor confirmed at laparotomy; the preoperative CEA value may have raised the probability of metastases being present.

majority were not receiving chemotherapy. The frequency of observation was whenever possible every 6 months, but in some it coincided with the annual visit. It is admitted that the frequency of observation is less than has been attained in some special referral centers, but it probably reflects the general result that would be obtained if the test were applied to a much larger cohort of patients.

Despite the advantages of the CEA test, in our experience it cannot detect all recurrences in advance of their presentation clinically, although a coincidental elevation of CEA and the detection of a suspicious mass may help to confirm this suspicion and be helpful to a clinician who is not a specialist in gastroenterology or oncology. Lesions in the liver and to a lesser extent in bones would appear to provide the best chance of early detection by CEA monitor-

Table 4. Principal Metastatic and Recurrent Sites of Colorectal Carcinoma[a]

Tissue	Plasma CEA: No change	Synchronous rise	Antecedent rise	Total
Liver	26	61	19	106
Lungs	1	1	2	4
Bone	2	3	1	6
Peritoneum	14	7	4	25
Pelvis	10	8	9	27
Other	13	9	2	24
Total	66	89	37	192

[a]These include patients diagnosed at laparotomy or preoperatively as well as postoperative recurrence.

ing. The behavior of metastases in the pelvis and on the peritoneal cavity is more variable depending on the rate of production and destruction of CEA. The site of the metastases may also influence the time when its presence is apparent clinically, so that a small but painful tumor in the perineum or a recurrence in the bowel wall causing intestinal obstruction can by chance present many months before a comparatively much larger mass growing asymptomatically elsewhere in the abdominal cavity or in the lungs.

The sequential measurements of plasma CEA show that its pattern of change of level after excision of the primary tumour is of two types. In the first, the level does not fall after surgery; if this event occurs after an apparently successful resection, it is of grave prognostic significance and is usually due to hepatic metastases that are too diffuse to be resolved by scanning or are not visible to the surgeon at laparotomy. Goligher in 1941 pointed out that from a postmortem study of perioperative deaths in rectal cancer it can be estimated that about one-sixth of cases treated by "curative resection" will be complicated by hepatic metastases that are readily demonstrable by histological examination of the liver, although Hogg and Pack (1956) have claimed that the surgeon is likely to miss about 2% of hepatic metastases by inspection of the liver.

The second pattern is typified by a period of normal CEA values preceding the eventual rise. In Tables 3 and 4 the analysis was based on the selection of a value of the CEA level as the discriminant to separate a positive test due to cancer from a false positive due to a variety of causes. A second approach is possible when there are a number of sequential values, i.e., examination of the slope of the values; provided that the quality of the assay is closely controlled, it should be possible to detect a change in the slope before the value reaches the arbitrary discriminant level, and this would be of value in finding lesions that make small amounts of CEA and have a slow growth rate. The evidence of a rising series of values against time would draw attention to the progression, a point that would be missed if the data were reported solely as positive or negative. The slope analysis would seem to be most valuable when the estimations of CEA are made frequently, say monthly, which is a simple matter to organize during the monitoring of chemotherapy (see below).

Perhaps it is wise to end this section with a word of warning: The interpretation of the results of postoperative CEA tests is strongly influenced by the amount of information available about the patient. Coincidental disease in the liver or gastrointestinal tract may interfere with the postoperative baseline and consequently reduce the sensitivity of the test; the smoking history and evidence of bronchitis are also relevant.

Random measurements of CEA, especially made some years after a resection for large bowel cancer done in another hospital, are difficult to interpret; only very high values can be said to be pathognomic of cancer, and even so they do not necessarily indicate that the lesion is a metastasis from an antecedent large bowel cancer as high values can be found in metastatic lung and breast cancer.

4. Multiparametric Tests in Assessing Colorectal Cancer

As shown above, CEA plays an essential role in the laboratory monitoring of colorectal cancer; despite its lack of specificity, it can provide information about the tumor and its growth which cannot be provided by other biochemical tests. However, it is now apparent that the information can be refined and amplified if other biochemical measurements are made on the patient's blood at the time of assaying the CEA. These factors are nonspecific, yet when taken in conjunction with the CEA level and in relation to one another they form a pattern and can provide additional evidence of the behavior of the tumor and the patient's reaction to the disease. These tests tend to fall into two main groups:

1. Those useful to call attention to the involvement of specific sites by distant metastases, liver, and bones.
2. Nonspecific reactions to the tumor that may be used as part of a monitoring system or as an aid in assessing prognosis.

5. Hepatic Metastases

Involvement of the liver by metastases from rectal and colonic cancer causes a progressive series of changes in the blood chemistry which can be monitored by standard biochemical techniques. There are still conflicting reports as to the incidence of hepatic metastases; this is mainly due to several papers in which the population under study has been biased in favor of patients who develop metastatic cancer in the liver. Goligher (1941) reported that the surgeon observed hepatic deposits in 103 of 893 (11.5%) cases of rectal cancer coming to laparotomy. Baden *et al.* (1971) reported an incidence of 16% with coincidental hepatic metastases in a series of 396 primary colorectal tumors; in Fischerman's series (Fischerman *et al.*, 1976) of 334 patients, 35 (10.5%) had hepatic metastases at presentation and 20 developed them later. Cass *et al.* (1976), reviewing 280 cases of large bowel cancer, observed a recurrence in 105 (37%). The tumor was local intraabdominal excluding the liver in 60%, in 14% there were concomitant local and distant metastases, and in 26% there were distant metastases only, of which half were in the liver. In these days when there is an increasing tendency to administer some form of chemotherapy, it is important to know what might have happened if the disease had been allowed to progress spontaneously. Although the average life span from the time of discovery of hepatic metastases when left to evolve untreated has been reported to be 4.5, 6.5, and 7.8 months by Jaffe *et al.* (1968), Fischerman *et al.* (1976), and Bengmark and Hafström (1969), respectively, the important feature from the point of view of a monitoring program is that the distribution about these means is 1–20 months. The sensitivity of routine hospital liver function tests for the detection of hepatic metastases is low. This is because their array of the levels of albumin, globulin, alkaline phosphatase (ALKP), transaminases (aspartate transaminase, more commonly referred to by its old name, "glutamic oxaloacetic transaminase"), and bilirubin provide a sound basis for general hepatological studies and differential diagnosis and are unaffected by the minor derangements of liver function in early metastatic cancer of the liver. γ-Glutamyltranspeptidase (GGT) is a serum enzyme whose level in the serum rises early in response to many types of liver injury, reflecting a disorder of the biliary pathway (Whitfield *et al.,* 1972); it is a nonspecific reaction and caution needs to be observed in interpreting the results of this test, especially in patients who are known or suspected to fortify themselves with alcohol prior to visiting their doctor (Schwartz, 1976). The GGT level can also be increased by barbiturates and phenytoin. In practice, we have found that the coincidental measurement of GGT and CEA is helpful, particularly during the postoperative monitoring of a case of large bowel cancer (Steele *et al.,* 1974; Cooper *et al.,* 1975), and this has been confirmed by others (Munjal *et al.,* 1976). The temporal sequence of biochemical disturbance in the blood in a patient with hepatic metastases is usually first an elevation of the CEA followed by a rise of GGT and then of the more specific markers of hepatobiliary disease such as 5′-nucleotidase (5′NT), then a rise of the transaminases as the parenchymal cells show evidence of disordered metabolism, and finally a rise of bilirubin. The 95th percentile of the distribution of GGT levels in patients without hepatic metastases is 30 IU/liter; recruitment of a rising 5′NT and ALKP can be expected when the GGT has reached somewhere between 100 and 150 IU/liter. The 5′NT is a specific marker for damage to the hepatobiliary tree, but ALKP can arise from liver, intestine, or bones. Hence the level of the GGT can act as a sensitive screen for biochemical disturbances produced by hepatic metastases. We do not measure the other parameters of liver function in patients whose GGT is <30 IU/liter, with the exception of ALKP, because this can occasionally be raised with a normal GGT level when there are bone metastases without evidence of the biliary tract being involved (Cooper *et al.,* 1976*b*), as confirmed by a coincidental lack of increase in the 5′NT.

The term "early" diagnosis of hepatic metastases is used in the sense that it can provide awareness of the condition several months ahead of routine follow-up examination, especially if the tumor is growing slowly. Comparison of the preoperative level of GGT and the findings at laparotomy during the treatment of a primary tumor of the colon or rectum indicates that the surgeon's eye is far better at detecting hepatic metastases than any chemical test. In our series of 29 patients in whom hepatic metastases were seen by the surgeon at laparotomy for the treatment of the primary tumor, the preoperative CEA was >100 ng/ml in 20 but the GGT was >100 IU/liter in only eight. In nine of 29, neither of these tests suggested the possibility of hepatic metastases. It will be noted that a GGT level of 100 IU/liter was chosen as the discriminant for preoperative patients; this was to avoid false positives due to reactions from local inflammatory conditions in the bowel and the problem of having to interpret the meaning of a single observation. Baden *et al.* (1971), using preoperative discriminant levels of 30 IU/liter for GGT and 80 IU/liter for ALKP, considered that these tests did not help the surgeon to predict likelihood of finding hepatic metastases. Hence, in the postoperative patient, by the time that the GGT has undergone a sustained rise for 1 or 2 months above the 30 IU/liter level, the metastases can be expected to be fairly extensive in the liver but may still be below the size that can be resolved by scintillating scanning or ultrasonography. Despite its limitations, the coincidental measurement of CEA and GGT has the distinct advantage of warning the clinician that the liver is the site of metastatic cancer, which may be an important factor in decision making about the most appropriate line of treatment of the recurrence. Prior knowledge of hepatic metastases would militate against second-look surgery, except when there is intestinal obstruction. Furthermore, this procedure may be valuable for the stratification of patients in chemotherapy trials since there are clearly two types of metastatic growth patterns, those where the tumor mass is essentially related to the area of the original operation site and those that involve distant organs, notably the liver; the evolution of these two forms of recurrent cancer will not necessarily be similar.

Our data suggest that it would be unwise to attempt to base an estimate of the survival of the patient with metastatic cancer on the level of CEA or GGT or both. They can be at very high levels for several months prior to death, especially after resection of the primary. However, we agree with Jaffe *et al.* (1968) that patients presenting with biochemical changes indicating an advanced hepatic lesions will tend to survive a shorter time than those in whom the metastases have made little or no change in the blood chemistry.

6. *Nonspecific Reaction to Cancer*

In the past prior to the discovery of tumor-related antigen, the nonspecific alteration of the activity of various serum enzymes and the amounts of proteins in the blood have been explored as possible aids to the diagnosis of cancer. Their lack of specificity made them unreliable, and they were never adopted for routine clinical use. However, the shift of emphasis in recent years toward biochemical aids to assessing prognosis and tumor recurrence has renewed interest in these older observations. There is a group of serum enzymes—phosphohexose isomerase, leucine aminopeptidase, and lactate dehydrogenase—which have been thought to have some potential for monitoring cancer. In practice, these offer no advantage compared to CEA, GGT, and 5′NT for monitoring large bowel cancer (Cooper *et al.,* 1975; Munjal *et al.*, 1976) as these enzymes tend to reflect involvement of the liver, for which there are other more efficient systems. At present, serum enzymology does not appear to be a fruitful source to fill gaps in the monitoring procedure when the CEA test is negative, as may happen in the earlier phases of recurrence in the region of the original tumor site.

It has been well known for many years that the electrophoretogram of the plasma proteins is often modified in cancer, especially in metastatic lesions.

The changes are predominantly in the α-globulins, which increase in relative and absolute amounts. Colorectal cancer exhibits this phenomenon (Cooper *et al.*, 1976*a*). The change is essentially due to alterations in the acute-phase reactant proteins (APRPs) that make up the bulk of the α-globulin fraction. The overall change is nonspecific, and similar elevations of α-globulins can occur in response to injury, acute and chronic infection, and various degenerative diseases (Koj, 1975; Bacchus, 1975). Modern protein technology enables many of the constituent individual APRPs to be identified and measured specifically, and a protein profile can be constructed. Typical members of the APRP's are α-antitrypsin, α_1-acid glycoprotein, haptoglobin, ceruloplasmin, and prealbumin. A detailed profile of these proteins does not give the same information as the erythrocyte sedimentation rate, dependent mainly on the ratio of albumin and fibrinogen, which can alter independently of the majority of the APRPs. These proteins are mainly synthesized and metabolized in the liver, although recently there has been a suggestion that α_1-antitrypsin may originate in tumor tissues. The levels in the blood are controlled by regulatory mechanisms that are still not understood, except that signals derived from several types of diseased tissue profoundly influence the levels of the proteins.

Two factors suggest that protein profiling may have a part to play in aiding cancer monitoring and assessing prognosis. The first is the stability of the protein profile in a healthy individual, although wide variation may be encountered between individuals. The second is the selection of a suitable array of APRPs; a series of progressive changes can resolve in the profile that are associated with the evolution of the cancer (Ward *et al.*, 1977). Examples of

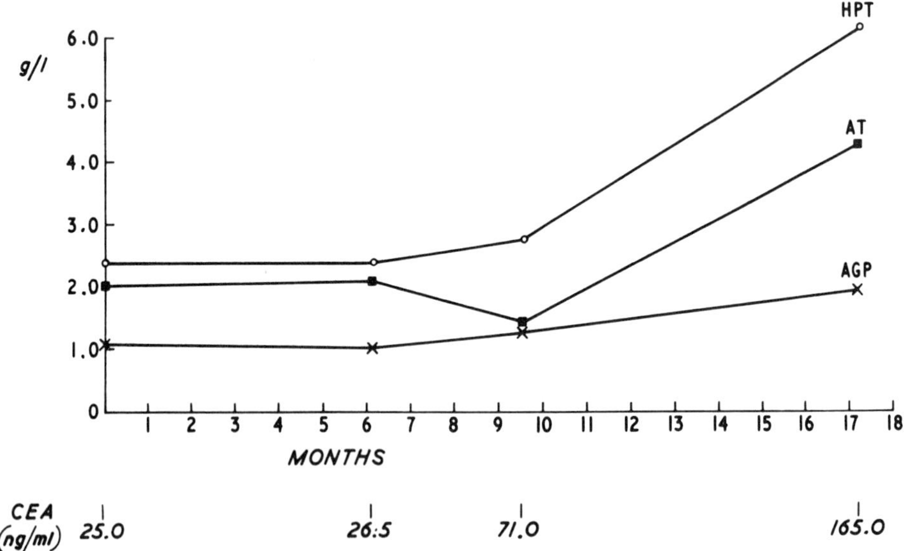

Fig. 1. Evolution of APRPs during the development of hepatic metastases. From Ward *et al.* (1977).

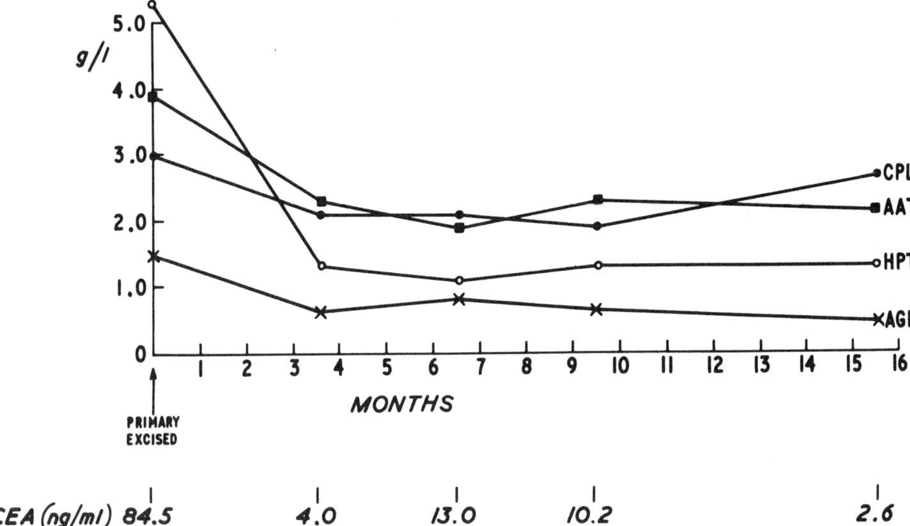

Fig. 2. Stability of the APRP profile in a patient who has remained free of recurrence. For convenience, the ceruloplasmin results are ×10 to fit the scale. From Ward *et al*. (1977).

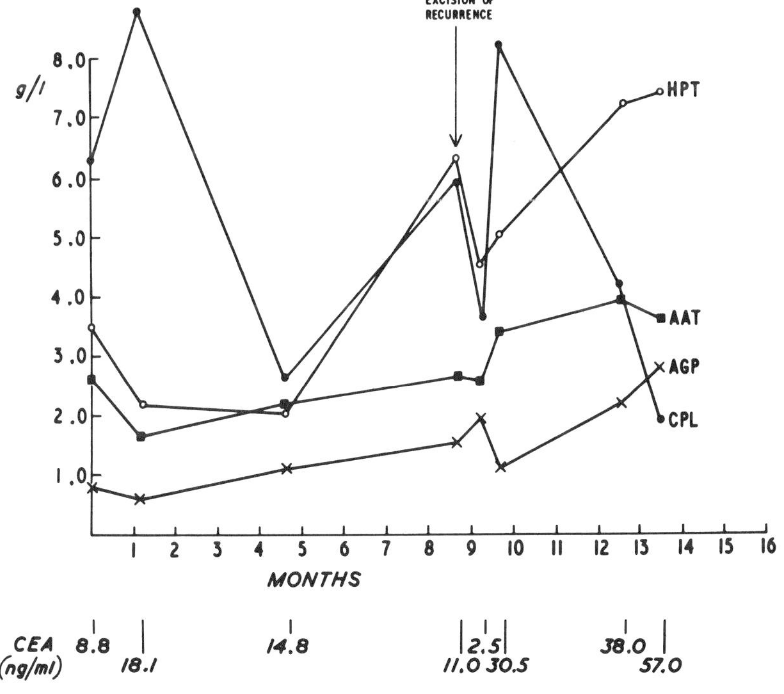

Fig. 3. Disturbance of the APRP profile caused by recurrent tumor localized to the pelvis requiring a second resection. Ceruloplasmin levels are ×10. From Ward *et al*. (1977).

changes of the APRPs in colorectal cancer are shown in Figs. 1–3; their application to clinical practice will be illustrated below.

7. Prognostic Indicators

As stated earlier, Dukes's classification and its more recent refinements (Kirklin *et al.*, 1949; Astler and Coller, 1954) provide a sound basis for making a decision on the probable chance of cure after "curative surgery." However, an experienced and careful pathologist is required if the opinion is going to carry much weight. It has been hoped that some form of independent laboratory measurement might help increase the precision of the prognosis and turn it from a group statistic into an assessment germane to the individual patient. The preoperative CEA level seemed an obvious parameter. However, it is only recently that sufficient time has lapsed after curative resection to see how this value might aid prognosis assessment.

Several authors have observed that a raised preoperative CEA increases the probability of recurrence within 3 years (LoGerfo and Herter, 1975; Zamcheck *et al.*, 1975). This led to our (Neville and Cooper, 1976) reexamination of the available data on 300 patients followed up for at least 2 years from presentation with a primary tumor: 131 have developed recurrences, of whom 85 had raised pre-operative CEA levels; 169 remain alive and well without demonstrable disease, of whom 59 had raised preoperative values. Data currently available as part of a national trial running in Yorkshire and London are shown in Table 3. While it is evident that a raised CEA carries a worse prognosis, the relationship is not simple. In looking for other factors that might help in assessing the prognosis, we have examined the preoperative data from 70 patients, 22 of whom had residual disease after surgery; of the remaining 48 patients, 11 had recurrences within 2 years. It was found that using a logistic discriminant analysis (Anderson, 1972) a function of the log CEA and the levels of α_1-antitrypsin and α_1-acid glycoprotein could be derived that predicted the outcome as follows: 19 of 22 of the cases in which residual disease remained after surgery had a negative index; of the potentially curative cases, eight of 18 (44%) with a negative index recurred within 1–2 years; while only three of 27 (11%) with a positive index recurred during the same time. In addition, there were three cases with an index of 0 which have remained without recurrence (Ward *et al.,* 1977). This approach using a combination of parameters and the stepwise addition of each factor to obtain the best separation of the groups would appear to offer a more powerful discriminant than CEA alone, although it must be stressed that its real power is seen when the CEA tends to be low or in the intermediate range. GGT levels were not contributing in this series of patients. There is no biological basis why this combination of factors can be made to produce an effective discriminant. Disturbances of CEA, α_1-antitrypsin, and acid glycoprotein are not unique to neoplastic conditions of the bowel, being found in various types of inflammatory disease (Booth *et al.*, 1974*b*; Marner *et al.*, 1975). However, this does not necessarily imply that it is the tissue response to inflammation that is critical. In the context of prognostic indicators it has been shown that the preoperative lymphocyte count is significantly related to the 5-year survival in colorectal cancer, Kim *et al.* (1976) reported that counts of 100 mm^3 were associated with a 30% 5-year survival. Likewise, in Dukes's B and C lesions with counts of $2000/^3$ there was a 81% survival compared to 50% for those with lower counts.

8. Monitoring Response to Chemotherapy

There are several reports that if a tumor is associated with a raised plasma CEA, this level may fall when there is a response to chemotherapy (for reviews, see Neville and Cooper, 1976; Go, 1976).

However, when this information is examined critically its value to the clinician may be not high. It must be borne in mind that the majority of patients on chemotherapy have advanced diseases and that tumors originating from the large bowel tend to produce an intraabdominal mass or hepatomegaly. The patient will be seen frequently by the physician so that he soon becomes aware of changes in the size of mass or deterioration of the patient's health. In this respect, the experience of the team at the Mayo Clinic is of interest (Ravry *et al.*, 1974). They found in gastrointestinal cancer that 75% of the responders to chemotherapy had a reduction of CEA value $\geqslant$35%; in all, 87% of the responders showed a reduction or unchanged CEA. Conversely, when there was tumor progression 65% showed a rise of CEA $\geqslant$ 35%. In some terminal patients there was a paradoxical fall of CEA in the presence of an increasing tumor load. Hence in the context of their clinical judgment, Ravry *et al.* (1974) did not find the monitoring of the CEA particularly helpful. Go (1976) has warned that it is possible that the direct action of various cancer chemotherapeutic compounds may alter the synthesis and secretion of CEA without affecting the tumor. Yet another source of misinterpretation could be a transient rise of CEA shortly after initiation of chemotherapy (Bagshawe *et al.*, 1973) which is probably due to tumor necrosis resulting in the release of CEA or CEA-like materials (Khoo and Mackay, 1973). Skarin *et al.* (1974) examined serial CEA levels in 38 patients with metastatic gastrointestinal cancer who were receiving chemotherapy; while a rising level usually coincided with tumor progression, stable elevated CEA could also accompany progression, and consistently low levels of CEA were a good prognostic sign but in their series were mainly patients with a minimal disease load. They were guarded about its value because of the disappointing effects of chemotherapy. In Leeds, we have examined the advantages given by sequentially measuring an array of markers during chemotherapy: CEA, GGT, ALKP, 5′NT, and four APRPs (Bullen *et al.*, 1976). The patients had either minimal residual disease or advanced indicator lesions; all survived more than 3 months. It was found that CEA gave the best indication of tumor progression, with a lead time averaging 4 months. Unfortunately, this was only in 40% of the 35 incidents of progression. By adding the other factors, changes in one or several of these indicators were found in more than 90%.

At present, it would seem that the biochemical monitoring of solid tumors has most to offer when the tumor cannot be detected clinically, as will happen in minimal residual disease or after a patient has responded favorably and the indicator lesion can no longer be felt. CEA emerges as the best marker, but sometimes it is negative despite an obvious recurrence. In these circumstances progressive increases in other nonspecific markers may alert the clinician that the treatment is failing to control the spread of the cancer.

9. Biochemical Studies of the Excised Tumor and Adjacent Bowel

Malignant tissues often show differences in the distribution of tissue enzymes compared to their normal counterparts. Interest has focused on three main groups of pathways: glycolytic metabolism, the biosynthesis and degradation of DNA precursors and metabolites, and the lysozomal enzymes. As yet, these approaches have not been sufficiently standardized to become a recommended procedure—nor has the information been evaluated to anywhere near the same extent as histopathology and serum chemistry. Schwartz (1975) has summarized the results of comparative studies of enzyme activities in colorectal cancer and the adjacent mucosa. The results are likely to be altered during tissue preparation, because the enzymes are very liable to leak from the cells (Dale, 1965). Schwartz was of the opinion that although changes in enzyme activity levels and the ratios of activity of associated enzymes alter in colon cancer, as yet this cannot be used for the early diagnosis of the disease. It had been hoped that such tests might be used on small biopsy specimens or bowel washings.

The lysozymal enzymes have been looked at as possible guides to the use of chemotherapeutic agents designed to have preferential release in the tissues. Double *et al.* (1977) in Leeds examined sulfatases A, B, and C, β-glucuronidase, and alkaline phosphatases in colorectal tumors. They found wide variations in the levels of these enzymes (up to fourfold), but there was no correlation with tumor stage; a similar variation has been observed in bladder cancer (Cooper, 1976). This variation raises the hope that alkylating agents presented as sulfates, phosphates, and glucuronides might have an increased release of the active moiety in the tumor tissue, if it exhibited a high level of the appropriate hydrolyase.

After a 2-year follow-up, analysis of the enzyme profiles in the colorectal cancers failed to predict the patients with potentially curative surgical excisions who had subsequently experienced recurrence or metastatic tumors. On the other hand, Langvad and Jemec (1975) reported that alterations of the lactic dehydrogenase isoenzyme ratios in the edge of the "normal" colonic mucosa can provide an indication of the probability of a patient's developing a local recurrence or a multicentric interval tumor. They found in 22 patients followed for 5–7 years after resection that a LDH_{iv}/LDH_{ii} ratio of 0.9 constituted a warning that recurrence was probable. In the tumor tissue, this ratio had a mean value of 1.67. This is an interesting application of the use of one of the field changes in the "healthy" bowel mucosa that have been observed in patients with colorectal cancer.

This chapter has attempted to show how a few specialized tests can provide the clinician with a basis for longer-range forecasting than is usually achieved with clinical biochemistry. At present, it would appear that the *regular sequential* measurement of CEA and GGT can play a role in reducing the period of uncertainty after a Dukes's B or C lesion resection. The clinician can have an early warning of recurrence or metastatic spread and can reassess his strategy while the patient is in a good state of health.

However, plasma CEA assays by themselves are still far from adequate indices of disease activity. While some unspecific reactants can in part fill this void, improved methods of measuring CEA production and secretion are needed together with the discovery of presently unrecognized colorectal tumor-associated products.

10. References

Anderson, J. A., 1972, Separate sample logistic discrimination, *Biometrika* **59:**19–35.

Astler, V. B., and Coller, F. A., 1954, The prognostic significance of direct extension of carcinoma of the colon and rectum, *Ann. Surg.* **139:**846–852.

Bacchus, H., 1975, Serum glycoproteins in cancer, *Progr. Clin. Pathol.* **6:**111–135.

Baden, H., Anderson, B., Augustenborg, G., and Hanel, H. K., 1971, Diagnostic value of γ glutamyl transpeptidase and alkaline phosphatase in liver metastases, *Surg. Gynal. Obstet.* **133:**769–773.

Bagshawe, K. D., Rogers, G. T., Searle, F., and Wilson, H., 1973, Blood carcinoembryonic antigen Regan Isoenzyme and human chorionic gonadotrophin in primary mediastinal carcinoma, *Lancet* **1:**210–211.

Bengmark, S., and Hafström, L., 1969, The natural history of primary and secondary tumours of the liver. I Prognosis for patients with hepatic metastases from colon and rectal carcinoma by laparotomy, *Cancer* **23:**198–202.

Booth, S. N., Jamieson, G. C., King, J. P. G., Leonard, J. C., Oates, G. D., and Dykes, P. W., 1974*a*, Carcinoembryonic antigen in management of colorectal cancer, *Br. Med. J.* **4:**183–187.

Booth, S. N., King, J. P. G., Leonard, J. C., and Dykes, P. W., 1974*b*, The significance of elevation of serum carcinoembryonic antigen (CEA) levels in inflammatory disease of the intestine, *Scand. J. Gastroenterol.* **9:**651–656.

Botsford, T. W., Aliapoulios, M. R., and Fogelson, F. S., 1971, Results of treatment of colorectal cancer at the Peter Bent Brigham Hospital from 1960 to 1965, *Ann. Surg.* **121:**398–402.

Bullen, B. R., Cooper, E. H., Turner, R., Neville, A. M., Giles, G. R., and Hall, R., 1976, Cancer markers in patients receiving chemotherapy for colorectal cancer, A preliminary report, *Med. and Ped. Oncology* **3:**289–300.

Carter, S. K., 1976, Large bowel cancer—The current status of treatment, *J. Natl. Cancer Inst.* **56:**3–10.

Cass, A. W., Million, R. R., and Pfaff, W. W., 1975, Patterns of recurrence following surgery alone for adenocarcinoma of the colon and rectum, *Cancer* **37:**2861–2865.

Cooper, E. H., 1967, Enzymes in bladder tumors, in: *Scientific Foundations of Virology* (D. I. Williams and G. D. Chisholm, eds.), pp. 322–325, Heinemann, London.

Cooper, E. H., Turner, R., Steele, L., Neville, A. M., and Mackay, A. M., 1975, The contribution of serum enzymes and carcinoembryonic antigen to the early diagnosis of metastatic colorectal cancer, *Br. J. Cancer* **31:**111–117.

Cooper, E. H., Turner, R., Geekie, A., Neville, A. M., Goligher, J. C., Graham, N. G., Giles, G. R., Hall, R., and MacAdam, W. A. F., 1976*a*, Alpha globulins in the surveillance of colorectal cancer, *Biomedicine* **24:**174–178.

Cooper, E. H., Eaves, G., Turner, R., Neville, A. M. and Ward, A. M., 1976*b*, Experience of multiparametric tests in the monitoring of large bowel cancer, *Bull. Cancer* **63:**541–550.

Dale, R. A., 1965, The activities of several enzymes of mucosa, carcinomata and polyps of human colon, *Clin. Chim. Acta* **11:**547–556.

Double, J. A., Cooper, E. H., and Goligher, J. C., 1977, Hydrolytic enzymes in colorectal cancer, *Biomedicine* **27:**11–13.

Dukes, C. E., 1932, The classification of cancer of the rectum, *J. Pathol. Bacteriol.* **35:**323–332.

Dukes, C. E., 1960, The pathology of rectal cancer, in: *Cancer of the Rectum* (C. E. Dukes, ed.), pp. 59–68, Livingstone, Edinburgh.

Egan, M. L., Lautenschleger, J. T., Coligan, J. E., and Todd, C. W., 1972, Radioimmunoassay of carcinoembryonic antigen, *Immunochemistry* **9:**289–299.

Fischerman, K., Patersen, C. F., Lindkaer Jensen, S., Christensen, K. Z., and Efsen, E., 1976, Survival among patients with liver metastases from cancer of the colon and rectum, *Scand. J. Gastroenterol. Suppl.* **37:**111–115.

Galen, R. S., 1975, Multiphasic screening and biochemical profiles: State of the art, *Progr. Clin. Pathol.* **6:**83–110.

Gérard, A., 1975, Carcinoma of the colon and rectum: Prognostic factors in cancer therapy, in: *Prognostic Factors and Criteria of Response* (M. J. Staquet, ed.), Raven Press, New York.

Go, V. L. M., 1976, Carcinoembryonic antigen, *Cancer* **37:**562–566.

Gold, P., and Freedman, S. O., 1965, Demonstration of tumor-specific antigens in human colonic carcinoma by immunological tolerance and absorption techniques, *J. Exp. Med.* **121:**439–462.

Goligher, J. C., 1941, The operability of carcinoma of the rectum, *Br. Med. J.* **2:**393–397.

Hogg, L., Jr., and Pack, G. T., 1956, Diagnostic accuracy of hepatic metastases at laparotomy, *Arch. Surg.* **72:**251–252.

Jaffe, B. M., Donegan, W. L., Watson, F., and Spratt, J. S., 1968, Factors influencing survival in patients with untreated hepatic metastases, *Surg. Gynecol. Obstet.* **127:**1–11.

Khoo, S. K., and Mackay, E. V., 1973, Carcinoembryonic antigen in cancer of the female reproductive system, *Aust. N.Z. J. Obstet. Gynecol.* **13:**1–7.

Kim, U. S., Papatestas, A. E., and Aufses, A. H., 1976, Prognostic significance of peripheral lymphocyte counts and carcinoembryonic antigens in colorectal carcinoma, *J. Surg. Oncol.* **8:**257–262.

Kirklin, J. W., Dockerty, M. D., and Waugh, J. W., 1949, The role of peritoneal reflection in the prognosis of carcinoma of the rectum and sigmoid colon, *Surg. Gynecol. Obstet.* **88:**326–331.

Koj, A., 1975, Acute phase reactants, in: *Structure and Function of Plasma Proteins,* Vol. I (A. C. Allison, ed.), pp. 73–132, Plenum, New York.

Langvad, E., and Jemec, B., 1975, Prediction of local recurrence in colorectal carcinoma: An LDH isoenzymatic assay, *Brt. J. Cancer* **31:**661–664.

Laurence, D. J., and Neville, A. M., 1972, Foetal antigens and their role in the diagnosis and clinical management of human neoplasm: A review, *Br. J. Cancer* **26:**335–355.

Laurence, D. R. J., Stevens, U., Bettelhiem, R., Darcy, D., Leesen, C., Tuberville, Co., Alexander, P., Jones, E. W., and Neville, A. M., 1972, Role of carcinoembryonic antigen, *Br. J. Med.* **3:**605–609.

LoGerfo, P., and Herter, F. P., 1975, Carcinoembryonic antigen and prognosis in patients with colon cancer, *Ann. Surg.* **181:**81–83.

Mach, J. P., Jaeger, P., Bertholet, M. M., Ruegsegger, C. H., Loosli, R. M., and Pettavel, J., 1974, Detection of recurrence of large bowel carcinoma by radioimmunoassay of circulating carcinoembryonic antigen (CEA), *Lancet* **2:**535–540.

Mackay, A. M., Patel, S., Carter, S., Stevens, U., Laurence, D. J. R., Cooper, E. H., and Neville, A. M., 1974, Role of serial plasma CEA assays in detection of recurrent and metastatic colorectal carcinomas, *Br. J. Med.* **4:**382–385.

Marner, I. L., Friborg, S., and Simonsen, E., 1975, Disease activity and serum proteins in ulcerative colitis: Immunochemical quantitation, *Scand. J. Gastroenterol.* **10**:537–544.

Munjal, D., Chawla, P. L., Lokich, J. J., and Zamcheck, N., 1976, Carcinoembryonic antigen and phosphohexose isomerase, gamma glutamyl transpeptidase and lactate dehydrogenase levels in patients with and without liver metastases, *Cancer* **37**:1800–1807.

Neville, A. M., and Cooper, E. H., 1976, Biochemical monitoring of cancer, *Ann. Clin. Biochem.* **13**:283–305.

Ravry, M., Moertel, C. G., Schutt, A. J., and Go, V. L. M., 1974, Usefulness of serial serum carcinoembryonic antigen CEA determinations during anti-cancer therapy or long term follow-up of gastrointestinal carcinoma, *Cancer* **34**:1230–1236.

Rhoads, J. E., 1975, The control of large bowel cancer, *Cancer* **36**:2314–2318.

Schwartz, M. K., 1975, Enzymes in colon cancer, *Cancer* **36**:2334–2336.

Schwartz, M. K., 1976, Laboratory aids to diagnosis—Enzymes, *Cancer* **37**:542–548.

Silverberg, E., and Hollet, A. I., 1974, Cancer statistics 1974—Worldwide epidemiology, *Cancer* **24**:1–64.

Skarin, A. T., Delwiche, R., Zamcheck, N., Lokich, J. J., and Frei, E. III, 1974, Carcinoembryonic antigen: Clinical correlation with chemotherapy for metastatic gastrointestinal cancer, *Cancer* **33**:1239–1245.

Sorokin, J. J., Sugarlaker, P. H., Zamcheck, N., Pisick, M., Kupchick, H., and Moore, F. D., 1974, Serial CEA assays: Use in detection of recurrence following resection of colon cancer, *J. Am. Med. Assoc.* **228**:49–53.

Steele, L., Cooper, E. H., Mackay, A. M., Losowsky, M. S., and Goligher, J. C., 1974, Combination of carcinoembryonic antigen and gamma glutamyl transpeptidase in the study of the evolution of colorectal cancer, *Br. J. Cancer* **30**:319–324.

Turner, M. D., 1975, Carcinoembryonic antigen, *J. Am. Med. Assoc.* **231**:756–758.

Ward, M. A., Cooper, E. H., Turner, R., Anderson, J. A., and Neville, A. M., 1977, Acute phase reactant protein profiles: An aid to monitoring of large bowel cancer by carcinoembryonic antigen and serum enzymes, *Br. J. Cancer* **35**:170–178.

Whitfield, J. B., Pounder, R. E., Neale, G., and Moss, D. W., 1972, Serum γ glutamyl transpeptidase activity in liver disease, *Gut* **13**:702–708.

Zamcheck, N., Doos, W. G., Prudente, R., Lurie, B. B., and Gottliet, L. S., 1975, Prognostic factors in colon carcinoma: Correlation of serum carcinoembryonic antigen and tumor histopathology, *Hum. Pathol.* **6**:31–45.

20

Enzymes of Normal and Malignant Intestine

M. Earl Balis

1. Introduction

The understanding of how the enzymatic balance in a eukaryotic cell leads to its function in the total organism, its mitotic activity, and on occasion malignancy is a goal many have sought. The differences in activities in similar tissues in slightly altered states could be highly indicative of their control. The cells of the intestinal mucosa undergo gradual changes and parallel these maturations with changes in location. In theory, at least, they provide an ideal model system to study.

The migration of cells from the crypts of the intestinal epithelium to the surface is accompanied by morphological and enzymatic changes. Some of these variations in the enzyme profile are qualitative; others are possibly only quantitative. It is difficult to say that those that appear to be only quantitative in nature are not also qualitative since few enzymes of the mucosa have been thoroughly analyzed. In the search for specific proof that a particular increase or decrease in activity is due to production of new enzyme or destruction of old, one must consider the possibility that changes are due to modification of existing enzyme in conformation or addition or loss of regulatory subunits.

2. Separation of Crypt and Villus

In view of the fact that the cells in the crypt that are undifferentiated and mitotically active are physically separated from the more highly differentiated nondividing cells, many investigators have felt that this was an ideal system in

M. Earl Balis • Memorial Sloan-Kettering Cancer Center, New York, New York 10021.

which to study the biochemical changes that accompany maturation and development. Several methods have been developed for physically separating and isolating the different kinds of cells. For some time, it has been known that trypsin (Harrer *et al.*, 1964) releases epithelial cells, as does hyaluronidase (Perris, 1966). Use of these enzymes, although of value in many kinds of studies, does not permit easy investigation of cells from the various parts of the crypt or villus. More recently, Weiser (1973*a*) has developed a method in which the small intestine is removed from the rat and incubated with sodium citrate and then treated with phosphate-buffered EDTA and dithiothreitol. In the latter medium, cells are released in sequential order from villus tip to crypt. The cells can then be collected by centrifugation and studied.

Other investigators have used a variety of physical methods of separation. One of these is based on low-amplitude, high-frequency vibrations of sections of gut (Harrison and Webster, 1969). Fortin-Magana *et al.* (1970) used a microtome to make sections of the small bowel. This permits alternate slices to be used for enzyme assay and for histological examination. Imondi *et al.* (1969) have demonstrated the suitability of a planing apparatus that cuts the stretched intestine and permits isolation of individual fractions of the villus down to the crypt of the small bowel. This apparatus has also been useful in separating flat mucosal cells from crypt cells of the colon. The validity of this method has been confirmed by showing that radioactive thymidine is incorporated into the DNA of cells which have been removed from the crypt fraction 30 min after labeling. As time after labeling increased, the radioactive cells were found in cuts nearer and nearer to the villus tip. In addition, the histological appearance of sections left behind after various fractions of epithelial cells had been removed seemed consistent with that predicted on the assumption that the planing apparatus removed discrete fractions, one at a time.

The several methods have individual characteristics which make them more or less useful in various kinds of biochemical and enzymatic studies. The frozen microtome method provides the best morphological control. The planing apparatus supplies the largest amount of material quickly after the sacrifice of the animal. The various buffers give easy and extensive separation, but the cells are in nonphysiological condition for a relatively long period of time before they can be isolated, and in some studies this can lead to extensive biochemical changes.

3. Enzymes of Crypts and Villi

3.1. Qualitative and Quantitative Differences

Using the various methods, several investigators have shown that in many cases, as might have been predicted, enzymes of the crypt are quite different from those of the villus. Folquis and Nordstrom, who had used the microtome method, showed that a variety of hydrolytic enzymes were located specifically in various parts of the small bowel (Nordstrom *et al.*, 1967). One of the most extensive studies was that carried out by Moog and her associates, who demonstrated that alkaline phosphatase occurs primarily in the crypt cells of the small intestines and furthermore that the enzyme found in the crypt is isozymatically distinct from that found in the tip. Chromatography of intestinal alkaline phosphatase on DEAE-cellulose had already shown the presence of three components (Grossberg *et al.*, 1961; Moss, 1963). Electrophoresis confirmed the presence of different enzyme forms. Moss (1965) felt that these were not true isozymatic differences but actually posttranscriptional variations and that there was in actuality only one native human intestinal phosphatase. In their investigation, Moog and her associates showed that in the mouse duodenum there exists an alkaline phosphatase that can be resolved into two forms by chromatography on DEAE-cellulose. One form has a higher preference for phenylphosphate and the other hydrolyzed β-glycerophosphate more extensively. In addition, Moog and associates showed that extracts from the distal portion of the duodenum and the jejunum contained relatively little of the form of alkaline phosphatase that preferentially hydrolyzed phenylphosphate. Electrophoresis revealed four phosphate bands in the intestinal extracts. Again, the authors showed that the makeup of the various enzyme forms was different in the distal and proximal ends of the duodenum. They further showed that the form that preferentially hydrolyzed the β-phosphate could be resolved into three bands on chromatography (Moog *et al.*, 1966).

Webster and Harrison (1969), using the vibration technique which they had developed, measured a variety of enzymes such as glucose-6-phosphate dehydrogenase, NAD-cytochrome oxidase, invertase, alkaline phosphatase, esterase, and leucine aminopeptidase. They found a large variety of patterns. Most of the enzymes they studied were found to increase in the villous cells relative to the activity in the crypts. Cytochrome oxidase and glucose-6-phosphate dehydrogenase appeared to remain at a constant level in all parts of the villus. The increases varied from four-fold with the esterase and leucine aminopeptidase to sixty-fold with the alkaline phosphatase. Thus no simple generalized change in pattern of enzyme concentration could be developed.

3.2. *Effects of Protein and RNA Inhibition*

Imondi *et al.* (1969) examined a series of enzymes related to the function of nucleic acid precursors and showed, not surprisingly, that thymidine kinase was found primarily in the crypt cells when simple assay of total homogenate was carried out. Thymidylate phosphatase and adenylate deaminase were found in a fairly uniform amount per cell through the entire mucosa of the small intestines. Adenosine deaminase and nucleoside phosphorylase were found to increase as cells migrated lumenward. Several possible explanations can be proposed for the changes observed in enzyme concentrations, as has been mentioned earlier. New enzymes could be made at an increased rate as cells move toward the villus tip, or there could be a change in the rate of destruction. Regulation of enzymes could be affected by changes in the stability of messenger RNA, or there could be changes in the rate and manner in which messengers were transcribed. There could also be changes in the rate of synthesis of messengers *per se*.

Attempts to analyze which of the factors were involved were carried out through the use of inhibitors of RNA and protein synthesis. From these studies, it was possible to deduce that all the possible mechanisms are operable. Each enzyme is regulated by one or more of these potential mechanisms (Hardman and Sutherland, 1969). In most of these cases, no evidence can be

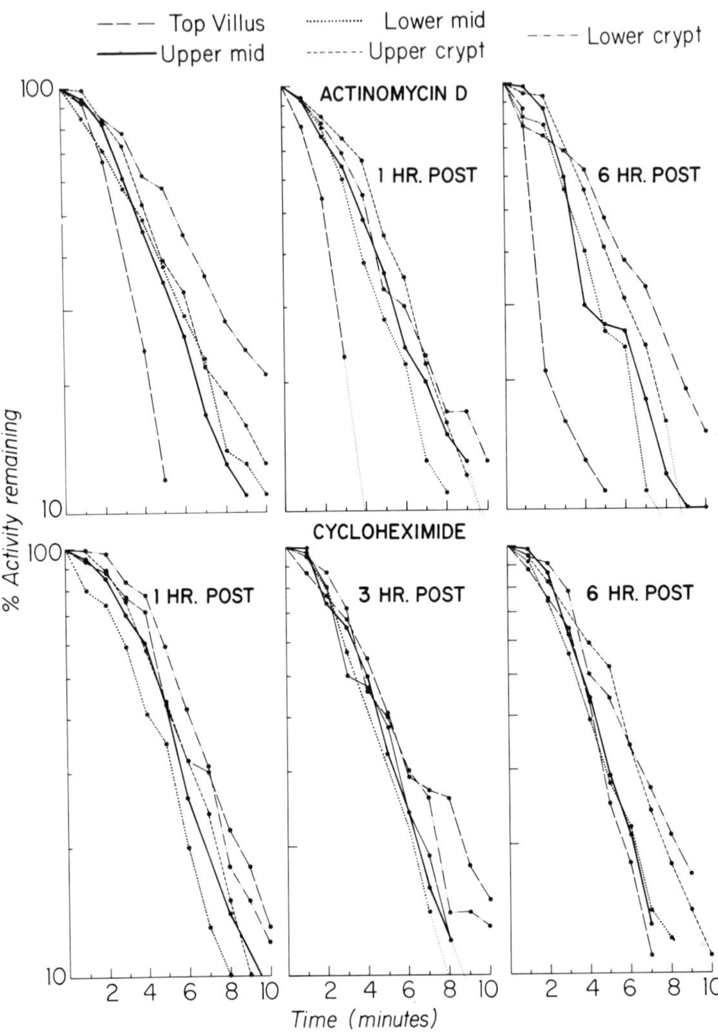

Fig. 1. Heat inactivation of APRTase. Animals were killed by cervical dislocation, a portion of the jejunum was removed and slit lengthwise, and the mucosal epithelial cells were separated with a planing apparatus. Activity was based on radioactivity of adenine, which was converted to a form not washed from DEAE-cellulose paper with 10^{-3} M $HCOONH_4$. Cycloheximide (1.5 mg/kg) and actinomycin D (1 mg/kg) were injected intraperitoneally. Aliquots were heated at 55°C for the indicated periods of time and then assayed. Results are expressed as fractions of initial values.

deduced indicating that there are any differences qualitatively in the enzymes. In some cases, however, it has been possible to show that there may be changes in the enzymes themselves. Adenylate pyrophosphorylase (adenine pyrophosphate phosphoribosyltransferase, APRT) is apparently able to exist in different forms. Examination of the enzyme from the various parts of the villus of the small bowel showed that the enzyme in the tip was more heat labile than that found in the crypt and the enzyme in the intermediate cuts was of intermediate heat stability. This was probably due to synthesis of a different variant or modification of the existing enzyme by the synthesis of a small regulatory polypeptide. Administration of cycloheximide, an inhibitor of protein synthesis, prevented the formation of the heat-labile form without greatly decreasing the amount of total enzyme (Balis *et al.*, 1971) (Fig. 1). Administration of actinomycin D, which prevents RNA synthesis, did not prevent the formation of the tip-specific form. These data suggested that no new RNA is required for the modification that occurs. It had been suggested that the increased activity found in the villus tip could be most economically produced by modification of existing enzyme and that since the cells have a relatively short life span there is no value in making a stable enzyme in this particular situation.

3.3. Cyclic Nucleotides

A large amount of work has been done on the regulation of cyclic AMP and cyclic GMP in the intestine and the physiological and pathological roles of these "second messengers." Cyclic AMP and adenylate cyclase have been particularly implicated in control of cell replication. Tissue culture cells in growth phases have low cyclase activity, but when the cells become confluent the cyclase (and the cyclic AMP concentration) increases sharply (Abell and Monahan, 1973). Like many other tissues, the intestine responds to a variety of exogenous stimuli via changes in the nucleotide cyclases and the cyclic nucleotide phosphodiesterase. Unfortunately, it is not easy to correlate all the data that have been published because some investigators have studied the jejunum, some the duodenum, and some, rather loosely, the small intestine.

Considerable interest has centered on the ileum because of its role in sodium transport. Direct application of dibutyryl cyclic AMP results in an inhibition of sodium transport and a stimulation of chloride secretion from serosa to mucosa (Field, 1971). A heat-labile moiety found in cell-free filtrates of *Vibrio cholerae* cultures produces a similar response (Greenough *et al.*, 1969; Shafer *et al.*, 1970). The nature of the response suggests that it is cyclic AMP mediated, and direct assay has shown that the enterotoxin does indeed cause an increase in mucosal cyclic AMP (Guerrant *et al.*, 1973; Al-Awqati *et al.*, 1970).

Prostaglandins and theophylline induce changes in secretion of water and electrolytes by intestinal mucosa presumably via changes in net cyclic AMP concentrations (Pierce *et al.*, 1971). The synergistic relationship between these two compounds suggests that a similar site of action is involved. However, studies of the interaction of several known effectors of cyclic AMP on ion fluxes and the concentration of the nucleotides *per se* have suggested that only a small fraction of the mucosal cyclic AMP is involved in ion transport (Field *et al.*, 1975). Of particular interest in this regard is the observation that villus cyclase was much more responsive than the crypt enzymes to cholera toxins (Weiser and Quill, 1975). The growth regulatory role of cyclic AMP and the influence of this function on differentiation and the development of malignancy can be independent of the transport phenomena. In view of the proposals that changes in the intestinal flora can be related to incidence of carcinomas of the colon, it is intriguing to note that some strains of *Escherichia coli* have the ability to provoke large changes in jejunal adenylate cyclase.

The analogous guanine derivative, cyclic GMP, has also been considered a "second messenger" and has been valued as a potential regulator of cell growth and differentiation. In view of the early studies of cyclic GMP, Ishikawa *et al.* (1969) assayed the content of this nucleotide in several tissues of the rat. In general, the levels were much lower that those seen with cyclic AMP. The increase seen following administration of the phosphodiesterase inhibitor theophylline suggested that the nucleotide is renewed at a rapid rate. In the small intestine, they also demonstrated the existence of an enzyme system capable of catalyzing the conversion of GTP to cyclic GMP. The enzyme was Mn^{2+}-requiring and was inhibited by ATP.

Ishikawa *et al.* divided the small bowel into distal and proximal halves with interesting disregard of the more conventional classification of its sections. They found twice as much cyclic GMP in the proximal half as in the distal. The contents of the lumen, on the other hand, contained 3–5 times as much cyclic GMP in the distal half.

Despite the fact that there is considerably more cyclic AMP than cyclic GMP in the bowel, the cyclase responsible for the formation of the two cyclic nucleotides is present in about the same concentrations. There are pronounced differences between the two cyclases, most strikingly the metal requirements, and the response to the presence of Triton in the assay mixture distinguishes the two activities. Triton activates cyclic GMP formation about 25-fold while exerting a strong inhibition of cyclic AMP synthesis. Other work has clearly shown that the two intestinal activities are due to completely independent enzymes (Hardman and Sutherland, 1969).

In many tissues there are two forms of guanylate cyclase, one soluble and one particulate. In heart (Kimura and Murad, 1974) and lung (Chrisman *et al.*, 1975), at least, the two forms of the enzyme differ in catalytic and physical properties. The soluble form is largely, if not entirely, missing from the tissues of the small bowel (Ishikawa *et al.*, 1969; Kimura and Murad, 1974). The major portion of the cyclase of the small bowel is associated with the microvilli of the brush border (de Jonge, 1975*b*). As a consequence of this specific membrane localization, the enzyme is primarily found in the villus cells, not in the crypts. Since the enzyme is highly concentrated in the brush border, the specific activity in this tissue is extremely high. AMP cyclase has about the same relative distribution in parts of the small bowel mucosa and is about 5 times as high in the various fractions as GMP cyclase (de Jonge, 1975*a*). GMP cyclase from the microvillus fractions behaves quantitatively differently from that from the brush border in response to Mn^{2+}.

4. Changes in Malignant Tissues

4.1. Cyclic Nucleotides

In a study designed to analyze the role of cyclic AMP and GMP in normal and malignant growth in the colon, DeRubertis *et al.* (1976) analyzed the cyclic nucleotides of surgical specimens of tumors and adjacent uninvolved mucosa. They reported that tumor levels were significantly lower than those of the normal tissue. There was, however, a wide range of values in the uninvolved mucosa of over four-fold and an almost eight-fold range per milligram of DNA in the tumors. Although statistical analysis indicated a highly significant difference, the great overlap of values and the range of normals indicate the great difficulty of working with labile substances in surgical specimens and make one a bit skeptical of extensive interpretation of such data without further support. No significent difference was seen between normal and malignant tissues in cGMP levels per cell, although they were seen on a wet weight basis, but here too variations among tissues were high.

The suggestion was made that the difference between tumors and normal mucosa was due to changes in adenylate cyclase. This was supported by the observation that incubation of mucosa and tumor slices with and without theophylline increased cyclic levels, but the tumor values remained lower than those of normal tissue. No significant differnces in phosphodiesterase were seen between normal and malignant tissue.

As a result of their studies and in context with other reports, DeRubertis *et al.* concluded that although absolute levels of cyclic nucleotides are not the sole determinants of malignancy they are interacting factors. The total impact of these regulators is exercised through other systems and is in turn modified by them. Many external stimuli act through these nucleotides, and alterations in them would modify the reaction to normal host regulators.

4.2. Polyamines and Ornithine Decarboxylase

Many investigators have reported correlations between polyamine synthesis and accumulation and new or increased cell growth (Domshke and Domshke, 1972; Russell, 1973*b*,*b*). The enzyme ornithine decarboxylase (ODC), which catalyzes the conversion of ornithine to putrescine and can therefore be considered the first enzyme of polyamine production, has also been shown to vary with the rates of cell growth. Low ODC levels are generally found in nongrowing tissues and high levels are found in fetuses and embryos of chicks, rats, and amphibians as well as regenerating liver and malignant cells (Hogan *et al.*, 1974; Russell and Snyder, 1968; Williams-Ashman *et al.*, 1972; Russell and Levy, 1971).

There is great clinical interest in the levels of polyamines and their metabolism as possible indicators of the severity of cancer and of the efficacy of various therapeutic regimens (Russell and Russell, 1975). In the case of gastric cancer, urinary polyamines have been reported to decrease from twice normal to normal following surgical intervention (Takeda *et al.*, 1975). Much more work is needed before it will be possible to assess fully the prognostic value of serum and urine polyamines in the therapy of cancer. It is not yet completely clear whether data are best presented as total amines or in terms of the ratios of the three compounds to themselves or some other parameter.

These correlations led to the analysis of ODC activity of the intestinal tract. It was felt that the enzyme should be very high in the rapidly dividing mucosa of all parts of the gut, but especially in the crypt cells.

4.2.1. *Age and Tissue Specificity*

The level of ODC in small bowel is extremely high and the enzyme appears to be similar if not identical to the form found in regenerating liver (Ball and Balis, 1976). Both enzymes have the same K_m and response to several effectors. Surprisingly, the value in the colon is much lower than that in the small intestines (Balis *et al.*, 1974). Despite the fact that the mitotic index is about half as great in the colon as in the ileum, the ODC value is 4 in the colon and more than 1000 in the ileum (Table 1). The stomach also has a low ODC value. It is striking that the two parts of the GI tract with the highest rates of malignancy should have this enormously reduced level of ODC. Analysis of the ODC level of several carcinogen-induced colon tumors showed a great increase (approximately fiftyfold) over that of normal mucosa.

The amount of ODC is related to the age of the rat in many tissues. In the small intestine, there is a high level in the early fetus followed by a rapid decrease. The level begins to increase again 15–20 days postpartum and becomes maximal at weaning or shortly after. The rapid increase that occurs during weaning parallels a rapid increase in crypt-to-villus migration and an increased differentiation of villous cells (Fig. 2). In view of the age-related

Table 1. ODC and Putrescine in Rat Tissues[a]

	ODC	Putrescine
Stomach	3	0.58 ± 0.10
Duodenum	541	0.57 ± 0.07
Jejunum	334	0.50 ± 0.06
Ileum	1063	0.52 ± 0.07
Colon	23	0.05 ± 0.01
Liver	7	0.03 ± 0.01
Brain	4	0.03 ± 0.02

[a]The ODC activity is given as pmol/mg protein/5C min. The enzymatic activity for fetal tissues is the average for three litter groups of animals. Six to eight separate determinations were made with 200-g animals. Values are average ± SEM. From Ball and Balis (1976).

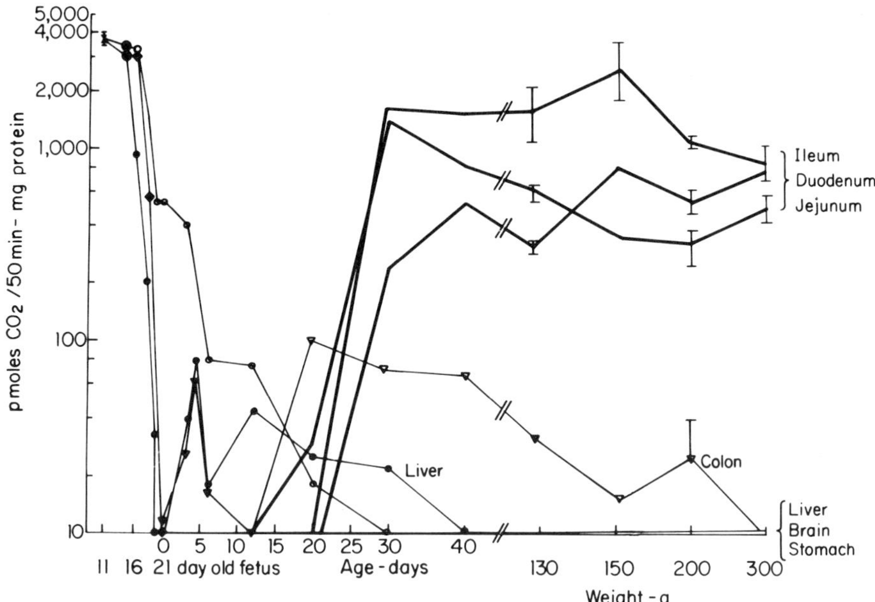

Fig. 2. Changes in ODC activity in rat tissues as a function of age. The first point on the chart represents the value for whole embryos (×); the next pair of points (●) represents head and body assayed separately (upper value is the head); by 15–16 days the brain (○), liver (•), and fetal intestines (◆) were separated. In newborn to weaning age (21 days) the rat intestine could be divided into stomach, duodenum, jejunum, ileum, and colon (△) sections. Only with 21-day and older animals were epithelial cells removed from the mucosal lining and then assayed. The results are the average of two to six separate determinations, and a few representative error ranges are shown (± SEM).

incidence of cancer of the colon, the changes in ODC in the colon with age are of particular interest. The colon activity becomes maximal at about 18 days and steadily decreases with age until it is barely detectable in rats 300 g or more in weight (about 7 months of age).

The function of ODC is, of course, the production of putrescine and from this spermine and spermidine. Thus the amount of the amines themselves is a critical measure of functioning ODC. In the intestine, the polyamine levels are not easily correlated with either ODC activities or cell growth rates. In adult rats, putrescine concentrations of the small intestine are about 10 times those of the colon mucosa. However, the stomach mucosa, which has little ODC activity, has a higher concentration of polyamines than any part of the small intestine. The primary increase is in the spermine, which is almost 4 times the spermidine value. The putrescine and spermidine of the stomach are essentially the same as in the small bowel. Despite the large increase in ODC seen in the carcinogen-induced tumors, only a sixfold increase in putrescine and a less trhan twofold increase in spermine and spermidine were noted.

It is not clear how polyamines are maintained in the rapidly migrating and turning-over colonic and stomach cells. These cells have little ODC activity, yet they have polyamine levels similar to or higher than those present in the small intestine. ODC may be the rate-limiting factor in polyamine biosynthesis, but probably other enzymes in the pathway play important roles in regulating polyamine levels. Probably, ODC levels in the small intestine not only are due to high proliferative activity of the epithelial cells but also are related to the unique metabolic function of the organ. In addition, changes in the relative amounts of the polyamines may be more important than the specific concentrations *per se*.

Despite the looseness of the correlations, it is intriguing to note that the colon and stomach, which have low ODC activity relative to the small intestine, also have a high incidence of tumor formation. O'Brien *et al.* (1975) have reported a rapid temporary increase in ODC in mouse epidermis as a consequence of exposure to carcinogen. Early studies with other organs suggest that this may be generally true. For example, in one investigation it was shown that a liver carcinogen had little effect on ODC of the stomach or large or small intestine but increased liver ODC from a value of 4 to over 300. In a parallel study dimethylhydrazine, a colon carcinogen, brought about a large increase in ODC in the colon but had little effect on liver, stomach, or small bowel.

4.2.2. Effects of Metabolic Inhibitors

The effects on ODC of four drugs that are known to act by inhibiting the synthesis of RNA and/or protein were analyzed in the duodenum (Table 2). The protein synthesis inhibitor cycloheximide caused a sharp drop of 80–90% in the ODC activity of all parts of the duodenal mucosa within the first hour after its administration. The extent of this decrease in activity and its rapid onset are consistent with the reported half-life of ODC, approximately 15 min (Russell and Snyder, 1969). In contrast, puromycin at levels essentially equal

Table 2. Effects of Drugs on ODC[a]

	ODC relative to control						
	Cycloheximide		But_2-cAMP	Cycloheximide + But_2-cAMP		Puromycin + But_2-cAMP	
	3 hr	5 hr	3 hr	3 hr	5 hr	1 hr	3 hr
Duodenum							
Villus tip	0.52	1.15	0.86	0.70	0.88	1.52	2.46
Midvillus	0.64	1.28	1.16	0.76	0.89	0.53	2.58
Villus–crypt junction	0.80	1.88	1.16	0.83	1.44	0.35	4.25
Crypt	0.54	1.39	0.39	0.57	1.31	0.04	1.35
Colon	14.51	19.83	1.57	14.03	8.18	0.72	5.07
Liver	2.14	18.85	20.42	6.28	45.14	0.14	156.64

[a]From Ball and Balis (1976, unpublished data).

in protein inhibitory potency produced a 62% decrease in crypt ODC in 1 hr but had no effect on the villus cell enzyme. Three hours after administration of puromycin, the ODC activity of all parts of the duodenal epithelium was increased by 20–100% in various fractions and the least increase was in the crypts.

Two RNA synthesis inhibitors that act by very different mechanisms gave similar results. Although at the dose used actinomycin was somewhat faster acting, both it and cordycepin caused slight increases in tip activity and reduced the crypt ODC to about one-half of the control value.

The decrease in ODC in all cells of the duodenum following cycloheximide treatment is consistent with the hypothesis that ODC activity is maintained in the mucosa by a continuing synthesis as the cells move lumenward. The half-life of the enzyme is less than 1% of the life span of the epithelial cell after it has begun to migrate up the villus. The fact that inhibition of RNA synthesis causes a tip–crypt differential suggests that turnover of ODC messenger RNA is more rapid in the dividing than in the more highly differentiated cells of the villi.

The fact that both ODC and nucleotide cyclase activities have been implicated in cell division, development, and malignancy makes the evaluation of the relationship between these two systems appear to be a fruitful area of investigation. As an initial step, the amount of ODC in crypts and villi of duodenum and jejunum was assayed. Although the activity per milligram of protein was higher in the crypts of both organs, the activity per cell (based on DNA) was essentially the same in crypt and villus of the duodenum. ODC of jejunal crypts was 3 times that of villous cells (Ball and Balis, 1976). The difference between these organs by this criterion is quite striking and emphasizes the danger in the indiscriminant lumping together of data on all parts of the small intestine.

4.2.3. Effects of Cyclic AMP

Studies of ODC in rat liver by Beck *et al.* (1973) showed that compounds that raise the level of cyclic AMP can alter ODC and that administration of puromycin can stimulate ODC and interact positively with dibutyryl cyclic AMP given concurrently. Similar studies of the duodenal enzyme showed that these compounds react analogously in the duodenum (Ball and Balis, 1976). Administration of dibutyryl cyclic AMP caused a modest temporary increase in the ODC of tip cells and a 60% decrease in the crypt cell activity. When puromycin was given together with the cyclic AMP derivative, the inhibition in crypt cell ODC at 1 hr was even more pronounced. The reduction in the crypts reached 96% and the increase in tip cell enzyme was about 50% at 1 hr. Three hours after administration of these two drugs in combination, all cells of the duodenal epithelium had ODC activities 2 1/2–3 1/2 times the control values. In a similar manner, theophylline, an inhibitor of cyclonucleotide phosphodiesterase, given in conjunction with dibutyryl cyclic AMP caused an initial decrease in activity over that seen with dibutyryl cyclic AMP alone.

Three hours after this combination of drugs was given, there was a generalized increase in the ODC of the duodenum. Theophylline alone caused an increase after 3 hr. Epinephrine, which acts by increasing cyclic AMP levels, produced an extremely rapid increase in ODC followed in 3 hr by a return to control values. All of these results suggest that cyclic AMP has a regulatory effect on the synthesis and maintenance of ODC in the duodenum and that the villus and crypt cells respond uniquely and individually to altered cyclic AMP levels.

The unusual baseline levels of ODC in the colon and the high incidence of colonic carcinomas suggest the possibility that the response to these drugs might be different in this organ. Very little short-term (1 hr) effect was noted, but many of the drug regimens resulted in strong increases 3 hr after their administration. The most potent effect was that produced by theophylline and theophylline plus dibutyryl cyclic AMP. These caused twenty- and thirtyfold increases in ODC. As was seen in the duodenum, the response to epinephrine was extremely rapid in the colon. None of the compounds studied had any *in vitro* effect on ODC activity.

The results of the ODC measurements correlate well with the *in vivo* cyclic AMP levels reported above. Thus several drugs—e.g., epinephrine, theophylline, and prostaglandin E_1—stimulate villus cAMP and ODC more than the crypt nucleotide. The mechanism by which normal and cyclic AMP-altered ODC are regulated is not clear. One proposal postulates that cyclic AMP-mediated induction of ODC is activated by a protein kinase that causes increased production of an ODC-specific messenger RNA rather than synthesis of a more active or more stable enzyme variant (Byus and Russell, 1975). Cycloheximide rapidly blocks the increase in ODC and also prevents the cyclic AMP-induced stimulation. This suggests that enzyme modification is now occurring but that new protein synthesis is required for the higher activity. Cycloheximide affects duodenal crypts and villus cells equally, and the rate of protein synthesis appears to be essentially constant in dividing and nondividing cells.

In addition, it has been generally assumed that altered ODC activity reflects changes in the level of enzyme protein and is not caused by changes in enzyme activity *per se*. Immunochemical work by Hölttä (1975) has shown that the previously reported changes in ODC activity that occur in the liver following partial hepatectomy or the administration of growth hormone are indeed accompanied by corresponding changes in antigen levels.

The response to actinomycin, cordycepin, puromycin, and actinomycin suggests that changes in ODC levels result from changes in messenger RNA synthesis or degradation. In the duodenum, the effect of the RNA synthesis inhibitors actinomycin D and cordycepin indicates that the ODC mRNA of the crypt cells is more labile than that of the villus cells. It also appears that transcriptional events are essential for the stimulation of ODC levels in nondividing cells. Cordycepin and actinomycin D largely prevented the dibutyryl cAMP plus theophylline-caused stimulation of ODC in the duodenal villus cells but not in the crypt cells. These compounds are also very effective in preventing the induction of the liver enzyme. They are less effective in the colon epithelium, but this may be the result of having isolated the villus and crypt cells together.

An unexplained finding is the observation that actinomycin D and cordycepin do not prevent the rebound in ODC activity of the crypt cells when they are administered along with dibutyryl cAMP and theophylline. It may be that cAMP reduces the effectiveness of actinomycin D in the crypt cells or that cAMP can temporarily prevent the utilization of the mRNA while at the same time increasing its stability. It is possible of course that these RNA synthesis inhibitors are affecting some RNA species other than messenger RNA, and inhibiting ribosome formation or protein synthesis. However, the data do seem to suggest that transcriptional events are regulating ODC levels and that the exact manner of this regulation is tissue specific and also related to the stage of cell development in a given organ.

4.3. Thymidine Kinase

In several systems the enzyme thymidine kinase (dTK) has been associated with cell division. Autoradiography of the intestine of normal animals following administration of labeled thymidine shows uptake in crypt cells only (Lipkin, 1973). On the other hand, it has been reported that normal-appearing cells of the flat mucosa of the colon adjacent to polyps are able to take up thymidine *in vivo* (Lipkin, 1973). In addition, homogenates from the nondividing cells of the villus tip contain considerable dTK when assayed *in vitro* (Salser and Balis, 1973).

In order to clarify the relationships between dTK and normal, abnormal, and fetal cell division, a comparison of certain properties of dTK in the surface and villus cells with those of the enzyme from crypt and that from placental cells and from intestinal tumors was undertaken. If the enzymes of intestinal tumor cells resemble those of the nondividing surface cells, it should be possible to design chemotherapeutic approaches to treatment of carcinoma of the colon in which tumor and surface cells would be preferentially destroyed while the stem cells of the crypt would remain viable. These surviving cells could serve to replenish in a short time the intestinal mucosa and permit the animal to survive. The currently used antimitotic drugs kill both tumor and crypt cells and can denude the gut.

Some, but not all, properties of the dTK in crude extracts resemble those of the dTK found in surface cells (Salser and Balis, 1974). Similarly, some properties of the tumor enzyme are like those of the dTK in extracts of fetal intestine, while others are not. Further exploration of these questions required pure enzyme preparations for study. dTK was purified from the colon of cadavers, and antisera to this enzyme were raised in rabbits.

When the antibody was reacted with extracts of total colon mucosa, two sets of lines of immunoprecipitin were apparent. Figure 3A is an idealized version of the plate. The center well contained the antibody. Well I contained an extract of an adenocarcinoma of the colon. Its line appeared to be essen-

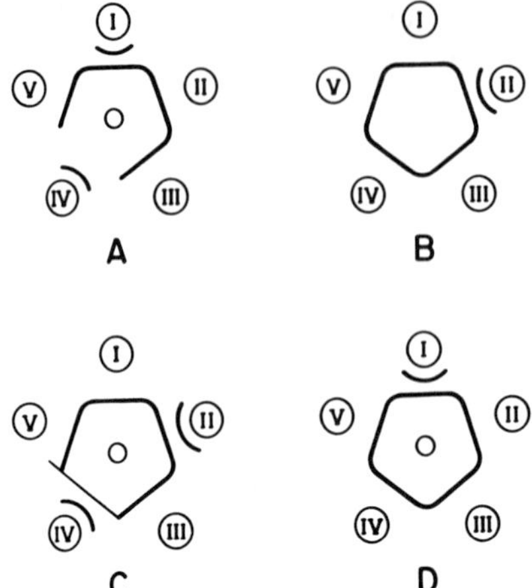

Fig. 3. Schematic representation of double-diffusion precipitin reactions in agar gels. Immune serum is in the center wells and antigen extracts are in the peripheral wells of micro-Ouchterlony plates. Based on data of Salser and Balis (1976).

tially the same as one of the lines seen with total normal colon. Scrapings of the colonic flat mucosa in well II yielded an immunoprecipitin line that also appeared to be identical to that formed by the tumor extract. An extract of colonic crypt cells in well III gave two lines, one of which formed a line of identity with that from the flat mucosa; the other resembled the line seen with total colon extracts. Since on some occasions similar scrapings gave primarily the outer line with little or no precipitin coincident with the tumor and surface extract, it appears that the double line seen here in crypt cell extracts was due, at least in part, to imperfect slicing. A placental extract in well V gave a line coincident with that given by the tumor and surface cell extracts. Stafford and Jones (1972) have demonstrated that dTK from rodent tumors is fetal-like in some of its properties.

Figure 3B shows a somewhat similar study with total colon extract in position I, placenta in II, a carcinoma of the rectum in position III, the same crypt as was used in A in position IV, and in well V an extract of an adenocarcinoma of the colon. All these tumors are essentially like the surface and placental material.

Figure 3C again shows the total colon extract in position I, an adenocarcinoma of the colon in position II, an osteogenic sarcoma metastatic to the lung in well III, a colonic polyp in well IV, and a placental extract in well V. The polyp extract reacts like the tumor, and the tumors all have a common antigen that appears to be found also in the surface.

In the Ouchterlony plate represented in Fig. 3D an adenocarcinoma was in position I, a total scrape in position II, and an ovarian carcinoma in position III. It is interesting to note that the ovarian carcinoma was the first tumor seen that contained both the dividing and nondividing cell froms of dTK. Position IV contained another adenocarcinoma of the rectum and position V a placental extract. All tumors except the ovarian had one antigen, and it was the one found in flat mucosa cells.

All these data suggest that there are two principal forms of dTK in the

Table 3. Neutralization of dTK by Rabbit Antiserum[a]

Tissue source	Percent neutralization		
	Undiluted serum	1:10	1:1000
Normal colon	92	73	63
Adenocarcinoma	46	33	14
Placenta	40	23	13

[a]Enzyme from tissue was mixed with antisera and kept at 4°C for 17 hr. Residual activity of the supernatant was then denatured. Based on data of Salser and Balis (1976).

colon. One is found in the surface cells, while total colon mucosal samples have both. The enzyme in the surface cells gives immunoprecipitin lines that suggest that it is immunologically the same as that found in all of the tumors of the colon that have been examined.

Examination of total colonic extracts suggests that the line corresponding to the surface cell material is a doublet. The significance of this is not readily apparent at the present time (Salser and Balis, 1976).

Further examination of these antibodies against the dTK activity of the tissue extracts was done by assaying residual activity after addition of antibody and removal of any precipitate that formed. Table 3 shows that partially purified dTK from normal colon was strongly inhibited by the antibody, while that from placental extracts and that from a tumor were only partially inhibited. This indicates some difference between the two enzyme forms, and a similarity between the dTK from the tumor and placenta. A crude extract of the ovarian carcinoma that had been studied by immunodiffusion was inhibited more than the colonic tumor or placental extracts, but less than that from normal colonic mucosa. This observation is consistent with the immunodiffusion patterns seen. Interestingly, the dTK activity of PHA-stimulated and leukemic lymphocytes was not inhibited by the antibody. It may also be worth noting that no precipitin line was seen on immunodiffusion with extracts of those lymphocytes.

These data strongly suggest that a placental form of dTK exists in man and that it has great similarity to the enzyme found in the nondividing cells. One might propose on this basis that tumors do in fact arise from the nondividing flat mucosa. This is consistent with the hypothesis proposed by others on the basis of thymidine uptake data (Cole, 1973; Lipkin, 1974).

Since the dTK of tumor cells differs from that of normal intestinal mucosa cells, changes in the properties of dTK of the intestines as animals mature and age might also occur. Furthermore, treatment of animals with carcinogens might be expected to cause changes that would lead to a dTK with properties more like those of the enzyme found in fetal intestines.

Table 4 presents data comparing dTK activity in the small intestine of normal rat fetuses and rats of various ages to that from some animals that have received dimethylhydrazine, an intestinal carcinogen. The intestine of

Table 4. Effects of Dimethylhydrazine of dTK[a]

Tissue	Enzyme activity
Fetal gut	400
Neonatal gut	117
Weanling jejunum	94
Adult jejunum	6
DMH-treated normal	5
DMH-treated abnormal	8–30
Tumors	67–223

[a]From J. S. Salser and M. E. Balis (unpublished).

the DMH-treated rats was further subdivided into two groups on the basis of an evaluation of the gross morphological appearance of the intestine. If it appeared abnormal, it was classified as such. The specific activity of the dTK decreases rapidly from the fetal to the adult rat. In addition, activity in tumors is high so that is is more like the fetal or neonatal bowel, and abnormal-appearing DMH-treated intestine has a somewhat higher than normal activity.

Earlier reports had noted that addition to the reaction mixture of phospholipase C (PC) stimulates dTK to varying degrees and that the mercaptans dithiothreitol (DTT) and glutathione (GSH) alter the activity of dTK (Salser and Balis, 1974). Fetal and tumor enzyme extracts are less stimulated by PC than are adult rat tissue extracts. DMH-treated intestine shows a pattern of response to PG intermediate between that shown by normal gut and that of tumors. Similar changes are seen with DTT and GSH. Although they are not very profound, the differences seen in the DMH-treated animals are suggestive that the fetal-like properties of the tumor enzyme begin to appear in the premalignant gut.

The specific activity of dTK undergoes a similar change in the colon, and here too, the DMH-treated animals begin to show higher specific activities than controls of the same age. The changes with the other effectors are much smaller than those seen in the small bowel.

4.4. DNA Repair

Following the demonstration that xeroderma pigmentosum cells do not have the capacity to repair DNA (Cleaver, 1968; Setlow *et al.*, 1969), several investigators have proposed a related role for repair of carcinogen-damaged DNA in chemical carcinogenesis (Damjanov *et al.*, 1973; Goodman and Potter, 1972). It is possible that excessive damage and repair or faulty repair could directly lead to the chromosomal changes that characterize malignancy. This hypothesis leaves unanswered the question of why certain alkylating agents cause DNA damage and subsequent repair without producing cancer and others cause tumor production. A further problem concerns the tissue specificities of alkylating carcinogens.

In view of the fact that the mucosal linings of the large and small intestine have similar rapid rates of cell division and yet have greatly different rates of spontaneous and chemically induced carcinogenesis, it was thought likely that the study of damage and repair of cellular DNA in the intestinal mucosa might shed light on both of these enigmas. This could be of significance in understanding the etiology of carcinoma of the colon since tumors are so often found at the surface, not in the crypts. This fact does not, however, suggest that they originate by transformation of a surface cell rather than a crypt cell.

In an attempt to evaluate the significance of repair, three compounds known to damage DNA and cause carcinoma of the colon and three noncarcinogenic compounds also able to damage DNA were administered to rats 24 hr after a tracer dose of [^{3}H]thymidine. The animals were killed at various times after the drugs were administered. Damage and subsequent repair of the DNA of the jejunal and colonic mucosal cells were evaluated by sedimentation in alkaline sucrose gradients (Kanagalingam and Balis, 1975). All the compounds caused breakdown of the DNA to lower molecular weight pieces. There was extensive cleavage both in dividing crypt cells and in mature nondividing cells that had been separated by use of a slicing apparatus. Repair occurred to varying extents in the jejunal and colonic cells. The surface cells of the colon were much less able to repair the damage resulting from insult by the carcinogens than were any other cells or the same cells when damaged by the noncarcinogens. These observations are summarized in Table 5. The results support the concept that damage to DNA and the quality and rate of subsequent repair play an intimate role in the carcinogenic action of these particular compounds.

In view of the general interest in tumor cell membranes, it is unfortunate that so little has been learned about the enzymes of glycolipid and glycoprotein synthesis in the intestine. It is readily understandable since they are

Table 5. Difference in the Repair of Rat Intestinal DNA Damaged in Vivo[a]

	Jejunum		Colon	
	Surface cells	Crypt cells	Surface cells	Crypt cells
Noncarcinogens				
HN2	+	+	++	++
MHS	+	+	++	++
MTC	++	+	++	++
Carcinogens				
MAM	−	++	−	++
DMAB	−	++	−	++
DMH	++	+	−	++

[a] ++, Complete repair; +, incomplete repair; −, absence or very poor repair. From Kanagalingam and Balis (1975).

difficult materials to work with. Several advances have resulted from the work of Kim and his associates, who have characterized several glycosyltransferases from rat intestinal mucosa (Kim *et al.*, 1971*a*,*b*). Weiser (1973*b*) attacked this problem using the method he had developed for removing mucosal cells stepwise in buffer and EDTA. He found a high capacity in villi to incorporate glucosamine into membranes. The incorporation was highest in the microvilli. The need for further work is emphasized not only by the current interest in membrane components and tumor-specific antigens but also by the finding that there is a cancerlike change in apparently normal mucosa adjacent to colon carcinomas in humans. This "transitional" mucosa (Filipe and Cooke, 1974) has increased amounts of total hexosamines and sialic acid that are reminscent of the changes seen in carcinoma of the colon (Barker *et al.*, 1959).

The enzyme composition in both absolute and relative terms determines the metabolic activity and function of cells. Thus the differences between dividing and functional parts of the various parts of the various organs of the gastrointestinal tract are defined by the functioning enzymes. The development and expression of malignancy also must be encoded in this same way. An understanding of the various enzymatic parameters should contribute to our understanding and eventual control of cancer.

5. References

Abell, C. W., and Monahan, T. M., 1973, The role of adenosine 3′,5′-cyclic monophosphate in the regulation of mammalian cell division, *J. Cell Biol.* **59:**549–558.

Al-Awqati, Q., Cameron, J. L., Field, M., and Greenough, W. B., III, 1970, Effect of prostaglandin E_1 on electrolyte transport in rabbit ileal mucosa, *J. Clin. Invest.* **49:**2a.

Balis, M. E., Brown, G. F., and Cappuccino, J. G., 1971, Heat stability of AMP pyrophosphorylase in differentiating intestinal epithelial cells, *Biochem. Biophys. Res. Commun.* **42(6):**1007–1011.

Balis, M. E., Ball, W. J., Salser, J. S., and Yip, L. C., 1974, Effects of drugs on cells at various stages of differentiation in the intestinal epithelium, in: *Perinatal Pharmacology* (J. Dancis and J. C. Hwang, eds.), pp. 27–47, Raven Press, New York.

Ball, W. J., and Balis, M. E., 1976, Ornithine decarboxylase activity in rat intestines: Changes during aging, *Cancer Res.* **36:**3312–3316.

Barker, S. A., Stacey, M., and Tipper, D. J., 1959, Some observations on certain mucoproteins containing sialic acid, *Nature (London)* **184:**68–90.

Beck, W. T., Bellantone, R. A., and Canellakis, E. S., 1973, Puromycin stimulation of rat liver ornithine decarboxylase activity, *Nature (London)* **241:**275–277.

Byus, C. V., and Russell, D. H., 1975, Ornithine decarboxylase activity: Control by cyclic nucleotides, *Science* **187:**650–652.

Chrisman, T. D., Garbers, D. L., Parks, M. A., and Hardman, J. G. 1975, Characterization of particulate and soluble guanylate cyclases from rat lung, *J. Biol. Chem.* **250:**374–381.

Cleaver, V. E., 1968, Defective repair replication in xerodermic pigmentosum, *Nature (London)* **218:**652–656.

Cole, V., 1973, Carcinogens and carcinogenesis in the colon, *Hosp. Pract.* **8:**123–130.

Damjanov, I., Cox, R., Sarma, D. S. R., and Farber, E., 1973, Patterns of damage and repair of liver DNA induced by carcinogenic methylating agents *in vivo, Cancer Res.* **33:**2122–2128.

de Jonge, H. R., 1975*a*, Properties of guanylate cyclase and levels of cyclic GMP in rat small intestinal villus and crypt cells, *FEBS Lett.* **55:**143–152.

de Jonge, H. R., 1975*b*, The localization of guanylate cyclase in rat small intestinal epithelium, *FEBS Lett.* **53:**237–242.

DeRubertis, F. R., Chayoth, R., and Field, J. B., 1976, The content and metabolism of cyclic adenosine 3',5'-monophosphate and cyclic guanosine 3',5'-monophosphate in adenocarcinoma of the human colon, *J. Clin. Invest.* **57**:641–649.

Domshke, S., and Domshke, W., 1972, Polyamines and the liver, *Acta Hepato-Gastroenterol.* **19**:212–217.

Field, M., 1971, Intestinal secretion: Effect of cyclic AMP and its role in cholera, *N. Eng. J. Med.* **284**:1137–1144.

Field, M., Sheerin, H. E., Henderson, A., and Smith, P. L., 1975, Catecholamine effects on cyclic AMP levels and ion secretion in rabbit ileal mucosa, *Am. J. Physiol.* **229**:86–92.

Filipe, M. I., and Cooke, K. B., 1974, Changes in composition of mucin in the mucosa adjacent to carcinoma of the colon as compared with the normal: A biochemical investigation, *J. Clin. Pathol.* **27**:315–318.

Fortin-Magana, R., Hurwitz, R., Herbst, J. J., and Kretchner, N., 1970, Intestinal enzymes: Indicators of proliferation and differentiation in the jejunum, *Science* **167**:1627–1628.

Goodman, J. I., and Potter, V. R., 1972, Evidence for DNA repair synthesis and turnover in rat liver following ingestion of 3',-methyl-4-dimethyl-aminoazobenzene, *Cancer Res.* **32**:766–755.

Greenough, W. B., III, Pierce, N. F., Al-Awqati, Q., and Carpenter, C. C. J., 1969, Stimulation of gut electrolyte secretion by prostaglandins, theophylline, and cholera exotoxin, *J. Clin. Invest.* **48**:32a.

Grossberg, A. L., Harris, E. G., and Schlamowitz, M., 1961, Enrichment and separation of alkaline phosphatase activities of human tissues by chromatography on cellulose ion-exchange adsorbents, *Arch. Biochem. Biophys.* **93**:267–277.

Guerrant, R. L., Ganguly, U., Casper, A. G. T., Moore, E. J., Pierce, N. F., and Carpenter, C. C. J., 1973, Mechanism and time-course with enterotoxin and whole bacterial cells, *J. Clin. Invest.* **52**:1707–1714.

Hardman, J. G., and Sutherland, E. W., 1969, Guanyl cyclase, an enzyme catalyzing the formation of guanosine 3',5'-monophosphate from guanosine triphosphate, *J. Biol. Chemis.* **244**:6363–6370.

Harrer, D. S., Stern, B. K., and Reilly, R. W., 1964, Removal and dissociation of epithelial cells from the rodent gastrointestinal tract, *Nature (London)* **203**:319–320.

Harrison, D. D., and Webster, H. L., 1969, The preparation of isolated intestinal crypt cells, *Exp. Cell Res.* **55**:257–260.

Herbst, J. J., Fortin-Magana, R., and Sunshine, P., 1970, Relationship of pyrimidine biosynthetic enzymes to cellular proliferation in rat intestines during development, *Gastroenterology* **59**:240–246.

Hogan, B. L. M., McIlhinney, A., and Murden, S., 1974, Effect of growth conditions on the activity of ODC in cultured hepatoma cells, *J. Cell. Physiol.* **83**:353–363.

Hölttä, E., 1975, Immunochemical demonstration of increased accumulation of ornithine decarboxylase in rat liver after partial hepatectomy and growth hormone induction, *Biochim. Biophys. Acta* **399**:420–427.

Imondi, A. R., Balis, M. E., and Lipkin, M., 1969, Changes in enzyme levels accompanying differentiation of intestinal epithelial cells, *Exp. Cell Res.* **58**:323–330.

Imondi, A. R., Lipkin, M., and Balis, M. E., 1970, Enzyme and template stability as regulatory mechanisms in differentiating intestinal epithelial cells, *J. Biol. Chem.* **245**:2194–2198.

Ishikawa, E., Ishikawa, S., Davis, J. W., and Sutherland, E. W., 1969, Determination of guanosine 3',5'-monophosphate in tissues and of guanyl cyclase in rat intestine, *J. Biol. Chem.* **244**:6371–6376.

Jänne, J., and Hölttä, E., 1973, Putrescine metabolizing enzyme activities in some rat tissues during postnatal development, *Acta Chem. Scand.* **27**:2399–2404.

Kanagalingam, K., and Balis, M. E., 1975, *In vivo* repair of rat intestinal DNA damage by alkylating agents, *Cancer* **36**:2364–2372.

Kim, Y. S., Perdomo, J., and Nordberg, J., 1971*a*, Glycoprotein biosynthesis in small intestinal mucosa, *J. Biol. Chem.* **246**:5466–5467.

Kim, Y. S., Perdomo, J., Bella, A., and Nordberg, J., 1971*a*, Glycoprotein biosynthesis in small intestinal mucosa, *J. Biol. Chem.* **246**:5466–5467.

Kim, Y. S., Perdomo, J., Bella, A., and Nordberg, J., 1971*b*, *N*-Acetyl-D-galactosaminyltransferase in human serum and erythrocyte membranes, *Proc. Natl. Acad. Sci. USA* **68:**1753–1756.

Kimura, H., and Murad, F., 1974, Evidence for two different forms of guanylate cyclase in rat heart, *J. Biol. Chem.* **249:**6910–6916.

Lipkin, M., 1973, Proliferation and differentiation of gastrointestinal cells, *Physiol. Rev.* **53:**891–915.

Lipkin, M., 1974, Phase 1 and phase 2 proliferative lesions of colonic epithelial cells in diseases leading to colonic cancer, *Cancer* **34:**878–888.

Moog, F., Vire, H. R., and Grey, R. D., 1966, The multiple forms of alkaline phosphatase in the small intestine of the young mouse, *Biochim. Biophys. Acta* **113:**336–349.

Moss, D. W., 1963, Heterogeneity of human intestinal alkaline phosphate, *Nature (London)* **200:**1206–1207.

Moss, D. W., 1965, Properties of alkaline phosphatase fractions in extracts of human small intestine, *Biochem. J.* **94:**458–462.

Nordstrom, C., Dahlqvist, A., and Josefsson, L., 1967, Quantitative determination of enzymes in different parts of the villi and crypts of rat small intestine, *J. Histochem. Cytochem.* **15:**713–721.

O'Brien, T. G., Simsiman, R. C., and Boutwell, R. K., 1975, Induction of the polyamine-biosynthetic enzymes in mouse epidermis by tumor-promoting agents, *Cancer Res.* **35:**1662–1670.

Perris, A. D., 1966, Isolation of the epithelial cells of the rat small intestine, *Can. J. Biochem.* **44:**687–693.

Pierce, N. F., Carpenter, C. C. J., Elliott, H. L., and Greenough, W. B., III, 1971, Effects of prostaglandins, theophylline, and cholera exotoxin upon transmucosal water and electrolyte movement in the canine jejunum, *Gastroenterology* **60:**22–32.

Russell, D. H., 1973*a*, in: *Polyamines in Normal and Neoplastic Growth* (D. H. Russell, ed.), p. 1, Raven Press, New York.

Russell, D. H. 1973*b*, Roles of the polyamines, putrescine, spermidine and spermine in normal and malignant tissues, *Life Sci.* **13:**1635–1647.

Russell, D. H., and Levy, C. C., 1971, Polyamine accumulation and biosynthesis in mouse L1210 leukemia, *Cancer Res.* **31:**248–251.

Russell, D. H., and Russell, S. D., 1975, Relative usefulness of measuring polyamines in serum, plasma, and urine as biochemical markers of cancer, *Clin. Chem.* **21:**860–863.

Russell, D. H., and Snyder, S. H., 1968, Amine synthesis in rapidly growing tissues: ODC activity in regenerating rat liver, chick embryo, and various tumors. *Proc. Natl. Acad. Sci. USA* **60:**1420–1427.

Russell, D. H., and Snyder, S. H., 1969, Amine synthesis in regenerating rat liver: Extremely rapid turnover of ornithing decarboxylase, *Mol. Pharmacol.* **5:**254–262.

Salser, J. S., and Balis, M. E., 1973, Distribution and regulation of deoxythymidine kinase activity in differentiating cells of mammalian intestines, *Cancer Res.* **33:**1889–1897.

Salser, J. S., and Balis, M. E., 1974, Enzymatic studies of normal and malignant intestinal epithelium, *Cancer* **34:**889–895.

Salser, J. S., and Balis, M. E., 1976, Fetal thymidine kinase in tumors and colonic flat mucosa of man, *Nature (London)* **260:**261–263.

Setlow, R. B., Regan, J. D., German, J., and Carrier, W. L., 1969, Evidence that xeroderma pigmentosum cells do not perform the first step in the repair of ultraviolet damage to their DNA, *Proc. Natl. Acad. Sci. USA* **64:**1035–1041.

Shafer, D. E., Lust, W. D., Sircar, B., and Goldberg, N. D., 1970, Elevated concentration of adenosine 3′,5′-cyclic monophosphate in intestinal mucosa after treatment with cholera toxin, *Proc. Natl. Acad. Sci. USA* **67:**851–856.

Stafford, M. A., and Jones, O. W., 1972, The presence of "fetal" thymidine kinase in human tumors, *Biochim. Biophys. Acta* **277:**439–442.

Takeda, Y., Tominaga, T., Kitamura, M., Taguchi, T., Takeda, T., and Miwatani, T., 1975, Urinary polyamines in patients with gastric cancer and their change after gastrectomy, *Gann* **66:**455–447.

Webster, H. L., and Harrison, D. D., 1969, Enzymic activities during the transformation of crypt to columnar intestinal cells, *Exp. Cell Res.* **56**:245–253.

Weiser, M. M., 1973*a*, Intestinal epithelial cell surface membrane glycoprotein synthesis. I. An indicator of cellular differentiation, *J. Biol. Chem.* **248**: 320–324.

Weiser, M. M., 1973*b*, Intestinal epithelial cell surface membrane synthesis, *J. Biol. Chem.* **248**:2536–2534.

Weiser, M. M., and Quill, H., 1975, Intestinal villus and crypt cell responses to cholera toxin, *Gastroenterology* **69**:479–482.

Williams-Ashman, H. G., Coppoc, G. L., and Weber, G., 1972, Imbalance in ornithine metabolism in hepatomas of different growth rates as expressed in formation of putrescine, spermidine, and spermine, *Cancer Res.* **32**:1924–1932.

21

Cancer in Inflammatory Bowel Disease: Risk Factors and Prospects for Early Detection

Paul Sherlock and Sidney J. Winawer

1. Introduction

Chronic inflammation or irritation has been considered responsible for the development of various cancers in man, although the etiology and mechanisms associated with the development of the neoplastic state have never been clarified. Examples include achalasia and lye strictures with carcinoma of the esophagus, atrophic gastritis with carcinoma of the stomach, cholelithiasis with cancer of the gallbladder, tobacco and alcohol with cancers of the oral cavity, *Clonorchis sinesis* infestation with cholangiocarcinoma, *Schistosoma haematobium* infestation with cancer of the urinary bladder, mucosal ulcerative colitis with carcinoma of the colon, and Crohn's disease with both carcinoma of the ileum and colon.

The purpose of this report is twofold: (1) to delineate risk factors thought to be responsible for the development of cancer superimposed on both ulcerative colitis and granulomatous colitis and (2) to consider some of the newer techniques which show promise in helping to diagnose superimposed cancer of the colon at the earliest possible time.

2. Ulcerative Colitis

Among chronic inflammatory states, ulcerative colitis is frequently associated with malignancy appearing at later times. The cancer usually origi-

Paul Sherlock and Sidney J. Winawer • Gastroenterology Service, Department of Medicine, Memorial Sloan-Kettering Cancer Center, New York, New York 10021, and Department of Medicine, Cornell University Medical College, New York, New York 10021.

nates in the epithelium, resulting in adenocarcinoma, but it may on rare occasions be of lymphoid origin (Cornes *et al.*, 1961). If ulcerative colitis is considered without reference to age at onset or duration of disease, there seems to be general agreement that the likelihood of carcinoma of the colon developing is between 3% and 5% (Edwards and Truelove, 1964; Morson, 1966), except in a recent study from continental Europe where no increase was noted (Binder *et al.*, 1973). If this figure is compared to the prevalence of cancer of the colon and rectum, the risk of malignant change in patients with ulcerative colitis is 5–10 times greater (Goldgraber and Kirsner, 1964). The risk of malignant change begins to rise after 10 years, with a more precipitous rise after 20 years, as high as 30% in some series. If ulcerative colitis has its onset before age 25, the risk of developing carcinoma may be doubled as compared to its development after age 25 (MacDougall, 1964). Michener *et al.* (1961) estimated that the chance of a child with chronic ulcerative colitis dying of carcinoma of the colon is 556 times that of a normal child.

Patients with colitis involving the entire colon are principally at risk for superimposed carcinoma. With only left-sided involvement the risk diminishes, and with localized proctosigmoiditis there may be no increased risk. Those who have had a clinically severe first attack and chronic continuous symptoms are also more likely to develop carcinoma. However, relative freedom from the symptoms of ulcerative colitis does not imply that cancer will not develop. There may be a symptom-free period for several years before the onset of cancer.

When cancer is superimposed on ulcerative colitis, it occurs at least one or more decades earlier than when it is not. The average age at onset of cancer superimposed on ulcerative colitis is 40–42 years. The cancer is more evenly distributed throughout the colon as compared to colorectal cancer without colitis. In ulcerative colitis, a significant percentage of tumors involve the transverse and right colon. The cancers are frequently multiple, colloid in type, infiltrating, and usually of a higher grade of malignancy than cancers of the colon arising in the general population without ulcerative colitis, perhaps accounting for the poor prognosis and rapid progression of the cancer usually reported for this group of patients (Morson, 1966). However, in series where lower grades of malignancy are present, 5-year survival may be as high as 75% (Hinton, 1966).

The poorer prognosis may be related to diagnostic difficulties, because symptoms of cancer of the colon may be similar to those of ulcerative colitis, and suspicious radiological findings are often difficult to evaluate in the presence of ulcerative colitis. Malignant polypoid change may look like pseudopolypoid areas which are almost never malignant, while strictures may be considered inflammatory but should be considered malignant until proven otherwise. In one series, six of 13 potentially diagnosable neoplastic lesions were missed radiographically because they were felt to be secondary to inflammatory change (Diaz *et al.*, 1965).

3. Granulomatous Bowel Disease

Granulomatous bowel disease (Crohn's disease) has not previously been considered a premalignant disorder. However, more cases are being reported with Crohn's disease of both small and large intestine associated with superimposed carcinoma. Carcinoma of the ileum is an extremely rare disease. When carcinoma does involve the small bowel in the general population without underlying Crohn's disease, it more often involves the proximal portion; when superimposed on Crohn's disease it more often involves the ileum in the area of the inflammatory involvement. The age at onset is about 15 years earlier than expected in the general population, and carcinoma has been seen in surgically bypassed segments of small intestine affected by Crohn's disease (Brown *et al.*, 1970).

Weedon *et al.* (1973), in agreement with findings of Perrett *et al.* (1968), demonstrated that patients with Crohn's disease of the large bowel have 20 times the risk of developing superimposed carcinoma of the large bowel. Most of the cancers were on the right side of the colon and most patients were under 40 years of age. We have reported the development of carcinoma in fistulous tracts associated with granulomatous colitis (Lightdale *et al.*, 1975). Since it appears that the association of cancer and granulomatous colitis is real, clinicians can no longer dismiss the possibility of a cancer risk in patients with this disease, and vigorous surveillance is needed just as in chronic mucosal ulcerative colitis.

4. Early Detection of Superimposed Cancer

Routine sigmoidoscopy, biopsy of suspicious lesions, and barium enema with air contrast are still important diagnostic techniques for following patients with colitis. Fiberoptic colonoscopy with direct brush cytology or lavage cytology is now being used to clarify suspicious areas, particularly strictures beyond reach of the standard sigmoidoscope. Exfoliative cytology is a vastly underutilized technique that may be very helpful in detecting *in situ* or early carcinoma of the colon in patients with ulcerative colitis, as it has in cervical cancer. Newer techniques of continued irrigation and lavage via the sigmoidoscope and colonoscope utilizing a pulsatile dental irrigating unit have made it possible to obtain samples for cytological analysis (Katz *et al.*, 1972) (Figs. 1 and 2).

Morson and Pang (1967) have suggested serial rectal biopsies for predicting which patients with universal ulcerative colitis for more than 10 years have cancer elsewhere in the colon. Random rectal biopsies were examined for precancer, which consisted of flattened rather than polypoid mucosa; stratified, hyperchromatic, and irregular nuclei with multiple mitotic figures; loss of parallelism; and lateral budding of the glands extending through the

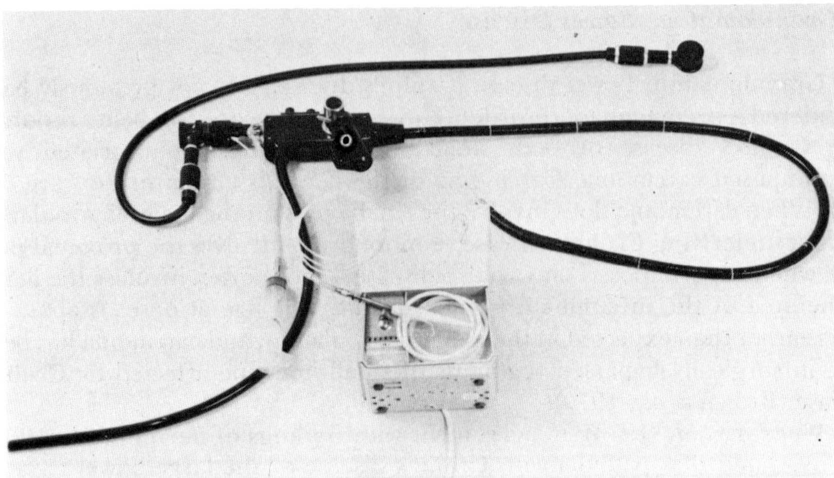

Fig. 1. Fiberoptic endoscope attached to pulsatile lavage apparatus (Water-pik) for obtaining exfoliative cytological specimens.

muscularis mucosa. When these patchy and diffuse changes were present in the rectum, about one-half of the patients had cancer elsewhere in the colon. Histological changes of precancer in conjunction with other factors such as duration and extent of disease and severity of symptoms may assist in selecting patients for colectomy. Not all pathologists agree, however, on which epithelial changes in the colon constitute precancer and have been cautious in

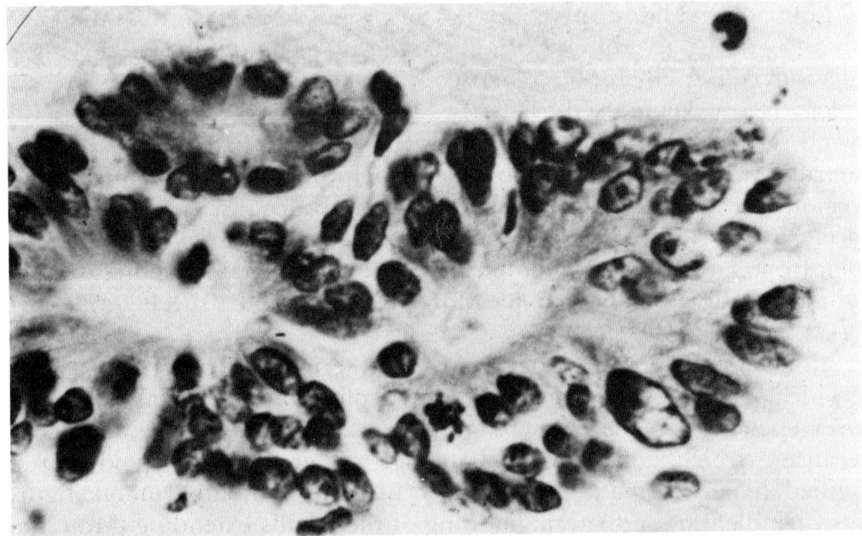

Fig. 2. Papanicolaou cytological preparation from a patient with chronic ulcerative colitis showing malignant cells having large nucleoli with coarsely granular chromatin. ×400.

making the diagnosis because of the problem of interpretation in the presence of severe inflammation.

In patients with precancer, lactic dehydrogenase (LDH) isoenzyme patterns of the rectal biopsies showed an increased ratio of LDH_4 and LDH_5 to LDH_1 and LDH_2. This increase in the isoenzyme ratio was highly significant in relation to both the control series and to the patients with ulcerative colitis who did not have rectal precancer (Lewis *et al.*, 1971). In another preliminary report a rare isoenzyme of alkaline phosphatase was identified in the serum of four patients with ulcerative colitis (Streifler *et al.*, 1972). This may have use as an indicator of the precancerous state but must be further evaluated. Assays of these or other tissue enzymes or enzymes in colonic secretions or washings may also be helpful. Certain lysosomal enzymes are elevated in tumors as compared to their normal counterpart tissue. This may be reflected in the secretion of the tumor tissue. For example, β-glucuronidase has been found to be elevated in vaginal washings from patients with cancer of the cervix (Muir and Valeris, 1969) and in the gastric juice in patients with cancer of the stomach (Kim and Plaut, 1965). One of the isoenzymes of the hydrolytic lysosomal enzyme arylsulfatase has been found to be elevated in cancer of the colon. Arylsulfatase was noted to be decreased in ulcerative colitis (Danovitch *et al.*, 1972). This suggests the potential value of enzyme determination if levels rise when superimposed carcinoma develops. Other enzyme abnormalities have been noted in neoplastic tissue, such as collagenase succinic dehydrogenase and cytochrome oxidase (Lesher *et al.*, 1973; Wattenberg, 1959). Collagenase activity was absent in rectal biopsies in 50 patients with carcinoma of the colon, compared to only four of 100 patients with minor anal conditions and three of 31 patients with inflammatory bowel disease (Lesher *et al.*, 1973).

Other biochemical measurements are being investigated in an attempt to detect early changes of colon cancer in ulcerative colitis. When normal colonic cells transform, a variety of abnormalities occur in nucleic acid metabolism and cell proliferation (Lipkin, 1973; Deschner *et al.*, 1963). The cells of precancerous colon lesions develop characteristics that enable them to continue to synthesize DNA and to proliferate. Metabolic pathways leading to continued DNA synthesis persist in these cells. The proliferative zone of rectocolonic epithelium normally is limited to the lower two-thirds of the crypt, but upward displacement of the proliferative zone develops (Deschner *et al.*, 1963). Eastwood and Trier (1973), using an *in vitro* organ culture analysis of ulcerative colitis biopsy specimens, observed labeled epithelial cells in the upper one-third of crypts and upward extension of the proliferative zone. Bleiberg *et al.* (1970) noted similar findings. Both studies indicated a larger percentage of labeled cells in the lower two-thirds of the crypt, suggesting increased proliferative activity. These findings are in conflict with those of Shorter *et al.* (1966), who described decreased epithelial cell proliferation in rectal mucosa in active ulcerative colitis.

Surface cells retrieved after pulsatile colonic lavage through the sigmoidoscope or colonoscope have demonstrated labeling with tritiated

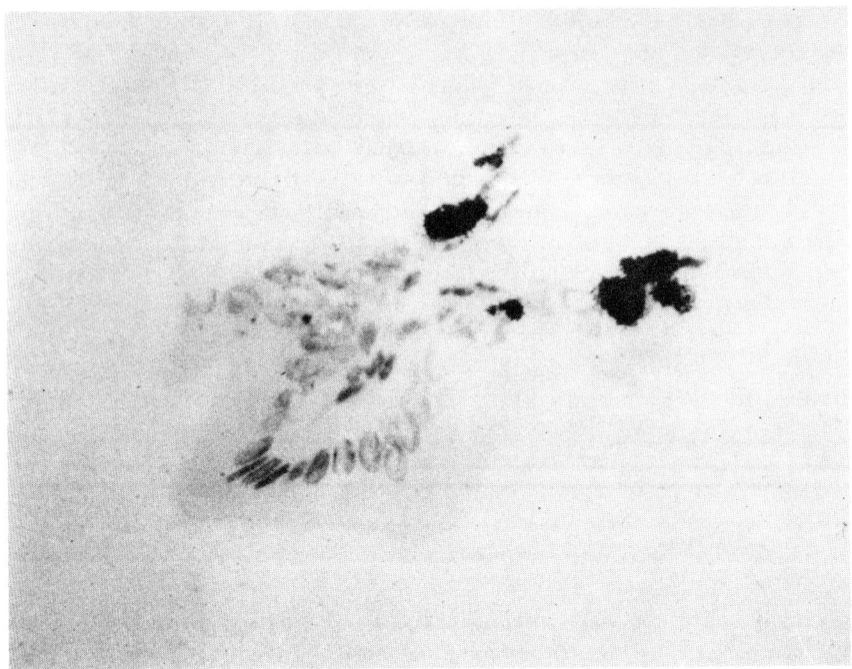

Fig. 3. Labeled nuclei in colon surface epithelial cells from colonic washings after *in vitro* incubation with tritiated thymidine (TdR^3H). ×250.

thymidine, thereby identifying an abnormal proliferative state (Deschner *et al.*, 1973) (Fig. 3). The utility of this technique in conjunction with other parameters is being studied in patients with chronic colitis to identify mucosal cells at risk.

Carcinoembryonic antigen (CEA) also is elevated in ulcerative colitis and in granulomatous bowel disease in 10–75% of various series, with the usual rate being about 30% (Dykes and King, 1972). More severe disease, more extensive anatomical involvement, a younger age, and shorter duration of disease are more likely to give elevation in CEA (Rule *et al.*, 1972), although this is not invariably so. There does not seem to be any consistent relationship between elevation in CEA and known risk factors for the development of carcinoma. In one series (Booth *et al.*, 1972) three patients had premalignant changes in the rectal mucosa similar to those noted by Morson and Pang (1967). One of these three patients had an elevated CEA level and two had normal levels. More studies are needed to correlate the CEA level with rectal mucosal biopsy. It would also be of interest to correlate CEA levels with LDH isoenzyme levels in the rectal mucosa which correlate with histological precancer changes (Lewis *et al.*, 1971).

Since patients with inflammatory bowel disease may have variations in levels of CEA during the course of their disease, following the CEA as an indicator of early superimposed carcinoma is not a helpful guide. Continued follow-up studies are needed to define the significance of these elevated levels.

The development of very sensitive radioimmunoassays has permitted the search for tumor antigens in other body fluids. CEA has been detected in the urine of a large percentage of patients with bladder carcinoma (Hall *et al.*, 1972) and in feces of patients with gastrointestinal cancer (Freed and Taylor, 1972). We have detected CEA in aspirated fluid following lavage of the colon with saline in patients with colon cancer and large colonic adenomas (Winawer *et al.*, 1974). Go *et al.* (1975), utilizing a technique of colon perfusion, have been able to determine CEA secretion in the human colon, suggesting the possibility of assaying CEA in patients with inflammatory bowel disease to determine whether the technique would be useful for the diagnosis of superimposed cancer (Molnar *et al.*, 1976).

Ulcerative colitis and Crohn's disease may both be in part genetically determined, probably on a multifactorial basis (Sherlock, 1967). Chromosomal abnormalities characterized principally by hyperploidy have been noted in carcinoma of the colon and in adenomatous polyps (Enterline and Arvan, 1967). Although chromosomal abnormalities are present, a consistent specific type of abnormality has not been reported. No chromosomal change comparable to the consistency of the Philadelphia chromosome in chronic granulocytic leukemia has been obtained.

A technique permitting direct cytogenetic studies of colon mucosa has been developed by Xavier *et al.* (1973) at the University of Chicago. The cellular material is collected via nylon brushing through a sigmoidoscope and processed in short-term cell culture for standard squash preparation. Profound abnormalities were demonstrated with carcinoma. In chronic ulcerative colitis, aneuploidy and chromatid breaks were seen in some patients with and without cancer. Further studies are needed to clarify whether this technique will have predictive value for the development of superimposed cancer in patients with inflammatory bowel disease.

Radioisotopic scanning may be used in attempting to diagnose colon cancer. Several interesting approaches are being investigated. Using a small Geiger counter through an open-tube sigmoidoscope following injection of ^{32}P, Nelson (1968) has demonstrated an overall accuracy of 88% in detecting cancer of the rectum. The procedure was particularly useful in diagnosing submucosal cancer, determining its extent, and selecting the best area for biopsy. The uptake of gallium-67 (^{67}Ga) was highest in biopsy specimens of undifferentiated carcinoma of the colon when compared to normal specimens (Nash *et al.*, 1972). Binding of radioactively tagged antibody to tumor antigen is in progress in several laboratories. Indium-111 is one isotope being investigated. Utilizing a tumor-bearing animal model, Goldenberg *et al.* (1974) have used isotope-scanning following the injection of iodine-125-tagged goat anti-CEA and have been able to localize the tumor. Further assessment of tumor scanning by all of these techniques seems indicated with the possibility that it may be a way of showing neoplastic change in patients with longstanding chronic ulcerative colitis.

Fluorescent and dye-binding endoscopic and cytological techniques utilizing tetracycline, declomycin, indigo carmine, atabrine, methylene blue, acridine orange, and hematoporphyrin should all be further investigated since previous information suggests that tumor can be localized. Much of the work in this area has been done with upper gastrointestinal tract tumors (Berk, 1967), and investigation along these lines is needed in the colon.

5. Conclusion

Prospects for improvement in survival from cancer superimposed on inflammatory bowel disease may depend on our advances in knowledge of biochemical and immunological alterations that occur in maligna cy. Intensive periodic selective investigation in these patients will make earlier diagnosis possible. The use of sigmoidoscopy, barium enema, rectal biopsy for histology, tissue enzymes and cytogenetics, colonoscopy, blood CEA and pulsatile lavage techniques for CEA in washings, cytology, fluorescent cytology, and enzymes and isotopic labeling offers promise for the future. If we are to salvage larger numbers of patients, very early diagnosis or diagnosis in the incipient stage of disease is needed.

6. References

Berk, J. E., 1967, Fluorescence techniques in the diagnosis of malignant lesions of the gastrointestinal tract, *Gastrointest. Endoscopy* **14:**102–105.

Binder, V., Bonnevic, O., Gertz, T., Krasilnikoff, P., Vestermock, S., Riis, P., 1972, Ulcerative colitis in children: Treatment, cause and prognosis, *Scand. J. Gastroenterol.* **8:**161–167.

Bleiberg, H., Mainguet, P., Galand, P., Chretian, J., and Dupont-Mairesse, N., 1970, Cell renewal in the human rectum: *In vitro* autoradiographic study on ulcerative colitis, *Gastroenterology* **58:**851–855.

Booth, S. N., King, J. P. G., Leonard, J. C., and Dykes, P. W., 1972, Serum carcinoembryonic antigen in clinical disorders, *Gut* **14:**794–799.

Brown, N., Weinstein, V. A., and Janowitz, H. D., 1970, Carcinoma of the ileum twenty-five years after by-pass for regional enteritis: A case report, *Mt. Sinai J. Med.* **37:**675–677.

Cornes, J. S., Smith, J. L., and Southwood, F. W., 1961, Lymphosarcoma in chronic ulcerative colitis, *Br. J. Surg.* **49:**50–53.

Danovitch, S. M., Galucci, A., and Shora, W., 1972, Colonic mucosal lysosomal enzyme activities in ulcerative colitis, *Am. J. Digest. Dis.* **17:**977–992.

Deschner, E. E., Lewis, C. M., and Lipkin, M., 1963, *In vitro* study of human rectal epithelial cells. I. Atypical zone of H^3 thymidine incorporation in mucosa of multiple polyposis, *J. Clin. Invest.* **42:**1922–1928.

Deschner, E. E., Long, F. C., and Katz, S., 1973, Autoradiographic method for an expanded assessment of colonic cytology, *Acta Cytol.* **17:**435–438.

Diaz, R. J., Farmer, R. G., and Brown, C. H., 1965, Carcinoma of the colon and ulcerative colitis, *Am. J. Digest. Dis.* **10:**643–656.

Dykes, P. W., and King, J., 1972, Progress report: Carcinoembryonic antigen, *Gut* **13:**1000–1013.

Eastwood, G. L., and Trier, S., 1973, Epithelial cell renewal in cultured rectal biopsies in ulcerative colitis, *Gastroenterology* **64:**383–390.

Edwards, F. C., and Truelove, S. C., 1964, Course and prognosis of ulcerative colitis. IV. Carcinoma of the colon, *Gut* **5:**15–22.

Enterline, H. T., and Arvan, D. A., 1967, Chromosome constitution of adenoma and adenocarcinoma of the colon, *Cancer* **20**:1746–1759.

Freed, D. L. G., and Taylor, G., 1972, Carcinoembryonic antigen in faeces, *Br. Med. J.* **1**:85–87.

Go, V. L. W., Ammon, H. V., Holtermuller, K. H., Krag, E., and Phillips, S. F., 1975, Quantification of carcinoembryonic antigen-like activities in normal human gastrointestinal secretions, *Cancer* **36**:2346–2350.

Goldenberg, D. M., Preston, D. F., Primus, F. J., *et al.*, 1974, Photoscan localization of GW-39 tumors in hamsters using radiolabeled anticarcinoembryonic antigen immunoglobulin G, *Cancer Res.* **34**:1–9.

Goldgraber, M. B., and Kirsner, J. B., 1964, Carcinoma of the colon in ulcerative colitis, *Cancer* **17**:657–665.

Hall, R. A., Lawrence, D. J. R., Darey, D., Stevens, U., James, R., Roberts, S., and Munro, N. A., 1972, Carcinoembryonic antigen in the urine of patients with urothelial carcinoma, *Br. Med. J.* **3**:604–611.

Hinton, J. M., 1966, Risk of malignant change in ulcerative colitis, *Gut* **7**:427–432.

Katz, S., Sherlock, P., and Winawer, S. J., 1972, Rectocolonic exfoliative cytology: A new approach, *Am. J. Digest. Dis.* **17**:1109–1116.

Kim, Y. S., and Plaut, A. G., 1965, β-Glucuronidase activity of gastric secretion from patients with gastric cancer, *Gastroenterology* **49**:50–57.

Lesher, T., Dilwari, J. B., and Hawley, P. R., 1973, Comparison between collagenase activity in rectal biopsies and plasma carcinoembryonic antigen (CEA) levels in patients with carcinoma of the colon and rectum (abstr.), *Gut* **14**:819.

Lewis, B., Morson, B. C., February, A. W., Jones, H. J., and Misiewicz, J. J., 1971, Abnormal lactic dehydrogenase isoenzyme patterns in ulcerative colitis with precancerous change, *Gut* **12**:16–19.

Lightdale, C. J., Sternberg, S. S., Posner, G., and Sherlock, P., 1975, Carcinoma complicating Crohn's disease: Report of seven cases and review of the literature, *Am. J. Med.* **59**:262–268.

Lipkin, M., 1973, Proliferation and differentiation of gastrointestinal cells, *Physiol. Rev.* **53**:891–915.

MacDougall, I. P. M., 1964, The cancer risk in ulcerative colitis, *Lancet* **2**:655–658.

Michener, W. M., Gage, R. P., Sauer, W. G., and Stickler, G. B., 1961, Prognosis of chronic ulcerative colitis in children, *N. Eng. J. Med.* **265**:1075–1079.

Molnar, I. G., Vandevoorde, J. P., and Gitnick, G. L., 1976, CEA levels in fluids bathing gastrointestinal tumors, *Gastroenterology* **70**:513–515.

Morson, B. C., 1966, Cancer in ulcerative colitis, *Gut* **7**:425–426.

Morson, B. C., and Pang, L. S. C., 1967, Rectal biopsy as an aid to cancer control in ulcerative colitis, *Gut* **8**:423–434.

Muir, G. G., and Valeris, G., 1969, Vaginal fluid enzyme pattern in benign and malignant lesions of the female genital tract, *J. Clin. Pathol.* **22**:593–597.

Nash, A. G., Dance, D. K., Macready, V. R., and Griffiths, J. D., 1972, Uptake of gallium-67 in colonic and rectal tumors, *Br. Med. J.* **3**:508–510.

Nelson, R. S., 1968, The detection of malignant neoplasms of the gastrointestinal tract by the use of radioactive phosphorus (^{32}P) and a miniature Geiger tube, *Gastrointest. Endoscopy* **15**:18–23.

Perrett, A. D., Truelove, S. C., and Massarella, G. R., 1968, Crohn's disease and carcinoma of the colon, *Br. Med. J.* **2**:466–468.

Rule, A. H., Goleski-Reilly, C., Sachar, D. B., Vandevoorde, J., and Janowitz, H. D., 1972, Circulating carcinoembryonic antigen (CEA): Relationship to clinical status of patients with inflammatory bowel disease, *Gut* **14**:880–884.

Sherlock, P., 1967, Genetics and gastrointestinal disease, *Gastroenterology* **53**:675–677.

Shorter, R. G., Spencer, R. J., and Hallenbeck, G. A., 1966, Kinetic studies of the epithelial cells of the rectal mucosa in normal subjects and in patients with ulcerative colitis, *Gut* **7**:593–596.

Streifler, C., Schnitzer, N., and Harell, A., 1972, A rare isoenzyme of alkaline phosphatase in 4 patients with ulcerative colitis, *Clin. Chim. Acta* **38**:244–246.

Wattenberg, L. W., 1959, A histochemical study of five oxidative enzymes in carcinoma of the large intestine in man, *Am. J. Pathol.* **35**:113–126.

Weedon, D. D., Shorter, R. G., Ilstrup, D. M., Huizenga, K. A., and Taylor, W. F., 1973, Crohn's disease and cancer, *N. Eng. J. Med.* **289:**1099–1103.

Winawer, S. J., Fleisher, M., Melamed, M., Sherlock, P., Deschner, E. E., and Schwartz, M. K., 1974, Cytological, immunological (CEA) and isotope labeling studies based on gastrointestinal endoscopic lavage (abstr.), *Gastroenterology* **66:**800.

Xavier, R. G., Prolla, J. C., Bemvenuti, G. A., and Kirsner, J. B., 1973, Further tissue cytogenic studies in inflammatory bowel disease (abstr.), *Gastroenterology* **64:**875.

22

Cytopathology of Human Gastrointestinal Cancers

Steven I. Hajdu

1. Introduction

Since the development of Papanicolaou's technique for cytological examination of vaginal smears for the diagnosis of uterine carcinoma, exfoliative cytological techniques have been successfully employed for the detection of uterine, pulmonary, and genitourinary tumors. Exfoliative cytological techniques can be applied to gastrointestinal tumors with more or less similar results to those for other anatomical sites (Ackerman, 1967; Brandborg and Wenger, 1968; Lemon, 1952; Raskin *et al.*, 1959; Rubin *et al.*, 1953; Sherlock *et al.*, 1972; Winawer *et al.*, 1976; Witte, 1970; Yamakawa *et al.*, 1971; Yoshii *et al.*, 1970, 1971).

Beale, in London, in 1858 was probably the first to perform microscopic examination of gastric secretion for the detection of gastric carcinoma (Hajdu and Hajdu, 1976). Marini, in Bologna, in 1909 introduced gastric lavage to obtain well-preserved neoplastic cells. By using a gastric tube and an alkaline solution to wash the stomach, he successfully demonstrated malignant cells in 32 of 37 gastric and esophageal carcinomas. The first report of using saline lavage and staining of smears of gastric washings for the detection of malignant cells was made by Loeper and Binet, in Paris, in 1911. Lyon, in 1919, extended the use of the gastric tube to the collection of biliary secretion, and Lemon and Byrnes, in 1949, collected duodenal secretion for cytological examination. The introduction of the fiberoptic gastroscope by Hirschowitz *et al.*, in 1958, and the first successful application of the direct-vision fibergastroscope for cytological examination by Kasugai and Kameya signified the

Steven I. Hajdu • Attending Pathologist, Memorial Sloan-Kettering Cancer Center, New York, New York 10021, and Associate Professor of Pathology, Cornell University Medical College, New York, New York 10021.

beginning of a new chapter in the history of gastroenterology (Kasugai, 1968). Complete integration of direct-vision fiberendoscopy and cytological techniques now appears to be the best approach to the examination of the esophagus, stomach, duodenum, and colon (Benvenuti *et al.*, 1975; Fukuda *et al.*, 1967; Kobayashi *et al.*, 1970; MacKenzie and Miller, 1949; Spjut *et al.*, 1963).

The most difficult step in gastrointestinal cytology is the collection of an adequate number of well-preserved cells for cytological examination.

All of the available techniques—including lavage, the abrasive and rotating balloon, various brushes, flexible scope, fiberscope, Water-pic, and enzymatic studies—are designed to obtain an adequate number of well-preserved cells for cytological examination. In obtaining satisfactory specimens, however, the actual technique used is less important than the care taken in the preparation of the patient and the promptness with which the specimen is processed to prevent degeneration and enzymatic digestion of the cells (Knoerschild *et al.*, 1961; Dreiling *et al.*, 1960; McNeer and Ewing, 1949, Simon and Caussade, 1914; Spjut *et al.*, 1963). It is beyond the scope of this chapter to describe the various collecting techniques. Interested readers are referred to published reports on the subject.

Once the material for cytological examination is obtained, it is of utmost important that it be properly fixed. After proper fixation, smears are prepared and stained according to the Papanicolaou technique (Hajdu and Hajdu, 1976).

Any material that remains in the bottom of the centrifuge tube after the smears have been prepared is processed for examination as a cell block (Hajdu and Hajdu, 1976).

2. *Papanicolaou Stain for Cytological Smears*

Solutions:

Formula for EA 65:

1. Eosin Y .... 10 g
2. Bismark Brown Y .... 10 g
3. Light Green SF .... 10 g
4. Distilled water .... 300 ml
5. 95% alcohol .... 2000 ml
6. Phosphotungstic acid .... 4 g
7. Saturated lithium carbonate solution (in distilled water) 20 drops

1. Stock Solution No. 1

Prepare separate 10% solutions of each of the stains as follows:

A. 10 g Eosin Y in 100 ml distilled water.

B. 10 g Bismark Brown Y in 100 ml distilled water.
C. 10 g Light Green SF in 100 ml distilled water.
2. MIX: (for 2000 ml of stain).
A. 45 ml Eosin Y stock No. 1.
B. 10 ml Bismark Brown Y stock No. 1.
C. 4.5 ml Light Green SF stock No. 1.
3. Take mixture up to 2000 ml with 85% alcohol.
4. ADD:
A. 4 g phosphotungstic acid.
B. 20 drops saturated lithium carbonate solution.
5. Mix well. Store solution in dark-brown stoppered bottles.

FOR USE: Use full strength, filter before using.

Formula for OG 6:

1. Orange G crystals .... 10 g
2. Distilled water .... 100 ml
3. 95% alcohol .... 1000 ml
4. Phosphotungstic acid .... 0.16 g

Procedure:

I. Stock solution No. 1
Prepare 10% aqueous solution as follows:
1. 10 g Orange G crystals in 100 ml distilled water.
2. Shake well and allow to stand for 1 week before using.

II. Stock solution No. 2
Orange G (0.5% solution) 50 ml stock solution No. 1 up to 1000 ml with 95% alcohol.

III. Final solution for 1000 ml stain
1. 1000 ml stock solution No. 2.
2. 0.15 g phosphotungstic acid.

IV. Mix well. Store in dark-brown stoppered bottles.

FOR USE: Use full strength, filter before using.

Formula for Hematoxylin Stain:

1. Hematoxylin .... 8 g
2. 95% alcohol .... 80 ml
3. Aluminium ammonium sulfate .... 160 g
4. Distilled water .... 600 ml

Procedure:

1. Dissolve aluminum ammonium sulfate in distilled water by heating.
2. Dissolve hematoxylin crystals in 95% alcohol.

3. Add hematoxylin solution to sulfate solution.
4. Bring mixture to 95°C.
5. Remove from flame and slowly add the mercuric oxide while stirring.
6. Immediately plunge into cold water bath.
7. When cool, filter.

FOR USE: Dilute with an equal part of distilled water, and filter again.

Procedure:

1.	80% ethyl alcohol	5 dips
2.	70% ethyl alcohol	5 dips
3.	50% ethyl alcohol	5 dips
4.	Distilled water	a few dips
5.	Harris's hematoxylin (without acetic acid)	5 min
6.	Distilled water	a few dips
7.	0.5% aqueous solution of HC1	5 dips
8.	Tap water	5 min
9.	50% ethyl alcohol	5 min
10.	70% ethyl alcohol	5 dips
11.	80% ethyl alcohol	5 dips
12.	95% ethyl alcohol	5 dips
13.	Orange G	2 min
14.	95% ethyl alcohol	5 dips
15.	95% ethyl alcohol	5 dips
16.	EA 65	2 min
17–19.	95% ethyl alcohol (3 changes)	5 dips in each
20–21.	Absolute ethyl alcohol (2 changes)	5 dips in each
22.	Equal parts of absolute ethyl alcohol and xylol	5 dips
23–26.	Xylol (4 changes)	5 dips in each

3. Processing and Staining of Cell Blocks

Neutral Buffered Formalin Solution:

1. 40% formalin .... 100 ml
2. Distilled water .... 900 ml
3. Sodium phosphate monobasic, monohydrate .... 4 g
4. Sodium phosphate dibasic, anhydrous .... 6 g

Processing of Cell Blocks:

1.	10% buffered formalin	1 hr
2.	10% buffered formalin	1 hr
3.	10% buffered formalin	1 hr
4.	95% ethyl alcohol	30 min
5.	95% ethyl alcohol	30 min
6.	100% ethyl alcohol	1 hr

7. 100% ethyl alcohol	1 hr
8. 100% ethyl alcohol	1 hr
9. Xylene	1 hr
10. Xylene	1 hr
11. Paraffin	1 hr
12. Paraffin	2 hr

Hematoxylin and Eosin Stain for Cell Block Sections:

Harris's hematoxylin solution (see Papanicolaou)

Eosin Solution:

Eosin Y	16 g
Potassium dichromate	8 g
Picric acid (saturated aqueous)	160 ml
95% ethyl alcohol	1280 ml

Procedure:

1. Xylene	5 min
2. Xylene	5 min
3. Absolute ethyl alcohol	5 dips
4. Absolute ethyl alcohol	5 dips
5. 95% ethyl alcohol	5 dips
6. 80% ethyl alcohol	5 dips
7. 70% ethyl alcohol	5 dips
8. Distilled water	5 dips
9. Harris's hematoyxlin	5 min
10. Tap water	5–10 dips
11. 70% ethyl alcohol	5–10 dips
12. Acid-alcohol	Until red
13. Tap water	5–10 dips
14. 70% ethyl alcohol	5–10 dips
15. Ammonia water	1 min
16. Tap water	5–10 dips
17. 50% ethyl alcohol	5–10 dips
18. Eosin	2 min
19. Tap water	5–10 dips
20. 95% ethyl alcohol	5 dips
21. 95% ethyl alcohol	5 dips
22. Absolute ethyl alcohol	5 dips
23. Absolute ethyl alcohol	5 dips
24. Xylene	5 dips
25. Xylene	5 dips
26. Xylene	5 dips
27. Mount in Permount.	

The value of cytological examination is best summarized by saying that malignant cells, in general, are not recovered from organs which are otherwise normal. Gastrointestinal cytological examination is no more difficult than that of other areas (Anthonisen and Riis, 1962; Belladonna *et al.*, 1974; Bowden and Papanicolaou, 1960; Winawer, *et al.*, 1976; Yoshii *et al.*, 1970). In experienced hands the highest positive yield (90%) should be expected in gastroesophageal malignant tumors (Gephart and Graham, 1959; Graham and Rheault, 1954; Winawer *et al.*, 1975). Malignant tumors of the colon and rectum may be identified by cytological techniques in about 80% of cases (Burn, 1961; Cameron, 1906; Heindenreich, 1961; Knoerschild and Cameron, 1963), and approximately 50% of pancreatobiliary tumors should be expected to exfoliate identifiable tumor cells (Bowden and Papanicolaou, 1960; Goldstein and Ventzke, 1968; Rosen *et al.*, 1968). Present techniques may fail to detect intramural tumors without mucosal invasion or ulcerated necrotic tumors with an overlying fibrin coat. There are several gastrointestinal lesions which may exfoliate bizarre cells and result in false-positive cytology (Boddington and Truelove, 1956; Boen, 1957; Enas *et al.*, 1972; Gardner, 1956). However, there are several well-documented so-called false-positive cytological cases which turned out later to be confirmed malignant neoplasms that were not detectable clinically (Kasugai, 1968; Katz *et al.*, 1972; Winawer *et al.*, 1974*b*).

The morphology of individual cells is not significantly altered by the technique used to obtain the specimen. The pertinent nuclear and cytoplasmic features which characterize exfoliated cells of carcinomas are summarized in Table 1. However, there is some variation in these criteria according to anatomical site and histological type of tumor.

The photomicrographs in this chapter were prepared from material obtained from various anatomical sites by the use of either the lavage or the brush technique.

Table 1. Cytological Criteria of Exfoliated Tumor Cells of Malignant Epithelial Gastrointestinal Tumors

Nuclear morphology
Hyperchromasia and abnormal clumping of chromatin
Pleomorphism and enlargement
Binucleation or multinucleation
Prominent nucleoli
Abnormal mitosis
Naked nuclei
Cytoplasmic morphology
Anisocytosis and enlargement
Cannibalism and inclusions
Intracytoplasmic vacuoles
Loss of cytoplasm
Loss of cytoplasmic cohesion
Change in color

4. Esophagus

Since even with improved therapeutic techniques there is little hope for survival with deeply invasive and metastatic esophageal carcinoma, earlier diagnosis at the *in situ* stage of the disease should be employed more. Esophageal washings have proven valuable in the diagnosis of such early lesions. There are a number of case reports in the literature documenting the value of cytological examination in the detection of suspected lesions when other diagnostic methods failed (Table 2).

The various techniques available to obtain diagnostic cytologic material from the esophagus require little equipment or preparation (Anthonisen and Riis, 1962; Cameron and Hajdu, 1977; Johnson *et al.*, 1955).

The majority of malignant tumors of the esophagus are epidermoid carcinomas. Cytologically, there are two distinct forms: well-differentiated (keratinizing squamous) carcinoma and poorly differentiated epidermoid carcinoma.

As a rule, well-differentiated epidermoid carcinomas exfoliate a large number of polygonal tumor cells. The nuclei are either pyknotic round or oval or elongated spindly. Occasionally, long "fiber cells" with elongated slender cytoplasm and darkly staining nuclei are intermixed with less well-differentiated, fairly uniform round or oval epidermoid cells. Keratotic epithelial pearls are seen only occasionally.

Poorly differentiated epidermoid tumor cells can be differentiated from malignant glandular epithelial cells only with great difficulty. Spreads of these round or oval cells, however, often contain occasional squamous-looking cells, which suggests the true identity of the poorly differentiated or undifferentiated cells. Both well-differentiated and poorly differentiated forms are found either singly or in loosely arranged clusters. Because of frequent erosion or ulceration of the tumor or adjacent squamous mucosa, the background of smears contains various amounts of inflammatory and reactive cells. It is not uncommon in bronchoesophageal fistula to find ciliated bronchial epithelial cells in smears prepared from esophageal washings.

Malignant tumors other than epidermoid carcinoma are quite uncommon. Most adenocarcinomas are located in the lower third of the esophagus, and they are often extensions of gastric adenocarcinoma rather than true primary neoplasms of the esophagus. Leiomyosarcoma is a rare primary neoplasm of the esophagus and does not exfoliate tumor cells readily. Malignant lymphoma, malignant melanoma, malignant thymoma, and car-

Table 2. Comparison of the Diagnostic Value of Tissue Biopsy vs. Cytological Examination in 30 Consecutive Cases of Esophageal Carcinoma

	Number of patients with positive findings
Tissue biopsy	20/30 (66%)
Cytological examination	29/30 (97%)

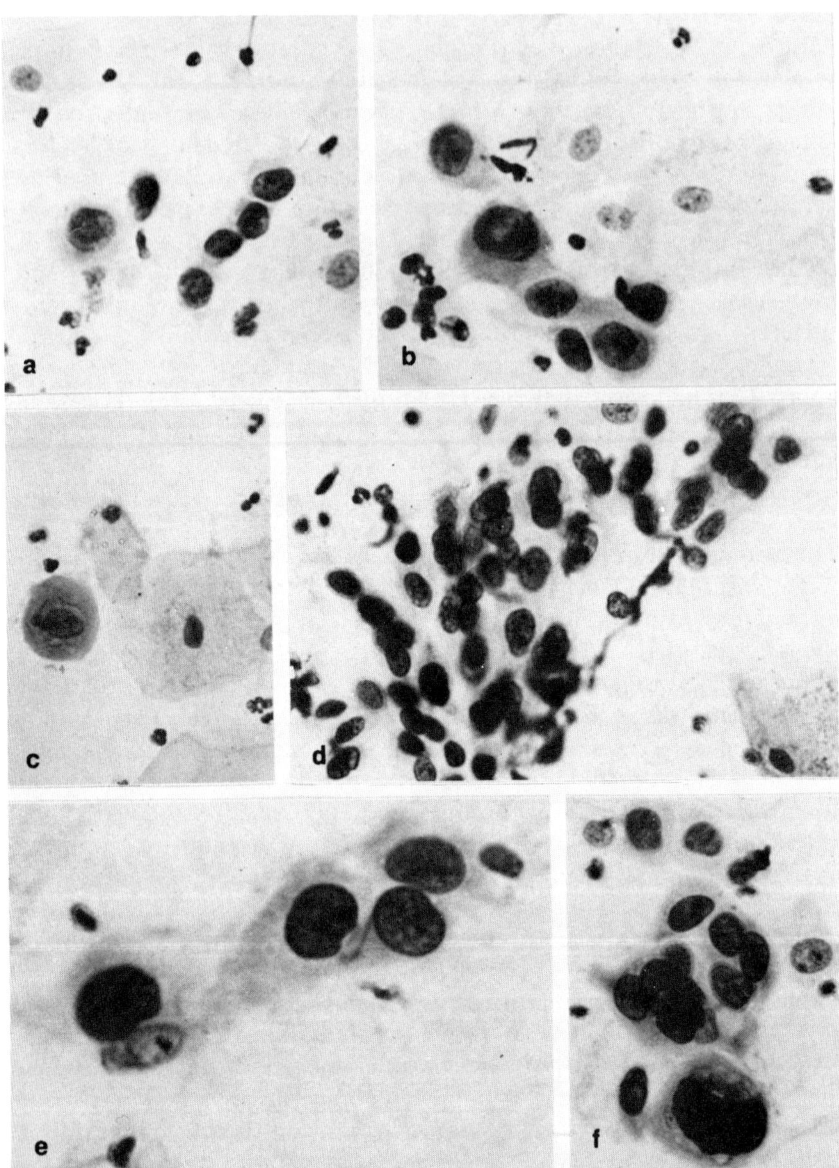

Fig. 1. Esophageal cytology. (a,b) Poorly differentiated malignant epithelial cells in esophageal washing. Note marked cohesion of the neoplastic cells. (c) Solitary keratinizing squamous cell adjacent to benign squamous epithelial cells. (d) Smear prepared from brushing of distal esophagus showing a cluster of undifferentiated benign epithelial cells from an ulcerated area. (e,f) Epidermoid carcinoma of the esophagus. These clusters of malignant cells are in smears prepared from a brush specimen. Note that the tumor cells in brush smears appear larger than the neoplastic cells in lavage specimens. Papanicolaou, ×570.

cinoma of the lung and larynx may all involve the esophagus occasionally (Messelt, 1960; Prolla *et al.,* 1965; Winawer *et al.*, 1975).

Bizarre mononuclear round cells, reparative epithelial cells, mimicking poorly differentiated neoplastic cells may exfoliate in esophagitis. A large number of inflammatory cells and occasional multinucleated histiocytic forms are considered suggestive of a benign rather than a malignant lesion (Fig. 1).

5. Stomach

It has been shown by several investigators that exfoliative cytology is more accurate than roentgenography or gastroscopy in determining whether a gastric lesion is benign or malignant (Benvenuti *et al.*, 1975; Foushee *et al.*, 1969; Papanicolaou and Cooper, 1947; Prolla *et al.*, 1969, 1970; Raskin *et al.*, 1959; Winawer *et al.*, 1976). A disturbing feature of gastric cytology is the occasional failure to obtain malignant cells from large fungating or ulcerating carcinomas. These lesions may cause obstruction or are frequently covered with a heavy lining of fibrin at the site of erosion and ulceration which prevents exfoliation of tumor cells (Ayre and Oren, 1953; Katz *et al.*, 1972; Prolla *et al.*, 1969; Seyboet *et al.*, 1951) (Table 3).

The vast majority of malignant gastric neoplasms are adenocarcinomas. Histologically, there are several types, ranging from well differentiated to poorly differentiated.

Well-differentiated tumor cells exfoliate readily in loose clusters. These are larger than normal gastric cells and contain prominent round or oval nuclei. The nuclei are often displaced to one side of the cytoplasm. Intrachytoplasmic vacuoles are demonstrable with mucicarmine stain (Fig. 2).

Tumor cells from poorly differentiated adenocarcinomas exfoliate in sheets, loose clusters, or singly. They are about the size of normal gastric cells, but their polymorphic, often bizarre nuclei make them easily identifiable. The most typical form of these undifferentiated cells is the signet-ring cell. This cell type contains solitary cytoplasmic vacuoles which often completely fill the cytoplasm and the periphery of the cell. The identification of signet-ring cells is important because they indicate the presence of an undifferentiated, commonly diffusely growing, linitis plastica type of tumor. Despite the relatively nonprominent nuclei of poorly differentiated carcinomas, the nucleoli are prominent. The cytoplasm can be very scanty in some cells and quite abundant in others. Single tumor cells and occasionally naked nuclei are invariably present, but most of the tumor cells are in sheets, glands, or clusters. The

Table 3. Positive Brush Cytology in 60 Patients with Gastric Adenocarcinoma

	Number of patients with positive findings
Adenocarcinoma, exophytic	24/26 (92%)
Adenocarcinoma, infiltrative	12/24 (50%)

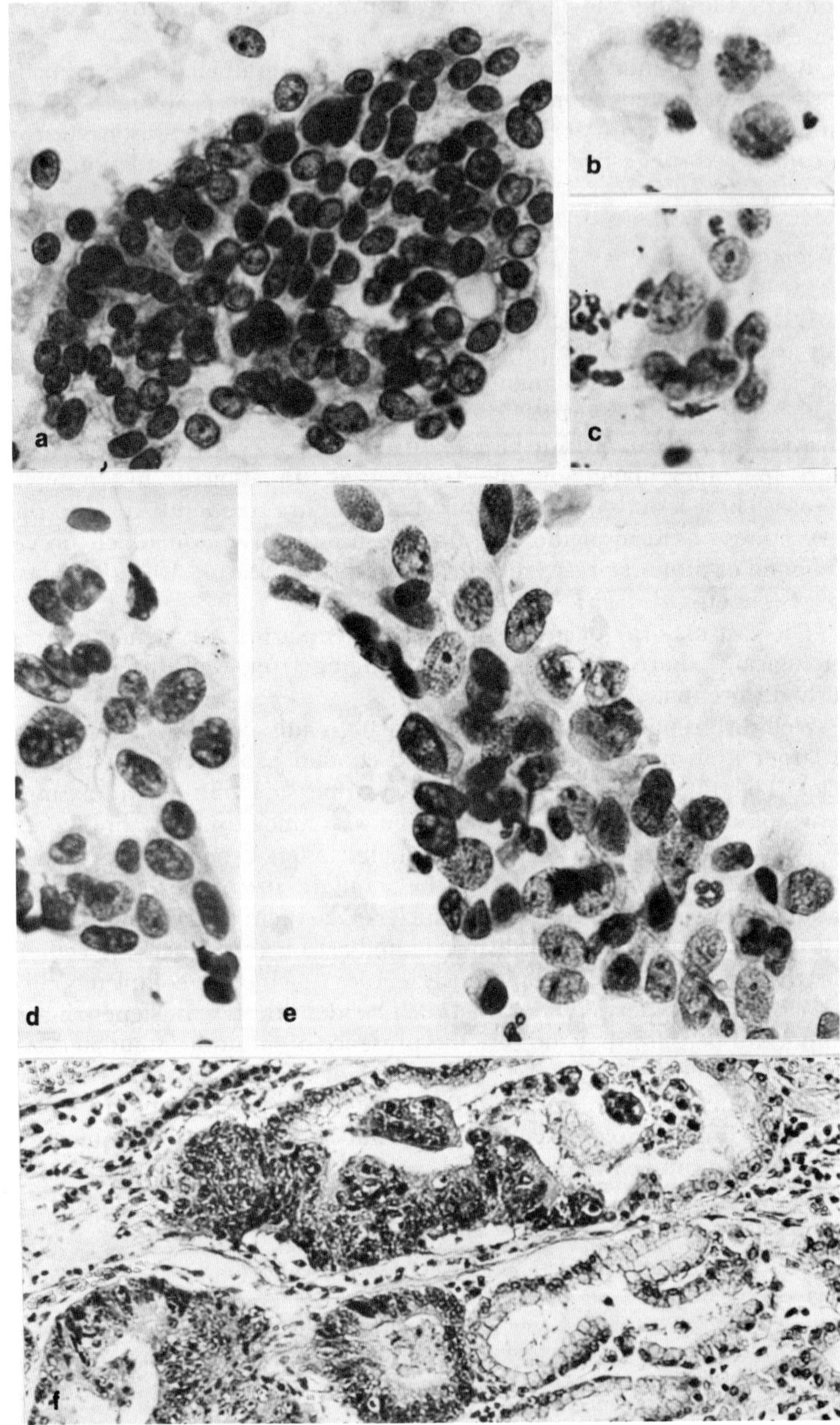
a
b
c
d
e
f

cohesive tendency of gastric epithelial cells makes it relatively easy to differentiate epithelial and lymphoreticular neoplasms in smears.

Cohesiveness of epithelial cells is especially preserved in smears prepared from material obtained by brush. In heavy and hypercellular clusters the preservation of the cells may be extremely poor. Technically poor fixation often results in enlargement and polymorphic distortion of the cells, and completely benign gastric epithelial cells may look atypical or neoplastic to the unexperienced cytologist. It is important in the evaluation of smears prepared from brush specimens that screeners and cytologists focus their attention on cells bordering cell clusters, cells in pairs, small groups of cells, and single cells.

Malignant lymphomas, particularly non-Hodgkin types, primary or metastatic, commonly involve the stomach. We and others (Katz *et al.*, 1972; Klayman *et al.*, 1955; Nelson and Lanza, 1974; Prolla *et al.*, 1970; Rubin and Massey, 1954) found cytological examination more rewarding in specific identification of malignant lymphomas than tissue biopsy. Tumor cells of lymphoreticular tumors do not have cytoplasmic cohesion; therefore, there is no cluster or sheet formation. Occasionally one may see exfoliated cells from primary leiomyosarcoma or leiomyoblastoma (Hajdu *et al.*, 1972) or extrinsic tumors such as malignant melanoma (Reed *et al.*, 1962), mammary carcinoma (Klein and Sherlock, 1972), and pancreatic carcinoma in gastric washing. The tumor cell morphologogy is similar to the well-known cytological morphology of identical tumors in malignant effusions.

Atrophic gastritis may exfoliate a significant number of pale, poorly preserved, so-called bland cells. Large numbers of inflammatory cells, lymphocytes and polymorphonuclear leukocytes, are present as a rule in this and other granulomatous (tuberculosis, sarcoidosis, syphilis, chronic peptic ulcer) diseases in the background of the smear (Bennington *et al.*, 1968; Hemmeter, 1889; Katz *et al.*, 1972; Winawer *et al.*, 1974*b*). Gastric washings in peptic ulcer and pernicious anemia in addition to various amounts of inflammatory cells may contain atypical, somewhat enlarged gastric epithelial cells (Boen, 1957; Graham and Rheault, 1954; Katz *et al.*, 1972; Papanicolaou and Cooper, 1947; Prolla *et al.*, 1970). Again, evaluation by experienced cytologists of the smear as a whole, epithelial as well as reactive elements, should guarantee proper identification (Fig. 3).

Fig. 2. Gastric cytology. (a) Benign gastric epithelial cells from a brush specimen. The cells are uniform with minute cytoplasm in a cohesive arranged pattern. (b,c) Tumor cells of adenocarcinoma of the stomach from gastric washing. These are hyperchromatic, somewhat pleomorphic cells with prominent nucleoli and poorly preserved cytoplasm. (d,e) Adenocarcinoma of the stomach in brush smears. Note that only occasional cells in the clusters show malignant features. (f) Admixture of benign and malignant epithelial cells in cytological specimens. This is occasionally due to side-by-side arrangement of benign and malignant glands in the area of the neoplasm or partial replacement of benign gastric epithelium by neoplastic cells, as is seen in this tissue section. (a–e) Papanicolaou, ×570; (f) hematoxylin and eosin, ×200.

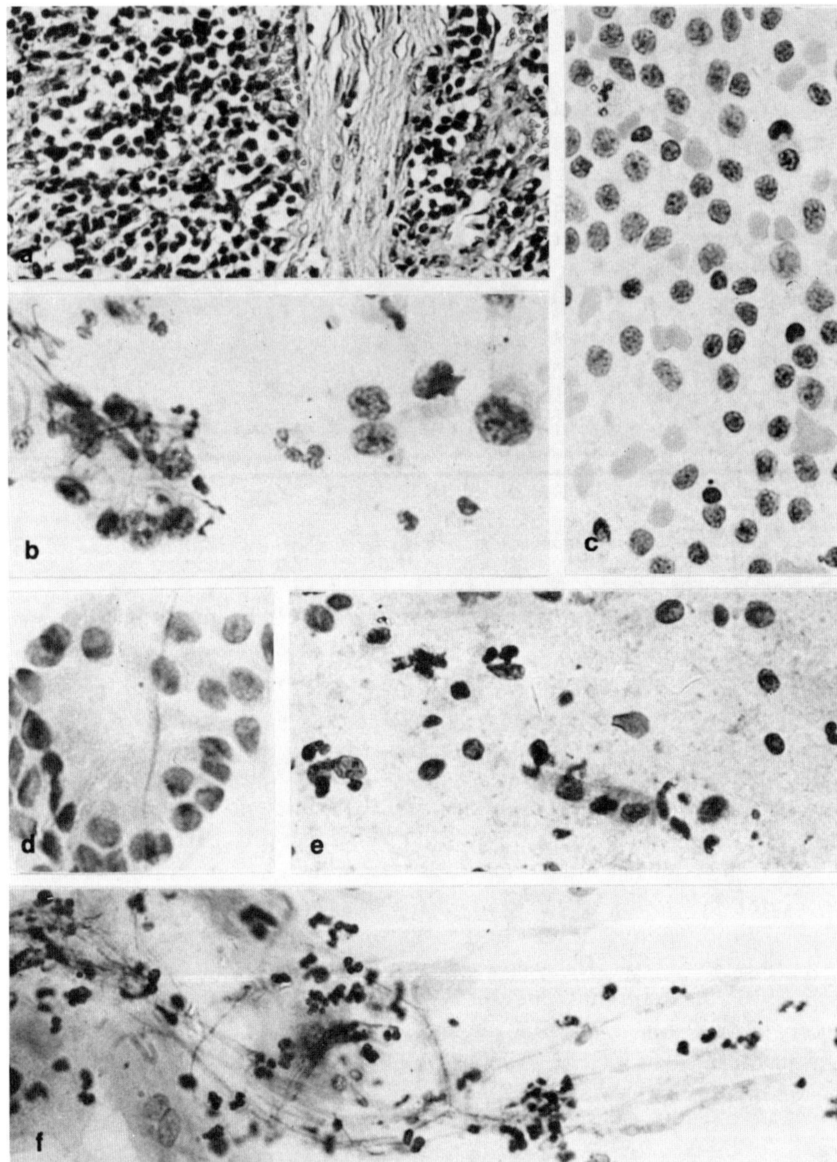

Fig. 3. Gastric cytology. (a) Tissue section of a poorly differentiated gastric adenocarcinoma. It is difficult to be certain whether this is an epithelial or a lymphoreticular neoplasm. (b) Smear prepared from gastric washing of the tumor illustrated in (a) clearly showing malignant glandular epithelial cells. (c) Isolated atypical lymphocytes in gastric washing of a gastric lymphoma. The cells are single, without cytoplasmic cohesion, which is a feature of malignant lymphoreticular neoplasms in smears. (d) A benign gastric gland as it appears in a smear prepared from gastric brushing. (e) Gastric washing from a patient with peptic ulcer. There are numerous poorly preserved epithelial cells in an inflammatory and necrotic background. (f) Gastric washing showing poorly preserved epithelial cells, inflammatory cells, and monilia, a common finding in treated cancer patients. (a) Hematoxylin and eosin, ×350; (b–f) Papanicolaou, ×570.

6. Duodenum

The usefulness of cytological examination of duodenal contents in the diagnosis of carcinoma of the duodenum, pancreas, and bile duct is well documented in the literature (Bowden and Papanicolaou, 1959, 1960; Dreiling *et al.*, 1960; Nieburgs *et al.*, 1962; Orell and Ohlsen, 1972). However, to obtain technically high-quality material from the duodenum is far more challenging and difficult than esophageal, gastric, or colonic lavages. The area is difficult to reach, and the collection of duodenal content without gastric secretion is also difficult.

The collection of pancreatic secretion induced by secretin and bile secretion following the administration of cholecystochinin is a delicate and time-consuming procedure.

At Memorial Hospital, we were unable to reach the 60% positive yield reported by others (Goldstein and Ventzke, 1968; Nieburgs *et al.*, 1962; Orell and Ohlsen, 1972; Rosen *et al.*, 1968). Our failure to obtain malignant cells, in many cases of carcinoma of the pancreas, is probably due to a combination of

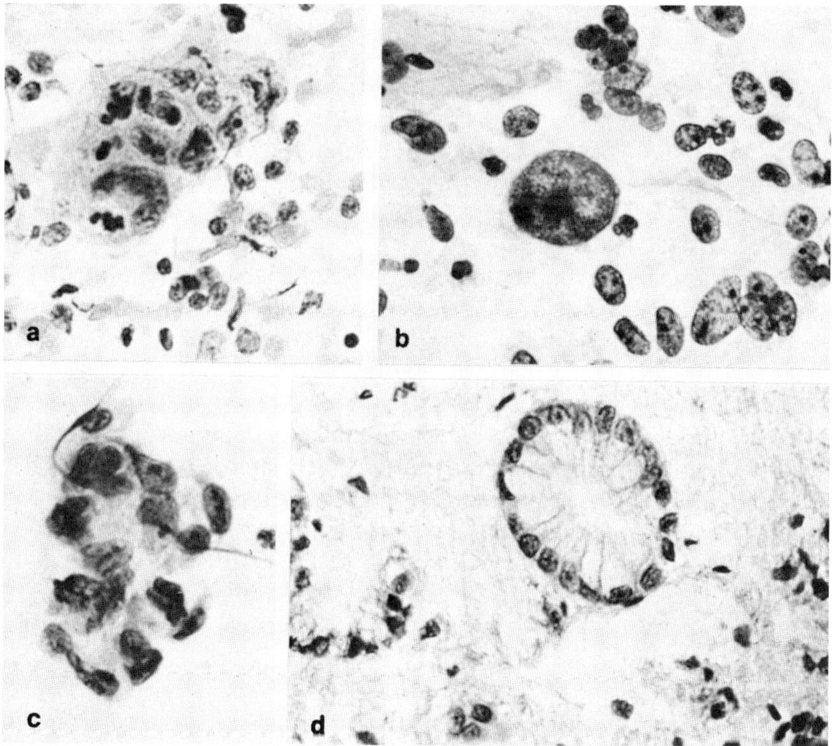

Fig. 4. Duodenal cytology. (a,c) Clusters of malignant glandular epithelial cells in smears from a patient with adenocarcinoma of the ampulla. (b) Smear of duodenal secretion showing a solitary malignant cell exfoliated from adenocarcinoma of the pancreas. (d) Clusters of benign duodenal epithelial cells, for comparison, in duodenal lavage. (a–c) Papanicolaou, ×570; (d) ×350.

several factors, e.g., obstruction of the pancreatic duct, no communication between the tumor and major ducts, or location of the tumor in the body or tail of the pancreas.

Cytologically, the identification of exfoliated malignant cells is not difficult, but routine light microscopic examination of Papanicolaou-stained smears often does not permit characterization of the neoplastic cells as to precise site of origin (Fig. 4). In general, smears prepared from duodenal aspirate are less cellular than aspirates of other sites.

It is of interest that cytological examination of duodenal aspirate can be complemented by determination of volume and concentration of bicarbonate. Reduced volume (less than 0.50 ml/kg/30 min) and low bicarbonate concentration (less than 50 mEq/liter) are common findings in pancreatitis, certain liver diseases, and carcinoma of the pancreas.

7. Colon

More than 50% of colonic cancers are within the reach of the examining finger or the sigmoidoscope. Others, tumors of the descending, transverse, and ascending colon, can be reached by the fiberoptic colonoscope. In spite of the fact that practically the entire colon is technically accessible to examination, cytology of the lower gastrointestinal tract does not enjoy the popularity of cytological examination of the stomach and esophagus. This is partly due to the fact that proper preparation of the patients is time consuming and requires the complete attention of the examining physician (Deschner *et al.*, 1973; Hajdu *et al.*, 1974*a*; Takenaka and Ayabe, 1970; Wiendl *et al.*, 1974; Winawer *et al.*, 1974*a*).

In our experience, more than 75% of the specimens are adequate for cytological evaluation. The most productive and representative specimens are usually the ones which were collected after vigorous cleansing enemas and purgation. It is mandatory that the specimen be free of heavy fecaloid and mucoid materials.

The cytological yield of number of tumor cells depends on the technique used to obtain the specimen and on the size and site of the tumor. There is some difference in the cytomorphology of tumor cells collected by lavage technique and by direct brush. Specimens obtained by various irrigation and lavage techniques usually contain tumor cells in small clusters, in pairs, and singly (Fig. 5). Smears prepared from brush specimens, on the other hand, contain a large number of cellular clusters and sheets of tumor cells. Malignant colonic epithelial cells in smears are strikingly similar to the tumor cells as they appear in histological sections. They are oval or short cigar-shaped cells with hyperchromatic nuclei, prominent nucleoli, and pale blue cytoplasm. The nuclei are usually eccentrically displaced in the cytoplasm and contain finely granular nuclear chromatin. The cytoplasm is sharply outlined and commonly elongated and spindly. Cytological diagnosis of colonic carcinomas is relatively easy because of highly distinct features of neoplastic cells.

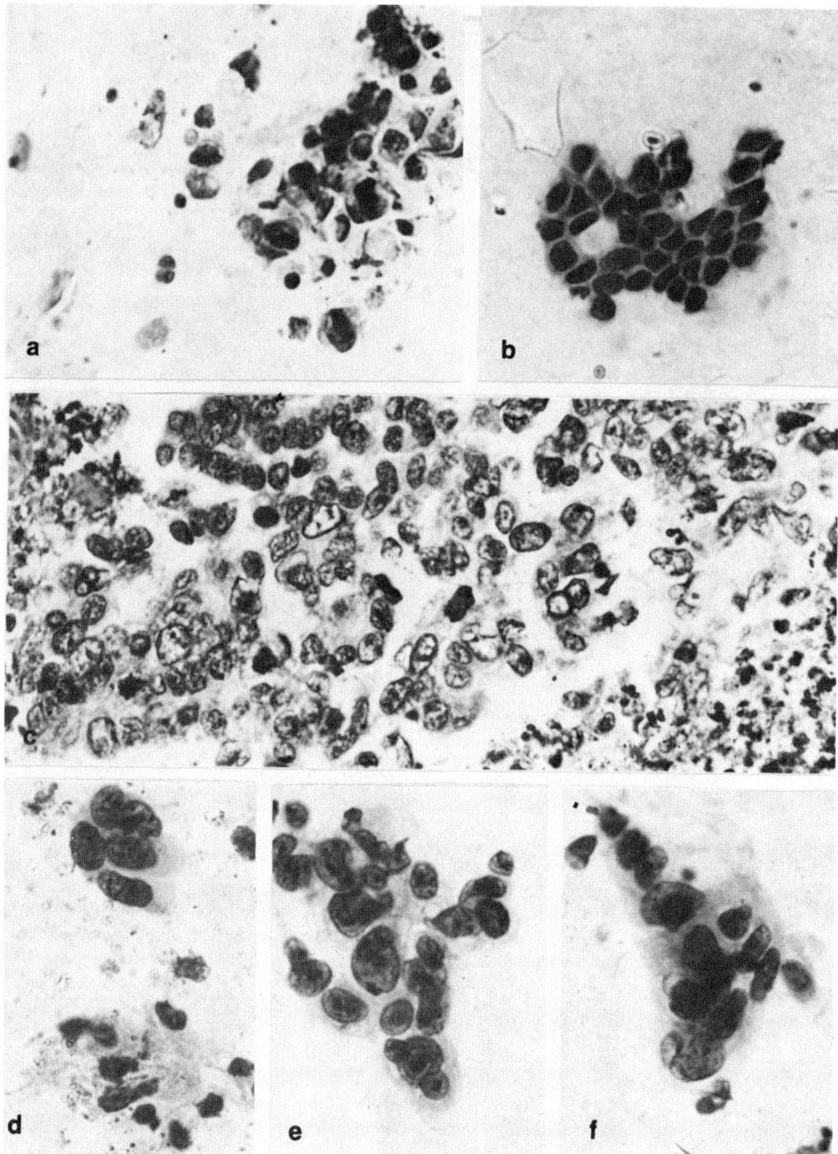

Fig. 5. Colonic cytology. (a) Poorly preserved epithelial and inflammatory cells in colonic lavage from a patient with ulcerative colitis. (b,c) Clusters of well-preserved uniform round cells with minute cytoplasm in smear (b) and in cell block (c) of colonic lavage from a patient with invasive carcinoid of the colon. (d,e,f) Clusters of malignant colonic epithelial cells in smears from colonic washings. These are round or oval cells with hyperchromatic nuclei and ill-defined cytoplasm. Note the variation of the size of the tumor cells and their tendency to form small clusters. (a–f) Papanicolaou, ×570; (c) hemetoxylin and eosin, ×400.

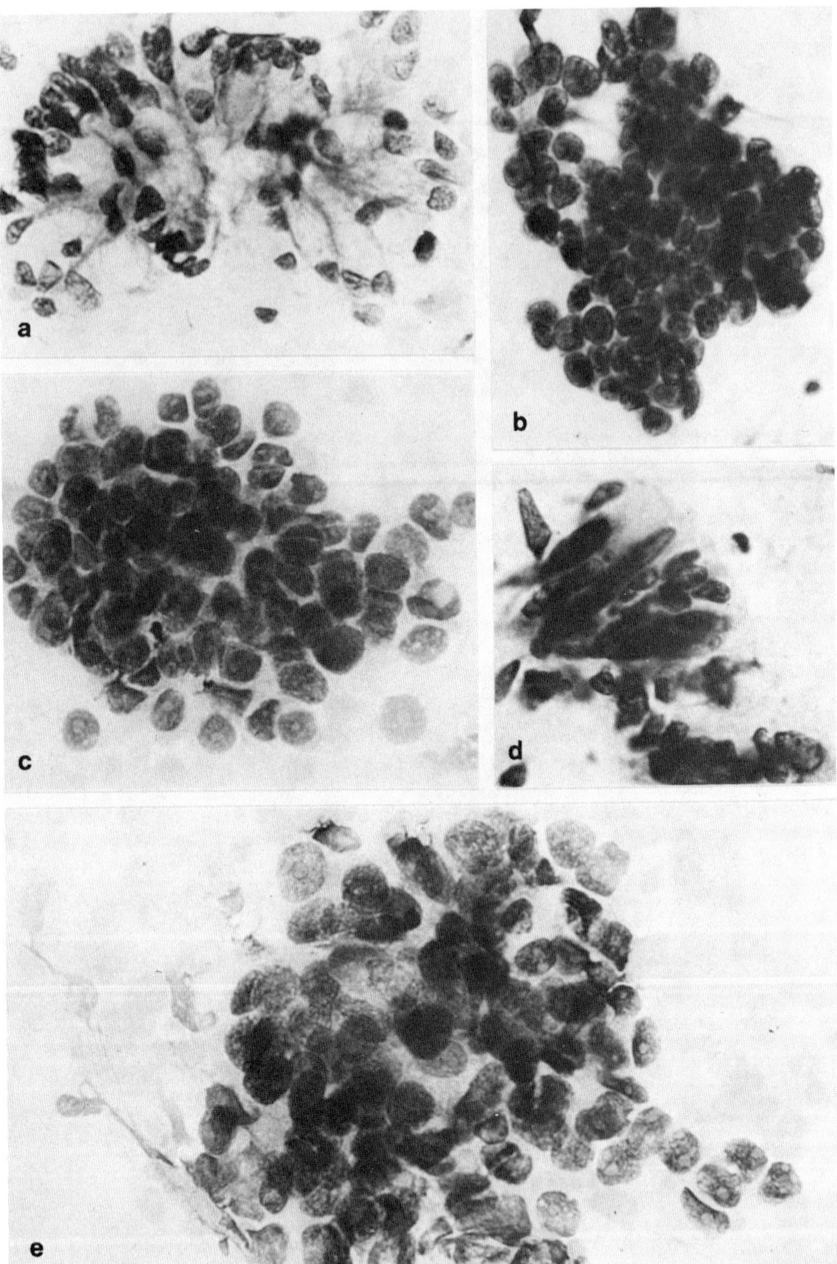

Fig. 6. Colonic cytology. These photomicrographs exemplify smears prepared from brush specimens. (a) A cluster of benign colonic epithelial cells. Note the small eccentrically placed nuclei in clear columnar cytoplasm. (b) A cluster of cells detached from a benign adenomatous polyp. (c) A cluster of atypical cells from an atypical adenomatous polyp. (d) A cluster of cells obtained from an atypical villous adenoma. (e) A cluster of neoplastic cells removed from a colonic adenocarcinoma. Most of the tumor cells are round, but there is marked variation in size. Also, note the prominent nucleoli and absence of well-preserved cytoplasm. Papanicolaou, ×570.

This is illustrated by the fact that we obtained diagnostic cytological material from 17 of 25 patients, in a series, with colonic adenocarcinoma (Fig. 6).

Various numbers of inflammatory cells, cell debris, and various amounts of acellular material are common findings in addition to neoplastic cells. Similar findings characterize inflammatory and granulomatous diseases, such as ulcerative colitis, diverticulitis, and Crohn's disease, and may cause diagnostic difficulties at the time of cytological evaluation. Benign polypoid lesions, adenomatous and villous polyps, may show characteristically arranged hyperplastic and atypical colonic cells short of clear-cut evidence of malignant features.

Tumor cells of carcinoid tumors, malignant lymphomas, and tumors of smooth muscle origin all have fairly typical morphology, and with experience it is not too difficult to identify them as neoplastic cells.

In conclusion, present cytological methods are valuable in the diagnosis of early as well as advanced gastrointestinal cancers. The clinical value of cytological examination is underlined by its accuracy and specificity. If the prognosis for patients with gastrointestinal cancers is to be improved, it is imperative that these neoplasms be detected early in the course of the disease. It is apparent that many gastrointestinal tumors are undetectable by present cytological techniques. It is hoped that in the near future new and improved endoscopic, cytological, biochemical, and immunological techniques will be available to assure earlier and better detection of all forms of gastrointestinal neoplasms.

8. References

Ackerman, N. B., 1967, An evaluation of gastric cytology: Results of a nationwide survey, *J. Chron. Dis.* **20**:621–626.

Anthonisen, P., and Riis, P., 1962, Cytology of colonic secretion in proctosigmoidal disease, *Acta Med. Scand.* **172**:375–381.

Attah, E. B., and Hajdu, S. I., 1968, Benign and malignant tumors of the esophagus at autopsy, *J. Thorac. Cardiovasc. Surg.* **55**:396–404.

Ayre, J. E., and Oren, B. G., 1953, A new rapid method for stomach cancer diagnosis: The gastric brush, *Cancer* **6**:1177–1181.

Ayre, J. E., and Oren, B. G., 1957, Colon brush: A new diagnostic procedure for cancer of the lower bowel, *Am. J. Digest. Dis.* **2**:74–80.

Bader, G. M., and Papanicolaou, G. N., 1952, Application of cytology in diagnosis of cancer of rectum, sigmoid and descending colon, *Cancer* **5**:307–314.

Belladonna, J. A., Hajdu, S. I., Bains, M. S., and Winawer, S. J., 1974, Adenocarcinoma *in situ* of Barrett's esophagus diagnosed by endoscopic cytology, *N. Engl. J. Med.* **291**:895–896.

Benvenuti, G. A., Hattori, K., Levin, B., Kirsner, J. B., and Reilly, R. W., 1975, Endoscopic sampling for tissue diagnosis in gastrointestinal malignancy, *Gastrointest. Endoscopy* **21**:159–161.

Bennington, J. L., Porus, R., Ferguson, B., and Hannon, G., 1968, Cytology of gastric sarcoid, *Acta Cytol.* **12**:30–36.

Blank, W. A., and Steinberg, A. H., 1951, Cytologic diagnosis of malignancies of the lower bowel and rectum, *Am. J. Surg.* **81**:127–131.

Boddington, M. M., and Truelove, S. C., 1956, Abnormal epithelial cells in ulcerative colitis, *Br. Med. J.* **1**:1318–1321.

Boen, S. T., 1957, Changes in nuclei of squamous epithelial cells in pernicious anemia, *Acta Med. Scand.* **159:**425–431.

Bowden, L., and Papanicolaou, G. N., 1959, Exfoliated pancreatic cancer cells in the duct of Wirsung, *Ann. Surg.* **150:**296–98.

Bowden, L., and Papanicolaou, G. N., 1960, The diagnosis of pancreatic cancer by cytology study of duodenal secretions, *Acta Un. Int. Cancr.* **16:**398–404.

Brandborg, L. L., and Wenger, J., 1968, Cytological examination in gastrointestinal tract disease, *Med. Clin. N. Am.* **52:**1315–1328.

Burn, J. I., 1961, Exfolative cytology of the colon, *Proc. R. Soc. Med.* **54:**726–729.

Cabre-Fiol, V., and Olo-Garcia, R., 1962, Citodiagnostico de las neoplasias gastricas malignas por biopsia exfoliativa, *Rev. Esp. Engerm. Apar. Dig.* **21:**571.

Cameron, A. B., 1960, A cytologic method of diagnosis of carcinoma of the colon, *Dis. Colon Rectum* **3:**230–236.

Cameron, A. B., and Thabet, R. J., 1959, Recovery of malignant cells from enema returns in carcinoma of colon, *Surg. Forum* **10:**30–33.

Cameron, J., and Hajdu, S. I., 1977, Cytology of esophageal and gastric carcinomas, in press.

Deschner, E. E., Long, F. C., and Katz, S., 1973, Autoradiographic method for an expanded assessment of colonic cytology, *Acta Cytol.* **17:**435–438.

Dreiling, D. A., Nieburgs, H. E., and Janowitz, H. D., 1960, The combined secretin and cytology test in the diagnosis of pancreatic and biliary tract cancer, *Med. Clin. N. Am.* **44:**801–815.

Eras, P., Goldstein, M. J., and Sherlock, P., 1972, Candida infection of the gastrointestinal tract, *Medicine* **51:**367–379.

Foushee, J. H. S., Kalnins, Z. A., Dixon, F. R., Girsh, S., Morehead, R. P., O'Brien, T. F., Pribor, H., and Tattory, C., 1969, Gastric cytology: Evaluation of methods and results in 1,670 cases, *Acta Cytol.* **13:**399–406.

Fukuda, T., Shida, S., Takita, T., and Sawada, Y., 1967, Cytologic diagnosis of early gastric cancer by the endoscope method with gastrofiberscope, *Acta Cytol.* **11:**456–459.

Galambos, J. T., 1962, Cytologic examination of benign colonic lesions, *Acta Cytol.* **6:**148–54.

Galambos, J. T., and Klayman, M. I., 1955, The clinical value of colonic exfoliative cytology in the diagnosis of cancer beyond the reach of the proctoscope. *Surg. Gynecol. Obstet.* **101:**673–679.

Gardner, F. N., 1956, Observations on the cytology of gastric epithelium in tropical sprue, *J. Lab. Clin. Med.* **47:**529–539.

Gephart, T., and Graham, R. M., 1959, The cellular detection of carcinoma of the esophagus, *Surg. Gynecol. Obstet.* **108:**75–82.

Goldgraber, M. B., Rubin, C. E., and Owens, F. J., 1953, The cytological diagnosis of duodenal sarcoma (polymorphic reticulosarcoma), *Ann. Intern. Med.* **39:**1316–1322.

Goldstein, H., and Ventzke, L. E., 1968, Value of exfoliative cytology in pancreatic carcinoma, *Gut* **9:**316–318.

Graham, R. M., and Rheault, M. H., 1954, Characteristic cellular changes in epithelial cells in pernicious anemia, *J. Lab. Clin. Med.* **43:**235–245.

Hajdu, S. I., and Hajdu, E. O., 1976, *Cytopathology of Sarcomas and Other Nonepithelial Malignant Tumors,* Saunders, Philadelphia.

Hajdu, S. I., Erlandson, R. A., and Paglia, M. A., 1972, Light and electron microscopic studies of gastric leiomyoblastoma, *Arch. Pathol.* **93:**36–41.

Hajdu, S. I., Bean, M. A., Fogh, J., Hajdu, E. O., and Ricci, A., 1974*a*, Papanicolaou smear of cultured human tumor cells, *Acta Cytol.* **18:**327–332.

Hajdu, S. I., Winawer, S. J., and Myers, W. P. L., 1974*b*, Carcinoid tumors: A study of 204 cases, *Am. J. Clin. Pathol.* **61:**521–528.

Heindenreich, A., 1961, Rectocolic exfoliative cytology, *Prensa Med. Argent.* **47:**2009–2019.

Hemmeter, J., 1889, The early diagnosis of cancer of the stomach, *Med. Rec. (N.Y.)* **46:**577.

Henning, N., Witte, S., and Bressel, D., 1964, The cytological diagnosis of tumors of the upper gastrointestinal tract (esophagus, stomach, duodenum), *Acta Cytol.* **8:**121–130.

Hirschowitz, B. I., Curtis, L. I., Peters, C. W., and Pollard, H. M., 1958, Demonstration of a new gastroscope, the "fibroscope," *Gastroenterology* **35:**50–53.

Johnson, W. D., Koss, L. G., Papanicolaou, G. N., and Seybolt, J. F., 1955, Cytology of esophageal washings: Evaluation of 364 cases, *Cancer* **8:**951–957.

Kasugai, T., 1968, Evaluation of gastric lavage cytology under direct-vision by the fibergastroscope employing Hands' solution as a washing solution, *Acta Cytol.* **12:**345–351.

Katz, S., Boyle, C. C., Sherlock, P., and Winawer, S., 1972, Gastric exfoliative cytology, a rapid method, *Gastroenterology* **62:**85.

Klayman, M. I., Kirsner, J. B., and Palmer, W. L., 1955, Gastric malignant lymphoma: Increasing accuracy in diagnosis, *Gastroenterology* **29:**536–547.

Klein, M. S., and Sherlock, P., 1972, Gastric and colonic metastases from breast cancer, *Am. J. Digest. Dis.* **17:**881–886.

Knoerschild, H. E., and Cameron, A. B., 1963, Mucosal smear cytology in the detection of colonic carcinoma, *Acta Cytol.* **7:**233–235.

Knoerschild, H. E., Cameron, A. B., and Zollinger, R. M., 1961, Millipore filtration of colonic washings in malignant lesions of the large bowel, *Am. J. Surg.* **101:**20–22.

Kobayashi, S., Prolla, J. C., and Kirsner, J. B., 1970, Brushing cytology of the esophagus and stomach under direct-vision by fiberscopes, *Acta Cytol.* **14:**219–223.

Lemon, H. M., 1952, The application of cytologic diagnosis to cancers of the stomach, pancreas and biliary system, *Ann. Intern. Med.* **37:**525–533.

Lemon, H. M., and Byrnes, W. W., 1949, Cancer of the biliary tract and pancreas: Diagnosis from cytology of duodenal aspiration, *Am. Med. Assoc. J.* **141:**254–257.

Loeper, M., and Binet, E., 1911, Le cytodiagnostic des affections de l'estomac, *Bull. Soc. Med. Hop. (Paris)* **31:**563–574.

MacKenzie, L. L., and Miller, H. B., 1949, Primary carcinoma of the duodenum: Report of a case in which malignant cells were recovered by duodenal drainage, *Gastroenterology* **12:**309–311.

Maimon, H. N., Dreskin, R. B., and Cocco, A. E., 1974, Positive esophageal cytology without detectable neoplasm, *Gastrointest. Endoscopy* **20:**156–59.

Marini, G., 1909, Ueber die Diagnose des Magencarcinomas auf Grund der Cytologischen des Spulwasser, *Arch. Verdaumgskrankh.* **15:**251–268.

McNeer, G., and Ewing, J. H., 1949, Exfoliated pancreatic cancer cells in duodenal drainage: Case report, *Cancer* **2:**643–645.

Messelt, O. T., 1960, Results of the cytologic diagnosis of esophageal cancer by smears from material obtained by esophagoscopy: Evaluation of 414 cases, *Acta Un. Int. Cancr.* **16:**1364–1367.

Nelson, R. S., and Lanza, F. L., 1974, The endoscopic diagnosis of gastric lymphoma, *Gastrointest. Endoscopy* **21:**66–68.

Nieburgs, H. E., Dreiling, D. A., Rubio, C., and Reisman, R., 1962, The morphology of cells in duodenal drainage smears: Histologic origin and pathologic significance, *Am. J. Digest. Dis.* **7:**489–505.

Oakland, D. J., 1961, The diagnosis of carcinoma of the large bowel of exfoliative cytology, *Br. J. Surg.* **48:**353–362.

Orell, S. R., and Ohlsen, P., 1972, Normal and post-pancreatic cytologic patterns of the duodenal juice, *Acta Cytol.* **16:**165–171.

Papanicolaou, G. N., and Cooper, W. A., 1947, The cytology of the gastric fluid in the diagnosis of carcinoma of the stomach, *J. Natl. Cancer Inst.* **7:**357–360.

Prolla, J. C., Taebel, D. W., and Kirsner, J. B., 1965, Current status of exfoliative cytology in diagnoses of malignant neoplasms of the esophagus, *Surg. Gynecol. Obstet.* **121:**743–752.

Prolla, J. C., Kobayashi, S., and Kirsner, J. B., 1969, Gastric cancer: Some recent improvements in diagnosis based upon the Japanese experience, *Arch. Intern. Med.* **124:**238–246.

Prolla, J. C., Kobayashi, S., and Kirsner, J. B., 1970, Cytology of malignant lymphomas of the stomach, *Acta Cytol.* **14:**291–296.

Raskin, H. F., Kirsner, J. B., and Palmer, W. L., 1959, Role of exfoliative cytology in the diagnosis of cancer of the digestive tract, *Am. Med. Assoc.* **169:**789–791.

Reed, P. I., Raskin, H. F., and Graff, P., 1962, Malignant melanoma of the stomach, *Am. Med. Assoc.* **182:**178–179.

Rosen, R. G., Garret, M., and Aka, E., 1968, Cytologic diagnosis of pancreatic cancer by ductal aspiration, *Ann. Surg.* **167**:427–432.

Rubin, C. E., 1955, The diagnosis of gastric malignancy in pernicious anemia, *Gastroenterology* **29**:563–587.

Rubin, C. E., and Massey, B. W., 1954, Preoperative diagnosis of gastric and duodenal malignant lymphoma by exfoliative cytology, *Cancer* **7**:271–288.

Rubin, C. E., Massey, B. W., and Kirsner, J. B., 1953, The clinical value of gastrointestinal cytology diagnosis, *Gastroenterology* **25**:119–138.

Seybolt, J. F., Papanicolaou, G. N., and Cooper, W. A., 1951, Cytology in diagnosis of gastric cancer, *Cancer* **4**:286–295.

Sherlock, P., Ehrlich, A. N., and Winawer, S. J., 1972, Diagnosis of gastrointestinal cancer: Current status and recent progress, *Gastroenterology* **63**:672–700.

Simon, P., and Caussade, L., 1914, Le cytodiagnostic du cancer de l'estomac, *Presse Med.* **22**:265–285.

Spjut, H. J., Margolis, A. A., and Cook, G. B., 1963, The silicone foam enema: A source for exfoliative cytologic specimens, *Acta Cytol.* **7**:79–84.

Takenaka, M., and Ayabe, M., 1970, Effect of carcinostatic agents on exfoliated cancer cells of the stomach, *Acta Cytol.* **14**:589–594.

Wiendl, H. J., Shwabe, M., Becker, G., and Kowatsch, J., 1974, Feulgen-cytophotometric studies of gastric mucosal smears in malignant and benign diseases of the stomach, *Acta Cytol.* **18**:222–230.

Winawer, S. J., Fleisher, M., Melamed, M. R., Sherlock, P., Deschner, E., and Schwartz, M., 1974*a*, Cytological, immunological (CEA) and isotope labeling studies based on gastrointestinal endoscopic lavage, *Gastroenterology* **66**:2–146/800.

Winawer, S. J., Mak, M. S., and Boyle, C., 1974*b*, Directed brush cytology in the diagnosis of recurrent gastric adenocarcinoma using a forward-viewing panendoscope, *Gastroenterology* **66**:2–176/830.

Winawer, S. J., Sherlock, P., Belladonna, J. A., Melamed, M. R., and Beattie, E. J., Jr., 1975, Endoscopic brush cytology in esophageal cancer, *Am. Med. Assoc.* **232**:1358.

Winawer, S. J., Sherlock, P., and Hajdu, S. I., 1976, Endoscopy in the diagnosis and management of patients with upper gastrointestinal cancer, *Cancer* **37**:440–448.

Witte, S., 1970, Gastroscopic cytology, *Endoscopy* **2**:88–93.

Yamakawa, T., Panish, J., Berci, G., Morgenstern, L., *et al.*, 1971, The correlation of target biopsy and contact smear cytology under direct visual control in malignant gastric lesions, *Gastrointest. Endoscopy* **17**:164–168.

Yoshii, Y., Takahashi, J., Yamaoka, Y., and Kasugai, T., 1970, Significance of imprint smears in cytologic diagnosis of malignant tumors of the stomach, *Acta Cytol.* **14**:249–253.

Yoshii, Y., Kobuyoshi, K., Yagi, M., and Kasugai, T., 1971, Endoscopy, biopsy and cytology in esophageal and gastric carcinoma with the fiberesophagoscope, *Gastrointest. Endoscopy* **17**:150–152.

23

The Skin and Gastrointestinal Malignancy

Janet Marks and Sam Shuster

1. Introduction

It is not uncommon for abnormalities of the skin and malignant disease of an internal organ to coexist, although the relationship between the two is not always of straightforward cause and effect. There are four possibilities:

1. The internal malignancy can be the cause of the skin disorder.
2. The skin disorder can cause the internal malignancy.
3. Skin disease and internal malignancy can occur as part of the same pathological process or in response to a common stimulus.
4. Skin disease and internal malignancy may be related not by cause and effect as in 1 and 2, nor by a common pathology as in 3, but indirectly as in the genetic cutaneosystemic syndromes.

Whatever the relationship may be, the skin signs may signal the presence of the malignancy, and it is therefore important to be able to recognize them and to appreciate their significance. Only rarely are they *early* signs of internal malignancy; consequently, any hope that through them one will be able to make an early diagnosis, and so effect a cure by early eradication of the cancer, is likely to be a forlorn one.

2. Skin Disease Caused by Internal Malignancy

A particular response of the skin can be the final common path for a number of different pathological processes, and so it is hardly surprising that

Janet Marks and Sam Shuster • University Department of Dermatology, Royal Victoria Infirmary, Newcastle upon Tyne NE1 4LP, England.

not all rashes which occur as a result of internal malignancy are specific. It is, for instance, possible for malignant disease, other chronic disease, infection, and drugs to produce an identical rash sometimes by very different mechanisms. However, some skin changes are more specifically associated with internal malignancy and a few even with a particular tumor. Often the causal relationship of the tumor to the rash is not proven, but individual cases in which removal of the tumor results in improvement of the skin suggest that the relationship is as stated. The mechanism is obscure more often than not. The following subgroups will be considered:

1. General effects of chronic disease and cachexia on skin appearance, structure, and function.
2. Skin metastases and infiltrations from internal malignant disease.
3. Skin effects of hormones and other pharmacologically active substances produced by internal tumors.
4. Rashes which are often caused by internal tumors.
5. Rashes which can be caused by internal tumors but usually have a less sinister cause.
6. Skin disorders no longer believed to be associated with systemic malignancy.

2.1. *General Effects of Chronic Disease and Cachexia on Skin Appearance, Structure, and Function*

2.1.1. *Skin Color*

The pallor of anemia has obvious associations with chronic disease and malignancy. The anemia of chronic disease is often associated with hypoferremia, although true iron deficiency is not always present. The combination of anemia, hypoferremia, and itch is said to be of bad prognostic significance in men because a large proportion of such patients have been found to develop internal malignancy in a 6-year follow-up (Vickers, 1974).

The other skin color change that occurs in malignant and other chronic diseases is hyperpigmentation due to melanin. This can be extremely gross and indistinguishable from that of Addison's disease, with involvement of mucosal surfaces as well as skin. It may be due to the ectopic production of MSH peptides. More often plasma MSH is normal; indeed, with the exception of ectopic production of MSH in tumors, Cushing's syndrome, Addison's disease, and chronic renal failure, pigmentation due to melanin in health and disease is not due to MSH peptides. In man, MSH peptides have lost their pigmentary function and appear to be mainly neurotropic.

2.1.2. *Change in Hair and Nails*

Fine lanugo hair can develop, and sometimes this is gross and involves the whole body. It is possibly a response to circulating cortisol, which stimulates lanugo hair growth. Various abnormalities of scalp hair can occur. Generally the hair is fine, sparse, and lusterless and the patient finds it difficult to manage. Follicular atrophy from protein deficiency is the likely mechanism, although changes in the hair cycle may also be involved. Diffuse thinning of hair occurs in iron deficiency, although most patients with thin, poor hair have neither iron deficiency nor chronic disease. Telogen effluvium (Kligman, 1961) is an acute hair loss from synchronous precipitation of large numbers of growing hairs into the resting or telogen phase and eventual shedding of these hairs usually as new hairs regrow. Thus the condition is usually noticed 2–3 months after the acute precipitating illness or operation and can follow an acute episode in malignant disease. Although it typically presents as an acute disorder, it can also occur as a chronic continuous hair loss easily confused with idiopathic diffuse hair loss in middle-aged women. We have seen colonic cancer present with this form of continuous telogen effluvium due to iron deficiency. Iron deficiency has also been associated with acute hair loss (Vickers, 1974). The diagnosis is easily confirmed by finding more than the usual 10–15% of club-shaped resting hairs (telogen) in a clump of hairs plucked from the scalp. Hair content of trace elements is a very sensitive index of their metabolism, but there has not yet been a systematic study of possible changes in malignant disease.

Slowing of the rate of growth of nails occurs and can result in brittleness. Beau's lines occur if interference with growth is more acute for any reason. White nails occur with hypoalbuminemia, and koilonychia or spooning of the nails has an association with iron deficiency. The iron content of fingernails is generally reduced in patients with iron deficiency (Jacobs and Jenkins, 1960), although the development of koilonychia cannot be correlated with iron deficiency *per se*.

2.1.3. *Changes in Skin Thickness and Elasticity*

The skin becomes thin in chronic disease; this is probably due to a decrease in collagen content. The cause of the spontaneous striae which occur in severely ill people is unknown but is likely to be due to changes in the intermolecular cross-linkage of collagen. In addition to its thinness the skin appears to be "too big for the patient" and does not have the ability of normal skin to spring back after stretching.

2.1.4. *Episodic Sweating*

The episodic sweating of patients with malignant disease may be due to hypermetabolism, pyrogens, or involvement of the central and autonomic nervous system. The role of pharmacologically active substances such as prostaglandins is unclear.

2.1.5. Dry Skin—Acquired Ichthyosis

The development of a dry scaly skin in adult life in someone whose skin was not previously dry is an indication for investigation to exclude an internal cause. This acquired ichthyosis has been described most often in lymphoreticular disorders such as Hodgkin's disease, but is it also seen in other malignancies including those of the bowel. It is likewise not specific to malignant disease and occurs in a variety of wasting disorders, particularly with intestinal malabsorption. We therefore proposed a common absorptive defect in patients with acquired ichthyosis (Shuster, 1967; Marks and Shuster, 1970). After bowel resection this defect has been defined as an essential fatty acid deficiency (Prottey *et al.*, 1975); it will now be interesting to see whether this is also found in patients with acquired ichthyosis of malignant disease. In extreme cases the appearance resembles that of autosomal dominant ichthyosis, and, on the lower legs particularly, inflammation of the cracks which go through the brittle keratin and epidermis leads to a "crazy-paving" appearance.

2.1.6. Itch

Itch is sensed by superficial ramifications of pain fibers in the skin: it has both a central and a peripheral modulating component, but whether one or both are involved in malignant pruritus is not clear. One of the causes of the itch of malignancy is the dryness of the skin common to any chronic wasting disease (see Section 2.1.5), and correction of the dryness by topical emollients is an important factor in relief of this type of itch. The pruritus of malignant disease, especially that due to lymphoreticular disease, may, however, predate other evidence of the disease by many years. Occasionally it is associated with hypoferremia, and this may be relieved in a matter of hours by intravenous iron (Vickers, 1974), although the mechanism of this is not understood. Occasionally it is due to bile salt retention. The most pruritic bile salts are the unconjugated dihydroxy salts, particularly chenodeoxycholate. It is not known whether specific retention of these salts is a cause of pruritus in malignancy other than with biliary obstruction. The commonest cause of itch is skin disease such as eczema, urticaria, or infestation, and only when this is absent and itch is persistent or severe is it necessary to search for a deeper cause.

2.2. Skin Metastases and Infiltrations from Internal Malignant Disease

Any carcinoma can metastasize to the skin, and the clinical lesions may be solitary or multiple nodules, ulcers, or soft vascular tumors which bleed easily. The scalp skin is a favorite site for metastases and stomach and colon tumors are among the commoner ones which metastasize there. Direct extension of gastrointestinal cancer to skin can occur, although for anatomical reasons this is less common than with carcinoma of the breast. Fistula and sinus formation can result.

Lymphedema is an obvious skin sign of lymphatic obstruction from lymphatic spread of internal cancer. Lymphangiosarcoma arising in chronically lymphedmatous skin (Stewart-Treves syndrome) is a rare complication, most cases occurring after radical mastectomy. Malignant lymphoma can result in skin "metastases" and infiltrations clinically identical with those of internal carcinoma.

Extramammary Paget's disease occurs in association with rectal or anal carcinoma. It presents as an eczematous or psoriasiform patch usually on the perianal skin but sometimes at a more distant site. There is invasion of the epidermis by large pale-staining ("Paget") cells which almost certainly migrate there from the underlying adenocarcinoma, although continuity can rarely be demonstrated. The condition is analogous to Paget's disease of the nipple associated with intraduct carcinoma of the breast.

2.3. Rashes Due to Hormones and Other Pharmacologically Active Substances Produced by Internal Tumors

The production of ACTH, ADH, MSH, parathormone, and other peptide hormones by nonendocrine tumors, usually of the bronchus, is well known. The commonest skin signs are those of Cushing's syndrome with acne, hirsutism, striae, purpura, and hyperpigmentation. The acne appears to be due to superficial obstruction of the sebaceous ducts, and the hirsutism is mostly a cortisol-induced lanugo.

Excessive production of hormones which are normally produced within the gastrointestinal tract will also give rise to skin changes. A number of such related polypeptides are known. Glucagon from the α cells of the pancreas is of special dermatological interest because of the characteristic rash that has been described in association with the glucagonoma by Mallinson *et al.* (1974). Increased levels of glucagon were found in the plasma of the patients in this particular study, and this, together with the fact that the rash regressed in the case in which resection of the tumour was possible, suggested that glucagon was the cause of the rash. In other cases the causal relationship has not been so obvious, and other polypeptides may also be responsible for the rash. The related vasoactive intestinal polypeptide (VIP) is a theoretically attractive possibility, although vasodilatation alone will not explain the characteristic skin signs. The rash is commonest in the flexures but may occur in other areas of friction; blisters, crusting, gyrate configuration of lesions, and hyperpigmentation are present clinically, and epidermal necrosis is a histological feature. The rash is sufficiently distinctive to enable a diagnosis of glucagonoma to be suspected from the presence of the rash alone. We have, however, seen one patient with this rash who also had a low serum zinc concentration. The rash appeared to respond to treatment with oral zinc sulfate, but the patient died of pneumonia. At postmortem examination there was no evidence of a tumor in the pancreas and none was found elsewhere in the gastrointestinal tract.

Carcinoid tumors produce widespread pharmacological effects of which flushing is the major dermatological sign. Metabolites released into the portal circulation from intestinal carcinoid tumors are not vasoactive by the time they reach the skin, and the skin effects of carcinoid are an indication that tumors from these sites have spread to the liver, usually with large deposits. Large amounts of serotonin are produced, and it is most exceptional not to find excess 5-hydroxyindoleacetic acid in the urine. Other vasoactive substances are produced, including kallikrein, bradykinin, prostaglandins, and histamine, and their possible role in the production of the flush is not fully worked out (Graham-Smith, 1970). The flush characteristically has a cyanotic tinge; it is initially episodic, but may later on be accompanied by chronic skin changes of telangiectasia and hyperpigmentation. A pellagralike rash most marked on light-exposed skin has been attributed to tryptophan deficiency associated with increased serotonin synthesis.

Porphyria with the characteristic signs of blistering and easily broken skin in light-exposed areas is a rare manifestation of internal tumors. Malignant liver tumors are the ones most likely to produce porphyrins, as for example in the case described by Thompson *et al.* (1970).

Acanthosis nigricans may well prove to be due to an epidermotropic peptide (see below).

2.4. *Rashes Commonly Associated with Internal Malignancy*

The two most important rashes associated with internal malignancy are the adult forms of dermatomyositis and acanthosis nigricans. Both diseases occur in children, and in them they have no association with malignancy. In adults a neoplasm should be assumed to be present until proved otherwise and, in general, the harder one looks the more often one finds it.

2.4.1. *Dermatomyositis*

Dermatomyositis is one of the collagen vascular diseases, and the only one with a definite association with malignancy. Although malignant disease is quoted as occurring in 7–52% of cases (Rowell, 1972), this is probably because of diagnostic inhomogeneity, and the more classical the clinical appearance the greater the incidence of cancer. The most commonly responsible cancers are those occurring most commonly, namely of the breast in women and of the bronchus in men. In the Chinese, where nasopharyngeal carcinoma is so prevalent, this is the usual tumor. Gastrointestinal cancers are not uncommonly involved. An immune response to a tumor antigen is the assumed but unproven mechanism, and if the tumor is operable its removal is followed by improvement in the dermatomyositis. However, as with acanthosis nigricans the likelihood of finding an operable tumor is low, and too rigorous a search is therefore unjustified. The skin signs which distinguish the condition are the distinctive livid blue color of the rash, which almost always involves the eyelids, and the tendency for it to be localized over the knuckles, elbows, and knees (possibly localized by trauma). Edema, which can occur in other collagen vascular diseases, is especially common in dermatomyositis and is a special feature of the eyelid involvement. Calcinosis cutis is a late sequela and is therefore most often seen in the juvenile (nonmalignant) form. It occurs in the hands, and deeper deposits are also found in affected muscles. The skin signs of small vessel blockage are indistinguishable from those in systemic lupus erythematosus and systemic sclerosis. They include dilated nailfold capillaries with thrombosis and hemorrhage, Raynaud's phenomenon, livedo reticularis, and gangrene, scarring, and spindling of the fingers. The myopathy affects predominantly proximal muscles. The various antinuclear factors so commonly found in systemic lupus erythematosus and systemic sclerosis are not found in dermatomyositis, and this may be helpful in making a diagnosis.

2.4.2. *Acanthosis Nigricans*

There are four distinct types of acanthosis nigricans:

1. Genetic–developmental, appearing in early life as part of a more general syndrome or as a local developmental ("nevoid") defect.
2. Obesity-related, due to friction–maceration, particularly in the axillae and inner thighs.
3. Endocrine, almost always in acromegaly and presumably due to an epidermotropic effect of growth hormone.
4. Neoplastic, almost invariably in an adult with acanthosis nigricans in the absence of causes 1–3. It is usually associated with a gastric carcinoma; other adenocarcinomas, e.g., of the bowel, are less common causes. Although the mechanism is unknown, it seems likely that it will prove to be due to an epidermotropic peptide hormone. In this respect the recently shown similarity of urogastrone and epidermal growth factor may prove to be important.

The pathological lesion is of increased epidermal activity, with increased thickness and production of keratin which is retained in warty folds. This gives rise to the clinical features which are a brown discoloration of the skin, especially of the flexures, a velvety feel to the skin, and an exaggeration of the fine folds which gives rise to the description "tripe hands." The mouth may also be affected. It is these lesions, away from the axillae and thighs, which help to distinguish the disorder from the nonmalignant varieties. As with dermatomyositis, the rash regresses if an operable tumor is removed, but the chances of finding an operable tumor are even less than with dermatomyositis, and so it is even less justifiable to prolong the search or use invasive diagnostic procedures such as laparotomy.

2.5. Skin Changes Which Can Be Due to Internal Malignancy But More Often Have a Less Sinister Cause

2.5.1. Urticarias and Erythemas

Urticarias and erythemas are among the commonest of rashes. Drugs, ingested foods, infections, infestations, and malignant disease are often blamed but are only occasionally proved to be responsible. Thus, in practice, most chronic urticarias remain unexplained and in the absence of other signs are not an indication for an extensive search for a tumour.

Cold urticaria, i.e., urticaria precipitated by cold, is a rare skin sign of malignant disease and here the mechanism is understood: any condition which leads to the production of cold agglutinins or cold-precipitating globulins may give rise to this clinical phenomenon.

Various ringed urticated erythemas with such names as "erythema annulare centrifugum" seem on occasion to be associated with internal tumors. They are believed to have an immunological explanation.

Erythema multiforme is a vasculitic rash with a distinctive clinical appearance of urticated erythematous rings arranged concentrically to form "target" or "iris" lesions. These are mostly on the peripheral parts of the limbs and may be accompanied by purpura, blister formation, and small skin infarcts. Severe erythema multiforme with fever, sore eyes and mouth, and genital ulceration is known as the Stevens-Johnson syndrome. Common causes are infection, including herpes simplex, and drugs; malignant disease, especially after treatment with radiotherapy, is a rare cause.

2.5.2. Blistering Diseases

The alleged association of pemphigoid with internal malignancy has not been substantiated by analysis of large series of patients. The previous case reports appear to be due to the association of two diseases occurring in the elderly (for pemphigoid is essentially a disease of 60-, 70-, and 80-year olds) and the tendency to report positive findings. The belief in a particular association with atypical pemphigoid (Sneddon, 1963) has likewise not been confirmed or refuted. The relationship of dermatitis herpetiformis to celiac disease and lymphoma will be discussed later. Pemphigus has been described in conjunction with thymoma (Stillman and Baer, 1972). The blistering dermatosis of glucagonoma has already been described.

2.5.3. Cutaneous Vascular Damage

Blockage of arteries and arterioles supplying the skin will produce the same physical signs of ischemia or cutaneous vasculitis, depending on the pattern of vessel involvement and nature of the underlying process, as already described in connection with dermatomyositis and the vasculitis or erythema multiforme. In malignant disease the abnormality is usually in the blood, as in the various hyperviscosity syndromes, cryoglobulinemia, immune complex disease, and the hypercoagulability syndrome.

Purpura in malignant disease has many possible causes including the hyperviscosity syndrome, thrombocytopenia, hypovitaminosis K and C, cutaneous amyloidosis, and disseminated intravascular coagulation associated with microangiopathic anemia.

Thrombophlebitis is usually due to varicose veins, trauma, or immobilization. More sinister causes are rare but important to recognize. Intraabdominal and pelvic tumors cause vein blockage by direct invasion or by pressure: superficial migratory thrombophlebitis has a special association with carcinoma, the pancreas being the site of the tumor in a third of these cases (Wormsley, 1964). It has been suggested that inferior vena caval involvement by the tumor is the mechanism.

2.5.4. *Jaundice*

Yellow skin is an obvious sign of obstructive and other jaundices, and primary and secondary tumors of the liver and pancreas feature in the long list of causes. The darker color of obstructive as compared with hepatocellular or hemolytic jaundice may in part be related to melanin pigmentation seen in the former. Its mechanism is unknown but it is not due to MSH, which is metabolized by the renal tubules and not by the liver. The intense itch of obstructive jaundice is sometimes helpful in differential diagnosis. It is due to unconjugated dihydroxy bile salts such as chenodeoxycholate in the skin. In the absence of jaundice it is unusual for itch to be due to liver or pancreatic tumors. The commonness of itch in malignant disease in general has already been discussed.

2.5.5. *Fat Necrosis*

Acute fat necrosis with painful subcutaneous nodules and ulcers occurs in association with a raised serum amylase and lipase in patients with pancreatic carcinoma and pancreatitis, but the majority of cases are not associated with pancreatic disease.

2.5.6. *Skin Signs of Immunosuppression*

The skin signs of immunosuppression are essentially the same whether the immunosuppression is the result of a genetically determined or developmental abnormality of the immune system, due to malignant disease, especially of the lymphoreticular system, or due to drugs and other agents used to treat malignant or nonmalignant disease.

a. Susceptibility to Infection. Widespread infections of skin and deeper organs with fungi, viruses, protozoa, and bacteria not normally pathogenic occur in patients with malignant disease, especially lymphoma. They are more common when immunosuppressive drugs are used in their treatment, although it is often difficult to apportion blame between disease and treatment. The mechanism is likewise unclear, and it is rare in malignant disease to find an isolated immunological defect especially in treated patients. Untreated chronic lymphatic leukemia with its suppression of T-cell function is said to be the reticulosis most likely to be associated with disseminated herpes zoster (Bluefarb, 1960), which is interesting in view of the fact that T cells are important in protecting against viral (and fungal) diseases. Impairment of T- and B-cell number and functions, helper activities, migration, and phagocytosis are some of the many factors whose contribution is uncertain. In immunosuppressed patients the clinical pictures of herpes simplex, herpes zoster, and vaccinia differ only in severity from those in the untreated patient. In herpes zoster it is unusual not to find a few lesions at sites distant from the main dermatomal rash, but in immunosuppressed patients the spread of the rash may be excessive. Herpes zoster involving a spinal root affected by malignant disease is uncommon. The herpes, vaccinia, and chickenpox viruses can be identified with little delay by methods involving electron microscopy, immunofluorescence, and culture. Occasionally there may be an excessive growth of viral warts.

Candida albicans infections are common in dermatological practice. Spread away from flexural sites, especially if extensive, systematized, or accompanied by granuloma formation, should give rise to suspicion of underlying disease such as malignancy, diabetes, and primary hypoparathyroidism. In the genetically determined diseases of cell-mediated immunity, candidiasis is often accompanied by hypoferremia (Higgs and Wells, 1973) and responds to a combination of anticandidal drugs and iron. Despite encouraging case reports, the therapeutic role of transfer factor remains uncertain. It is not known whether in malignant disease hypoferremia and susceptibility to *Candida* infection are related.

Pityriasis versicolor is a superficial fungal infection of the shoulders and upper trunk, where it is associated with scaling and hypo- or hyperpigmentation. It is common in Cushing's syndrome and in immunosuppressed patients.

"Synergistic gangrene" is destructive skin ulceration apparently due to dual infection by a nonhemolytic *Streptococcus* and *Staphylococcus pyogenes;* it can occur in immunosuppressed patients, presumably because of impaired resistance to the bacteria.

b. Impairment of Tissue Growth and Healing. Hair and nail growth are depressed. X rays and cytotoxic drugs affect hair in anagen (growing phase), producing alopecia, and this is most noticeable after intravenous injections of cytostatic drugs. Because of the rapid tissue fixation of these drugs, alopecia can be minimized by putting a tight band around the scalp at the time of the injection.

c. Acne. Acne occurs with cytostatic drugs, probably by reducing cell proliferation in the pilosebaceous ducts and so causing blockage. The corticosteroids often given in conjunction with cytostatics produce acne by the same mechanism.

d. Neoplasia. Skin neoplasms have been reported in immunodeficiency diseases (noted in Chapter 3 of this volume).

2.5.7. *Nonspecific Rashes in Lymphoma*

A variety of papular and other eruptions occur in patients with lymphomas. In leukemia they have been named "leukemids" to distinguish them from rashes which are due to infiltration of the skin by leukemic deposits, but similar rashes occur in other reticuloses. In some cases their presence is probably coincidental and in others they are probably explicable on the basis of phenomena already described, e.g., unusual infections in immunosuppressed patients. The lymphomas which complicate celiac disease are particularly difficult to diagnose early, partly because they start in intraabdominal lymph nodes. Thus skin signs which serve as a pointer are useful in diagnosis. Austad *et al.* (1967) found "ulcers, nodules and skin rashes" in five of seven patients with celiac disease when they developed their malignant lymphoma. It is unfortunate that these skin lesions remain poorly defined in dermatological terms. Until they are more clearly defined, it is obviously worth considering a diagnosis of malignant lymphoma when a dermatosis appears *de novo* in a patient with celiac disease, especially if the patient is deteriorating and especially if the celiac disease is untreated or unresponsive. We have seen one patient in whom the cutaneous disorder was a progressive and deeply destructive pyoderma gangrenosum. The other skin abnormalities which occur in celiac disease and which may give rise to confusion will be described later.

2.5.8. *Erythroderma (Exfoliative Dermatitis)*

Erythroderma is commonly due to eczema or psoriasis which has spread and become generalized. For various reasons it has been thought in the past to be an external manifestation of internal malignancy, often of the reticuloendothelial system. The occasions where it is due to leukemia or lymphoma are in our experience excessively rare. More often, but still rarely, some patients develop a lymphoreticular disorder after many years of erythroderma, and in these it is likely that chronic antigenic stimulation from the skin disease is the *cause* of the change (see below). As a rule, however, the abnormal findings in patients with erythroderma which have been attributed to an underlying reticulosis are in fact due to the skin disease and return to normal after treatment of the skin (Shuster and Marks, 1970). The causes of confusion include the following:

1. Dermatopathic lymphadenopathy (lipomelanic reticulosis) is a generalized lymphadenopathy that is usual in extensive skin disease. The condition regresses after the rash has cleared. Histologically the condition is distinctive.
2. Hepatomegaly is common in erythroderma. Heart failure from a

high-output state is the usual explanation (Shuster, 1963; Shuster and Marks, 1970).

3. Skin histology may show cells identical with the mycosis fungoides and Sézary cell (see below). The existence of these "malignant" cells in clinically benign conditions is well described (Flaxman *et al.*, 1971) and occurs particularly in sun-exposed skin.
4. Leukocytosis and a high erythrocyte sedimentation rate are common in erythoderma (Shuster and Marks, 1970) and return to normal when the skin is treated.
5. The "Sézary syndrome" erythroderma is accompanied by abnormal cells in the skin and blood. These are identical with mycosis fungoides cells; that is, they are mononuclear cells of T-cell origin, with a large folded nucleus and a polyploid DNA content. They appear to occur as a cutaneous lymphoreticular response to a chronic dermatosis (e.g., eczema or psoriasis) with overspill into the blood and not as a primary lymphoreticular disorder. Thus we have had cases where the abnormal cells disappeared when the skin was treated, and we suspect that this is the usual course of events. The confusion appears to be the rare occurrence of the Sézary syndrome in patients with Hodgkin's disease, lymphosarcoma, or reticulum cell sarcoma (Winkelmann and Linman, 1973). It is probably due to the same lymphoreticular response to extensive skin inflammation in these diseases. This also occurs in mycosis fungoides where episodes of erythroderma may evoke overspill of Sézary cells into the blood which disappear when the skin is treated.

Thus erythroderma is rarely due to internal malignancy; more often erythroderma will stimulate a lymphoreticular response and possibly ultimately a malignancy.

2.5.9. *Skin Lesions in Ulcerative Colitis*

Ulcerative colitis is a premalignant condition and as such will be discussed here. Most of the skin lesions that are seen in ulcerative colitis are related to the activity of the disease, and, although occasionally they are the presenting symptom, it is usual even then to find active disease on sigmoidoscopy or barium enema examination. There is, as far as we know, no special relationship of the skin lesions to the development of intestinal malignancy.

Pyoderma gangrenosum is the skin lesion most characteristically associated, half of the patients with this disease having ulcerative colitis. The appearance is of one or more ulcers at any site on the skin. These ulcers often start as small pustules which become necrotic and enlarge rapidly. There is no association with specific bacteria and no primary vasculitis; the pathogenesis is unknown, although there is assumed to be an abnormal immunological response to infection or to injury. The disorder is controlled by treatment of the bowel and if not severe by topical corticosteroids.

Perianal abscesses and fissures occur in ulcerative colitis but are much commoner in Crohn's disease. Mouth ulcers are a feature of both these diseases as well as of celiac disease, and patients with chronic mouth ulceration without obvious cause should always be investigated with these diseases in mind. Lesions resembling pemphigus vegetans with vegetative lesions in the flexures, perianal region, and mouth are seen in ulcerative colitis. They appear to be a hypertrophic response to chronic infection, the pemphiguslike separation of epidermal cells being due to bacterial products.

In other rashes seen in ulcerative colitis it is often difficult to be certain whether the disease or the drugs used in treatment, especially salazopyrine, are to blame: erythema nodosum, erythema multiforme (Edwards and Truelove, 1964), and rashes resembling lichen planus (Wyatt, 1975) come into this category. "Toxic erythemas" and hemorrhagic skin manifestations of the hypercoagulability state occur in patients severely ill with ulcerative colitis, and skin signs of cachexia occur in those with chronic wasting.

2.5.10. *Unproven and Disproven Associations*

Many bizarre unclassifiable and atypical rashes are reported in association with a systemic malignancy. Whether these represent a true association is mostly unknown, and most reports appear to reflect the age of the patients, the duration and intensity of the diagnostic search, and the tendancy to report positive findings. Thus statistically adequate studies refute a correlation of malignancy with pemphigoid, Campbell de Morgan spots, Bowen's disease, punctate keratoses, and seborrheic warts.

3. *Internal Malignancy Caused by Skin Disease*

3.1. *Tumors Arising in the Skin*

Tumors arising in the skin can spread to internal organs. Examples include squamous cell carcinoma of epidermis and adnexae, sarcomas of vascular and other dermal tissue, and malignant melanoma. Spread to the liver occurs with malignant melanoma, and this tumor has also been reported as metastazing.to stomach, intestine, and pancreas (Fraser-Moodie *et al.*, 1976). Normally there will be no great diagnostic difficulty in patients presenting with lymphadenopathy or hepatomegaly will have an obviously malignant skin tumor. Occasionally a malignant melanoma can metastasize without itself looking clinically malignant, or distant metastases can arise a long time after removal of the primary tumor; amelanotic melanoma occasionally causes clinical difficulty, too. Kaposi's sarcoma is particularly prone to metastasize to the gastrointestinal tract with gastrointestinal hemorrhage many years after the slow-growing vascular tumors appear on the limbs.

Mycosis fungoides is a primary cutaneous reticulosis of T cells characterized by the presence in skin of the "mycosis" or Sézary cell, which is an atypical mononuclear cell with a convoluted, polyploid nuecleus containing an excess of DNA. Spread to lymph nodes, liver, and spleen may occur late in the disease when skin nodules, plaques, and fungating ulcers are found; systemic spread does not occur at an early stage where skin lesions are less tumid, nor at the even earlier stage of the "premycotic" eruption. In the past the rapid appearance and growth of fungating skin tumors with systemic spread were thought to be a variant of mycosis fungoides, but this syndrome is now known to be part of a primary systemic lymphosarcoma presenting in the skin.

3.2. Chronic Antigenic Stimulation

There is a theoretical possibility that in longstanding eruptions such as chronic erythroderma, parapsoriasis, and mycosis fungoides (Tan *et al.*, 1974) a systemic lymphoreticular malignancy will arise through prolonged lymphoreticular stimulation, but it is not clear from case reports whether this has actually happened.

4. Common Pathology or Common Cause of Skin Disease and Internal Malignancy

4.1. Mastocytosis

Mastocytosis is a relatively uncommon disease, and in the majority of cases the skin only is involved in the pathological process, although pharmacological effects even then may be more widespread. Occasionally there is widespread infiltration of a large number of internal organs by mast cells. All types of mast cell disease can occur in children as well as adults.

4.1.1. *Mast Cell Nevus*

Mast cell nevus is usually solitary and is pinkish brown in color. It is commonest in very young children and regresses spontaneously.

4.1.2. *Urticaria Pigmentosa*

The skin lesions of urticaria pigmentosa vary in extent, but usually there is eventual widespread involvement. The lesions are pink macules or papules which urticate or swell on rubbing and are followed by telangiectasia and by hyperpigmentation. Spontaneous remission can occur, especially in children. The degree of systemic involvement is variable.

4.1.3. *Diffuse Infiltration*

Diffuse infiltration is the rarest form of mast cell disease. There is yellowish thickening of the skin with nodule formation, and spontaneous remission is unusual. Systemic involvement is common.

In mast cell disease there is release of histamine and heparinlike substances from the cells. This usually occurs on trauma and is accompanied by mast cell degranulation. The skin lesions of all types of mast cell disease have, in consequence of the histamine they release, the tendency to itch, to urticate on rubbing, and to blister. Pharmacological effects of the histamine release are most marked in extensive disease but can be noticeable even with a solitary tumor. In extensive skin disease, bathing and rubbing down with a towel can result in massive histamine release with hypotension, flushing, diarrhea, and bronchospasm (Brett *et al.*, 1967). The release of heparinlike substances seems only exceptionally to be associated with coagulation defects (Brett *et al.*, 1967), but an osteoporosis (Sagher and Schorr, 1956) similar to that seen after long-term heparin treatment (Griffith *et al.*, 1965) does occur. There is also an association with myelofibrosis and sclerosis. When there is systemic involvement, spleen, liver, bones, and lymph nodes are most commonly involved; the pancreas (Berlin, 1955) and small bowel (Sagher and Even-Par, 1967) have been reported to be involved in some cases. Gastrointestinal involvement without skin involvement is rare (Scott *et al.*, 1975*b*). Mast cell disease usually runs a benign, slowly progressive course but can behave in a malignant fashion and even end in a mast cell leukemia.

4.2. *Other Lymphoreticular Disorders*

A number of lymphoreticular diseases are apparently multicentric and arise in the skin and internal organs simultaneously. After mastocytosis the commonest is probably plasmacytoma. In reticuloses other than mycosis fungoides it is often difficult to know whether there is multicentric origin of skin and internal tumors or whether the skin lesions represent metastases. Diseases of the histiocytosis X group affect both skin and internal organs. It is not known whether these are storage diseases or whether they are true neoplasms.

4.3. *Neoplasia Following Inorganic Arsenic Ingestion*

Environmental exposure and medicinal use of inorganic (but not organic) arsenic give rise to neoplastic change in skin and other organs. This may not occur for many years after the treatment, and in some patients it has occurred after relatively small doses of arsenic. Thus there is a statistically significant correlation between carcinoma of the bronchus and previous arsenic ingestion (Robson and Jelliffe, 1963), and a personal series contains two patients, one with a squamous cell carcinoma of the tongue and one with a squamous cell carcinoma of the esophagus, both of whom have skin signs of chronic arsenic poisoning from ingestion of liquor arsenicalis many years ago. The main skin sign of inorganic arsenic poisoning is the appearance of a number of malignant and premalignant lesions. Intraepidermal carcinoma, squamous cell carcinoma, and basal cell carcinoma occur, but the most characteristic lesions are the keratoses of the palms and soles. These are hard wartlike lesions which, unlike certain other warty lesions, are not easy to remove with a fingernail or with a curette; some of them progress to squamous cell carcinomas. The much described "raindrop" pigmentation of the back in arsenic poisoning is not seen in these patients with skin cancer and keratoses; presumably it is an earlier sign. Whether the risk of producing tumors is greater with inorganic arsenic than with the contemporary cytostatic drugs time alone will tell. When the choice between the two arises, as for example occasionally in the treatment of intractable psoriasis, most dermatologists would not use inorganic arsenic other than in the elderly.

4.4. Tumors and Radiation

Both X irradiation and chronic exposure to ultraviolet light can produce multiple skin tumors. Ultraviolet light is especially damaging in those with fair skin, the 290–320 nm sunburn wavelength being the most active in this respect. The skin tumors produced are basal cell carcinoma, squamous cell carcinoma, intraepidermal carcinoma, and solar keratoses. Chronic exposure to sunlight is a less important factor in the production of malignant melanoma. X ray and radiation cancers have occurred in those working with the X rays as well as those undergoing treatment. Multiple tumors are still being seen in people who years ago were treated with X rays for ringworm of the scalp and ankylosing spondylitis of the spine, although both forms of treatment were stopped many years ago. The tumors, which are basal cell carcinomas, squamous cell carcinomas, or intraepidermal carcinomas, are usually confined very clearly to the areas of irradiation and are accompanied by the atrophy, telangiectasia, and scarring of "radiodermatitis." Systemic cancer does not of course follow exposure to sunlight, but lymphoreticular disease has been described in those exposed to X rays, and carcinoma of the thyroid in patients treated with X rays for benign skin conditions such as acne (Albright and Allday, 1967).

4.5. Xeroderma Pigmentosum

Xeroderma pigmentosum is a genetically determined disease in which there is an inability to achieve normal excision-repair of DNA dimers after exposure to ultraviolet radiation at 290–320 nm. Eventually a variety of skin tumors including basal and squamous epithelioma and malignant melanoma develop and patients die young from metastases. The defect of DNA repair is not confined to the skin, and so the possibility that the patient may develop internal malignant disease if he or she lives long enough has to be considered.

4.6. Immunosuppression and Malignancy

Internal malignant disease occurs with increased frequency in those on immunosuppressive drugs, and malignancy is a feature of some of the syndromes in which there is a congenital immunological defect (e.g., the Wiskott-Aldrich syndrome, ataxia-telangiectasia, and the Chédiak-Steinbrinck-Higashi syndrome).

4.7. Iron Deficiency and Postcricoid Carcinoma

The skin, hair, and nail changes associated with iron deficiency have already been described, as has the association of these changes with sore tongue and dysphagia in the Plummer-Vinson or Kelly-Paterson syndrome. The precise relationship of these changes to iron deficiency is not known, but the severe mucosal abnormalities and the carcinoma following the postcricoid web are apparently less common now that iron deficiency is diagnosed and treated earlier than it was in the past.

5. Skin Disease and Internal Malignancy Occurring Together in the Cutaneosystemic Syndromes and Other Genetically Related Defects

Skin disease and internal malignancy that occur together in cutaneosystemic syndromes and other genetic defects will be discussed on an anatomical basis according to the part of the gastrointestinal tract involved.

5.1. Mouth and Jaw

5.1.1. Basal Cell Nevus Syndrome

The basal cell nevus syndrome (Gorlin and Goltz, 1960) is a dominantly inherited condition in which any of the following can occur:

1. Multiple basal cell carcinomas of skin. These start earlier in life than basal cell carcinoma as a rule. They are often locally malignant but in some cases behave clinically in a benign fashion even though the histology is indistinguishable from that of invasive basal cell carcinoma.
2. Cysts of the jaw. These are lined with stratified squamous epithelium and sometimes undergo malignant change.
3. Small pits in the skin of the palms and soles. These represent local defects in keratin formation.
4. Skeletal abnormalities including bifid ribs, spina bifida, and hypertelorism.
5. Endocrine abnormalities, especially hypogonadism in the male and pseudohypoparathyroidism.
6. Neurological abnormalities including medulloblastoma and mental deficiency.

5.1.2. *Medullary Carcinoma of the Thyroid*

Calcitonin produced from tumors of parafollicular C cells is associated with neuromas of the tongue, lips, and eyelids and ganglioneuromas of the bowel. The mucosal neuromas are easily biopsied and have a characteristic histopathology (Cunliffe *et al.*, 1970).

5.1.3. *Primary Amyloidosis*

Primary amyloidosis may antecede other evidence of myeloma or lymphoreticular disease. The macroglossia may be diagnostic and so is the periorbital purpura. This purpura resembles that of corticosteroid-induced and senile purpura (Shuster and Scarborough, 1961). We have shown it to have the general features of the supportive purpuras where a defect in the connective tissue allows vessel rupture by shear and excessive spread of the extravasated blood.

5.2. **Esophagus**

5.2.1. *Tylosis*

Tylosis is a warty condition of the palms and soles associated in only a few families with carcinoma of the esophagus (Howel-Evans *et al.*, 1958). The skin lesions, which present in childhood, serve as a useful marker of the carcinoma, which does not present until the fourth or fifth decade, for it is found only in those members of the family who have the tylosis. The skin lesion must be distinguished from other similar syndromes of tylosis of the palms and soles, some of which are also inherited as autosomal dominant traits. The tylosis in the common forms usually has a later onset than that in the excessively rare families with carcinoma.

5.2.2. *Celiac Disease*

There is an increased incidence of carcinoma of the esophagus in celiac disease (Harris *et al.*, 1967). Dermatitis herpetiformis occurs in patients with celiac disease and their families probably on a genetic basis (see below). Thus it would not be surprising if there were an increased incidence of carcinoma of the esophagus in patients with dermatitis herpetiformis, although this has not to our knowledge been described. The diagnosis of dermatitis herpetiformis will be dealt with elsewhere.

5.3. Stomach

5.3.1. Pernicious Anemia

The association of carcinoma of the stomach with pernicious anemia makes it likely that any skin disease that is associated with this anemia might be useful as a skin marker for carcinoma of the stomach. These skin diseases include: vitiligo, alopecia areata, premature graying of hair, lichen sclerosus, and dermatitis herpetiformis.

a. Vitiligo. Howitz and Schwartz (1971) found pernicious anemia to be about 50 times as common in patients with vitiligo as in a control population, and autoantibodies to gastric parietal cells are significantly increased in patients with vitiligo (Cunliffe *et al*; 1968). The white patches of skin in vitiligo are associated with destruction of melanocytes, and—in view of the association with other autoimmune conditions like Addison's disease, diabetes, and thyroiditis, as well as with pernicious anemia—it is suggested, but not proved, that the basis of this cell destruction is autoimmune, too. Familial vitiligo and pernicious anemia are common, and some patients with vitiligo have a family history of pernicious anemia, although they do not have the disease themselves; this relationship may have a genetic basis.

b. Alopecia Areata. Alopecia areata is a clinically distinct form of baldness similar to vitiligo in its association with pernicious anemia and other autoimmune diseases as well as with vitiligo itself. As in vitiligo there may be some destruction of melanocytes so that as hair regrows it may be white for a time. More often alopecia areata affects pigmented but not white hair and a diffuse alopecia areata causing loss of pigmented but not white hair is the cause of hair going white "overnight."

c. Premature Graying of Hair. Premature hair graying has an association with pernicious anemia and is presumably a genetically related abnormality.

d. Lichen Sclerosus. Patients with lichen sclerosus have an increased incidence of autoantibodies to parietal cells and, to a lesser extent, to intrinsic factor (Goolamali *et al.*, 1974), although frank pernicious anemia has not yet been described. The disease presents clinically as vulval atrophy, and the lesions on other parts of the skin consist of small spots or plaques, white in color and studded with horny plugs.

e. Dermatitis Herpetiformis. Pernicious anemia (Kumar and Dawson, 1973), atrophic gastritis, and achlorhydria (Lancaster-Smith and Kumar, 1974) seem to be quite common in dermatitis herpetiformis, although in a study of a series of patients with this disease the apparent increase in the incidence of gastric parietal cell antibodies did not reach statistical significance (Fraser, 1970). One patient in a personal series of 120 patients with dermatitis herpetiformis has recently developed carcinoma of the stomach, although this may be coincidental.

5.3.2. *Polyposis*

Gastric polyposis occurs as part of several syndromes and can occur with and without polyposis of the intestine. Malignant change in gastric polyps has been reported in the following:

1. Peutz-Jeghers syndrome (Achord and Proctor, 1963). The dermatological and other features of this syndrome will be discussed below.
2. Neurofibromatosis (Levy and Khatib, 1960). This is a disease with an autosomal dominant inheritance in which skin tumors and patchy hyperpigmentation are the commonest features, but tumors of spinal and cranial nerves occur. Tumors of other organs including the gastrointestinal tract are rare. The pathognomic skin change is axillary freckling, although the "cafe au lait" patches containing giant melanosomes and pedunculated skin tumors are perhaps more well known.

5.4. *Intestine*

5.4.1. *Polyposis*

The causes of polypoid tumors of the intestine are hamartoma formation, adenomatosis, inflammation, lymphoid hyperplasia, and rare tumors including neurofibromas. Skin abnormalities can occur, particularly in association with hamartomas and adenomas and may thus be helpful in diagnosis. Early diagnosis is important, especially in familial adenomatosis where prophylactic colectomy is commonly practiced to prevent carcinoma of the colon.

A relatively small number of patients with familial adenomatous polyposis of the large intestine, or Gardner's syndrome (Gardner, 1951), have in addition epidermoid cysts and other skin tumors, multiple osteomas, and less often tumors of other organs.

Peutz-Jeghers syndrome (Jeghers *et al.*, 1949) is a disease transmitted as an autosomal dominant character in which disturbances of pigmentation are associated with hamartomatous polyposis. The polyps can occur anywhere in the gastrointestinal tract but are usually in the small intestine. Local malignant change in the polyps may be difficult to assess histologically, but metastases occur occasionally and there is probably an increased risk of carcinoma of the upper gastrointestinal tract in patients with the syndrome (Bussey, 1970). The characteristic skin changes are brown or black macules due to melanin deposition around the mouth, on the lips and bucal mucosa, and on the dorsal aspects of the fingers and toes.

The skin and other manifestations of neurofibromatosis have already been described. Intestinal polyposis, like gastric polyposis, is a rare clinical manifestation.

In the Cronkhite-Canada syndrome there is a generalized gastrointestinal polyposis associated with a protein-losing enteropathy. There are a diffuse alopecia and a characteristic nail deformity.

5.4.2. *Gastrointestinal Hemorrhage and the Skin*

The cause of gastrointestinal bleeding is occasionally apparent from an examination of the skin, e.g., gastric carcinoma and acanthosis nigricans and the various syndromes of polyposis. In addition, there are two other groups of cutaneous syndromes associated with bleeding but without malignancy:

1. Vascular: (a) developmental, e.g., hemorrhagic telangiectasia and multiple hemangiomas, (b) neoplastic, e.g., Kaposi's sarcoma, (c) vasculitic, e.g., leukocytoplastic vasculitis (Henoch-Schoenlein purpura).
2. Connective tissue disorders, e.g., pseudoxanthoma elasticum and Ehlers-Danlos syndrome.

5.4.3. *Celiac disease*

The increased incidence of malignant lymphoma of the small intestine and carcinoma of the esophagus in patients with celiac disease has already been mentioned. The explanation is uncertain, although in lymphoma at least it is possible that prolonged immunological stimulation from years of chronic disease plays a role. An alternative explanation is that celiac disease and susceptibility to malignancy are genetically related. One of the most important rashes associated with celiac disease, and one in which small intestinal lymphoma has been reported, is dermatitis herpetiformis. There is evidence that the skin disease and the bowel disease are genetically related, although the rash occurs only occasionally. The skin associations of celiac disease have been reported to occur in 10–20% of patients (Cooke *et al.*, 1953; Badenoch, 1960). They will now be summarized, and then dermatitis herpetiformis will be described more fully.

a. Signs of Weight Loss and Cachexia. When weight loss occurs in celiac disease, the skin manifestations are indistinguishable from those of cachexia in malignant disease and other chronic wasting disease and have already been mentioned.

b. Signs of Vitamin and Other Deficiencies. Vitamin and other deficiencies occur in severe malabsorption of whatever cause. Vitamin K deficiency with hemorrhage into the skin is one example.

c. Mouth Ulcers. Mouth ulcers are common in celiac disease, Ferguson *et al.* (1975) quoting an incidence as high as 20%. This work highlights the importance of carrying out small intestinal mucosal biopsy in the investigation of patients with unexplained intractable mouth ulcers.

d. Signs of Small Bowel Reticuloses. Skin signs can herald malignant change of small bowel reticuloses, although their usefulness is lessened by the fact that they are nonspecific and poorly defined (see above).

e. Eczematous and Psoriasiform Rashes. Eczematous and psoriasiform rashes that occur in celiac diseases are not clinically or histologically distinct from other eczematous or psoriasiform rashes, but since an underlying celiac disease is only rarely found in patients presenting with these dermatoses, routine screening for celiac disease is not indicated in patients with eczema and psoriasis. Patients with extensive eczema and psoriasis do, however, have steatorrhea which we have named "dermatogenic enteropathy" (Shuster and Marks, 1965), but this is due to the skin disease and recovers once the rash is cleared. It has none of the diagnostic features of celiac disease (Marks and Shuster, 1970) and a gluten-free diet should not be given. The much rarer eczematous and psoriasiform rashes due to celiac disease usually occur in patients with other clinical and biochemical manifestations of malabsorption and at a stage when the small intestinal mucosa is extensively involved, and they disappear when the celiac disease is treated with a gluten-free diet. The mechanism of their production is not known, but they occur in other forms of malabsorption such as tropical sprue and so they are most unlikely to be due to gluten "sensitivity." The possibility that they are due to deficiency of essential fatty acids or zinc has not so far been investigated.

f. Dermatitis Herpetiformis. Dermatitis herpetiformis is a distinctive skin disease which can affect both adults and children. It runs a chronic course, with relapses and remissions, but can undergo spontaneous cure (Wyatt *et al.*, 1971). The rash consists of itchy blisters and papules, often grouped and often situated on extensor surfaces; it responds to treatment with sulfonamides and sulfones, especially dapsone. Histologically the blisters are subepidermal, but the histology of a papule is more specific and therefore more helpful in diagnosis showing microabscesses in the dermal papillary tips (Pierard and Whimster, 1961). The most useful single diagnostic criterion is the presence of IgA deposits (Cormane, 1967) in the dermal papillae in clinically unaffected skin.

In 1966 we found that two-thirds of patients with this disease had flattening of their upper small intestinal mucosa which was "indistinguishable from that of celiac disease" (Marks *et al.*, 1966), and it is now accepted that the small intestinal lesion is that of celiac disease (Fry *et al.*, 1967; Shuster *et al.*, 1968; Marks and Whittle, 1969). There may be minimal or no clinical or biochemical evidence of small bowel disease even in the presence of a completely flat mucosa. This is probably related to the small length of bowel involved by the disease process. Thus the rash is a skin marker for a subgroup of celiac diseases, some severe, but mostly mild and subclinical, which might not otherwise come to light.

We totally disagree with those who claim that *all* patients with dermatitis herpetiformis have celiac disease. Attempts to extend the diagnosis of celiac disease have been made by measuring the number of intraepithelial lymphocytes in the small intestinal mucosa (Fry *et al.*, 1972), by taking multiple small intestinal mucosal biopsies (Brow *et al.*, 1971), and by feeding massive amounts of gluten to people with an apparently normal bowel (Weinstein, 1974). There is no evidence, however, that any of these maneuvers define the celiac population more closely, and even with them we still find that about 20% of our patients with dermatitis herpetiformis do not have celiac disease (Scott *et al.*, 1975*a*; Marks, 1977).

As we predicted (Shuster and Marks, 1969), malignant lymphoma has been found in patients with dermatitis herpetiformis. So far, cases seem to have been confined to those who have had celiac disease and clinical malabsorption (Gjone and Nordöy, 1970; Anderson *et al.*, 1971; Goodwin and Fry, 1973), although documentation with regard to small intestinal mucosal biopsy in some of these cases is not as full as one would like. In any case we cannot assume that the risk is confined to those with severely affected bowel; nor do we yet know whether the 20% of patients with dermatitis herpetiformis who do not have celiac disease are also at risk, although on present evidence it seems unlikely.

Genetically, celiac disease and dermatitis herpetiformis are related, and the incidence of HLA-B8 (Gebhard *et al.*, 1973; White *et al.*, 1973; Scott *et al.*, 1975*a*; Seah *et al.*, 1976; Reunala *et al.*, 1976; Thomsen *et al.*, 1976) and the MLC determinant HLA-DW3 (Thomsen *et al.*, 1976; Solheim *et al.*, 1976) in dermatitis herpetiformis is of the same order as previously reported in celiac disease. Whether the susceptibility to malignant disease in dermatitis herpetiformis will prove to be more closely related to these and other gene loci than to an associated celiac disease is not yet clear.

A practical point in treatment concerns the use of gluten-free diet in the treatment of dermatitis herpetiformis. There is no doubt that patients with clinical celiac disease should be on a gluten-free diet to correct their malabsorption and possibly also to lessen the risk of malignancy (Harris *et al.*, 1967). It is still not clear whether patients with subclinical celiac disease should follow a gluten-free diet to forestall problems from malabsorption which might develop in the future. Nor do we know whether the risk of developing malignant lymphoma will also be reduced by gluten withdrawal in this subclinical group. In spite of opinion to the contrary (Fry *et al.*, 1973) a gluten-free diet has not in our hands proved to be a very effective treatment of the rash of dermatitis herpetiformis, although the dose of dapsone may decrease.

In summary, the association of dermatitis herpetiformis with celiac disease is so common that all general physicians and gastroenterologists should be able to make the diagnosis from the appearance of the rash and simple tests on the skin. Dermatologists should recognize that all patients with the rash should have a small intestinal mucosal biopsy, for this is the only way of making the diagnosis of celiac disease, especially in the milder and subclinical cases which are common in dermatitis herpetiformis. Dermatitis herpetiformis has an association with malignant lymphoma, probably through its association with celiac disease. Obviously, patients with celiac disease producing clinical and significant biochemical changes should be on a gluten-free diet, for a number of reasons. At present, there is no good evidence that patients with dermatitis herpetiformis who do not have celiac disease, or have it in subclinical form, should be subjected to a gluten-free diet.

6. References

Achord, J. L., and Proctor, H. D., 1963, Malignant degeneration and metastasis in Peutz-Jeghers syndrome, *Arch. Intern. Med.* **111**:498–502.

Albright, E. C., and Allday, R. W., 1967, Thyroid carcinoma after radiation therapy for adolescent acne, *J. Am. Med. Assoc.* **199**:280–281.

Anderson, H., Dotevall, G., and Mabacken, H., 1971, Malignant mesenteric lymphoma in a patient with dermatitis herpetiformis, hypochlorhydria and small bowel abnormalities, *Scand. J. Gastroenterol.* **6**:397–399.

Austad, W. I., Cornes, J. S., Gough, K. R., McCarthy, C. F., and Read, A. E., 1967, Steatorrhoea and malignant lymphoma, *Am. J. Digest. Dis. N.S.* **12**:475–490.

Badenoch, J., 1960, Steatorrhoea in the adult, *Br. Med. J.* **2**:879–887.

Berlin, C., 1955, Urticaria pigmentosa as a systemic disease, *Arch. Dermatol.* **71**:703–712.

Bluefarb, S. M., 1960, *Leukemia Cutis,* Thomas, Springfield, Ill.

Brett, E. M., Ong, B. H., and Friedmann, T., 1967, Mast-cell disease in children, *Br. J. Dermatol.* **79**:197–209.

Brow, J. R., Parker, F., Weinstein, W. M., and Rubin, C. E., 1971, The small intestinal mucosa in dermatitis herpetiformis, *Gastroenterology* . **60**:355–361.

Bussey, H. J. R., 1970, Gastrointestinal polyposis, *Gut* **11**:970–978.

Cooke, W. J., Peeney, A. L. P., and Hawkins, C. F., 1953, Symptoms, signs and diagnostic features of idiopathic steatorrhoea, *Q. J. Med. N.S.* **22**:59–77.

Cormane, R. H., 1967, Immunofluorescent studies of the skin in lupus erythematosus and other diseases, *Pathol. Eur.* **2**:170–180.

Cunliffe, W. J., Hall, R., Newell, D. J., and Stevenson, C. J., 1968, Vitiligo, thyroid disease and autoimmunity, *Br. J. Dermatol.* **80**:135–139.

Cunliffe, W. J., Hudgson, P., Fulthorpe, J. J., Black, M. M., Hall, R., Johnston, D.D.A., and Shuster, S., 1970, A calcitonin-secreting medullary thyroid carcinoma associated with mucosal neuromas Marfanoid features, myopathy and pigmentation, *Am. J. Med.* **48**:120–126.

Edwards, F. C., and Truelove, S. C., 1964, The course and prognosis of ulcerative colitis, *Gut* **5**:1–15.

Ferguson, R., Basu, M. J., Asquith, P., and Cooke, W. T., 1975, Recurrent aphthous ulceration and its association with coeliac disease, *Gut* **16**:393.

Flaxman, B. A., Zelazny, G., and Van Scott, E. J., 1971, Non-specificity of characteristic cells in mycosis fungoides, *Arch. Dermatol.* **104**:141–147.

Fraser, N. G., 1970, Autoantibodies in dermatitis herpetiformis, *Br. J. Dermatol.* **83**:609–613.

Fraser-Moodie, A., Hughes, R. G., Jones, S. M., Shorey, B. A., and Snape, L., 1976, Malignant melanoma metastases to the alimentary tract, *Gut* **17**:206–209.

Fry, L., Kier, P., McMinn, R. M. H., Cowan, J. D., and Hoffbrand, A. V., 1967, Small-intestinal structure and function and haemotological changes in dermatitis herpetiformis, *Lancet.* **2**:729–734.

Fry, L., Seah, P. P., McMinn, R. M. H., and Hoffbrand, A. V., 1972, Lymphocytic infiltration of epithelium in diagnosis of gluten-sensitive enteropathy, *Br. Med. J.* **3**:371–374.

Fry. L., Seah, P. P., Riches, D. J., and Hoffbrand, A. V., 1973, Clearance of skin lesions in dermatitis herpetiformis after gluten withdrawal, *Lancet* **1**:288–291.

Gardner, E. J., 1951, A genetic and clinical study of intestinal polyposis, a predisposing factor for carcinoma of the colon and rectum, *Am. J. Hum. Genet.* **3**:167–176.

Gebhard, R. L., Katz, S. I., Marks, J., Shuster, S., Trapani, R. J., Rogentine, G. N., and Strober, W., 1973, HL-A antigen type and small-intestinal disease in dermatitis herpetiformis, *Lancet* **2**:760–762.

Gjone, E., and Nordöy, A., 1970, Dermatitis herpetiformis, steatorrhoea and malignancy, *Br. Med. J.* **1**:610.

Goodwin, P., and Fry, L., 1973, Reticulum-cell sarcoma complicating dermatitis herpetiformis, *Proc. R. Soc. Med.* **66**:625–626.

Goolamali, S. G., Barnes, E. W., Irvine, W. J., and Shuster, S., 1974, Organ-specific antibodies in patients with lichen sclerosus, *Br. Med. J.* **4:**78–79.

Gorlin, R. J., and Goltz, R. W., 1960, *N. Eng. J. Med.* **262:**908–912.

Graham-Smith, D. D., 1970, The carcinoid syndrome, *Gut* **11:**189–191.

Griffith, G. C., Nichols, G., Asher, J. D., and Flanagan, B., 1965, Heparin osteoporosis, *J. Am. Med. Assoc.* **193:**85–88.

Harris, O. D., Cooke, W. T., Thompson, H., and Waterhouse, J. A. H., 1967, Malignancy in adult coeliac disease and idiopathic steatorrhoea, *Am. J. Med.* **42:**899–912.

Higgs, J. M., and Wells, R. S., 1973, Chronic mucocutaneous candidiasis: New approach to treatment, *Br. J. Dermatol.* **89:**179–190.

Howel-Evans, W., McConnell, R. B., Clarke, C. A., and Sheppar, P. M., 1958, Carcinoma of the oesophagus with keratosis palmaris et plantaris (tylosis), *Q. J. Med.* **27:**413–429.

Howitz, J., and Schwartz, M., 1971, Vitiligo, achlorhydria and pernicious anaemia, *Lancet* **2:**1331–1335.

Jacobs, A., and Jenkins, D. J., 1960, Iron content of finger nails, *Br. J. Dermatol.* **72:**145–148.

Jeghers, H., McKusick, V. A., and Katz, K. H., 1949, Generalized intestinal polyposis and melanin spots of the oral mucosa, lips and digits, *N. Eng. J. Med.* **241:**993–1005.

Kligman, A. M., 1961, Telogen effluvium: Pathologic dynamics of human hair loss, *Arch. Dermatol.* **83:**175–198.

Kumar, P. J., and Dawson, A. M., 1973, Dermatitis herpetiformis with pernicious anaemia and thyrotoxicosis, *Proc. R. Soc. Med.* **66:**1128–1129.

Lancaster, Smith, M. J., and Kumar, P. J., 1974, Atrophic gastritis and dermatitis herpetiformis, *Lancet.* **3:**777.

Levy, D., and Khatib, R., 1960, Intestinal neurofibromatosis with malignant degeneration: Report of a case, *Dis. Colon Rectum* **3:**140–144.

Mallinson, C. N., Bloom, S. R., Warin, A. P., Salmon, P. R., and Cox, B., 1974, A glucagonoma syndrome, *Lancet* **2:**1–5.

Marks, J., 1977, Dogma and dermatitis hepatiformis, *Clin. Exp. Dermatol.* **2:**189–207.

Marks, J., and Shuster, S., 1970, Dermatogenic enteropathy, *Gut* **11:**292–298.

Marks, J., Shuster, S., and Watson, A. J., 1966, Small bowel changes in dermatitis herpetiformis, *Lancet* **2:**1280–1282.

Marks, J., Birkett, D., Shuster, S., and Roberts, D. F., 1970, Small intestinal mucosal abnormalities in relatives of patients with dermatitis herpetiformis, *Gut* **11:**493–497.

Marks, R., and Whittle, M. W., 1969, Results of treatment of dermatitis herpetiformis with a gluten-free diet after one year, *Br. Med. J.* **4:**772–775.

Pierard, J., and Whimster, I., 1961, The histological diagnosis of dermatitis herpetiformis, *Br. J. Dermatol.* **73:**253–266.

Prottey, C., Hartop, P. J., and Press, M., 1975, Correction of the cutaneous manifestations of essential fatty acid deficiency in man by the application of sunflower seed oil to the skin, *J. Invest. Dermatol.* **64:**228–234.

Reunala, T., Salo, O. P., Tiilikainen, A., and Mattla, M. J., 1976, Histocompatability antigens and dermatitis herpetiformis with special reference to jejunal abnormalities and acetylator phenotype, *Br. J. Dermatol.* **94:**139–143.

Robson, A. O., and Jelliffe, A. M., 1963, Medicinal arsenic poisoning and lung cancer, *Br. Med. J.* **2:**207–209.

Rowell, N. R., 1972, Lupus erythematosus, scleroderma and dermatomyositis, in: *Textbook of Dermatology* (A. Rook, D. S. Wilkinson, and F. J. G. Ebling, eds)., p. 1126, Blackwell, Oxford.

Sagher, F., and Even-Par, Z., 1967, *Mastocytosis and the Mast Cell*, Karger, Basel.

Sagher, F., and Schorr, S., 1956, Bone lesions in urticaria pigmentosa, *J. Invest. Dermatol.* **26:**431–434.

Scott, B. B., Young, S., Rajah, S. M., Marks, J., and Losowsky, M. S., 1975*a*, The incidence of coeliac disease and HL-A8 in dermatitis herpetiformis, *Gut* **16:**845.

Scott, B. B., Hardy, G. J., and Losowsky, M. S., 1975*b*, Involvement of the small intestine in systemic mast cell disease, *Gut* **16:**918–924.

Seah, P. P., Fry, L., Kearney, J. W., Campbell, E., Mawbray, J. F., Stewart, J. S., and Hoffbrand, A. V., 1976, A comparison of histocompatibility antigens in dermatitis herpetiformis and adult coeliac disease, *Br. J. Dermatol.* **94:**131–138.

Shuster, S., 1963, High-output cardiac failure from skin disease, *Lancet* **1:**1338–1340.

Shuster, S., 1967, The gut and the skin, in: *Third Symposium on Advanced Medicine*, pp. 349–361, Pitman Medical, London.

Shuster, S., and Marks, J., 1965, Dermatogenic enteropathy—A new cause for steatorrhoea, *Lancet* **1:**1367–1368.

Shuster, S., and Marks, J., 1969, Dermatitis herpetiformis and the coeliac syndrome, *Proc. R. Soc. Med.* **62:**985–986.

Shuster, S., and Marks, J., 1970, *Systemic Effects of Skin Disease,* Heinemann, London.

Shuster, S., and Scarborough, H., 1961, Senile purpura, *Q. J. Med.* **30:**33–40.

Shuster, S., Watson, A. J., and Marks, J., 1968, Coeliac syndrome in dermatitis herpetiformis, *Lancet* **1:**1101–1106.

Sneddon, I. B., 1963, The skin markers of malignancy, *Br. Med. J.* **2:**405–409.

Solheim, B. G., Ek, J., Thune, P. O., Baklien, K., Bratlie, A., Rankin, B., Thoresen, A. B., and Thorsby, E., 1976, HLA antigens in dermatitis herpetiformis and coeliac disease, *Tissue Antigens* **7:**57–59.

Stillman, M. A., and Baer, R. L., 1972, Pemphigus and thymoma, *Acta Dermato-Venereol.* **52:**393–397.

Tan, R. S.-H., Butterworth, C. M., McLaughlin, H., Malka, S., and Samman, P. D., 1974, Mycosis fungoides—A disease of antigen persistence, *Br. J. Dermatol.* **91:**607–616.

Thompson, R. P. H., Nicholson, D. C., Farnan, T., Whitmore, D. N., and Williams, R., 1970, Cutaneous porphyria due to a malignant primary hepatoma, *Gastroenterology* **59:**779–783.

Thomsen, M., Platz, P., Marks, J., Ryder, L. P., Shuster, S., Svejgaard, A., and Young, S. H., 1976, Association of LD-8a and LD-12a with dermatitis herpetiformis, *Tissue Antigens* **7:**60–62.

Vickers, C. F. H., 1974, Nutrition and the skin, in: *Tenth Symposium on Advanced Medicine* (J. G. G. Ledingham, ed.), Pitman Medical, London.

Weinstein, W. M., 1974, Latent coeliac sprue, *Gastroenterology* **66:**489–493.

White, A. G., Barnetson, R. St. C., Da Costa, J. A. G., and McClelland, D. B. L., 1973, The incidence of HL-A antigens in dermatitis herpetiformis, *Brit. J. Dermatol.* **89:**133–136.

Winkelmann, R. K., and Linman, J. W., 1973, Erythroderma with atypical lymphocytes (Sézary syndrome), *Am. J. Med.* **55:**192–198.

Wormsley, K. G., 1964, *The Skin and Gut in Disease,* Pitman Medical, London.

Wyatt, E. H., 1975, Lichen planus and ulcerative colitis, *Br. J. Dermatol.* **93:**465–468.

Wyatt, E. H., Shuster, S., and Marks, J., 1971, A postal survey of patients with dermatitis herpetiformis, *Br. J. Dermatol.* **85:**511–518.

V

Future Directions in Therapy

24

Early and Definitive Surgical Therapy for Colonic and Rectal Cancer

Maus W. Stearns, Jr.

1. Prophylactic Surgery

1.1. Premalignant Adenoma

The term "prophylactic surgery" in regard to cancer is not applicable to many anatomical sites. However, it is increasingly clear that the detection and removal of adenomas substantially reduces the incidence of colonic and rectal cancer.

There is still considerable discussion regarding the adenoma-adenocarcinoma relationship. Respected authorities can be found denying any importance of the relation (Spratt *et al.*, 1958). Other authorities affirm this sequence of pathogenesis (Fenolio and Lane, 1975; Grinnell and Lane, 1958; Morson, 1974). Our concept is that a substantial proportion, probably the majority, of all adenocarcinomas of the large bowel arise in preexisting adenomas. Pathologists generally have accepted as a precursor of cancer the histological variant described as papillary adenomas. This has often been equated with the clinical entity villous adenoma, which is a sessile lesion. These villous adenomas may be small, or they may encompass the entire circumference of the bowel mucosa. However, papillary features may be found in pedunculated lesions as well. Many of the smaller polyps either sessile or pedunculated are found on careful histological study to contain both adenomatous and papillary features (Redentor *et al.*, 1965; Wychulis *et al.*, 1967).

Maus W. Stearns, Jr. • Chief, Rectal and Colon Service, Memorial Sloan-Kettering Cancer Center, New York, New York 10021.

A valid and persistent clinical observation has been that a 2–3 mm *de novo* mucosal carcinoma is either nonexistent or an extreme rarity (Stearns, 1963), whereas 2 or 3 mm foci of adenocarcinoma in preexisting adenomas or papillary adenomas are frequent. Since carcinoma must be small initially and since the small lesion is seen only in adenomas, it would seem logical to conclude that this is the site of origin of most adenocarcinomas of the bowel.

The most convincing clinical data relating to the possibility of prophylactic treatment of carcinoma of the bowel have been provided by Gilbertson (1974), who has reported on a 25-year follow-up of 18,000 patients examined at the University of Minnesota cancer prevention clinic. These patients had had routine sigmoidoscopies and any polyps detected were removed. In the follow-up there were only 11 cancers found in this portion of the bowel subsequently, whereas statistically on the basis of age and distribution of the patients 75–80 should have been found. All were early cancers, and none of the patients died as a result of these cancers. Moreover, in the colon above this visualized area, the same incidence of cancer was found as was anticipated statistically.

Thus we feel confident that the detection and irradication of adenomas in the bowel constitute true cancer prophylaxis and can reduce the incidence of large bowel cancer more than can any other existing or foreseeable measure.

1.1.1. Detection

Effective detection of adenomas, to be truly useful, demands not only adequate examination of all patients with bowel symptoms but also a program for screening all patients in the age group where the incidence of adenomas becomes significant, i.e., those over 40 years old.

Adequate examination of patients with bowel symptoms includes abdominal examination, digital-rectal examination, proctosigmoidoscopy, barium enema with air contrast, and often flexible colonoscopy. To these we must add screening for occult blood, according to the method described by Greegor (1969). It should be emphasized that these are complementary examinations. Each has its advantages and limitations. Digital examination is limited by length of the examining finger. It has the advantage of palpation of the area immediately above the sphincter posteriorly, in which good-sized lesions are often not seen by sigmoidoscopy. Sigmoidoscopy again has the limitation of length, usually 25 cm, but affords excellent visualization of even very small abnormalities. Barium enema with air-contrast provides shadow examination of the remaining colon. However, small rectal lesions are missed even with special techniques. It is unreliable for lesions smaller than 1 cm. Lesions located in flexures may be missed, as overlapping bowel may obscure small lesions. Flexible colonoscopy has been a very useful addition to our diagnostic methods, as it provides direct visualization of the mucosa. It has the drawback that there are a limited number of skillful colonoscopists. Even the most able are able to pass the instrument to the caecum in only 70–80% of all cases. The accuracy of the examination depends on the cleanliness of the bowel, particularly in the right colon, and the assurance that small lesions do not lie behind redundant folds. The detection of blood by Hemoccult slides after a meat-free, high-bulk diet in spite of all other negative studies alerts the examiner to the probability that a lesion is present and indicates a need for continued evaluation of the patient.

Obviously, adequate examination of any symptomatic patient will reveal any cancer that is present as well as premalignant adenomas.

As demonstrated by Gilbertson, routine proctosigmoidoscopy of all patients past 40 with removal of any polyps found will be effective in reducing the incidence of subsequent cancer in that portion of the bowel screened. Cancer detection clinics have for 30 years included sigmoidoscopy as a screening test for cancer of the bowel. The yield for asymptomatic cancer for these efforts has been very low, averaging 0.12% (Moertel *et al.*, 1966). However, a 6–8% pickup of "polyps" has been generally found, and when these are removed a significant number of cancers have undoubtedly been avoided. There are considerations associated with routine sigmoidoscopy as a screening method which have limited wider use then is currently practiced. There are only so many trained physicians and facilities to provide this examination for all patients, even if the patients could be persuaded to prepare themselves and take time for the examination. Furthermore, the method provides examination only of the distal 25 cm of the bowel. Previously it was calculated that 70% of all large bowel cancer lay within this region, but in recent years colonic cancer is becoming relatively more frequent. Thus as a screening procedure sigmoidoscopy has limited value, although it fills a role for those patients who are willing to undergo it.

The only currently available method that even approximates a true screening method is the Hemoccult slides method of Greegor. This is an inexpensive test which requires only a meat-free, high-bulk diet for 4 days. The patient takes two samples from each stool with a provided spatula and puts these on slides. This is repeated on 3 successive days. The slides are mailed to his physician. The patients loses no time, takes no laxatives, has no discomfort, and does not have to handle unsightly containers, and the test has proved highly acceptable to patients and physicians. If blood is found, appropriate diagnostic studies are carried out. Our own, and others', previous experience with routine examination of stool for occult blood was unrewarding and had been generally abandoned. The advantage of Greegor's method which has already been amply demonstrated is that there are very few false positives, so that not many unrewarding examinations to determine the source are required. As well as we can tell at this time, there have been very few false negatives, probably because the test is done on 3 successive days. In a significant number subsequently found to have adenomas or carcinomas, only one of the six specimen showed blood.

Currently the major problem is to convince physicians that this is probably as useful and less demanding of time and efforts and expertise than the Papanicolaou smear in reducing the incidence of cancer of clinical significance.

1.1.2. Treatment

With respect to treatment, the clinical presentation of the polyp, i.e., whether it is pedunculated or sessile, is a more important consideration than the pathological classification as of adenoma or papillary adenoma.

Pedunculated adenomas are in almost all instances adequately treated by local excision. Lesions of the rectum, sigmoid, and descending colon have for years been removed by an electric wire snare through rigid scopes of varying lengths up to 50 cm. With these longer instruments lesions up to the splenic flexure could be removed without laparotomy. These procedures for the lesions in the proximal sigmoid and descending colon often involved general anesthesia with necessary hospitalization and expensive operating room time. The lower sigmoidal and rectal lesions visualized with the 25-cm scope were removed as simple outpatient procedures requiring no hospitalization and no anesthesia. Lesions proximal to the splenic flexure of sufficient size in the appropriate clinical setting required laparotomy for their removal by colotomy and excision by ligation of the pedicle. The remainder of the bowel was inspected through sterile scopes and any additional polyps found were removed. There was considerable difference of opinion as to what circumstances justified removal of pedunculated lesions when laparotomy was required.

The introduction of flexible colonoscopes with continued improvement of them and the snares used to remove the polyps has greatly simplified the removal of these polyps. Almost total elimination of the need for laparotomy has largely silenced the objections to treatment. Laparotomy is advocated now only where for technical reasons the colonoscope cannot be passed to the site of the lesion, or where the lesion for various technical reasons cannot be removed.

Many of these pedunculated adenomas contain foci of adenocarcinoma. Although the foci vary greatly in size, rarely do they indicate the need for additional resective surgery. In earlier years we often did resections when we found carcinoma in these lesions. However, we found so little additional pathology in the way of either residual or regional nodal metastatic cancer that we adopted the following criteria for resection: (1) cancer extending to the line of excision, (2) highly anaplastic carcinoma, (3) foci of metastatic cancer demonstrated in lymphatics or veins of the pedicle. It is our current practice that when our pathologists report cancer in one of these pedunculated lesions, we discuss the pathology together and unless one of the above criteria is met we inform the patient of the finding but do not urge further treatment.

Sessile lesions are a more difficult problem. Technically they are harder to remove. If carcinoma is present, there is no protective pedicle to delay invasion of the muscle wall of the bowel. Most of the larger villous tumors are found in the rectum, usually in older persons. They are also found in the caecum and ascending colon, where detection by X ray is difficult. Sessile nonmalignant lesions are infrequent in other parts of the colon.

Sessile lesions in the caecum and other parts of the colon generally do not lend themselves to local removal through the colonoscope. However, if they are not too large this type of removal occasionally can be accomplished by highly skilled colonoscopic operators. Generally, however, these lesions should be resected and bowel continuity restored. If the lesion is completely soft, without any induration or ulceration, segmental resection is adequate treatment. If there is any suggestion of induration or clinical infiltration, then they should be regarded as cancer and an appropriate resection for cancer carried out. We do not rely on frozen section study of these polyps as our pathologists prefer permanent sections.

Most of the large villous lesions are found in the rectum of older patients where highly individualized consideration of all factors becomes essential to proper management (Quan and Castro, 1971). A number of methods should be in the armamentarium of any surgeon who undertakes their treatment. Removal of the tumor in single or multiple stages by cautery snare with a fine wire has proved very effective over the years. It is especially useful in elderly patients where operative procedures involving anesthesia are undesirable. Transanal full-thickness excision through either the dilated or transected anal sphincter is used for lesions in the mid and distal rectum. Posterior proctotomy with removal of the coccyx is another approach. We have used this less frequently in recent years as we have had undetected cancer at the depth of the lesion result in seeding of cancer in the pelvis, which made subsequent curative resection impossible. These lesions can also be treated by fulguration.

Annular villous lesions are very difficult to remove locally. They usually require some type of resection. In the mid or upper rectum, anterior resection with restoration of continuity can be done. In the low rectum if no clinical infiltration is present, a pull-through type of abdominoperineal resection may be indicated. If there is any question of clinical infiltrating cancer being present in the low rectum, then a Miles-type abdominoperineal resection offers the patient the best chance of long-term survival.

No matter what type of local removal has been used, if infiltrating cancer is found by the pathologist extending to the line of removal, then additional resection must be considered and weighed against other clinical factors such as age, condition of the patient, wishes of the patient after being fully informed of the findings, and the available alternatives. These are very difficult decisions and all those involved must participate in the final choice.

1.1.3. *Multiple Polyps*

The various syndromes of multiple polyps have been described and given a multitude of names, sometimes indicating significantly different problems (Yonemoto, *et al.*, 1969). From a purely clinical standpoint, "multiple" polyps vary from two to literally thousands, which may involve the entire rectal and colonic mucosa. Those occurring in the small bowel and stomach generally are not premalignant, although a number of cancers are being reported in association with them (Reid, 1974; Ross and Mara, 1974). Those which involve the colon, except for the juvenile type (hamartomas), are premalignant, and the chance of cancer rises with the duration and number. Many of these occur in patients in whose families other polyps or colonic cancers are found. This relationship is useful in initiating casefinding in other relatives. However, in almost half of our patients who had more than ten colonic polyps no familial history regarding gastrointestinal polyps or cancer could be obtained. In some families with a strong history of polyposis, the manifestations in individual patients vary from a few polyps scattered throughout the large bowel to thousands of colonic polyps to polyps of the right colon and hyperplastic polyps of the ileum.

From a therapeutic standpoint patients with multiple polyps present a number of problems. If there is literal replacement of the entire colonic mucosa with adenomas, subtotal colectomy with ileoproctostomy is a minimal procedure. At the time of resection or preceding it, enough rectal mucosal should be freed of polyps to allow an anastomosis that does not necessitate incorporation of polyps in it. As much of the rectosigmoid should be removed as consistent with a good anastomosis, usually to the upper rectum 10–12 cm from the anal verge. Remaining polyps can be removed by a cautery snare in the early postoperative period. Careful follow-up is essential to detect and remove recurrent polyps as they appear. This approach is feasible only if infiltrating cancer is not already present in the rectal segment. In such event, total colectomy with abdominoperineal resection and permanent ileostomy is mandatory.

The wisdom of retaining the rectal segment which contains many polyps has been questioned, particularly since the publication of a follow-up from Mayo Clinic on the high incidence of cancer in the rectal stump developing over a long period of time (Moertel *et al.*, 1970). However, this has not been the experience at St. Mark's (Morson, 1972) or at Memorial Hospital, where we have seen only two such cases and in one the cancer developed in a blind stump. We believe that the conservative approach is justified as long as the patient will return for periodic examinations and the polyps that do appear can be removed promptly.

Cole and Holden (1959) have reported the spontaneous regression of rectal polyps after subtotal colectomy. While we have seen several such cases, we have found that in some the polyps reappeared after several years. We believe that these patients must all be followed with the expectation that subsequent polyps will appear and should be removed.

It should be noted that especially in Gardner's syndrome the associated stigmata, specifically the fibrosarcoma, may cause more problems than the original polyposis of the colon (Watne *et al.*, 19[illegible]).

1.2. Longstanding Colitis

Patients who have had colitis over 10 years, especially with onset in their teens, become high risks for the development of carcinoma. For some time after the separation of ulcerative (mucosal) from granulomatous (transmural) forms of colitis it was believed that carcinoma occurred only in the ulcerative form. However, it is becoming apparent that it occurs in either manifestation. While we have not yet arrived at the conviction that we should advocate prophylactic colectomy in a patient who has lived succesfully with colitis more than 10 years, we do monitor that patient very carefully. The most generally useful diagnostic method is barium enema. However, the usual radiographic characteristics of carcinoma often are not found until late with carcinomas associated with ulcerative colitis. These lesions are often submucosal with relatively little mucosal ulceration. They present as segmental narrowing. Thus areas of narrowing are viewed with great suspicion and should be examined by colonoscopy, biopsy, brush cytology, and/or pulsatile washing cytology.

Mucosal biopsy of the rectum, biopsy of the rectum, according to Morson and Pang (1967), show changes that suggests developing carcinoma higher up. This appears to require a great deal of experience by the pathologist and has not been widely used by other pathologists to date.

In a number of patients with narrowing it is impossible to establish a preoperative diagnosis of carcinoma so that it has been our policy to advise resection when strictures appear.

The surgery carried out is basically that for the underlying disease, except that the segment under suspicion should have a resection as one does for cancer.

1.3. Obstructing Diverticular Disease

There is no apparent etiological relationship between diverticular disease and colonic carcinoma, but they both can and do occur in the same patient. Patients who present with bowel symptoms, either acute or chronic, and in whom subsequent barium enema reveals an obstructed segment of the colon present difficult diagnostic problems. In some instances with diverticula and a long narrowed segment with intact mucosa the radiologist can with reasonable assurance state that diverticulitis is the diagnosis. However, in a number of instances the differential from carcinoma cannot be made with assurance. Flexible colonoscopy with specimens obtained by a brush or pulsatile lavage is conclusive when positive but not when negative.

Surgery is often warranted in the asymptomatic patient with a narrowed colonic segment where the differential between diverticulitis and carcinoma cannot be established preoperatively. Inasmuch as biopsies are generally contraindicated on the intact bowel, the diagnosis may not be established at laparotomy until the resected specimen is examined. Under these circumstances, one should do a resection as one would do for carcinoma.

2. Definitive Surgery

2.1. Principles of Colon Surgery

The essentials of definitive surgery for cancer as applied to the colon and rectum are (1) wide removal of the cancer-bearing bowel segment, (2) widest feasible excision of the lymphatics draining the cancer-bearing bowel segment to remove regional nodal metastases that may be present, (3) the accomplishment of these with a minimum of cancer cell contamination and embolization. In general, the adequate accomplishment of excision of the lymphatic drainage pathways also effects a wide local removal of the cancer-bearing bowel segment.

Thus operations for cancer of the colon depend on the lymphatic drainage. The lymphatics of the colon and rectum were well described by Rouviere (1938), and our surgical procedures have been based on these descriptions. In summary, the lymphatic drainage of the right colon and transverse follows the vascular tree derived from the superior mesenteric vessels. In the cecal and ascending colon the drainage is along the ileocolic and right colic systems down to their origins from the superior mesenteric. The transverse colon drains along the midcolic to the superior mesenteric. Similarly, the left colon from the splenic flexure downward drains toward the root of the mesentery as defined by the inferior mesenterics. The entire rectum drains along the superior hemorrhoid to the inferior mesenteric. In addition, from the low rectum, i.e., the low 6–7 cm from the anal verge, lymphatic drainage may also be distal along the inferior hemorrhoids or laterally along the middle hemorrhoid.

2.2. *Specific Application to Rectum and Colon*

For right colon lesions a right hemicolectomy is performed. When the lesion is near the ileal cecal valve, a substantial segment of the terminal ileum (10–12 cm) with its mesentery should be removed because of the lymphatics along the ileocolic vessels. When the lesion is in the hepatic flexure or mid-transverse colon, not so much ileum need be removed but a meticulous dissection of the mesentery to the root of the midcolic from the superior mesenteric is considered essential. With any left colon lesion, left hemicolectomy is done with dissection to the root of the mesentery as defined by the origin of the inferior mesenterics. An exception to this would be a lesion in the redundant mid or lower sigmoid, where sigmoidectomy with dissection to the root of the inferior mesenteric would remove as much of the lymphatic drainage as does a left hemicolectomy since the lymphatic drainage does not go along the marginal vessels away from the root of the mesentery.

All of the lesions which lie in the intraperitoneal colon can be removed by resection which allows restoration of bowel continuity.

In the upper rectum, where the lymphatic drainage is cephalad, some kind of a sphincter-preserving type of resection is theoretically possible and, in our experience, justified (Stearns, 1974). Here we add little to the excision of lymphatic drainage by removing the distal rectum, sphincters, and perineal structures by a combined abdominoperineal resection.

In practice, when we have a patient with a lesion in the upper rectum he is told preoperatively that while we expect to do a procedure that allows him to move his bowels through the normal location, we may find it necessary to perform a permanent colostomy. At laparotomy after thorough abdominal exploration the operative field is isolated. Peritoneal incisions made parallel to the ureters are carried down into the pelvis and upward to the level of the duodenum. The mesorectum and mesosigmoid are freed from the common iliac vessels across the aorta by blunt and sharp dissection. The mesentery and the contained vascular pedicle are freed in good-risk patients up to the origin from the inferior mesenteric or in poor-risk or elderly patients to the left colic. The vessels are isolated and divided. The mesorectum is then freed from the hollow of the sacrum posteriorly. Inferiorly the periureteral peritoneal incisions are connected across the midline on the posterior aspect of the seminal vesicles or vagina and these structures are freed by blunt and sharp dissection from the lateral wall of the pelvis. The lateral ligments containing the midhemorrhoidal vessels are transected close to their origin without prior clamping. By retracting the rectum anteriorly, Waldeyer's fascia extending from the posterior aspect of the rectum to the sacrum is identified and incised, and further mobilization of the rectum is accomplished by additional blunt dissection in this space. When moblization has been completed, then the decision as to what type of resection is indicated is made. If at least two fingers can be placed below the palpable border of the tumor, if a clamp can be placed across the bowel below them without stretching the rectum, and if after the bowel is transected below the clamp there will be adequate distal bowel for anastomosis, an anterior resection with end-to-end anastomosis is done (Dixon, 1939). If there is two fingerbreaths free margin without tension but insufficient room for a clamp and an adequate stump after transection, then we will consider a pull-through type of abdominoperineal resection (Babcock and Bacon, 1949; Bacon, 1971). If the tumor cannot be mobilized with adequate margin above the levators, then a Miles-type abdomino perineal resection is done (Miles, 1908).

In the distal rectum, i.e., in the lower 6 cm of the large bowel, a Miles-type abdominoperineal resection is done for the usual clinically infiltrating rectal carcinoma. In addition to the abdominal and pelvic dissection described for lesions in the upper rectum, the perineal phase is as extensive as possible, limited only by the bony structures of the pelvis. Wide excision of the perineal skin to the ischial tuberosities and back to the tip of the coccyx defines the extent of resection. The contents of the ischiorectal fossa are removed by deepening the incision down to the levator muscles. The pelvis is entered at the tip of the coccyx. While the levator muscles are retracted medially they are transected at their attachment to their bony pelvis. The pelvic peritoneal floor is usually closed during the abdominal phase and the perineum is closed temporarily over a pelvic pack which is removed after 4–5 days, but no primary closure of the perineum is attempted.

2.2.1. *Protection against Cancer Cell Contamination, Implantation, and Embolization*

A number of authors, particularly Warren Cole (1952), have directed surgeons' attention to the danger of spreading and implanting cancer cells during operations for cancer. We perform our operations with concern for this possibility. Cancer operations are treated as one would an operation in an infected field. Protection of wound edges and adjacent viscera by laparotomy pads is stressed. The abdomen is thoroughly explored before the tumor is approached. The operative field should be isolated before examination of the tumor. While we do examine the tumor sufficiently to determine operability and any associated problems, we do not manipulate it unnecessarily. Traction on the proximal or distal bowel to provide exposure can be substituted for handling of the tumor. We wash contaminated gloves and change contaminated packs frequently. After the tumor has been resected, the operative field is irrigated with sterile distilled water to provide mechanical flushing. Although crushing clamps are placed across the bowel at points selected for subsequent transection before any manipulation of the tumor is done, surprisingly large tumor fragments lying free in the lumen proximal or distal to the isolated segment are not infrequently found. Prior to performing anastomosis we excise the crushed ends of the bowel, aspirate the contents of the proximal and distal bowel, and swab the mucosa liberally with whatever skin antiseptic we are currently using.

2.2.2. *Colostomies*

Most temporary colostomies are satisfactorily constructed as a simple loop of colon exteriorized over a rod. When done for obstruction, a site near the point of obstruction allows subsequent concomitant resection of the colostomy with resection of the tumor. A colostomy at some distance may result in an unnecessary three-stage procedure.

Temporary colostomies done in conjunction with anterior resection are usually transverse colostomies. These can be closed whenever satisfactory healing of the anastomosis has occurred, usually 3–4 weeks. Only about 20–30% of anterior resections involve temporary colostomies. They should be considered in the following circumstances. Elderly patients do not tolerate infection well. With low anastomosis in these patients a protective diverting colostomy may be life saving. If in a patient who has had an obstructing lesion an inadequately cleansed bowel is found at resection, a colostomy should be considered. A colostomy should be done if a low anastomosis is less than ideal technically. When a hysterectomy has been done in conjunction with an anterior resection, the closure of the vaginal stump at the same level as the bowel anastomosis invites a rectovaginal fistula with any breakdown of the anastomosis and again a temporary colostomy should be considered.

Temporary colostomies, even though temporary, should be located where they can be easily managed. Since patients with temporary colostomies are seldom taught to manage them by irrigation, this means that they should be situated where a proper-fitting colostomy bag can be applied satisfactorily. Permanent colostomies usually are formed with a Miles-type abdominoperineal resection. We prefer to bring them out through the midline located between the umbilicus and the symphysis pubis. Any redundancy of the bowel should be eliminated by bringing the sigmoid out as a gentle curve from its junction with the descending colon, removing the excess bowel.

Usually patients with permanent colostomies are taught to irrigate as part of their management. There are several reasons for irrigation. First and foremost, many patients consider a colostomy degrading, mainly because they have no control over when bowel function occurs. Irrigations done every other day usually restore to the patient the ability to have the bowel function when he wishes. Patients are instructed in the management of their colostomy before leaving the hospital. These instructions include not only demonstration of the methods of irrigation but also discussion of sensible diets, stressing the well-rounded diet with omission only of those foods patients may find to cause trouble, such as constipation, diarrhea, or odor. They are urged to resume their normal business and social activities as rapidly as returning strength and vigor permit. They are advised to avoid only the most strenuous lifting and straining.

2.2.3. *Limited Procedures for Cancer of the Rectum*

Since a colostomy is not something patients want to have unless it offers the only possiblity for cure, a number of procedures to avoid a colostomy have been advocated as treatment for cancer of the rectum. There are a number of lesions which can be adequately treated by these means. As described earlier, the villous adenoma with histological cancer in it can be adequately removed by local methods unless cancer is found infiltrating the bowel wall at the base of the line of excision. In these circumstances, more adequate resection should be considered.

Some forms of cancer present as exophytic polypoid projection without clinical invasion of the muscle of the bowel wall. These can be removed locally provided that careful follow-up surveillance for signs of local recurrence is carried out. If there is no invasion of the muscle, the chance of regional nodal metastases is very small. This is probably true of minimal invasion of the muscle propria. However, with invasion through the entire muscle wall the chance of nodal metastases rises to 35–40%. Thus deeply infiltrating ulcerated lesions, even if small, have a significant number of regional nodal metastases. These are not adequately treated by local methods which do not remove them and thereby do not offer a possible control.

Even in patients with cancer clinically infiltrating the bowel wall, local methods are useful in management. A patient with significant distant metastases, particularly hepatic and/or peritoneal, who has a suitable nonobstructing lesion is probably better managed by local control of the primary than by a major debilitating resection and a permanent colostomy added to his problems. However, the lesion has to be amenable to local methods. Thus an annular lesion will usually be better treated with an abdominoperineal resection as local methods are inadequate to control such extensive lesions. Some patients because of mental or physical disabilities are unable to care for a colostomy. If the lesion is amenable to local methods of control, palliative local management may well be preferable to the permanent incapacitation or institutionalion of such patients because of their inability to cope with or manage a colostomy.

A number of local methods have been used to control rectal cancer locally. Our experience is limited to local surgical excision and electrosurgical methods. Papillon (1974) has used high-dose, low-voltage radiation therapy with excellent reported results in selected patients. Deddish (1974) has reported his personal experience with local excision of infiltrating cancer. The survival in 86 such patients was about 83% for 5 years and 72% for 10 years. While the criteria he used to select these patients are not clear in his report, he has stated that the patients were those with highly selected lesions. This group of 86 was selected by him over a 25-year period and hence constituted a very small portion of patients with rectal cancer seen by him during this time.

Electrosurgical methods have been vigorously promoted by Madden and Kandalaft (1971) and Crile and Turnbull, (1972). Each team uses somewhat different techniques for electrocoagulation. Madden reintroduced this method in 1967 as the "primary and preferred method for treatment of cancer of the rectum." There have been too few patients treated by electrocoagulation with a long-term follow-up to permit valid statistical comparison with the results obtained by the major types of resection. However, in view of its failure to remove regional nodal metastases and thereby offer these patients at least a potential chance of cure, it does not warrant the claims that it should replace resection for the usual infiltrating rectal cancer.

One unfortunate result of the efforts to popularize electrocoagulation has been the assumption by some that this is an office procedure which spares the patient not only colostomy but also hospitalization, anesthesia, and operating room costs. Madden has rightly pointed out that it must be done properly and is the equivalent of a major operative procedure taking 1½–2 hr in the operating room under anesthesia with substantial complications resulting. We see a number of patients who have been treated in doctors' offices on a weekly basis until they arrive in a hopelessly inoperable condition.

Since local methods do have a limited role in the management of rectal cancer, surgeons should be able to pick the local method most suited to the clinical condition of the patient and the local characteristics of the cancer. Thus in some instances local transanal excision can effect wide local removal simply. In others which are not as approachable, electrocoagulation is more applicable.

2.2.4. *Adjuvant Therapy for Cancer of the Colon and Rectum*

For at least 20 years there has been great interest in adjuvant therapy following curative resection to improve the survival in these patients. To date, no single-agent adjuvant chemotherapy program has been proved effective in improving survival. Great interest exists at present in combined chemotherapy programs with and without immunotherapy. The results will be followed with great interest.

Preoperative radiation therapy for cancer of the rectum has also been studied, with equivocal results. A retrospective review of our experience with relatively low-dose preoperative radiation from 1939 to 1951 (Stearns *et al.*,

1959) indicated substantial improvement in survival of those found to have regional nodal metastases. We began a new series in 1957 which was continued through 1967. On analysis we could no longer show any benefit (Stearns *et al.*, 1974). However, the Veterans Administration has studied a series using essentially the same radiation dosage (Higgins *et al.*, 1975) and has concluded that there was definite advantage in those having abdominoperineal resection as primary treatment. In reviewing our own material, we could not corroborate this conclusion.

Additional studies utilizing higher doses preoperatively are in progress. Cooperative efforts are being carried out to determine the usefulness of postoperative radiation therapy.

3. References

Babcock, W. W., and Bacon, H. E., 1949, Carcinoma of the large bowel, *Phila. Med.* **44**:1931.

Bacon, H. E., 1971, Present status of the pull-through sphincter-preserving procedure, *Cancer* **28**:196–203.

Cole, J. W., and Holden, W., 1959, Post colectomy regression of adenomatous polyps of the rectum, *AMA Arch. Surg.* **79**:385–392.

Cole, W. H., 1952, Recurrence in carcinoma of colon and rectum following resection for carcinoma, *AMA Arch. Surg.* **65**:264–270.

Crile, G. J., and Turnbull, R. B., Jr., 1972, The role of electrocoagulation in the treatment of carcinoma of the rectum, *Surg. Gynecol. Obstet.* **135**:391.

Deddish, M. R., 1974, Local excision, *Surg. Clin. N. Am.* **54**:877–880.

Dixon, C. F., 1939, Surgical removal of lesions occurring in the sigmoid and rectosigmoid, *Am. J. Surg.* **46**:12.

Fenolio, C. M., and Lane, N., 1975, The anatomic precursor of colorectal carcinoma, *J. Am. Med. Assoc.* **231**:640–642.

Gilbertson, V., 1974, Proctosigmoidoscopy and polypectomy in reducing the incidence of rectal cancer, *Cancer* **34**:936–939.

Greegor, H., 1969, Detection of silent colon cancer in routine examination, *Ca* **19**:330–337.

Grinnell, R. S., and Lane, N., 1958, Benign and malignant adenomatous polyps and papillary adenomas of the colon and rectum: An analysis of 1,856 tumors in 1,335 patients, *Int. Abst. Surg.* **106**:519–538.

Higgins, G. A., Jr., Conn, J. H., Jordan, P. H., Jr., Humphrey, E. H., Roswit, B., and Keehn, R. J., 1975, Preoperative radiotherapy for colorectal cancer, *Ann. Surg.* **181**:624–631.

Madden, J. L., and Kandalaft, 1971, Clinical evaluation of electrocoagulation in the treatment of cancer of the rectum, *Am. J. Surg.* **122**:347–352.

Miles, W. E., 1908, A Method of performing abdomino-perineal excision for carcinoma of the rectum and of the terminal portion of the pelvic colon, *Lancet* **2**:1812.

Moertel, C. G., Hill, J. R., and Dockerty, M. B., 1966, The routine proctoscopic examination: A second look, *Mayo Clin. Proc.* **41**:368–374.

Moertel, C. G., Hill, J. R., and Adson, M., 1970, Surgical management of multiple polyposis: The problem of cancer in the retained bowel segment, *AMA Arch. Surg.* **100**:521–526.

Morson, B. C., 1972, *Gastrointestinal Pathology*, p. 535, Blackwell, London.

Morson, B. C., 1974, Evolution of cancer in the colon and rectum, *Cancer* **34**:845–849.

Morson, B. C., and Pang, L. S. C., 1967, Rectal biopsy as an aid to cancer control in ulcerative colitis, *Gut* **8**:423–434.

Papillon, J., 1974, Endocavitary irradiation in the curative treatment of eary rectal cancer, *Dis. Colon Rectum* **17**:172–180.

Quan, S. H. Q., and Castro, E. B., 1971, Papillary adenomas (villous tumors): A review of 215 cases, *Dis. Colon Rectum* **14**:267–280.

Redentor, J. G., Pagtalunan, M. D., Dockerty, M. B., Jackman, R. J., and Anderson, M. J., 1965, The histopathology of diminutive polyps of the large intestine, *Surg. Gynecol. Obstet.* **120:**1259–1265.

Reid, J. D., 1974, Intestinal carcinoma in the Peutz-Jeghers syndrome, *J. Am. Med. Assoc.* **229:**833–834.

Ross, J. E., and Mara, J. E., 1974, Small bowel polyps and carcinoma in multiple intestinal polyposis, *AMA Arch. Surg.* **108:**736–738.

Rouviere, H., *Anatomy of the Human Lymphatic System: A Compendium,* pp. 188–192, translated by M. J. Tobias, Edwards Brothers, Ann Arbor, Mich.

Spratt, J. S., Jr., Ackerman, L. V., and Moyer, C. A., 1958, Relationship of polyps of the colon to colonic cancer, *Ann. Surg.* **148:**682–698.

Stearns, M. W., Jr., 1974, The choice among anterior resection, the pull-through and **116:**625.

Stearns, M. W., Jr., 1974, The choice among anterior Resection, the pull-through and abdomino-perineal resection of the rectum, *Cancer* **34:**969–971.

Stearns, M. W., Jr., 1975, The cancer patient with a colostomy, in: *Cancer Epidemiology and Prevention* (D. Schottenfeld, ed.), pp. 502–510, Thomas, Springfield, Ill.

Stearns, M. W., Jr., Deddish, M. R., and Quan, S. H. Q., 1959, Preoperative roentgen therapy in cancer of the rectum, *Surg. Gynecol. Obstet.* **109:**225–229.

Stearns, M. W., Jr., Deddish, M. R., Quan, S. H. Q., and Leaming, R. H., 1974, Preoperative roentgen therapy for cancer of the rectum and rectosigmoid, *Surg. Gynecol. Obstet.* **138:**584–586.

Watne, A. L., Johnson, J. G., and Chang, C. H., 1969, The challenge of Gardner's syndrome, *CA* **19:**267–275.

Wychulis, A. R., Dockerty, M. B., Jackman, R. J., and Beahrs, O. H., 1967, Histopathology of small polyps of the large intestine, *Surg. Gynecol. Obstet.* **124:**87–92.

Yonemoto, R. H., Slayback, J. B., Byron, R. L. J., and Rose, R. B., 1969, Familial polyposis of the entire gastrointestinal tract, *AMA Arch. Surg.* **99:**427–434.

25

Chemotherapy of Colorectal Cancer: A Critical Analysis of Response Criteria and Therapeutic Efficacy

Alan Yagoda and Nancy Kemeny

1. Introduction

Large bowel cancer afflicts more patients in the United States than any other malignant neoplasm excluding skin cancer, is second only to lung cancer as a cause of cancer death, and accounts for 15% of all cancer deaths (Silverberg and Holleb, 1971). During the past 30 years there has been little change in the overall 5-year survival, 30% (Cutler, 1968), in patients who undergo "curative" surgical resection for colorectal cancer. These statistics are not surprising since almost half the patients with colorectal carcinoma have evidence of metastatic lymph node involvement at the time of surgery (Coller, 1956). While pre- and postoperative radiation therapy has permitted an increase in surgical resectability and overall palliation, it has not influenced 5-year survival rates. Obviously, other therapeutic modalities are needed.

Almost two decades ago a new antineoplastic chemotherapeutic agent, 5-fluorouracil (5FU), was introduced for the treatment of gastrointestinal cancers. In the early trials 5FU appeared to offer significant improvement in response rates in advanced disease, and there was hope it would be still more effective in patients with a minimal tumor burden. When additional clinical studies with 5FU noted a huge variability of 8–85% (Moertel and Reitemeier, 1969) in objective response rates, considerable controversy ensued regarding

---

Alan Yagoda and Nancy Kemeny • Assistant Attendings, Solid Tumor Service, Department of Medicine, Memorial Sloan-Kettering Cancer Center, New York, New York 10021.

the optimal dosage, schedule, and route of administration. Therefore, nonrandomized and later randomized trials examined the efficacy of 5FU when given orally or intravenously; daily, weekly, twice weekly, monthly, or intermittently; with a high or a low loading dose; and as an intravenous bolus or a continuous 2-, 8-, 24-, or 120-hr infusion. The results of these preliminary studies led some oncologists to express the view that no patient with colon cancer, regardless of the stage, should be denied 5FU as the initial form of therapy (Zubrod, 1966; Lemon and Foley, 1966).

The promise of 5-fluorouracil to achieve a significant increase in survival in patients with large bowel cancer has never materialized. Eighty to eighty-five percent of patients treated with the drug obtain no benefit; rather, a significant number experience only its toxic side effects. While 15–20% show some objective improvement, responses are rarely complete and many partial remissions are probably nothing more than "very transient shrinkages of vaguely defined lumps which frequently may be more reflective of human error in measurement than of actual reduction in tumor size" (Moertel, 1975).

Phase II and III drug- or disease-oriented trials generally demand objective parameters which are readily measurable and can be repeatedly followed with relative precision. Colon cancer seems ideally suited for such studies since the pattern of dissemination indicates a propensity to metastasize to a variety of easily measurable sites, such as liver, lungs, and lymph nodes (Golbey *et al.*, 1960). Other criteria which can be accurately monitored include various biochemical parameters such as abnormal liver function tests produced by hepatic metastases and biological markers such as carcinoembryonic antigens. Since there are measurable parameters, marked differences in response rates to 5FU are not easily explained unless investigators are interpreting the term "response" differently.

2. *Response Criteria*

2.1. *Complete Remission*

During the past 20 years many schemata have been devised to assist clinicians in determining clinically useful responses. The most frequently employed ones are outlined in Table 1.

Complete remission (CR) generally denotes total disappearance of all objective disease. This definition requires investigators to document, utilizing all available diagnostic tools, the complete regression of macroscopic disease. Obviously, the frequency of so-called complete remissions will depend on how hard investigators look for residual disease. Unfortunately, some older studies have not detailed a vigorous search for evidence of remaining disease and have assumed "complete" osseous, intraabdominal, or hepatic tumor regression. Recent reports, however, are beginning to include histological examination of material from previously known sites of metastatic involvement obtained by aspirations, biopsies, and even second-look operations. This approach should assist physicians in comparing results between various clinical trials.

Response not only should be an objective volumetric improvement of measurable lesions for a minimum duration, but also should result in some subjective benefit to the patient. Karnofsky (1961; Karnofsky *et al.*, 1962) realized the need for meaningful response categories to include a patient's subjective improvement when defining responses and thus, for example, required in his I-C category—complete remission for 1 year—"complete relief of symptoms." Symptoms include general malaise, anorexia, nausea, weight loss, fever, pain, and an increase in performance status. Although complete objective regression of tumor may be rapidly obtained, concomitant improvement in subjective parameters may be delayed or even prevented because of residual damage persisting from a prior carcinomatous process or toxic side effects produced by chemotherapy. Unfortunately, recent schemata used in defining response tend to disregard subjective signs altogether and focus only on objective regression of disease.

2.2. Partial Remission

Most clinical trials today define partial remission (PR) as greater than 50% reduction in the sum of the products of two perpendicular diameters of a lesion(s) without simultaneous increase in other lesions. This category can include mixed responses since all lesions do not need to show regression. It assumes, indirectly, that other lesions which do not regress are still favorably affected by chemotherapy and are stabilized. In this PR category, metastatic deposits in such sites as bone, abdomen, pelvis, and rectum are often included and these cannot be measured with a reasonable degree of accuracy. Therefore, some investigators have devised other objective PR response criteria for these sites. Since the pattern of dissemination in colon cancer frequently is to these four sites, differences in objective response rates in the literature may be due to the manner in which some investigators define PR status in these sites.

2.2.1. *Evaluation of the Liver*

Although liver metastases from colon cancer appear at first glance to be easily measurable and reproducible by physical examination, radioisotopic scanning, and biochemical tests, accuracy is lacking. Many investigators (Moertel and Reitemeier, 1962) use a modification in evaluating objective changes in malignant hepatomegaly, i.e., a 30% reduction in the sum of measurements below the xyphoid and each costal margin at the midclavicular line. Let us assume that an enlarged liver measures 5 cm below the costal margin at the xyphoid and 5 cm below the costal margin at the right midclavicular line. The sum is 10. After treatment the liver now measures 4 cm below the costal margin at the xyphoid and 3 cm at the right midclavicular line. The reduction, 10 cm to 7 cm, is 30% and represents an objective response as long as abnormal liver function tests, such as serum bilirubin, glutamic oxaloacetic trans-

Table 1. Categories of Response[a]

	Karnofsky	MSKCC	Frei and Holland	Moertel	Western Cooperative Cancer Chemotherapy Group
CR[b]	↓ All manifestations of active disease >1 year; no recurrence between courses of therapy; complete relief of symptoms (I-C)	No evidence of disease; PS = 100	No evidence of tumor (0); no abnormality in subjective status (0)	Complete regression of measurable disease	100% ↓ and subjective improvement for *>1 month* (I-C)
PR	Objective ↓ of *all* palpable or measurable disease >1 month in a relatively *asymptomatic* patient; tumor regression should be unequivocal; all lesions reduced >50% (I-B) [Distinct subjective benefit with favorable objective change in *all* measurable criteria >1 month (I-A)]	>50% ↓ in measurable disease for 1 month Hepatomegaly: *>50%* in *sum* of *all* measurements below costal margins and improvement in liver function tests	>50% ↓ in *product* of largest diameter of *several* representative tumor masses; mild abnormality in performance (1)	>50% ↓ in the *product* of largest perpendicular diameters of most clearly measurable primary *indicator* lesion; no ↑ in other lesions; no new lesions [>50% ↓ of lesions <5 cm; *>30% ↓ of lesions •5 cm*]; hepatomegaly: *>30%* ↓ in the *sum* of measurements below *xyphoid* and each costal margin at the midclavicular line *without deterioration* of liver function tests (objective response)	>50% ↓ and subjective improvement for >1 month (I-B)
MR	Subjective benefit and favorable objective changes in measurable criteria <1 month (O-C) [Favorable objective changes without subjective benefit (O-B)]	>25% to <50% ↓ in measurable disease, or >50% ↓ for <1 month	>25% to <50% ↓ in measurable lesions		>25% to <50% ↓ for >1 month and subjective improvement (I-A)
STAB	Interruption or slowing in progression of disease without definite evidence of subjective or objective improvement (II)	Same as Karnofsky	≤25% ↓ or ↑ in measurable lesions; symptoms unchanged or markedly relieved	—	—
PROG	Disease progresses; no objective or subjective benefit (O-O) [Subjective benefit without objective changes (O-A)]	Same as Karnofsky	>25% ↓ in measurable lesions	None of the above	None of the above

[a]( ), Abbreviations used to denote response category. [ ], Other definitions which are approximately similar to response categories CR, PR, MR, STAB, or PROG, or variations which have been used to define a category of response in recent or past clinical trials.
[b]See text.

Table 1. Continued

Southwest Oncology Group	Israel	Falkson	American Oncologic Hospital	Roswell Park
Complete disappearance of all measurable lesions and all symptoms >1 month	—	—	Disappearance of all lesions >2 months	Complete disappearance of disease >1 month
>50% ↓ in sum of products of 2 diameters of *all* measurable lesions by physical X-rays or isotopic scans for >1 month Hepatomegaly: same as Moertel	>50% ↓ in *product* of 2 perpendicular diameters *without* simultaneous ↑ in *any other lesions*	>50% ↓ of *all* measurable lesions	>50% ↓ for >2 months	>50% ↓ sum of products of 2 perpendicular diameters of measurable lesions, or >50% ↓ of nonmeasurable evaluable disease for >1 month; no new lesions; hepatomegaly: same as Moertel but >50% ↓ in sum of measurements
—	—	Good tumor shrinkage (IMP)	—	—
≂50% ↓ or ↑ in sum of products of 2 perpendicular diameters of *all* lesions (no change) [<50% ↑ to <25% ↓]	>25% ↑ in *product* of 2 perpendicular diameters	—	<50% ↓ to 0% ↑ and subjective improvement >2 months	<50% ↓ *of evaluable disease •1 month, or o50, √ measurable lesions; no new lesions; no progression of nonmeasurable disease*
>50% ↑ in size of measured lesions or new lesions	All variations between <50% ↓ and >25% ↑ of *product* of 2 perpendicular diameters	None of the above	>25% ↑ tumor	⋝25% ↓ sum of the products of 2 perpendicular diameters

aminase, and alkaline phosphatase, do not increase. Interestingly, this definition does not even demand a decrease in any abnormal values. Since the anatomical location of the midclavicular or mammary line is variable and poorly reproducible (Rytand, 1968), and some studies show as high as a 50% error by multiple investigators in judging the extent of hepatomegaly (Ariel and Briceno, 1976), a different approach is utilized at Memorial Sloan-Kettering Cancer Center (MSKCC). The liver is measured during quiet respiration with the patient in the supine position with arms at the sides. Marks are made on the chest horizontally across the rib cage at the xyphoid and 5, 10, and 15 cm to its left and right. That portion of the enlarged liver which extends below the costal margin at these designated marks is recorded. An objective partial remission is defined as 50% reduction in the sum of all available measurements. In addition, a 50% reduction in all abnormal biochemical parameters or in all filling defects on radioisotopic scans must be achieved or PR status is reduced to a minor response.

2.2.2. *Evaluation of Pelvic and Intraabdominal Masses*

Generally, measurements of rectal, pelvic, or intraabdominal lesions are inaccurate, too. Pelvic lesions tend to have indistinct margins because of surrounding areas of induration, edema, and fibrosis. Intraabdominal masses may be relatively mobile within the abdominal cavity, and their apparent size may be influenced by ascites, feces, or gaseous distention. Lesions in both of these sites are not infrequently composed of nonhomogeneous masses because of asymmetrical lobulations and necrotic areas which further hinder uniform assessment by different examiners. Moertel and Hanley (1976) tested 16 experienced oncologists who measured 12 simulated tumor masses without knowledge that two of the masses were identical in size. When the same investigators, using a 25% reduction in size as the criterion of response, evaluated identical masses repetitively, a 19% error ensued. When different investigators measured the same mass, there occurred a 25% chance of error. This study suggests the need for stricter PR response criteria, such as 75% regression of lesions in these metastatic sites. Unfortunately, radiological contrast studies used to corroborate possible responses in these difficult areas have been of limited utility; perhaps computerized transaxial tomography may be more helpful.

2.3. *Minor Responses*

The category minor remission (MR) is used to denote 25–50% tumor regression. In the past, the category stabilization indicated changes of less than 25% decrease and not greater than 25% increase in tumor size. However, this category recently has been enlarged by some clinicians to permit the inclusion of lesions showing an increase in size up to 50%, thereby minimizing its clinical significance. These categories, MR and stabilization, should always be reported separately from the combined CR plus PR categories, since they represent an antitumor effect of far lesser magnitude. While there is room for recognition of MR and stabilization categories when the quality and duration of response are meaningful to the patient, inclusion of these minor categories in the overall response rates is to be deplored.

2.4. *Duration of Response*

Duration of response can be reported differently. Some investigators record responses from the start of therapy while others use the time at which a 25–50% tumor decrease is achieved. Although the former definition is more precise, either can be used. When evaluating results between various clinical trials, physicians need to know that the definitions of the durations of response are comparable.

2.5. *Conclusion*

These differences in defining response, particularly PR status, may explain much of the variations found in response rates when similar agents were evaluated in phase II–III studies in colon cancer. Moertel and Reitemeier (1969) recognized this fact when they noted a significantly lower response of pulmonary metastases to 5FU compared to the higher response rates found at other sites: "It is tempting to state that this difference may be completely artificial since pulmonary metastasis is usually easily demonstrable, easy to measure and rather vulnerable to review; for most other sites, one must rely much more on the objectivity and accuracy of the investigator."

All data in this chapter have been reevaluated in terms of the categories of response presently employed at MSKCC. Obviously, our interpretations and conclusions relative to many reported studies may not parallel those of previously published reviews (Livingston and Carter, 1970).

3. *5-Fluorouracil*

3.1. *Pharmacology*

5-Fluorouracil has been the backbone of the chemotherapeutic approach to the treatment of gastrointestinal neoplasms. It has the same structure as one of the two main pyrimidine bases, uracil, except for a fluorine atom attached to the carbon-5 portion of the ring. This fluorinated pyrimidine was created in the laboratory following very specific predictions of the properties it was expected to have: inhibition of tumors because of their need for uracil as a precursor of tumor nucleic acid; incorporation in place of uracil in RNA with no direct incorporation in DNA; and blockage of DNA synthesis indirectly by inhibition of the enzyme thymidylate synthetase, which catalyzes the attachment of the methyl group to the carbon-5 of uracil (Bosch *et al.*, 1958). 5FU is itself inactive and must be metabolized to the active component, 5 fluoro-2′-deoxyuridylate or FdUMP. One alternative pathway for conversion of 5FU to FdUMP is through 5-fluoro-2′-deoxyuridine or FUdR, another fluorinated pyrimidine used extensively in intrahepatic infusions.

^{14}C-labeled FU and FUdR have a serum radioactive half-life of approximately 20 min and are rapidly metabolized to respiratory carbon dioxide. Some drug, 16%, is excreted in urine. The method of administration is important since the largest respiratory excretion, 90%, follows oral or continuous 24-hr intravenous administration, while the lowest, 63%, is found after a single intravenous injection. Prolonged infusion of 5FU leads to lower blood levels and less toxicity, and favors a change in the catabolic pathways with urinary excretion of only 1.8–4.5% of the drug. However, when FUdR is given as a continuous infusion, the opposite effect occurs: only 45% is excreted as CO_2 and 9% is found in urine in 24 hr. Administered as a bolus, FUdR shows 67% excretion as CO_2 and 25% in urine. Therefore, FUdR appears to be degraded to a greater extent after rapid intravenous administration and is more toxic when infused continuously (Mukherjee *et al.*, 1963; Clarkson *et al.*, 1964).

3.2. Clinical Data

3.2.1. Standard Regimen

Initial studies with 5FU employed 15 mg/kg for 4–5 consecutive days followed by one-half this dose every other day until toxicity appeared (Livingston and Carter, 1970; Ansfield *et al.*, 1962). Severe toxicity included diarrhea, 64%; stomatitis, 48%; nausea and vomiting, 30%; and moderate (2000–3000 cells/mm^3) and severe (less than 2000 cells/mm^3) leukopenia, 22% and 32%, respectively. Clinical responses were found in 15% (Ansfield *et al.*, 1962). Less toxic schedules were developed using 12 mg/kg for 5 consecutive days. Response rates were similar but toxicity became more manageable, with only 7% of patients having severe leukopenia (Moertel and Reitemeier, 1969). After many clinical trials, criteria were established for good- and poor-risk patients resulting in modifications of 5FU dosages. Lower doses, 8–10 mg/kg for 5 days, should be used in elderly patients more than 70 years of age and in patients who have extensive prior pelvic irradiation or chemotherapy (particularly with alkylating agents), diffuse osseous involvement, liver metastases with obstructive jaundice, negative nitrogen balance, low performance status, significant intercurrent infection, and (possibly) a previous adrenalectomy or hypophysectomy (Ansfield *et al.*, 1962). This new "standard" loading regimen produced objective responses varying between 15% and 21% (Moertel, 1976; Carter and Friedman, 1974). At MSKCC, using the response criteria previously outlined, only 12% of patients with colorectal cancer responded (Young *et al.*, 1960; Krakoff, 1972).

3.2.2. *Oral*

5FU by the oral route was tried because data indicated that more drug would be delivered directly to the liver via the portal circulation and would possibly be more effective in treating hepatic metastases. Initial reports (Khung *et al.*, 1966; Lahiri *et al.*, 1971) described a 50% remission rate for all disease sites and 79% for hepatic metastases. Bateman *et al.* (1971) at first also found higher responses with 5FU when given orally, 40% compared to the intravenous route, 21% with identical doses of 15 mg/kg for 4 days. However, as additional patients were entered, they (Bateman, 1974) obtained 23% responses with the intravenous route and only 12% with the oral route. An older study with 5FU indicated erratic and unpredictable absorption when administered as a tablet or in a solution (Clarkson *et al.*, 1964). Douglass and Mittleman (1974) demonstrated increased concentrations of 5FU in the portal system after oral administration, but Hahn *et al.* (1975) and Cohen *et al.* (1974) have again documented the variable gastric and small bowel absorption of 5FU.

A randomized double-blind study in 100 patients with colorectal cancer by Hahn *et al.* (1975) comparing the intravenous vs. the oral route revealed no statistically significant difference in response rates when patients were initially stratified for performance status, site of metastases, and histological grade. In this study 5FU was given for 5 days every 5 weeks at an oral dose of 20 mg/kg/day or 13.5 mg/kg/day intravenously. These doses were comparable since gastrointestinal, mucocutaneous, and hematological toxicities were equivalent. Hepatomegaly was assessed separately in 45 patients, and all patients were evaluated at 5 and 10 weeks. Overall objective response at 10 weeks was 26% for patients treated intravenously compared to 13% for patients treated orally. The average duration of response favored the intravenous group, 20 weeks to 11 weeks. Regression of hepatomegaly at 10 weeks was again in favor of the intravenously treated group, 32% vs. 17%. The average duration of response was 22 weeks for the i.v. group vs. 10 weeks for the orally treated patients. Therefore, oral administration of 5FU was distinctly inferior, yielding fewer remissions of shorter durations.

3.2.3. *Weekly*

A different schedule, 5FU administered weekly, was tried in an attempt to decrease toxicity and frequency of outpatient visits, and to increase patient acceptance (Ramirez *et al.*, 1969). The Western Cooperative Cancer Chemotherapy Group (Jacobs *et al.*, 1971) used 15–20 mg/kg of 5FU weekly in 94 patients and found an overall CR plus PR rate of 16%. Responses rose to 28% if MR status was included. Only 1 CR and 6 MR were obtained in 36 patients with rectosigmoid lesions. Eighty five percent of patients had mild to moderate toxicity while 11% had "hazardous" toxicity. The Eastern Cooperative Oncology Group (Horton *et al.*, 1970) compared weekly intravenous doses of 7.5, 15, and 20 mg/kg. Objective regression of colorectal cancer at these doses was noted in 6%, 20%, and 25%, respectively. At the 15 mg/kg dose only 6% had severe leukopenia (less than 2000 cells/mm^3) and 24% moderate leukopenia (2000–3500 cells/mm^3). They suggested that the optimal weekly dose of 5FU was 15 mg/kg since 20% responded and toxicity was relatively mild. The Central Oncology Group (Ansfield, 1975) also initiated a randomized trial in 270 patients to evaluate the influence of 5FU schedules and routes in colorectal cancer. 5FU was administered (1) in a "standard" regimen, 5 consecutive days followed by alternate days until toxicity; (2) weekly, intravenously; (3) weekly, orally; and (4) at a "standard" low dose for 4 consecutive days and weekly thereafter. The response rates for these schedules were 38%, 12%, 18%, and 18%, respectively. While results appeared better with the "standard" regimen, toxicity was substantially less with the other three schedules. The response rate of 38% with the "standard" schedule was higher than normally reported with 5FU administered as a single agent, thereby raising questions concerning the evaluation of response and equal patient stratification.

3.2.4. Continuous Administration

Additional information concerning 5FU and FUdR metabolism indicated potential therapeutic advantage with continuous infusion. Clarkson *et al.* (1964) using a continuous 24-hr infusion found a twofold decrease in toxicity with 5FU and a thirtyfold increase in toxicity with FUdR. However, Mukherjee *et al.* (1963) giving smaller doses of labeled 5FU noted a much lower tumor uptake of drug with continuous rather than with rapid intravenous administration. Various clinical trials were started evaluating continuous infusion of 5FU for 2–8 to as long as 120 hr (Moertel *et al.*, 1972). In one randomized study (Moertel and Reitemeier, 1969) 5FU was administered either as a bolus at a dose of 15 mg/kg for 5 consecutive days, followed by 7.5 mg/kg every other day for 4 additional doses, or in an 8-hr infusion at a dose of 22.5 mg/kg. Objective tumor regression occurred in 11% of 45 patients infused with 5FU compared to 20% of 45 patients given a single injection. Toxicity and responses showed that these two schedules were not comparable, since 14% of patients failing infusion obtained objective regression when treated to toxicity with the other schedule.

The effects of various diluents were evaluated by Lemon (1960), who noted a decrease in 5FU toxicity when 5% dextrose solutions were used. Seifert *et al.* (1975) studied this question in a randomized fashion in 70 patients and found a higher response rate, 44% with continuous infusion compared to 22% with bolus administration. Durations of response were similar, 5–6 months. The patients were not stratified and "signal" lesions were not similar, since 53% of the infusion group had pelvic, perineal, osseous, or intraabdominal metastases compared to only 32% of the "bolus" group. The more readily measurable "signal" lesions, lung and superficial nodes, were the parameters used in 55% of the bolus group compared to only 32% of the infusion group. This study indicates again the difficulties in evaluating responses in patients with poorly defined masses and stresses the need to stratify equally for both easily and poorly measurable lesions prior to randomization.

3.2.5. Hepatic Infusion

A different approach was tried for the hepatic pattern (Golbey *et al.*, 1960) of colon cancer dissemination. This metastatic pattern normally results in progressive liver failure with survival of 150–270 days (Bengmark and Hafstrom, 1969; Pestana *et al.*, 1964; Galante *et al.*, 1967). Although the average survival in most reported series is 6 months or less, some patients are alive 3+ years after documentation of liver metastases (Wood, *et al.*, 1976). The extent of liver involvement is important since patients with a solitary or a few metastases have an average survival of 16.7–18 months (Neilsen *et al.*, 1971; Wood *et al.*, 1976). If metastases are localized to only one segment or lobe, the average survival is 9–10.6 months, while patients presenting with widespread metastases involving both lobes survive only 3.1–5.0 months (Wood *et al.*, 1976; Wilson and Adson, 1976).

Hepatic metastases obtain 70–90% of their blood supply from the hepatic artery and little from the portal system (Breedis and Young, 1954). Surgical techniques developed for hepatic artery ligation proved somewhat effective in reducing the size of hepatic lesions (Bengmark and Hafstrom, 1969; Almersjo *et al.*, 1966) but produced no significant prolongation of survival in patients with hepatic metastases from colorectal cancer. Further extension of hepatic artery ligation led to infusion of the liver with antineoplastic drugs through either a surgically or a percutaneously placed intraarterial catheter. The major agents and doses used in infusions have been 5FU, 25–30 mg/kg daily for 7–10 days, and FUdR, 20 mg/kg/day (Ansfield *et al.*, 1971). Some type of objective response was reported in 40–60% of patients, with responders achieving a median survival of 12–15 months compared to 4–8 months for nonresponders (Cady and Oberfield, 1974; Watkins *et al.*, 1970). As previously noted by Wood *et al.* (1976), minimal liver involvement can result in 18 months' survival in untreated patients.

Although proponents of this procedure feel they have demonstrated increased efficacy in treating hepatic metastases by a regional chemotherapeutic approach, the differences in overall survival data for responders vs. nonresponders are not statistically signigficant. Hepatic artery infusion is not a simple procedure; it is expensive and cumbersome, frequently requires hospitalization, and has a distinct morbidity and mortality associated with it. Since systemically administered 5FU results in a 4.5–9 month increase in survival for patients who respond, hepatic artery infusion appears, at this time, to be of no significant benefit.

3.3. Summary

An analysis of multiple trials of 5FU or other fluorinated pyrimidines as single agents in the treatment of colorectal cancer yields partial remissions in

11–20% (Krakoff, 1972) by the "standard" or 5-day regimens. While other schedules probably result in similar or fewer responses, the oral route may not be of any therapeutic value. Complete remissions are uncommon and most responses are listed as PRs lasting 4–9 months. However, this PR category may really include patients attaining only MR status when the primary "indicator" lesion is hepatomegaly. Claims of minimal responses or stabilization of disease with 5FU are of questionable significance, particularly when such categories are applied to patients with poorly evaluable lesions.

5FU singly produces regressions in metastatic lesions of the abdomen, 32%; peripheral nodes, 24%; and cutaneous and subcutaneous areas, 16%. Pulmonary metastases have the lowest response rate, 6–8%. Responders are generally those with a high performance status, ECOG 0, 1, 2 or Karnofsky's 70, 80, 90 (Moertel *et al.*, 1974), at the start of chemotherapy and those who have a relatively long interval, greater than 12 months, between initial diagnosis and the appearance of metastases. Patients who have a comprised hematopoietic reserve because of age or extensive prior irradiation or chemotherapy frequently cannot tolerate full therapeutic doses. When full doses are administered, they tend to induce a significant incidence of severe leukopenia which apparently results in fewer responses. The average survival after diagnosis of "incurable" colon cancer is 20 months for 5FU responders and 10 months for both nonresponders and untreated patients (Moertel and Reitemeier, 1969). It is doubtful that any further manipulations of doses, schedules, or routes of administration of 5FU alone will produce any major therapeutic advance in colorectal cancer.

4. Other Single Agents

4.1. Cyclophosphamide

The use of other antineoplastic agents in the treatment of colorectal cancer has been equally disappointing. Although modest successes have consistently been reported in early phase I and II trials, subsequent studies, particularly randomized ones, have failed to confirm any significant benefit. Many alkylating agents have been evaluated, and response rates have varied between 0% and 25% (Livingston and Carter, 1970). Although comparative trials between alkylating agents have not been reported, cyclophosphamide at a dose of 30 mg/kg every 3 weeks used as primary therapy has produced response rates as high as 39% in 13 patients (Schutt *et al.*, 1973). Duration of responses was exceedingly short, 1–2 months. When cyclophosphamide was used in patients who had failed prior chemotherapy, response rates were very low, 0–8%.

4.2. Mitomycin C

Although initial clinical trials with mitomycin C reported significant objective tumor regression, dosage schedules were extremely toxic (Frank and

Osterberg, 1960). Subsequent modifications of mitomycin C dosages and schedules resulted in an acceptable level of toxicity, and two separate studies (Moertel *et al.*, 1968; Moore *et al.*, 1968) noted partial remission in 10–23% of patients treated with daily administration. A weekly schedule using 0.25 mg/kg yielded 17% responses (Hum *et al.*, 1974) but 43% developed thrombocytopenia below 100,000 cells/mm^3. Although the overall response in colorectal cancer to mitomycin C, 18% (Crooke and Bradner, 1976), is probably similar to that obtained with the fluorinated pyrimidines, the average duration appears to be distinctly shorter, 3–4 months, and the margin between the therapeutic dose and toxicity remains narrow.

4.3. *Methotrexate*

The therapeutic efficacy of methotrexate in some tumors seems to depend on the method of administration. This drug has been evaluated when given orally or intravenously; at low or high dose; on a daily, weekly, twice weekly, or monthly schedule, or by continuous infusion; as a single, divided, or intermittent dose; and with or without leucovorin rescue. Response rates have varied between 8% (Moertel *et al.*, 1970) and 41% (Sullivan *et al.*, 1967). A randomized study compared 5FU and intravenous methotrexate, the latter at a dose of 0.4 mg/kg for 4 consecutive days followed by one-half that dose every other day for 4 additional days, and found PR plus MR response rates of 29% and 10%, respectively (ECOG, 1967). Cumulative data for methotrexate indicate a remission rate of 17% (Carter and Friedman, 1974) in colorectal cancer. Probably less than 10% of patients achieve PR status (Moertel and Reitemeier, 1969).

4.4. *Nitrosoureas*

One of the more promising groups of drugs in the treatment of colorectal cancer are the nitrosoureas: BCNU, 1,2-bis(2-choloroethyl)-1-nitrosourea; CCNU, 1-(2-chloroethyl)-3-cyclohexyl-1-nitrosourea; and, more recently, MeCCNU, 1-(2-chloroethyl)-3-*trans*-4-methylcyclohexyl-1-nitrosourea. BCNU in single or divided intravenous doses of 250–375 mg/m^2 produces 13% overall (17/128) response rate and up to 18% in patients with no prior chemotherapy. CCNU at a dose of 130 mg/m^2 orally every 6 weeks achieves 9% objective remissions (Wasserman *et al.*, 1975). However, CCNU is felt to be inferior to BCNU because of the same 9% remission rate in previously untreated patients (Moertel, 1973). MeCCNU at doses of 175–250 mg/m^2 orally yields 11% (11/168) response and up to 25% in previously untreated patients. In previously treated patients Cedermark *et al.* (1976) obtained 9% remissions while Engstrom *et al.* (1976) found no responses in 26 patients. While there appears to be, at first glance, no significant advantage of one nitrosourea over another, MeCCNU is preferred because of (1) the convenience of oral administration, (2) the higher response rate, 25%, in untreated patients, (3) the long duration of response, 5.5 months, compared to CCNU, 4.5 months, and BCNU, 2 months, and (4) the 10% incidence of "complete" remissions (Moertel, 1973). Randomized trials with nitrosoureas vs. 5FU confirm their therapeutic efficacy and suggest, because of their delayed hematopoietic toxicity, their potential usefulness in combination chemotherapy regimens.

4.5. Other Drugs

Many other chemotherapeutic agents have been evaluated but none has shown significant activity against colorectal cancer. Adriamycin, which has produced significant responses in other gastrointestinal neoplasms such as hepatoma and adenocarcinoma of the stomach and gallbladder, yields only 9% remissions in colorectal cancer (Carter and Friedman, 1974). In one randomized study in untreated patients, adriamycin was inferior to 5FU, 13% vs. 24%, respectively (Frytak *et al.*, 1975). Other agents producing less than 10% remissions in patients with this tumor include streptozotocin, 6-thioguanine, procarbazine, DTIC [5-(3,3-dimethyl-1-triazeno)imidazole-4-carboxamide], and diamine dichloride platinum II (Kovach *et al.*, 1973; Horton *et al.*, 1975; Slavik, 1976).

5. Combination Chemotherapy

No currently available cytotoxic drug when used alone consistently produces responses above 25% or significantly prolongs survival. Combination chemotherapy has induced higher remission rates in acute leukemias, lymphomas, testicular tumors, and some soft tissue sarcomas and has also been tried in the treatment of colorectal cancer. These regimens generally combine drugs which can be used in almost full doses because of different nonadditive toxicities and yet have actions at multiple points in the cell cycle which may result in additive or synergistic therapeutic effect. Only four combination chemotherapy regimens in the treatment of colorectal cancer are worthy of further discussion, and these include schedules which combine 5FU with mitomycin C or one of the nitrosoureas.

Reitemeier *et al.* (1970) conducted a seven-arm stratified, randomized trial in 132 patients of the three most active drugs, 5FU, mitomycin C, and BCNU, alone and in a two- or a three-drug combination. Of particular note in this study was the definition of PR status: lesions less than 5 cm in diameter still needed a 50% decrease in the sum of perpendicular diameters but lesions 5 cm or greater in diameter required only a 30% decrease. It was hoped that one of these combinations would be additive therapeutically since the hematological nadirs of the agents are different. However, 5FU produced the highest response rate, 25%, while the other drugs alone or in combination yielded 5–18% response rates. Two studies (Vaughn *et al.*, 1975; Kim *et al.*, 1975) suggest higher responses with the combination of mitomycin C and 5FU when the latter is administered by continuous infusion. Confirmation of these results is needed.

Ota *et al.* (1972) combined mitomycin C, 5FU, and cytosine arabinoside and reported 60% responses in 16 patients with colorectal cancer. However, two nonrandomized studies from MSKCC (DeJager *et al.*, 1974; Yagoda *et al.*, 1974) using equivalent doses and schedules found no therapeutic advantage to this combination. In addition, Gailani *et al.* (1972) in a randomized study of 5FU vs. 5FU and cytosine arabinoside noted no statistical difference in response rates between the two treatment groups.

Falkson *et al.* (1974) evaluated the four-drug regimen of 5FU, BCNU, DTIC, and vincristine in a randomized trial against 5FU alone in patients with large bowel-excluding rectal cancer. This combination was used in spite of a reported 8% and 0% response rate in this tumor to DTIC (Horton *et al.*, 1975) and vincristine (Carter and Friedman, 1974), respectively. Of 28 patients treated with the combination, 43% responded compared to 25% with 5FU. Surprisingly, 8% of patients treated with 5FU and 14% with the combination attained CR status, yet the overall duration of remissions was short, 3.3–4.5 months.

Moertel *et al.* (1975) combined MeCCNU, 175 mg/m^2 p.o. every 10 weeks, and 5FU, 10 mg/kg i.v. or p.o. for 5 consecutive days, with vincristine, 1 mg/m^2 on day 1 (MOF) every 5 weeks. In a stratified, randomized study of this combination vs. 5FU alone, 43% responded to MOF and 19% to 5FU. While these data suggested a significant improvement in induction rates, the durations of remission and survival were not increased. Falkson and Falkson (1976) tried the same combination, MOF, but reduced the dose of MeCCNU to 100 mg/m^2 and repeated courses at monthly intervals. In a randomized study, they obtained 37% remissions with MOF vs. 22% with 5FU. In calculating the median duration of response, they included patients achieving MR status, which resulted in an overall duration of only 3.8–5.0 months. Those patients, 12% achieving complete remissions, responded for 18–22 months. However, there was no significant improvement in the median survival, which approximated 7 months for both groups. The Southwest Oncology Group (Baker *et al.*, 1976) compared 5FU, 400 mg/m^2 i.v. weekly, vs. the same dose and schedule of 5FU plus MeCCNU, 175 mg/m^2 p.o. every 6 weeks, in a prospective randomized trial in which patients were stratified for the presence or absence of liver metastases. Hepatic involvement was present in 59%. The criteria for response employed for evaluating changes in hepatomegaly utilized Moertel's modification. A statistically significant difference, $p = 0.009$, was found for the combination, with 32% of 152 patients responding compared with only 10% of 42 patients treated with 5FU alone. The average durations of remission, however, were only 138 and 77 days, respectively, with a range of 28–455 days. Woolley *et al.* (1976) also evaluated the MOF combination and found in 23 patients a 43% remission rate. The median duration of response was only 4.5 months.

At MSKCC previously untreated patients with colorectal carcinoma were randomized to one of two MOF regimens, A or B. The same total dose of MeCCNU, 150 mg/m^2 repeated every 10 weeks, was used in each arm, but administered as a single dose in MOF A or in equally divided doses for 5 consecutive days in MOF B. In both arms, 5FU, at a dose of 300 mg/m^2 for 5 consecutive days, and vincristine, at a dose of 1.0 mg/m^2 on day 1, were administered intravenously every 5 weeks. Prior to randomization patients were stratified for (1) performance status (Karnofsky, 1961) greater or less than 60, (2) the presence of lung metastases, and (3) an interval from diagnosis to metastases greater or less than 12 months. There were 69 patients randomized and 86% had an adequate trial. Partial remissions, using the criteria previously defined, occurred in 11% of patients in MOF A and 12% in MOF B. An additional 11% of patients in MOF A and 22% in MOF B attained MR status. The average duration of response for both groups was 5 months. Age, sex, and performance status were comparable in A and B and not significantly different for responders vs. nonresponders. Toxicity was greater with MOF A since 40% of patients experienced nausea and vomiting and 30% severe thrombocytopenia, less than 50,000 cells/mm^3, compared with only 3% and 7%, respectively, with MOF B.

The 12% PR response rate to these MOF combinations is exactly the same as that obtained in a previous study at MSKCC (Young *et al.,* 1960), with 5 FU. If patients attaining MR and PR status are combined, then the number of responders in this study approximates the range of "response" reported by Moertel *et al.* (1975), Woolley *et al.* (1976), Falkson and Falkson (1976), and Baker *et al.* (1976). Since all five MOF studies show responses lasting only 4–6 months, which is identical to or less than the duration of the remissions described for 5FU used singly, any apparent benefit to this drug combination is clearly minimal and of no practical significance.

6. *Adjuvant Therapy*

The use of chemotherapy or immunotherapy in conjunction with primary curative surgery in asymptomatic patients who have a high risk for recurrence is conceptually appealing and some adjuvant studies in solid tumors indicate efficacy with this approach. One of the first adjuvant studies in colorectal cancer was by Holden *et al.* (1967), who randomized patients following curative surgery to placebo or thiotepa. No statistical difference between the two groups was shown except in women older than 55 years, in whom a 33% increase in survival was seen. Mackman and co-workers (Mackman and Curreri, 1968; Mackman *et al.*, 1974) administered 5FU to patients after curative surgery for colon cancer and combined this approach with a second-look operative procedure. This protocol, which was nonrandomized, was felt to be beneficial in selected patients. Rousselot *et al.* (1968) in another nonrandomized study administered 5FU intraluminally at the time of surgery followed by two additional doses of 5FU intravenously and reported a 58% survival in patients with Dukes's C lesions at 8 years (Rousselot *et al.*, 1972). Lawrence *et al.* (1975) coobined the technique described by Rousselot *et al.* (1968) with the adjuvant protocol of Mackman and Curreri (1968) in a randomized trial, but gave monthly courses of 5FU orally instead of intravenously; no difference was found between the two groups at 6 years. Li and

Ross (1976) using 5FU as adjuvant therapy reported 5-year survivals of 82% to 58% for patients with Dukes's B and C lesions, respectively, and compared these results to those with an unmatched group of patients from the preceding 5 years from the same institution showing survivals of 59% with Dukes's B and 24% with Dukes's C lesions. Although the chemoprophylaxis and the control group were relatively similar, the proportion of patients presenting with rectal lesions was 50% in the 5FU-treated group compared with only 10% in the controls. Their results therefore were impressive, since the survival for rectal cancer has been consistently inferior to that of the large bowel cancers from other sites (Schottenfeld, 1971). However, the lack of concomitant controls with adequate stratification prevents definitive conclusions.

The importance of randomized controls in adjuvant studies in colon cancer is eloquently discussed by Higgins *et al.* (1976). In two separate randomized trials, actually representing five studies, no statistical difference is discernible between treated and untreated cases. Although small differences exist which tend to favor the treated group, the stratification used for patient selection and the variations in the placebo arms negate any definitive conclusions. The hazard of using historical controls was illustrated by an increase in survival at 18 months in the placebo group from 16% in 1971 to 27% in 1976. In fact, the 18-month survival in the 1971 trial of 30% in the 5FU-treated group is equivalent to the 27% survival obtained by the placebo group in the 1976 study. If a sequential chemotherapy trial had used 1971 historical controls for comparison with the 5FU-treated cases in the 1976 trials, it would have been concluded that there had been a statistically significant improvement from the use of 5FU.

Prospective randomized adjuvant studies by three separate groups(Grage *et al.*, 1975; Dwight *et al.*, 1973; Higgins *et al.*, 1971, 1976) fail to demonstrate any statistically significant therapeutic effect. In the next few years the results of randomized national protocols using chemotherapy, immunotherapy, and chemoimmunotherapy as adjuvant treatment in colorectal cancer will be available. Until such data are available, any conclusion regarding adjuvant treatment must be held in abeyance. Interpretation of nonrandomized chemotherapy (Li and Ross, 1976) or chemoimmunotherapy (Mavligit *et al.*, 1976) trials is hazardous, and conclusions from such trials may be considered only testimonial in nature.

7. Conclusion

Probably more chemotherapeutic agents, used singly and in combination, have been evaluated in colon cancer than in any other solid tumor. Response rates have varied so greatly that one must conclude that criteria for response change, at times, to fit the investigators' prerogatives. The ultimate test of a drug's efficacy is the attainment of complete remissions or "cure." In the interim, however, it is necessary to accurately record PR status. Since the inherent inaccuracies of measuring partial remissions in colorectal cancer are great, it is important for investigators to decide on and utilize one set of response criteria. Downgrading the criteria of partial remission or including MR and stabilization categories in sequential studies has the effect of artificially increasing overall response rates and does a disservice to physicians as well as to patients. Combination chemotherapy regimens which result in higher induction response rates of shorter duration than those produced by any of their component drugs suggest the lack of any real progress.

Undoubtedly, some patients respond, and a few for prolonged periods, to available antineoplastic agents, but the vast majority of patients with this tumor continue to die without obtaining therapeutic benefit. Since the survival for untreated patients with advanced colon cancer, e.g., with liver metastases, averages 6–9 months, and responders to some combination chemotherapy programs may survive for an identical period of time, any therapeutic benefit may be illusory. The most "effective" agent in advanced disease, albeit minimal, remains 5FU, and potentially the most "active" combination is 5FU and MeCCNU. In minimal disease states no evidence yet exists for any therapeutic benefit with adjuvant therapy. Thoughtful investigators using carefully devised randomized trials will continue to build upon their previous experience and eventually change the present bleak outlook for patients with this tumor.

8. *References*

Almersjo, O., Bengmark, S., Engevik, L., Hafstrom, L. O., and Nilsson, L. A. V., 1966, Hepatic artery ligation as pretreatment for liver resection of metastatic cancer, *Rev. Surg.* **23**:377–380.

Ansfield, F., 1975, A randomized phase III study of four dosage regimens of 5-fluorouracil—A preliminary report (abstr. 1014), *Proc. Am. Soc. Clin. Oncol.* **16**:224.

Ansfield, F., Schroeder, J. M., and Curreri, A. R., 1962, Five years experience with 5-fluorouracil, *J. Am. Med. Assoc.* **181**:295–297.

Ansfield, F., Ramirez, G., Skibba, J. L., Byran, G. T., Davis, H. L., Jr., and Wirtmen, G. W., 1971, Intrahepatic arterial infusion with-fluoruracil, *Cancer* **28**:1147–1158.

Ariel, I. M., and Briceno, M., 1976, The disparity of the liver size as determined by physical examination and by hepatic gammascanning in 504 patients, *Med. Pediatr. Oncol.* **2**:69–73.

Baker, L. H., Talley, R. W., Matier, R., Lehane, D. E., Ruffner, B. W., Jones, S. E., Morrison, F. S., Stephens, R. L., Gehan, E. A., and Vaitkevicius, V. K., 1976, Phase III comparison of the treatment of advanced gastrointestinal cancer with bolus weekly 5-FU vs. methyl CCNU plus bolus weekly 5-FU, *Cancer* **38**:1–6.

Bateman, J. R., 1974, Oral vs. intravenous administration of fluoro *J. Am. Med. Assoc.* **229**:1109.

Bateman, J. R., Pugh, R. P., Cassidy, E. R., Marshall, G. J., and Irwin, L. E., 1971, 5-Fluorouracil given once weekly: Comparison of intravenous and oral administration, *Cancer* **28**:907–913.

Bengmark, S., and Hafstrom, L., 1969, The natural history of primary and secondary malignant tumors of the liver, *Cancer* **23**:198–202.

Bosch, L., Harbers, E., and Heidelberger, C., 1958, Studies of fluorinated pyrimidines vs. effects on nucleic acid metabolism *in vitro, Cancer Res.* **18**:335–343.

Breedis, C., and Young, C., 1954, The blood supply of neoplasms in the liver, *Am. J. Pathol.* **30**:969–974.

Cady, B., and Oberfield, R. A., 1974, Regional diffusion chemotherapy of hepatic metastases from carcinoma of colon, *Am. J. Pathol.* **127**:220–227.

Carter, S. K., and Friedman, M., 1974, Integration of chemotherapy into combined modality treatment of solid tumors. II. Large bowel carcinoma, *Cancer Treat. Rev.* **1:**111–129.

Cedermark, B. J., Didolkar, M. S., and Elias, E. G., 1976, MethylCCNU (NSC-95441) in advanced colorectal carcinoma after failure of 5-fluorouracil (NSC-19893) therapy, *Cancer Treat. Rep.* **60:**235–238.

Clarkson, R. B., O'Connor, A., Winston, L., and Hutchinson, D., 1964, The physiologic disposition of 5-fluorouracil and 5-fluoro-2′ deoxyuridine in man, *Clin. Pharmacol. Ther.* **5:**581–610.

Cohen, J. L., Irwin, L. E., Marshall, G. J., Darvey, H., and Bateman, J. R., 1974, Clinical pharmacology of oral and intravenous 5-fluorouracil (NSC-19893), *Cancer Chemother. Rep.* **58:**723–731.

Coller, F. A., 1956, *Cancer of the Colon and Rectum,* p. 100, American Cancer Society, Inc., New York.

Crooke, S. T., and Bradner, W. T., 1976, Mitomycin C: A review, *Cancer Treat. Rev.* **3:**121–139.

Cutler, S. J., 1968, *End Results in Cancer*, p. 47, Report No. 3, National Institutes of Health Publication No. 30, Washington, D.C.

DeJager, R., Magill, G. B., Golbey, R. B., and Krakoff, I. H., 1974, Mitomycin C, 5-fluorouracil and cytosine arabinoside (MFC) in gastrointestinal cancer (abstr. 776), *Proc. Am. Soc. Clin. Oncol.* **15:**178.

Douglass, H. O., Jr., and Mittleman, A., 1974, Metabolic studies of 5-fluorouracil-II influence of the route of administration on the dynamics of distribution in man, *Cancer* **34:**1878–1881.

Dwight, R. W., Humphrey, E. W., Higgins, G. A., and Keehn, R. J., 1973, FUDR as an adjuvant to surgery in cancer of the large bowel, *J. Surg. Oncol.* **5:**243–249.

Eastern Cooperative Group in Solid Tumor Chemotherapy, 1967, Comparison of antimetabolites in the treatment of breast and colon cancer, *J. Am. Med. Assoc.* **200:**770–778.

Engstrom, R., Catalano, R. B., and Creech, R. H., 1976, Phase II study of MeCCNU (NSC-95441) in advanced gastrointestinal cancer, *Cancer Treat. Rep.* **60:**285–287.

Falkson, G., and Falkson, H., 1976, Fluorouracil, methyl-CCNU and vincristine in cancer of the colon, *Cancer* **38:**1468–1470.

Falkson, G., van Eden, E. B., and Falkson, H., 1974, Fluorouracil imadizole carboximide dimethyl triazeno, vincristine and bis-cholorethyl nitrosourea in colon cancer, *Cancer* **33:**1207–1209.

Frank, W., and Osterberg, A. E., 1960, Mitomycin C (NSC-26980): An evaluation of the Japanese reports, *Cancer Chemother. Rep.* **9:**114–119.

Frytak, S., Moertel, C. G., Schutt, A. J., Hahn, R. G., and Reitmeier, R. J., 1975, Adriamycin (NSC-123127) therapy for advanced gastrointestinal cancers, *Cancer Chemother. Rep.* **59:**405–409.

Gailani, S., Holland, J. F., Falkson, G., Leone, L., Burmingham, R., and Larsen, V., 1972, Comparison of treatment of metastatin gastrointestinal cancer with 5-fluorouracil (5-FU) to a combination of 5-FU with cytosine arabinoside, *Cancer* **29:**1308–1314.

Galante, M., Dunphy, J. E., and Fletcher, W. S., 1967, Cancer of the colon, *Ann. Surg.* **165:**732–744.

Golbey, R. B., Streeter, B., and Karnofsky, D. A., 1960, Clinical observations on patterns of cancer, *Acta Un. Int. Cancr.* **16:**1469–1472.

Grage, T., Cornell, G., Strawitz, J., Jonas, K., Frelick, R., and Metter, G., 1975, Adjuvant therapy with 5-FU after surgical resection of colorectal cancer (abstr. 1149), *Proc. Am. Soc. Clin. Oncol.* **15:**258.

Hahn, R. G., Moertel, C. G., Schutt, A. J., and Bruckner, H. W., 1975, A double-blind comparison of intensive course 5-fluorouracil by oral vs. intravenous route in the treatment of colorectal carcinoma, *Cancer* **35:**1031–1035.

Higgins, G. A., Swight, R. W., Smith, J. V., and Keehn, R., 1971, Fluorouracil as a adjuvant to surgery in carcinoma of the colon, *Arch. Surg.* **102:**339–343.

Higgins, G. A., Humphrey, E., Juler, G. L., LeVeen, H. H., McCaughan, J., and Keehn, R. J., 1976, Adjuvant chemotherapy in the surgical treatment of large bowel cancer, *Cancer* **38:**1461–1467.

Holden, W. D., Dixon, W. J., and Kuzma, J. W., 1967, The use of triethylenethiophosphoramide as an adjuvant to the surgical treatment of colorectal carcinoma, *Ann. Surg.* **165:**481–503.

Horton, J., Olson, K. B., Sullivan, J., Reilly, C., and Shnider, B., 1970, The Eastern Cooperative Oncology Group, 1970, 5-fluorouracil in cancer: An improved regimen, *Ann. Intern. Med.* **73:**897–900.

Horton, J., Mittleman, A., Taylor, S. G., III, Jurkowitz, L., Bennett, J. M., Ezlini, E., Colsky, J., and Hanley, J. A., 1975, Phase II trials with procarbazine (NSC-77213), streptozotocin (NSC-85998), 6-thioguanine (NSC-752), and CCNU (NSC-79037) in patients with metastatic cancer of the large bowel, *Cancer Chemother. Rep.* **59:**333–340.

Hum, G. J., Bogdon, D. L., and Bateman, J. R., 1974, Phase I–II evaluation of weekly mitomycin C (NSC-26980) for patients with metastatic GI and breast malignancies, *Oncology* **30:**236–243.

Jacobs, E. M., Reeves, W. J., Wood, D. A., Pugh, R., Braunwald, J., and Bateman, J. R., 1971, Treatment of cancer with weekly intravenous 5-fluorouracil, *Cancer* **27:**1302–1305.

Karnofsky, D. A., 1961, Meaningful clinical classification of therapeutic responses to anticancer drugs, *Clin. Pharmacol. Ther.* **2:**709–721.

Karnofsky, D. A., Ellison, R. R., and Golbey, R. B., 1962, Selection of patients for evaluation of chemotherapeutic procedures in advanced cancer, *Cancer Chemother. Rep.* **16:**73–77.

Khung, C. L., Hall, T. C., Piro, A. J., and Dederick, M. M., 1966, A clinical trial of oral 5-fluorouracil, *Clin. Pharmacol. Ther.* **7:**527–553.

Kim, P. N., DeMattia, M., Buroker, T., and Vaitkevicius, V. K., 1975, Mitomycin C alone and in combination with infused 5-fluorouracil in treatment of disseminated gastrointestinal carcinomas (abstr. 1039), *Proc. Am. Soc. Clin. Oncol.* **15:**230.

Kovach, J. S., Moertel, C. G., Schutt, A. J., Reitmejer, R. G., and Hahn, R. G., 1973, Phase II study of *cis*-diamminedichloroplatinum (NSC-119875) in advanced carcinoma of the large bowel, *Cancer Chemother. Rep.* **57:**357–360.

Krakoff, I. H., 1972, Chemotherapy of gastrointestinal cancer, *Cancer* **30:**1600–1603.

Lahiri, S. R., Bioleau, G., and Hall, T. C., 1971, Treatment of metastatic colorectal carcinoma with 5-fluorouracil by mouth, *Cancer* **28:**902–906.

Lawrence, W. Jr., Terz, J. J., Horsley, J. S., II, King, R. E., Lovett, W. L., Brown, P. W., Ruffner, B. B., and Regelson, W., 1975, Chemotherapy as an adjuvant to surgery for coloraectal cancer, *Ann. Surg.* **181:**616–623.

Lemon, H. M., 1960, Reduction of 5-fluorouracil toxicity in man, with retention of anticancer effects by prolonged intravenous administration in 5% dextrose, *Cancer Chemother. Rep.* **8:**97–101.

Lemon, H. M., and Foley, J. F., 1966, Antimetabolite therapy of advanced carcinoma and sarcoma, in: *Controversy in Internal Medicine* (F. J., Ingelfinger, A. S. Relman, and M. Finland, eds.), pp. 575–590, Saunders, Philadelphia.

Li, M. C., and Ross, S. T., 1976, Chemoprophylaxis for patients with colorectal cancer—Prospective study with five-year follow-up, *J. Am. Med. Assoc.* **235:**2825–2828.

Livingston, R. B., and Carter, S. K., 1970, *Single Agents in Cancer Chemotherapy*, Plenum, New York.

Mackman, S., and Curreri, A. R., 1968, The second-look operation for cancer of the colon after administration of 5-fluorouracil, 1968, *Am. J. Surg.* **115:**227–230.

Mackman, S., Ansfield, F. J., Ramirez, G., and Curreri, A. R., 1974, A second look at the second-look operation in colonic cancer after the administration of 5-fluorouracil, *Ann. J. Surg.* **128:**763–766.

Mavligit, G. M., Gutteramn, J. U., Burgess, M. A., Khankanian, N., Seibert, G. B., Speer, J. F., Jubert, A. V., Martin, R., McBride, C. M., Copeland, E. M., and Gehan, E. A., 1976, Prolongation of post-operative disease-free interval and survival in human colorectal cancer by BCG or GCG plus 5-FU, *Lancet* **1(7965):**871–876.

Moertel, C. G., 1973, Therapy of advanced gastrointestinal cancer with the nitrosoureas, *Cancer Chemother. Rep. Part 3* **4(3):**27–34.

Moertel, C. G., 1975, Chemotherapy of gastrointestinal cancer: State of the art in 1975, *Int. J. Radiat. Oncol. Biol. Phys.* **1:**169–171.

Moertel, C. G., 1976, Gastrointestinal cancer—Treatment with fluorouracil-nitrosourea combinations, *J. Am. Med. Assoc.* **235:**2135–2136.

Moertel, C. G., and Hanley, J. A., 1976, The effect of measuring error on the results of therapeutic trials in advanced cancer, *Cancer* **38:**388–394.

Moertel, C. G., and Reitemeier, R. J., 1962, Experience with 5-fluorouracil in the palliative management of advanced carcinoma of the gastrointestinal tract, *Proc. Mayo Clin.* **37:**520–526.

Moertel, C. G., and Reitemeier, R. J., 1969, *Advanced Gastrointestinal cancer—Clinical Management and Chemotherapy,* Harper and Row, New York.

Moertel, C. G., Reitemeier, R. J., and Hahn, R. G., 1968, Mitomycin C therapy in advanced gastrointestinal cancer, *J. Am. Med. Assoc.* **204:**1045–1048.

Moertel, C. G., Reitemeier, R. J., and Hahn, R. G., 1970, Oral methotrexate therapy of gastrointestinal carcinoma, *Surg. Gynecol. Obstet.* **130:**292–294.

Moertel, C. G., Schutt, A. J., Reitemeier, R. J., and Hahn, R. G., 1972, A comparison of 5-fluorouracil administered by slow infusion and rapid injection, *Cancer Res.* **32:**2717–2719.

Moertel, C. G., Schutt, A. J. Hahn, R. G., and Reitmeier, R. J., 1974, Effects of patient selection on results of phase II chemotherapy trials in gastrointestinal cancer, *Cancer Chemother. Rep.* **58:**257–259.

Moertel, C. G., Schutt, A. J., Hahn, R. G., and Reitmeier, R. J., 1975, Brief communication: Therapy of advanced colorectal cancer with a combination of 5-fluorouracil, methyl-1,2 *cis*(2-chlorethyl)-1-nitrosourea, and vincristins, *J. Natl. Cancer Inst.* **54:**66–71.

Moore, G. E., Bross, I. D. J., Ansman, R., Nadler, S., Jones, R., Jr., Slack, N., and Rimm, A. A., 1968, Effects of mitomycin C in 346 patients with advanced cancer, *Cancer Chemother. Rep.* **52:**675–684.

Mukherjee, K. L., Boohar, J., Wentland, D., Ansfield, F. J., and Heidelberger, C., 1963, Studies on fluorinated pyrimidines. XVI. Metabolism of 5-fluorouracil-2-C and 5-fluor-2-deoxyuridine-2-C in cancer patients, *Cancer Res.* **23:**49–66.

Neilsen, J., Balsley, J., and Jensen, H. E., 1971, Carcinoma of the colon with liver metastasis, *Acta Chir. Sismol.* **137:**463–471.

Nilsson, L. A. V., 1966, Therapeutic hepatic artery ligation in patients with secondary liver tumors, *Rev. Surg.* **374:**6.

Ota, K., Kurita, S., Nishimura, M., Kamei, Y., Imai, K., Ariyoshi, Y., Kataoka, K., Murakami, M., Oyama, A., Hoshino, A., Amo, H., and Kato, T., 1972, Combination therapy with mitomycin D, 5-fluorouracil, and cytosine arabinoside for advanced cancer in man, *Cancer Chemother. Rep.* **56:**383–385.

Pestana, C., Reitmeier, R. J., Moertel, C. G., Judd, E. S., and Dockerty, M. B., 1964, The natural history of carcinoma of the colon and rectum, *Am. J. Surg.* **108:**826–829.

Ramiraz, G., Korbitz, B. C., Davis, H. L., Jr., and Ansfield, F. J., 1969, *Cancer Chemother. Rep.* **53:**243–247.

Reitemeier, R. J., Moertel, C. G., and Hahn, R. G., 1970, Combination chemotherapy in gastrointestinal cancer, *Cancer Res.* **30:**1425–1428.

Rousselot, L. M., Cole, D. R., Grosse, C. E., Conte, A. J., Gonzelez, E. M., and Pasternak, B. S., 1968, A five year progress report on the effectiveness of intraluminal chemotherapy (5-fluorouracil) adjuvant to surgery for colorectal cancer, *Am. J. Surg.* **115:**140–147.

Rousselot, L. M., Cole, D. R., Grossi, C. E., Conte, A. J., Gonzalez, E. M., and Pasternack, B. S., 1972, Adjuvant chemotherapy with 5-fluorouracil in surgery for colorectal cancer: Eight-year report, *Dis. Colon Rectum* **15(3):**169–174.

Rytand, D. A., 1968, The midclavicular line: Where is it?, *Ann. Intern. Med.* **70:**329–330.

Schottenfeld, D., 1971, *Statistical Report of End Results 1949–1954, 1955–1959, 1960–1964,* pp. 32–33, 38–39, Memorial Hospital for Cancer and Allied Diseases, New York.

Schutt, A. J., Hahn, R. G., Reitmeier, R. J., and Moertel, C. G., 1973, A phase II study of intermittent high-dose cyclophosphamide therapy of advanced gastrointestinal cancer, *Cancer Res.* **33:**2218–2220.

Seifert, P., Baker, L. H., Reed, M. L., and Vaitkevicius, V. K., 1975, Comparison of continuously infused 5-fluorouracil with bolus injection in treatment of patients with colorectal adenocarcinoma, *Cancer* **36:**123–138.

Silverberg, E., and Holleb, A. I., 1971, Cancer statistics, *Cancer* **21:**13–31.

Slavik, M., 1976, Clinical studies with DTIC in various malignancies, *Cancer Treat. Rep.* **60:**213–214.

Sullivan, R. D., Miller, E., Zurek, W. Z., Oberfield, R. A., and Ojima, Y., 1967, Re-evaluation of methotrexate as an anticancer drug, *Surg. Gynecol. Obstet.* **127:**819–824.

Vaughn, C. B., Chinn, B. J., Deversa, B., and Parzuchowski, J., 1975, Comparison of combination chemotherapy in advanced gastrointestinal malignancy: 5-Fluorouracil plus mitomycin C vs. 5-fluorouracil plus 1-(2 1-(2 chloroethyl) 3-(4 methylcyclohexyl)-1-nitrosourea, 1975 (abstr. 1126), *Proc. Am. Soc. Clin. Oncol.* **16:**252.

Wasserman, T. H., Slavik, M., and Carter, S. K., 1975, Clinical comparison of the nitrosoureas, *Cancer* **36:**1258–1268.

Watkins, E. Jr., Khazei, A. M., and Nahra, K. S., 1970, Surgical basis for arterial infusion chemotherapy of disseminated carcinoma of the liver, *Surg. Gynecol. Obstet.* **130:**581–605.

Wilson, S. M., and Adson, M. A., 1976, Surgical treatment of hepatic metastases from colorectal cancers, *Arch. Surg.* **111:**330–334.

Wood, C. B., Gillis, C. R., and Blumgart, L. H., 1976, A retrospective study of the natural history of patients with liver metastases from colorectal cancer, *Clin. Oncol.* **2:**285–288.

Woolley, P. V., III, MacDonald, J. S., and Schein, P. S., 1976, Chemotherapy of colorectal carcinoma, *Sem. Oncol.* **3:**415–420.

Yagoda, A., Lippman, A., Winn, R., Rosenberg, A., and Schulman, P., 1974, Mitomycin C, 5-FU and cytosine arabinoside (MiFuCa) in adenocarcinomas (abstr. 826), *Proc. Am. Soc. Clin. Oncol.* **15:**190.

Young, C. W., Ellison, R. R., Sullivan, R. D., Levick, S. N., Kaufman, R., Miller, E., Woldow, I., Escher, G., Li, M. C., Karnofsky, D. A., and Burchenal, J. H., 1960, The clinical evaluation of 5-fluorouracil and 5-fluoro-2′-deoxyuridine in solid tumors in adults: A progress report, *Cancer Chemother Rep.* **6:**17–19.

Zubrod, C. G., 1966, The limited usefulness of 5-fluorouracil (5-FU) and 5-fluorodeoxyuridine (5-FUDR) in the management of patients with adenocarcinoma, in: *Controversy in Internal Medicine* (F. J. Ingelfinger, A. S. Relman, and M. Finland, eds.), pp. 591–600, Saunders, Philadelphia.

26

Adjuvant Chemotherapy and Immunotherapy in Colorectal Cancer

G. M. Mavligit, J. U. Gutterman, and E. M. Hersh

1. Introduction

Colorectal cancer appears to be an ever-growing epidemic with an all-time high incidence of approximately 100,000 new cases estimated in the United States during 1977. This disease, which seems to affect males and females equally, has been subjected to numerous surgical therapeutic approaches during the past two decades. Unfortunately, these exhaustive conventional approaches have failed to improve the overall prognosis (Donaldson and Welch, 1974).

Radiotherapeutic trials in certain stages of the disease have been iniated both before and after surgery, some of which appear to be promising, while others have been disappointing (Roswit *et al.*, 1975; Stearns *et al.*, 1974).

The medical aspects of the management of colorectal cancer have emerged as a new field of therapeutic cancer research with the introduction of chemotherapeutic agents in general and 5-fluorouracil (5FU) in particular. It was quickly learned that the latter was effective in controlling the continued growth of metastatic colorectal cancer in approximately 15–20% of the cases. Numerous studies designed to improve the route of administration, dose, and schedule of this drug have resulted in little improvement in its efficacy when given as a single therapeutic agent.

More recently, 5FU has been combined with other chemotherapeutic agents, which also have some degree of efficacy against colorectal cancer (such

---

G. M. Mavligit, J. U. Gutterman, and E. M. Hersh • Section of Immunology, Department of Developmental Therapeutics, The University of Texas System Cancer Center, M. D. Anderson Hospital and Tumor Institute, Houston, Texas 77030.

as nitrosourea compounds) and the results obtained are encouraging, but certainly far from being satisfactory in terms of a major breakthrough in the treatment of this dreadful disease (Falkson *et al.*, 1974; Moertel *et al.*, 1975*b*).

It became obvious that in order to achieve a better control of colorectal cancer a major thrust of therapeutic research must be directed toward administration of systemic therapy in combination with surgical extirpation of the primary lesions during early stages of the disease, when tumor burden is small and the likelihood of controlling its continued growth by medical measures is perhaps the greatest. This concept has led to the emergence of immunotherapy, the latest therapeutic modality of a medical nature to be utilized in patients with colorectal cancer. This therapeutic tool is currently being investigated in a number of human cancers. The rationale and scientific basis for its use have been discussed at length elsewhere (Hersh *et al.*, 1973). Suffice it to say, at this junction, that immunotherapy is currently believed to correct or reverse some of the immunological deficiencies associated with human cancer in general, and colorectal cancer in particular.

In addition to the various specific and nonspecific immunological reactivities which have been demonstrated among patients with colorectal cancer, a growing body of evidence clearly indicates that serial determination of plasma levels of carcinoembryonic antigen (CEA) in patients with colorectal cancer can serve as a useful monitoring tool in the clinical follow-up and treatment evaluation of patients with colorectal cancer. Such a sophisticated monitoring system appears to be indispensable for an adjuvant therapeutic trial, where a delicate balance seems to exist between the host and the tumor following a surgical procedure of a potentially curative nature. This balance in the host–tumor relationship is perhaps best reflected by immunological parameters in patients with colorectal cancer which have been extensively correlated with some biological characteristics in growth patterns of the tumor, and with prognostic factors which can frequently predict the outcome of the postoperative course of the disease. These immunological parameters in the host–tumor relationship are additionally important since they form the scientific basis and the rationale for the use of immunological intervention (immunotherapy) intended to tip the aforementioned balance in favor of the host.

2. Immune Reactions in Colorectal Cancer Patients

The general abundance of studies reporting on the immunological aspects in cancer patients includes substantial information concerning patients with colorectal cancer. It is convenient to arbitrarily divide the immune reactivity observed in cancer patients into two components: (1) nonspecific reactivity, which usually reflects and quantitates the capacity of the host to respond to an immunological stimulus (immunocompetence); (2) tumor-directed immune reactivity, which implies a more specific response by presensitized host immune cells to antigens associated with growing tumor cells.

2.1. Nonspecific Immune Reactions

By far the most useful *in vitro* test to evaluate immunocompetence in cancer patients is lymphocyte stimulation with the mitogen phytohemagglutinin. Numerous studies have been done with this assay in patients with colorectal cancer, and the results vary considerably, as best summarized by Kaplan *et al.* (1975). While some reports indicate impaired lymphocyte reactivity to PHA among colorectal cancer patients compared to healthy controls, others clearly show no significant difference in lymphocyte reactivity. A careful study by Lauder and Bone (1973) has emphasized the importance of using various stimulatory doses of PHA in order to detect significant differences between lymphocyte reactivity of cancer patients and that of normal healthy donors. Equally controversial is the finding of a serum factor(s) capable of inhibiting the lymphocyte reactivity to PHA (Kaplan *et al.*, 1975). This controversy may be related to the intriguing finding of an inhibitory factor in the portal venous blood of patients with colorectal cancer (Edwards *et al.*, 1973). Such a finding strongly suggests that the inhibitory factor may indeed be liberated by the growing tumor. However, its access to the peripheral circulation may be hampered by the liver and depend, to a large extent, on the degree of the physiological portacaval blood shunting.

Another parameter of general immunocompetence which has been useful to characterize patients with colorectal cancer is the delayed hypersensitivity skin reaction to DNCB. The studies by Bone and Lauder (1974) clearly distinguish between patients with early, locally invasive, primary lesions (Dukes's A, B), in whom the reactivity to DNCB is usually vigorous, and patients with regional or distally advanced lesions (Dukes's C, D), in whom the reactivity to DNCB is usually poor. This finding may indicate the more urgent need among patients with advanced colorectal cancer (Dukes's C, D) for therapeutic immunological intervention intended to restore the impaired immunocompetence to a more effective level.

These investigators have laso drawn attention to the correlation between the number of circulating lymphocytes and the stage of disease (Bone and Lauder, 1974). Thus the absolute number of circulating lymphocytes was almost within normal limits in patients with early, less invasive disease, and reached significantly lower values in patients with metastatic widespread colorectal carcinoma. Preliminary data suggest that a thymus-dependent lymphocyte subpopulation is reduced in patients with colorectal carcinoma (Seitanides and Georgoulis, 1975), but further studies of other subclasses of lymphocytes are needed to ascertain the precise defect in lymphocyte function which is associated with colorectal cancer. Such information may be crucial for designing better immunotherapeutic approaches to this disease.

2.2. Tumor-Directed Immune Reactions

Any discussion of tumor-associated antigens and the various manifestations of immune reactivity against them in patients with colorectal cancer must begin with the original discovery by Gold and Freedman (1965) of a substance which they called carcinoembryonic antigen (CEA). Its current clinical use will be discussed later in this chapter, but at this junction suffice it to say that this substance which is commonly found in fetal tissues is produced by the growing tumor, perhaps as a result of fetal genome derepression, and is released into the circulation in abnormally large quantities. However, the question of its antigenicity, at least in man, is still unresolved (MacSween, 1975). While the existence of anti-CEA antibodies in man is controversial (Gold 1967; Collatz *et al.*, 1971; LoGerfo *et al.*, 1972), two studies, thus far, have also failed to demonstrate any evidence that CEA evokes any autologous cellular immune response in the human (Lejtenyi *et al.*, 1971; Straus *et al.*, 1975) despite its heterologous immunogenicity in other mammals. This heterologous immunogencity played a cardinal role in the development of a radioimmunoassay for diagnostic detection of plasma levels of CEA (Thompson *et al.*, 1969). It is noteworthy that a CEA-like material was isolated from tumor extracts and found to elicit delayed-type hypersensitivity skin reaction among patients with colorectal cancer (Hollinshead *et al.*, 1970).

2.3. *Mononuclear Cell Cytotoxicity against Cultured Tumor Target Cells*

The original finding by Hellström *et al.* (1968) that peripheral blood mononuclear cells obtained from 40–60% of patients with colorectal cancer are capable of destroying cultured colorectal carcinoma cells was further confirmed by the same authors (Hellström and Hellström, 1972) and by others (Baldwin *et al.*, 1973*a*; Nind *et al.*, 1975). Additional information suggests that this cellular immune reactivity is mainly mediated by thymus-dependent lymphocytes (Nind *et al.*, 1975). However, cytotoxicity was absent among lymphocytes extracted from regional lymph nodes draining the primary tumor sites (Nind *et al.*, 1973), indicating a state of compartmentalized anergy or immune paralysis. The possible role of tumor antigen in inducing this paralysis is supported by the finding of Baldwin *et al.* (1973*b*) that blood mononuclear cell cytotoxicity can be inhibited by pretreating these cells with solubilized tumor membrane fractions. Also, an inverse relationship was shown between mononuclear cell cytotoxicity and the stage of disease in colorectal cancer (Pihl *et al.*, 1975), suggesting that an excess of tumor antigen released from a widely spread tumor may be responsible for the development of immune paralysis.

In addition to its cellular cytotoxicity, serum obtained from some patients with colorectal cancer was found to be cytotoxic to cultured tumor cells (Schultz *et al.*, 1975).

2.4. *Inhibition of Leukocyte Migration*

Since the demonstration of its usefulness (Mavligit *et al.*, 1972; Bull *et al.*, 1973), the inhibition of leukocyte migration, an assay of cellular immunoreactivity to antigens associated with colorectal cancer, has received a great deal of attention (McIllmurray *et al.*, 1974; Lurie *et al.*, 1975; House *et al.*, 1975; Elias and Elias, 1975). It is noteworthy that no difference in reactivity was found between lymphocytes derived from peripheral blood and those from regional lymph nodes (Guillou *et al.*, 1975). Reactivity was transient and usually disappeared within a few weeks after surgical removal of the primary tumor (House *et al.*, 1975; Lurie *et al.*, 1975). Lymphocytes from patients with Dukes's class C lesions were more reactive to tumor antigens than lymphocytes from patients with Dukes's B or D lesions (Elias and Elias, 1975).

2.5. Lymphocyte Blastogenesis to Tumor-Associated Antigens

Studies conducted in our laboratory have demonstrated the usefulness of 3 M KCl extracts of colon carcinoma in the stimulation of blastogenesis among autologous lymphocytes (Mavligit *et al.*, 1972). We have also shown the state of relative anergy among lymphocytes from regional lymph nodes (Ambus *et al.*, 1974) and the varying degrees of the activity among lymphocytes from the appendix and terminal ileum of patients with carcinoma arising in the right colon (Mavligit *et al.*, 1974).

2.6. Humoral Immunity in Colorectal Cancer

The role of antibodies in the natural defense against colorectal cancer is as unclear as it is in cancer patients in general. As already mentioned above, the existence of circulating antibodies against CEA is controversial. Cytotoxic antibodies against cultured tumor cells have been found in serum derived from patients with colorectal cancer (Schultz *et al.*, 1975). This certainly needs to be further explored and confirmed before a more definitive statement can be made about it. It is possible that an interaction between antibodies and cellular components of the immune system may be of great importance and perhaps result in augmented or sometimes inhibited antitumor reactivity, depending on the circumstances. The isolation of facilitatory humoral factors and their separation from those which are inhibitory will be instrumental for better understanding of the complex of immune response against cancer in general and colorectal cancer in particular.

3. Biological Characteristics and Prognostic Factors in Colorectal Cancer

Carcinoma may arise in each portion of the large bowel from the caecum to the rectum. The question of whether all carcinoma lesions invariably arise from benign polyps undergoing malignant transformation or whether the two types of lesions develop independently is still controversial (Enterline, 1975). Once arisen, carcinoma of the large bowel continues to grow in a predictable fashion: from its origin in the mucosa the tumor will invade the muscular layer of the bowel wall and penetrate the serosa into the pericolic fat. During this process it may also invade blood vessels and lymphatic channels, which may culminate in metastatic disease in regional draining lymph nodes and the liver and/or the lungs. From the pericolic fat, the tumor may also invade adjacent organs and structures, as will be discussed below.

Since in most patients with colorectal cancer the first treatment is surgical, it is most desirable to accurately determine the extent of disease in a particular patient at the time of primary surgery whether it is considered a "curative" procedure with total removal of the primary lesion or only a palliative procedure, solely intended to relieve an impending or already established bowel obstruction in a patient with obvious metastatic disease. Information obtained during this initial surgical procedure coupled with a sound pathological report is invaluable for a judicious medical management thereafter.

3.1. *Disease Staging and Patient Classification*

For practical purposes, it is convenient to divide carcinoma of the large bowel into four major clinical pathological stages according to the slightly modified classification originally proposed by Dukes over 30 years ago. According to this classification, a patient belongs to Dukes's class A if his primary lesion of adenocarcinoma is limited in its invasive process to the mucosa and submucosa without penetrating the muscular layer of the bowel wall. In Dukes's class B lesions, the primary carcinoma has penetrated through the entire bowel wall, the serosa, and/or the pericolic fat. An intermediate phase may be encountered where the tumor has penetrated the muscular layers but not through the entire wall. However, in our experience, these intermediate cases are relatively rare and should be perhaps included under Dukes's class B, based on their similar natural history in terms of disease-free interval and survival following "curative" surgical procedures.

In a patient who belongs to Dukes's class C, the primary lesion not only has penetrated through all the bowel wall layers, including the serosa and the pericolic fat, but also has already invaded the regional draining lymph nodes, which can be proximal or distal to the tumor-bearing bowel segment. Not infrequently, what appears to be a Dukes's class C lesion is compounded by additional, usually microscopic, involvement by tumor of adjacent organs or structures such as urinary bladder, ureters, ovaries, uterus, vagina, prostate, small bowel segment, or abdominal wall structures. Consequently, despite what in the surgeon's mind was a total resection of all discernible tumor, these particular patients' postoperative survival is almost identical to that of patients who belong to the Dukes's class D, i.e., patients with widespread metastases who are already beyond any potentially curative surgical procedures. We therefore look upon the former as a subgroup of the latter and lump them together as a single treatment group representing advanced colorectal cancer.

3.2. *Operable and Inoperable Primary Carcinoma of the Large Bowel*

The major reason why many a patient with carcinoma of the large bowel can be cured is the high incidence of operable lesions (Dukes's A, B, C) which are encountered at surgery. The experience at M. D. Anderson Hospital is approximately 60% operable and 40% inoperable cases. Since it might have biological implications, we have addressed ourselves to the question of why some cases are operable and others are not, and what are the factors which may play a role in this distribution of patients.

We first noticed that operable and inoperable lesions were equally distributed along the various portions of the large bowel with one exception, i.e., a significantly higher incidence of Dukes's A lesions was found in the rectosigmoid portion. This finding should not be too surprising since this type of lesion is usually found in polyps which are easily accessible at this anatomical site by means of the sigmoidoscope, and therefore diagnosis of early-stage lesions is much easier.

The duration of symptoms prior to diagnosis can also be of value in understanding the biological behavior of the tumor. It would seem logical to assume that patients found to have inoperable lesions would have symptoms of longer duration, reflecting a delay in establishing the diagnosis, which will allow the tumor to grow further. We found virtually no difference in the duration of symptoms between operable and inoperable cases. The duration of symptoms in patients with Dukes's D lesions was if anything somewhat shorter than in patients with operable stages. This strongly suggests that progression of tumor growth and state of operability in colorectal cancer are less dependent on delays in establishing the diagnosis (patient's and/or doctor's fault) and more dependent on the intrinsic biological characteristics of the particular tumor itself, as also suggested by Welch and Burke (1962).

In contrast to duration, the type of presenting symptom appears to be of major prognostic importance. In a retrospective analysis, we have shown that a change in bowel habits as a single presenting symptom is associated with operable lesions (Dukes's A, B, C) in 96% of the cases while abdominal pain is a herald of 60% inoperability and gross rectal bleeding signals 60% operability. In any combination of symptoms the presence of a change in bowel habits tends to increase the percentage of operability while abdominal pain decreases it. These findings may suggest that a change in bowel habits is a manifestation of an early lesion, only minimally compromising bowel motility, whereas abdominal pain is a manifestation of a more advanced tumor, already causing a considerable degree of mechanical bowel obstruction or nerve involvement.

3.3 Tumor-Free Interval and Overall Survival

3.3.1. *Relationship to Stage of Disease*

The two clinical parameters which are most commonly used to evaluate cancer treatment in general and surgical treatment of colorectal cancer in particular are the tumor-free interval, i.e., the time from surgery to recurrence of tumor, and overall survival. By a computer-assisted retrospective analysis of 495 patients operated on at M. D. Anderson Hospital during a period of 10 years (1963–1973), we were able to show a clear-cut inverse relationship between these two parameters and the stage of disease by the Dukes classification, as was also previously reported by a number of investigators (Turnbull, 1970; Falterman *et al.*, 1974; Murray *et al.*, 1975). Thus, while the median tumor-free interval for all surgically treated patients with Dukes's B lesions at M. D. Anderson Hospital is approximately 85 months, the value for all patients with Dukes's C lesions is approximately 21 months. Similarly the overall median survival of the patients with Dukes's B is 86+ months, while that of patients with Dukes's C is approximately 40 months. The median survival of patients with Dukes's D is 10 months (regardless of chemotherapy).

Further analysis disclosed puzzling data. For instance, in patients with Dukes's B the presence of blood vessel or lymphatic invasion by tumor did not necessarily coincide with poor prognosis as suggested by other investigators. Both tumor-free interval and overall survival were, if anything, somewhat better among those with vascular invasion than among those without it.

Among patients with Dukes's C lesion the prognosis was inversely correlated to the number of lymph nodes involved by tumor. Thus patients with five or fewer positive nodes had a better prognosis than those with six or more positive nodes. This was also reported by other investigators (Spratt and Spjut, 1967; Gunderson and Sosin, 1974; Murray *et al.*, 1975).

The close relationship between the original stage of disease (by the Dukes classification) and prognosis continues to exist even after tumor recurrence. Thus postrelapse survival is longest in patients with Dukes's A, intermediate with Dukes's B, and shortest with Dukes's C. Furthermore, the survival of all patients with metastatic disease who originally presented with operable lesions (Dukes's A, B, C) is longer than that of patients whose lesions were originally inoperable (Dukes's D). This suggests that some of the biological characteritics of the tumor which determine thedegree of invasiveness in its original presentation continue to play a distinct role even at times when the host defense seems to have been completely broken down.

3.3.2. Relationship to Anatomical Site of Primary Tumor

In the surgical literature, one can find reports indicating no significant differences in prognosis among patients with colorectal cancer arising at various anatomical sites (Beahrs and Sanfelippo, 1971; Welch and Donaldson, 1974). Our retrospective analysis tends to confirm the previous reports, with a few apparent exceptions: (1) When the primary lesion arises in the hepatic flexure–right transverse colon area, the tumor-free interval and overall survival are worse than in any other anatomical site. (2) A primary Dukes's B lesion arising in the caecum carries a better prognosis than an equivalent lesion in the rectosigmoid area. (3) An opposite trend, i.e., better prognosis in rectosigmoid area than in caecum, exists for Dukes's C lesions. (4) There is an exceptionally high incidence (approximately 50%) of local and regional tumor recurrence in patients with primary carcinoma of the rectosigmoid colon as opposed to any other anatomical site. The last may be as a result of technical difficulties encountered during surgery, leading to inadvertently excessive tumor mass manipulation with spillage of tumor cells.

3.3.3. Relationship to Age and Sex of Patients

No significant differences in prognosis were found between various age groups except in those few patients who were 40 years old or younger, who seem to almost invariably have a grave prognosis. No significant difference in prognosis was found between males and females.

3.3.4. Relationship to Inflammatory Cell Infiltration, Abscess Formation, and Sinus Histiocytosis

Inflammatory cell infiltration, abscess formation, and sinus histocytosis were shown to be associated with good prognosis in cancer of the breast (Black *et al.*, 1955) and cancer of the colon (Spratt and Spjut, 1967; Murray *et al.*, 1975; Patt *et al.*, 1975) and are currently considered morphological (immunological and nonimmunological) manifestations of host defense and resistance against tumor growth. One study, however, claims that sinus histiocytosis does not independently correlate with survival, and prognosis is predominantly determined by the stage of disease according to the Dukes classification (Tsakraklides *et al.*, 1975).

3.3.5. Relationship to Preoperative Plasma Level of CEA

There are conflicting reports on the prognostic value of preoperative plasma levels of CEA. In some reports, the authors claim that higher levels correlate with poor prognosis and a high incidence of tumor recurrence as compared to low levels (LoGerfo and Herter, 1975), while other investigators find that only excessively high preoperative levels of over 100 ng/ml can be correlated with grave prognosis (Booth *et al.*, 1974).

4. Concept of Micrometastases and Rationale for Adjuvant Therapy in Colorectal Cancer

The high incidence of surgical failures among patients with Dukes's C lesions, and the lesser incidence among those with Dukes's B and A lesions, who subsequently present with local recurrence or distant metastasis must be accounted for by undetectable foci of micrometastases in adjacent tissues or distant organs, already present at the time of surgery. For the most part, a continued growth of these micrometastases seems to be independent of the primary tumor, although further delay in their growth may be anticipated following resection of the latter, perhaps because of the elimination of tumor antigen excess, which is currently believed to paralyze the immune system

(Bowen *et al.*, 1975). Systemic antitumor adjuvant therapy must therefore be administered in order to achieve a better control of the disease.

Considerations based on cell growth kinetics indicate that cell-cycle-specific chemotherapeutic agents can be expected to be more effective against small numbers of rapidly proliferating residual tumor cells than against bulky tumors with a low growth fraction (Schabel, 1975). However, since most chemotherapeutic agents act by first-order tumor cell kill kinetics and probably would not kill the last remaining cell(s), it would seem logical to combine this mode of therapy with immunotherapy. The latter would augment immune mechanisms which are curently believed to operate by second-order tumor cell kill kinetics and therefore might eradicate the last remaining tumor cell(s).

One may argue that immunosuppressive chemotherapy may interfere with effective antitumor immune mechanisms. However, studies in animal models have shown that small doses of intermittent chemotherapy tend to selectively spare cellular immune mechanisms, whereas humoral antibody production is usually suppressed (Heppner *et al.*, 1974). In addition to this selective immunosuppression by chemotherapy, there is recent evidence to suggest a synergistic effect between chemotherapy and immune mechanisms of tumor cell killing in that pretreatment with chemotherapeutic agents can condition the tumor cells and render them more susceptible to killing by antibody and complement (Segerling *et al.*, 1975).

5. *Experimental Design for Adjuvant Therapy Trials in Colorectal Cancer*

Before embarking on a study of adjuvant therapy trial, one has to have clearly defined objectives which one wants to achieve considering the limitation of the therapeutic agents one intends to use. It would therefore seem almost irrational to include, in an adjuvant therapy trial, patients who fall under the category of Dukes's A. The vast majority of these patients can be safely considered as cured by surgical extirpation alone, and no additional, currently available therapy can be anticipated to improve the surgical results in this group of patients.

The need for adjuvant therapy in patients with Dukes's B lesions is more debatable because the median tumor-free interval in these patients is approximately 7 years, so that more than 50% of the patients can be considered cured by surgery alone. The clinician is therefore left with a dilemma; he can either indiscriminately subject all patients with Dukes's B to an adjuvant therapy trial, ignoring half the population which clearly does not need it, or make an effort to further characterize prognostic factors which will eventually allow him to separate those patients in a poor prognostic subgroup who may benefit from adjuvant therapy from those in the better prognostic group who will not.

In such an attempt, we have recently failed to isolate a subgroup of patients with Dukes's B lesions who, we presumed (based on published reports), would be suitable for an adjuvant trial because of the presence of vascular invasion. Our analysis suggests that these Dukes's B patients are not only doing as well as those without vascular invasion, but perhaps even better. However, our series may be too small to allow a definite conclusion at this time. Be that as it may, in the absence of any major and characteristic prognostic factor which can allow a clear-cut separation between subgroups of patients with Dukes's B lesions, the solution must be a study which would include concurrently randomized "no treatment" controls. Such a study would obviously take years and require a large number of patients before results could be evaluated.

One exception may be a group of patients with Dukes's B lesions arising in the rectosigmoid area, where the incidence of local recurrence is excessively high for reasons which were discussed in a previous section of this chapter. In these cases the primary goal should be an improvement in the surgical technique, and, perhaps, the application of radiotherapy intended to control the tumor bed, although the use of chemo- and/or immunotherapy may also have a place.

The situation in patients with Dukes's C lesions appears to be more desperate, and clearly calls for more aggressive intervention than what was heretofore advocated. Since surgical failure can be ultimately anticipated in approximately 70–75% of the patients with Dukes's C lesions, it makes a great deal of sense to subject all patients to a form of adjuvant therapy without using "no-treatment" controls which may be even considered unethical under these circumstances. Patients should be stratified according to the number of mesenteric lymph nodes involved by tumor, which was found to be a major prognostic characteristic in a number of studies, as previously mentioned. Clinical results should be compared to those with historical controls who had surgery alone for this condition. These surgical controls must be carefully screened to ensure that both pathological and operative reports will clearly indicate that the lesion was indeed of the Dukes's C class.

Arguments claiming that surgical results have improved in recent years can be easily tempered (Welch and Donaldson, 1974). We found that from 1963 to 1973 the best results by the same surgical team at M. D. Anderson Hospital were obtained between 1964 and 1966. Results were, if anything, somewhat poorer between 1970 and 1972. Furthermore, we found that results of surgery performed at M. D. Anderson Hospital were practically identical to those of surgery performed elsewhere by referring doctors in other institutions. This finding lends further support to our conviction that in colorectal cancer the biological behavior of the tumor and the host–tumor relationship may play a more important role than differences in surgical manipulation in determining the natural history of the disease.

6. *Clinical Results of Adjuvant Therapy Trials*

Since adjuvant chemotherapy, and more so immunotherapy, trials in colorectal cancer have emerged as a result of longstanding frustration with the lack of improvement from surgery alone, the results of such studies are in most part preliminary and certainly need more confirmation. Nevertheless, there are already substantial, albeit controversial, data on the use of 5-fluorouracil as a surgical adjuvant in patients with Dukes's C lesions. Following the initial report by Higgins *et al.*, (1971), who claimed no more than a marginal benefit for patients treated postoperatively with 5FU, came a report by Rousselot *et al.*, (1972), who injected 5FU into the lumen of the tumor-bearing segment of the large bowel and demonstrated, with an 8-year follow-up, a dramatic improvement in 5-year survival among treated patients. More recent reports, using both historical and concurrently randomized controls, show quite convincingly the advantage of adjuvant 5FU in patients with Dukes's C lesions (Mackman *et al.*, 1974; Grage *et al.*, 1975; Li and Ross, 1976), although Lawrence *et al.* (1975) found no apparent benefit.

Our own trial began in April 1973, and the most recent analysis performed in August 1975 includes 83 patients with Dukes's C lesions who were randomized to receive adjuvant immunotherapy either with BCG alone or in combination with 5FU. BCG was given by scarification in a dose of 6×10^8 viable units weekly for 3 months and every other week thereafter. 5FU was given by mouth in a dose of 150 mg/m^2 daily for 5 days, every 28 days for a period of 2 years. With the longest follow-up of 30 months and results compared to those for historical controls, a statistically significant prolongation of both tumor-free interval and overall survival was observed in 50 patients who received the combination of BCG plus 5FU ($p = 0.03$, $p = 0.01$, respectively, Mavligit *et al.*, 1976). Somewhat similar results were observed among 33 patients who received BCG alone. However, while the efficacy of BCG plus 5FU was independent of the number of involved lymph nodes, BCG given alone appears to be effective only among patients with six or more positive nodes and ineffective in patients with five or fewer positive nodes. Obviously, more patients and longer follow-up will be necessary in order to substantiate these preliminary results.

7. *CEA: Role of Serial Determination in Adjuvant Therapy Trials*

The controversy over the diagnostic role of CEA in cancer in general, and that arising in the large bowel in particular, has been somewhat tempered since the independent demonstration, by different laboratories, that serial determination of CEA following surgery for colorectal cancer can frequently be an important auxiliary tool for diagnosing recurrence of tumor. More specifically, it was found that elevated preoperative levels of CEA usually declined within 3 months from the time of surgery (Booth *et al.*, 1974; Holyoke *et al.*, 1975). The CEA level would stay low as long as the patient remained in a state of NED (no evident disease), but would usually rise in a persistent and progressive manner even weeks to months before clinical relapse became evident (MacKay *et al.*, 1974; Zamcheck and Pusztaszeri, 1975).

Our own experience with serial determination of CEA in patients receiving adjuvant therapy is in complete agreement. CEA played a cardinal role in establishing the secondary diagnosis of recurring tumor in eight of 14 patients who had relapsed while receiving adjuvant therapy. Persistent and progressive elevation of CEA was found at the time of relapse in 12 of 14 patients. In six patients, the diagnosis of tumor recurrence was made at laparotomy when elevated CEA served as the only clinical indication for recurring disease. In one patient, CEA began to rise 3 months after the diagnosis of tumor recurrence was made, when the disease became widespread. In another patient who had a small perineal recurrence, CEA remained normal. The tumor was resected and the patient was rendered NED. The lack of rising CEA in patients with small local perineal recurrences has also been observed by Holyoke *et al.* (1975). We therefore strongly feel that serial determination of plasma CEA must be an integral part of any adjuvant therapy trial in colorectal cancer.

8. New Approaches and Prospects for the Future

The preliminary reports suggesting a synergistic antitumor effect between 5FU and nitrosourea compounds in metastatic colorectal cancer (Falkson *et al.*, 1974; Moertel *et al.*, 1975*b*) may ultimately lead investigators to apply this combination, perhaps in a less toxic regimen, as an adjuvant therapy based on the evidence that a smaller tumor burden will be even more susceptible to destruction by chemotherapy (Magrath *et al.*, 1974). However, one should bear in mind the remote possibility that excessive immunosuppression, induced by too much chemotherapy, may tip the delicate balance which exists between the host and the tumor in favor of the tumor and culminate in disastrous results.

New immunopotentiating and immunorestorative agents are currently being investigated in various human cancers in addition to BCG. It has been suggested that the methanol-extracted residue (MER) of BCG is a very potent stimulant of various immunological parameters in patients with metastatic colorectal cancer (Moertel *et al.*, 1975*a*). A study in melanoma using BCG by mouth (MacGregor *et al.*, 1975) may raise the question of whether this mode of BCG administration will be advantageous over the scarification method as an adjuvant in colorectal cancer.

Clinical trials with thymic extract, transfer factor, immune RNA, and interferon have been initiated in human cancer. Levamisole—an antihelminthic with immunorestorative capacity—is now being used in our institution in combination with chemotherapy in advanced colorectal cancer. *Corynebacterium parvum* has also received a great deal of attention as a potent immune-stimulant which can be given intravenously and is currently being used in combination with chemotherapy in metastatic melanoma and other malignancies.

Since one of the major problems in the management of patients with colorectal cancer is metastatic disease to the liver, an effort must be specifically directed to bolster the resistance of the liver. One possible way would be an adjuvant regional infusion through the hepatic artery of either 5FU, *C. parvum,* or even BCG. The last cannot be safely injected intravenously because the organisms are viable, and generalized, life-threatening granulomatous disease will almost undoubtedly develop. However, if injected into the hepatic artery, the BCG organisms may be trapped by the reticuloendothelial system of the liver and systemic infection may be avoided, while the presence of local BCG infection within the liver may be all that is necessary to prevent the establishment and development of metastatic disease from foci of micrometastases. Finally, attention must also be paid to the exceptionally high incidence of pelvic tumor recurrence in patients with carcinoma of the rectosigmoid. It may be necessary to include radiotherapy, either before or after surgery, in future studies of systemic adjuvant therapy. This would effectively minimize the incidence of local recurrence and improve the overall results of such studies.

ACKNOWLEDGMENTS

This work was supported by PHS Grant 1 R26 CA 15458-01 and in part by Hoffman-La Roche Grant 168196. Drs. Mavligit and Gutterman are the recipients of Career Development Awards CA 1 KO 4 CA 00130-01 and CA 71007-01, respectively, from the National Institutes of Health.

9. *References*

Ambus, U., Mavligit, G. M., Gutterman, J. U., McBride, C. M., and Hersh, E. M., 1974, Specific and non-specific immunologic reactivity of regional lymph-node lymphocytes in human malignancy, *Int. J. Cancer* **14**:291–300.

Baldwin, R. W., Embleton, M. J., Jones, J. S. P., and Langman M. J. S., 1973*a*, Cell-mediated and humoral immune reactions to human tumours, *Int. J. Cancer* **12**:73–83.

Baldwin, R. W., Embleton, M. J., and Price, M. R., 1973*b*, Inhibition of lymphocyte cytotoxicity for human colon carcinoma by treatment with solubilized tumour membrane fractions, *Int. J. Cancer* **12**:84–92.

Beahrs, O. H., and Sanfelippo, P. M., 1971, Factors in prognosis of colon and rectal cancer, *Cancer* **28**:213–218.

Black, M. M., Opler, S., and Speer, F., 1955, Survival in breast cancer cases in relation to the structure of the primary tumor and regional lymph nodes, *Surg. Gynecol. Obstet.* **100**:543–551.

Bone, G., and Lauder, I., 1974, Cellular immunity, peripheral blood lymphocyte count and pathological staging of tumours in the gastrointestinal tract, *Br. J. Cancer* **30**:215–221.

Booth, S. N., Jamieson, G. C., King, J. P. G., Leonard, J., Oates, G. D., and Dykes, P. W., 1974, Carcinoembryonic Antigen in management of colorectal carcinoma, *Br. Med. J.* **4**:183–187.

Bowen, J. G., Robins, R. A., and Baldwin, R. W., 1975, Serum factors modifying cell mediated immunity to rat hepatoma D23 correlated with tumour growth, *Int. J. Cancer* **15**:640–650.

Bull, D. M., Leibach, J. R., Williams, M. A., and Helms, R. A., 1973, Immunity to colon cancer assessed by antigen-induced inhibition of mixed mononuclear cell migration, *Science* **181**:957–959.

Collatz, E., Von Kleist, S., and Burtin, P., 1971, Further investigations of circulating antibodies in colon cancer patients: On the autoantigenticity of the carcinoembryonic antigen, *Int. J. Cancer* **8**:298–303.

Donaldson, G. A., and Welch, J. P., 1974, Management of cancer of the colon, *Surg. Clin. N. Am.* **54:**713–731.

Edwards, A. J., Lee, M. R., and Rowland, G. F., 1973, Reduction of lympocyte transformation by a factor produced by gastrointestinal cancer, *Lancet* **1:**687–689.

Elias, E. G., and Elias, L. L., 1975, Some immunologic characteristics of carcinoma of the colon and rectum, *Surg. Gynecol. Obstet.* **141:**715–718.

Enterline, H. T., 1975, Management of polypoid lesions, *J. Am. Med. Assoc.* **231:**967–969.

Falkson, G., van Eden, E. B., and Falkson, H. C., 1974, Fluorouracil, imidazole carboximide dimethyl triazeno, vincristine, and bis-chlorethyl nitrosourea in colon cancer, *Cancer* **33:**1207–1209.

Falterman, K. W., Hill, C. B., Markey, J. C., Fox, J. W., and Cohn, I., Jr., 1974, Cancer of the colon, rectum, and anus: A review of 2313 cases, *Cancer* **34:**951–959.

Gold, P., 1967, Circulating antibodies against carcinoembryonic antigens of the human digestive system, *Cancer* **20:**1663–1667.

Gold, P., and Freedman, S. O., 1965, Specific carcinoembryonic antigens of the human digestive system, *J. Exp. Med.* **122:**467–481.

Grage, T., Cornell, G., Strawitz, J., Jonas, K., Frelick, R., and Metter, G., 1975, Adjuvant therapy with 5-FU after surgical resection of colo-rectal cancer, *Proc. Am. Soc. Clin. Oncol.* **16:**258.

Guillou, P. J., Brennan, T. G., and Giles, G. R., 1975, A study of lymph nodes draining colorectal cancer using a two-stage inhibition of leucocyte migration technique, *Gut* **16:**290–297.

Gunderson, L. L., and Sosin, H., 1974, Areas of failure found at reoperation (second or symptomatic look) following "curative surgery" for adenocarcinoma of the rectum, *Cancer* **34:**1278–1292.

Hellström, I., and Hellström, K. E., 1972, Newer concepts of cancer of the colon and rectum: Cellular immunity to human colonic carcinomas, *Dis. Colon Rectum* **15:**100–105.

Hellström, I., Hellström, K. E., Pierce, G. E., and Yang, J. P. S., 1968; Cellular and humoral immunity to different types of human neoplasms, *Nature (London)* **220:**1352–1354.

Heppner, G. H., Griswold, D. E., Di Lorenzo, J., Poplin, E. A., and Calabresi, P., 1974, Selective immunosuppressive by drugs in balanced immune responses, *Fed. Proc.* **33:**1882–1885.

Hersh, E. M., Gutterman, J. U., and Mavligit, G., 1973, *Immunotherapy of Cancer in Man: Scientific Basis and Current Status,* p. 141, Thomas, Springfield, Ill.

Higgins, G. A., Dwight, R. W., Smith, J. V., and Keehn, R. J., 1971, Fluorouracil as an adjuvant to surgery in carcinoma of the colon, *Arch. Surg.* **102:**339–343.

Hollinshead, A., Glew, D., Bunnag, B., Gold, P., and Herberman, R., 1970, Skin-reactive soluble antigen from intestinal cancer-cell-membranes and relationship to carcinoembryonic antigens, *Lancet* **1:**1191–1195.

Holyoke, E. D., Ming Chu, T., and Murphy, G. P., 1975, CEA as a monitor of gastrointestinal malignancy, *Cancer* **35:**830–836.

House, A. K., Wisniewski, S., and Woodings, T. L., 1975, Immunity in colonic tumor patients after operation: Determination by leukocyte-migration inhibition, *Dis. Colon Rectum* **18:**100–106.

Kaplan, M. S., Mino, F. O., Kummerfeld, K. B., and Lundak, R. L., 1975, Phytohemmagglutinin-stimulated immune response, *Arch. Surg.* **110:**1217–1220.

Lauder, I., and Bone, G., 1973, Lymphocyte transformation in large bowel cancer, *Br. J. Cancer* **27:**409–413.

Lawrence, W., Jr., Terz, J. J., Horsley, S., III., Donaldson, M., Lovett, W. L., Brown, P. W., Ruffner, B. W., and Regelson, W., 1975, Chemotherapy as an adjuvant to surgery for colorectal cancer, *Ann. Surg.* **181:**616–623.

Lejtenyi, M. C., Freedman, S. O., and Gold, P., 1971, Response of lymphocytes from patients with gastrointestinal cancer to the carcinoembryonic antigen of the human digestive system, *Cancer* **28:**115–120.

Li. M. C., and Ross, S. T., 1976, Chemoprophylaxis for patients with colorectal cancer, *J. Am. Med. Assoc.* **235:**2825–2828.

LoGerfo, P., and Herter, F. P., 1975, Carcinoembryonic antigen and prognosis in patients with colon cancer, *Ann. Surg.* **181:**81–84.

LoGerfo, P., Herter, F. P., and Bennett, S. J., 1972, Absence of circulating antibodies to carcinoembryonic antigen in patients with gastrointestinal malignancies, *Int. J. Cancer* **9:**344–348.

Lurie, B. B., Bull, D. M., Zamcheck, N., Steward, A. M., and Helms, R. A., 1975, Diagnosis and prognosis in colon cancer based on a profile of immune reactivity, *J. Natl. Cancer Inst.* **54:**319–325.

MacGregor, A. B., Falk, R. E., Landi, S., Ambus, U., and Langer, B., 1975, Oral bacille Calmette Guérin immunostimulation in malignant melanoma, *Surg. Gynecol. Obstet.* **141:**747–754.

MacKay, A. M., Patel, S., Carter, S., Stevens, U., Laurence, D. J. R., Cooper, E. H., and Neville, A. M., 1974, Role of serial plasma CEA assays in detection of recurrent and metastatic colorectal carcinomas, *Br. Med. J.* **4:**382–385.

Mackman, S., Ansfield, F. J., Ramirez, G., and Curreri, A. R., 1974, A second look at the second look operation in colonic cancer after the administration of fluorouracil, *Am. J. Surg.* **128:**763–766.

MacSween, J. M., 1975, The antigenicity of carcinoembryonic antigen in man, *Int. J. Cancer* **25:**246–252.

Magrath, I. T., Lwanga, S., Carswell, W., and Harrison, N., 1974, Surgical reduction in tumour bulk in management of abdominal Burkitt's lymphoma, *Br. Med. J.* **2:**308–312.

Mavligit, G., Gutterman, J. U., McBride, C. M., and Hersh, E. M., 1972. Multifaceted evaluation of human tumor immunity using a salt extracted colon carcinoma antigen, *Proc. Soc. Exp. Biol. Med.* **140:**1240–1245.

Mavligit, G. M., Jubert, A. V., Gutterman, J. U., McBride, C. M., and Hersh, E. M., 1974, Immune reactivity of lymphoid tissues adjacent to carcinoma of the ascending colon, *Surg. Gynecol. Obstet.* **139:**409–412.

Mavligit, G. M., Gutterman, J. U., Burgess, M. A., Khankhanian, N., Seibert, G. B., Speer, J. F., Jubert, A. V., Martin, R. C., McBride, C. M., Copeland, E. M., Gehan, E. A., and Hersh, E. M., 1976, Prolongation of post operative disease free interval and survival in human colorectal cancer by bacillus-Calmette-Guérin (BCG) or BCG plus 5-fluorouracil, *Lancet* **1:**871–876.

McIllmurray, M. B., Price, M. R., and Langman, M. J. S., 1974, Inhibition of leucocyte migration in patients with large intestinal cancer by extracts prepared from large intestinal tumours and from normal colonic mucosa, *Br. J. Cancer* **29:**305–311.

Moertel, C. G., Ritts, R. E., Jr., Schutt, A. J., and Hahn, R. G., 1975*a*, Clinical studies of methanol extraction residue fraction of bacillus Calmette-Guérin as an immunostimulant in patients with advanced cancer, *Cancer Res.* **35:**3075–3083.

Moertel, C. G., Schutt, A. J., Hahn, R. G., and Reitemeier, R. J., 1975*b*, Brief communication: Therapy of advanced colorectal cancer with a combination of 5-flourouracil, methyl-1,3-*cis*(2-chlorethyl)-1-nitrosourea, and vincristine, *J. Natl. Cancer Inst.* **54:**69–71.

Murray, D., Hreno, A., Dutton, J., and Hampson, L. G., 1975, Prognosis in colon cancer, *Arch. Surg.* **110:**908–913.

Nind, A. P. P., Nairn, R. C., Rolland, J. M., Guli, E. P. G., and Hughes, E. S. R., 1973, Lymphocyte anergy in patients with carcinoma, *Br. J. Cancer* **28:**108–117.

Nind, A. P. P., Matthews, N., Pihl, E. A. V., Rolland, J. M., and Nairn, R. C., 1975, Analysis of inhibition of lymphocyte cytotoxicity in human colon carcinoma, *Br. J. Cancer* **31:**620–629.

Patt, D. J., Brynes, R. K., Vardiman, J. W., and Coppleson, L. W., 1975, Mesocolic lymph node histology is an important prognostic indicator for patients with carcinoma of the sigmoid colon: An immumorphologic study, *Cancer* **35:**1388–1397.

Pihl, E., Hughes, E. S. R., Nind, A. P. P., and Nairn, R. C., 1975, Colonic carcinoma: Clinicopathological correlation with immunoreactivity, *Br. Med. J.* **3:**742–743.

Roswit, B., Higgins, G. A., Jr., and Keehn, R. J., 1975, Preoperative irradiation for carcinoma of the rectum and rectosigmoid colon: Report of a national Veterans Administration randomized study, *Cancer* **35:**1597–1602.

Rousselot, L. M., Cole, D. R., Grossi, C. E., Conte, A. J., Gonzales, E. M., and Pasternack, B. S., 1972, Adjuvant chemotherapy with 5-fluorouracil in surgery for colorectal cancer; eight year progress report, *Dis. Colon Rectum* **15:**169–174.

Schabel, F. M., 1975, Concepts for systemic treatment of micrometatases, *Cancer* **25:**15–24.

Schultz, R. M., Woods, W. A., and Chirigos, M. A., 1975, Detection in colorectal carcinoma patients of antibody cytotoxic to established cell strains derived from carcinoma of the human colon and rectum, *Int. J. Cancer* **16:**16–23.

Segerling, M., Ohanian, S. H., and Borsos, T., 1975, Chemotherapeutic drugs increase killing of tumor cells by antibody and complement, *Science* **188:**55–57.

Seitanides, B., and Georgoulis, B., 1975, Rosette-forming-lymphocyte counts in cancer of the colon, *Lancet* **1**:461.

Spratt, J. S., Jr., and Spjut, H. J., 1967, Prevalence and prognosis of individual clinical and pathologic variables associated with colorectal carcinoma, *Cancer* **20:**1976–1985.

Stearns, M. W., Jr., Deddish, M. R., Stuart, H. Q., and Leaming, R. H., 1974, Preoperative roentgen therapy for cancer of the rectum and rectosigmoid, *Surg. Gynecol. Obstet.* **138:**584–586.

Straus, E., Vernace, S., Janowitz, H., and Paronetto, F., 1975, Migration of peripheral leukocytes in the presence of carcinoembryonic antigen: Studies in patients with chronic inflammatory diseases of the intestine and carcinoma of the colon and jancreas, *Proc. Soc. Exp. Biol. Med.* **148:**494–497.

Thompson, D., Krupey, W., Freedman, S., and Gold, P., 1969, The radioimmunoassay of circulating carcinoembryonic antigen of the human digestive system, *Proc. Natl. Acad. Sci. USA* **64:**161–167.

Tsakraklides, V., Wanebo, H. J., Sternberg, S. S., Stearns, M., and Good, R. A., 1975, Prognostic evaluation of regional lymph node morphology in colorectal cancer, *Am. J. Surg.* **129:**174–180.

Turnbull, R. B., Jr., 1970, Cancer of the colon: The five-and ten-year survival rates following resection utilizing the isolation technique, *Ann. R. Coll. Surg. Eng.* **46:**243–250.

Welch, C. E, and Burke, J. F., 1962, Carcinoma of the colon and rectum, *N. Eng. J. Med.* **266:**211–219.

Welch, J. P., and Donaldson, G. A., 1974, Recent experience in the management of cancer of the colon and rectum, *Am. J. Surg.* **127:**258–266.

Zamcheck, N., and Pusztaszeri, G., 1975, CEA, AFP and other potential tumor markers, *CA* **25:**204–214.

Index